T0259145

Āyurveda

The Divine Science of Life

For Bronwen.

For Elsevier
Commissioning Editor: Karen Morley
Development Editor: Louise Allsop
Project Managers: Caroline Horton, Morven Dean
Design Direction: Jayne Jones
Illustration Buyer: Gillian Murray
Illustrator: Jonathan Haste

Āyurveda

The Divine Science of Life

Todd Caldecott Cl.H., RH (AHG)
Consultant Clinical Herbalist, Ayurvedic Practitioner, Vancouver, Canada

Foreword by

Michael Tierra L.A.C., O.M.D.
Founder of the American Herbalists Guild, California, USA

MOSBY
ELSEVIER

EDINBURGH LONDON NEW YORK OXFORD PHILADELPHIA ST LOUIS SYDNEY TORONTO 2006

MOSBY
ELSEVIER

An imprint of Elsevier Limited

© Elsevier Ltd 2006. All rights reserved.

The right of Todd Caldecott to be identified as the author of this work has been asserted in accordance with the Copyright, Designs and Patents Act 1988.

No part of this publication may be reproduced, stored in a retrieval system, or transmitted in any form or by any means, electronic, mechanical, photocopying, recording or otherwise, without the prior permission of the publishers. Permissions may be sought directly from Elsevier's Health Sciences Rights Department, 1600 John F. Kennedy Boulevard, Suite 1800, Philadelphia, PA 19103-2899, USA. Phone: (+1) 215 239 3804, fax: (+1) 215 238 3805, email: healthpermissions@elsevier.com. You may also complete your request on-line via the Elsevier homepage (http://www.elsevier.com), by selecting 'Support and Contact' and then 'Copyright and Permission'.

First published 2006 ISBN-10 0-723
ISBN-10 0-723-43410-7
ISBN-13 978-0-7234-3410-8

British Library Cataloguing in Publication Data
A catalogue record for this book is available from the British Library

Library of Congress Cataloging in Publication Data
A catalogue record for this book is available from the Library of Congress

Notice
Knowledge and best practice in this field are constantly changing. As new research and experience broaden our knowledge, changes in practice, treatment and drug therapy may become necessary or appropriate. Readers are advised to check the most current information provided (i) on procedures featured or (ii) by the manufacturer of each product to be administered, to verify the recommended dose or formula, the method and duration of administration, and contraindications. It is the responsibility of the practitioner, relying on their own experience and knowledge of the patient, to make diagnoses, to determine dosages and the best treatment for each individual patient, and to take all appropriate safety precautions. To the fullest extent of the law, neither the publisher nor the author assumes any liability for any injury and/or damage to persons or property arising out of, or related to, any use of the material contained in this book. **The publisher**

Working together to grow libraries in developing countries
www.elsevier.com | www.bookaid.org | www.sabre.org
ELSEVIER BOOK AID International Sabre Foundation

ELSEVIER your source for books, journals and multimedia in the health sciences
www.elsevierhealth.com

Printed and bound in the United Kingdom
Transferred to Digital Print 2009

The Publisher's policy is to use **paper manufactured from sustainable forests**

Contents

Part 3: Appendices

APPENDIX 1: Dietary and lifestyle regimens   301

APPENDIX 2: Āyurvedic formulations   305

Note. Colour plate Section begins after page **296**.

Foreword

The two oldest extant and expounded systems of traditional medicine are East Indian Traditional Medicine, known as Āyurveda and dating back five to ten thousand years, and Traditional Chinese Medicine (TCM) whose history arguably is known to extend as much as 5000 years into antiquity. While Western medicine owes its origins to the Egyptian, Greek, Roman and Arabic cultures, it has been hopelessly fragmented several times over the last 2000 years due to the disintegration of the Roman Empire, then the early suppression by the church of any physical healing methods, and more recently, the development of pharmaceutical drugs.

It has been argued that Āyurveda is the basis for traditional Tibetan medicine, TCM and later Greek, Roman and Arabic (or Unani) medicines. All these traditional healing methods share a common unified body-mind-spirit orientation, meaning that disease and health are the result of the interaction of all three aspects of being. As well, all of them are energetic medicines based on their heating and cooling energies, for instance, of food, herbs, diseases and constitutions.

Just as there is a close relationship between Chinese martial arts and related physical disciplines and Traditional Chinese Medicine (TCM), there is also a healing relationship between the disciplines of yoga and Āyurveda. Today yoga continues to grow in popularity as it is increasingly accepted into the mainstream of the West. During the 1970s some of these same spiritual Indian teachers bringing yoga to the West were also responsible for introducing Āyurveda.

Because Āyurveda was first introduced by spiritual teachers along with other intended moral practices such as vegetarianism, it is seen by many as a harmonious system of medical support for vegetarianism rather than the distinct holistic healing system that it truly is.

My personal introduction, in 1974, was by Hari Das Baba who may have been one of the first teachers in the West, although Yogi Bhajan was another who informally taught Āyurveda to his followers. In 1980 the Maharishi, founder of Transcendental Meditation, began to popularise Āyurveda in the West and eventually incorporated a line of Āyurvedic products as I had done previously.

Since its introduction to the West, a number of Āyurvedics and Westerners trained in Āyurveda have conducted clinical practice, taught, written books and developed training courses in Āyurveda. One of the first was Robert Svoboda, then David Frawley, a Westerner who took it upon himself to master Sanskrit and is now recognised throughout the world, including India, as one of the foremost Vedic scholars. The West owes a great debt to the dedicated and pioneering efforts of Dr. Vasant Ladd, an Indian medical doctor as well as Āyurvedic doctor. Now, the Canadian, Todd Caldecott, has created a milestone in the evolution of Āyurveda in the West through his years of teaching and now the authorship of this definitive book.

Apart from its association with spiritual and yogic practices, Āyurveda is as relevant today for all people throughout the world as it was when the first classic texts were compiled between the first and sixth centuries. Its recommendations and prescriptions are not limited to any single class of people, neither to any specific religious belief nor any particular dietary regime since its origins as elucidated in the classic texts predate Buddhist influence in India and include various animal parts for food and medicine.

Just as Sanskrit is considered a root language whose influence can be found in most of the languages of Europe, Āyurveda is known by some as 'the mother of healing'. Because we live in a world where the wisdom of all people and times are at once available, it is possible to supplement the deficiencies of understanding from one system of thought by looking through the prism of another. This means that semantic differences aside, aspects of Āyurveda – its theory, principles, herbs, therapies – are to be found in all major world healing systems.

Therefore, an understanding of Āyurvedic medicine is bound to enhance and deepen the understanding of a conventional Western medical doctor as well as a TCM practitioner. In fact many of the treatments and even the medicines used in Āyurveda are found in Western medicine, such as *Rauwolfia serpentina* for high blood pressure. In addition, a large number of herbs used in Āyurveda are also used as part of the medical armamentarium of both Western and Chinese herbalists.

As another example, the three body types (somatypes) developed by the psychologist William Sheldon (1898–1977) during the 1940s closely corresponds to one of the cornerstones of Āyurveda, called 'tridosha'. The difference is that Sheldon only described and used the body types for their psychological temperament while Āyurveda uses them as a cornerstone guiding lifestyle, dietary and treatment modality.

The author of this book has absorbed many of the dominant alternative healing systems known in the West and has chosen to specialise in the practice and teaching of Āyurveda. For the Western student this means that much of the confusion between Western herbal medicine, scientific herbalism and TCM has been integrated by the author and the result is a text that is persuasive and immediately communicable to the Western mind without losing the flavour and integrity of its origin.

I have known Todd Caldecott as a colleague and respected professional member of the American Herbalists Guild (AHG) and have seen him grow in stature as one of the country's leading herbalists and one who is able to bridge the divide between various systems of traditional medicine and Western medical science. His book offers a clear and comprehensive elucidation of Āyurveda that will guide the serious student in acquiring the skills needed to become an effective practitioner.

Michael Tierra
California, 2006

Preface

The genesis of the present work began in 1992 after I returned from my first trip to India and West Asia, where I spent a year travelling overland from Sri Lanka to Western Turkey on only a few dollars a day. After several months of staying in the cheapest guest houses and eating at roadside stalls I unfortunately contracted a very serious case of dysentery that I only partially recovered from when I spent a month among the Hunza people in Northern Pakistan. Upon my return to Canada I sought treatment for what was now a chronic digestive disorder, and after undergoing a variety of treatments, including naturopathic and homeopathic medicine, finally received relief under the care of Āyurvedic physician Dr T. Sukumaran. The wise counsel given to me by the Kerala-born Dr Sukumaran impressed me greatly, and incited a passion to learn all I could about Āyurveda. Although there were some good texts available at the time, there were none I found that could deepen my interest in Āyurveda. During this time I enrolled in a 3-year clinical programme in Western herbal medicine, and continued to study Āyurveda with Dr Sukumaran as well as other teachers. When I completed my studies in Western herbal medicine my thirst for Āyurveda remained unquenched, and in 1996 I left for India with my pregnant wife and 1-year-old son where I studied at the Arya Vaidya Chikitsalayam in Coimbatore, India. Here I not only had the opportunity to study under the venerable Dr V. Vasudevan, but other Āyurvedic physicians as well, sitting with them in clinic and in the hospital, observing the skills they used in assessment and treatment. While I was India I began to synthesise all of this wonderful knowledge I had learned into the framework of a text that would serve as the kind of reference text I had sought a few years earlier. After the happy birth of my second son in India, my family and I returned to Canada where I opened a clinical practice, using my skills as a Western herbal and Āyurvedic practitioner. I continued to work on the text, and made a significant investment to acquire English translations of all the classical Āyurvedic texts available, as well as texts on Indian botany, which I digested with a voracious appetite. In 1999 I relocated to Calgary, Alberta, and in addition to seeing patients began to offer an introductory course in Āyurvedic medicine at the Wild Rose College of Natural Healing. In 2001 I became the Director of Clinical Herbal studies at Wild Rose College, where I developed a 3-year clinical programme in Western herbal medicine. During this time I continued to work on my text, rewriting large sections of the book and adding the appendices found in the current version, and converted all the Sanskrit terms into Unicode-compatible diacritical format. Although the present text is far from perfect, I believe that the almost 10 years I have spent working on it has come close to my original vision. It is my sincerest hope that this text is worthy of the serious student of the divine science that is Āyurveda.

Todd Caldecott
Vancouver, BC, Canada, 2005

Acknowledgements

There are so many people to acknowledge:

First, I give thanks to my adoring family and loving friends, to whom I am indebted for their patience, inspiration and profound love.

Secondly, I thank the many colleagues, teachers and friends that assisted me with their support, encouragement and wisdom, including Dr T. Sukumaran, Jaisri Lambert, K.P. Singh Khalsa, Dr Terry Willard, Chanchal Cabrera, Christopher Hansard, Dr V. Vasudevan, Dr S. Kumar, Dr D. Anandakusumam, Paul Bergner, Michael Tierra, David Winston, Alan Tillotson, Madhu Bajracharya and Vinod Haritwal.

Thirdly, I give my deepest veneration to the Āyurvedic physicians and scholars of Āyurveda that have illuminated the world with their wisdom, as well as the holy rishis who think to benefit all humanity when they reveal these sacred teachings.

Lastly, I give thanks to Mother Earth and the healing medicines that arise from Her body, and Great Spirit that infuses them with divine essence.

> *om bhaiṣajye bhaiṣajye mahā bhaiṣajye samudgate svāhā in divine recognition of you, the great medicine!*
>
> (Aṣṭāṅga Hṛdaya, Sūtrasthāna, 18:17)

Notes on transliteration

Sanskrit is a complex language that originated in India several thousand years ago, considered by modern scholars to be a remote cousin of the ancient European languages, including Ancient Greek and Latin. It evolved from an earlier language found in the ***Ṛg veda*** and was refined into its present form by the grammarian Pāṇini in the 4th century BCE (BCE = before common era). Since then the rigid grammatical structure laid out by Pāṇini has represented the 'perfected' (***saṃskṛta***) form of the language, as opposed to the many 'unperfected' (***prākṛtas***) regional dialects that evolved before, during and after the time of Pāṇini. Today Sanskrit is primarily a language of religion and scholarship, and like Latin is used in modern science, serves to standardise traditional Indian knowledge into a unified whole. The present text attempts to preserve this precedent, and uses many of the original Sanskrit terms found in the extant Āyurvedic literature.

To best achieve a fluency in Sanskrit terms without requiring the reader to learn the ***devanāgarī*** script in which it is written, Western scholars use a system of diacritics to transliterate these terms. It is important to note that Sanskrit contains many more sounds than does English, 49 letters in all as opposed to the 26 letters in English, and thus this system of diacritics is used to represent these different sounds, some of which are difficult for the Western ear to detect.

In the pronunciation of Sanskrit letters there are five possible regions from which a sound can be produced: (1) guttural, (2) palatal, (3) cerebral, (4) dental and (5) labial. *Guttural sounds* are produced by constricting the throat at the back of the tongue; *palatal sounds* are produced by pressing the tongue flat against the palate; *cerebral sounds* are produced by turning up the tip of the tongue against the hard palate; *dental sounds* by touching the upper teeth with the tongue; and *labial sounds* by pursing the lips.

Vowels

If language can be viewed as a living organism, Sanskrit considers vowels to be the life-force that awakens a language and gives it meaning. In total, there are 14 vowels, consisting of simple vowels (one vowel sound) and diphthongs (combined vowel sounds):

Vowels simple

	Short (one beat)	Pronounced like:	Long (two beats)	Pronounced like:
Guttural	*a*	'a' in 'america'	*ā*	'a' in 'calm'
Palatal	*i*	'i' in 'bit'	*ī*	'i' in 'machine'
Labial	*u*	'u' in 'book'	*ū*	'u' in 'rule'
Cerebral	*ṛ*	'ri' in 'rip'	*ṝ*	A long ṛ sound
Dental	*ḷ*	'tle' in 'bottle'	*ḹ*	Not used in practice

Vowels : dipthongs

Palatal	e	Pronounced like 'e' in 'prey'
Palatal	*ai*	Pronounced like 'ai' in 'aisle'
Labial	o	Pronounced like 'o' in 'road'
labial	*au*	Pronounced like 'ow' in 'cow'

In addition to the vowels described above, there are two special supporting vowels used in Sanskrit, called visarga and anusvāra:

visarga	*ḥ*	Occurs at the end of a word or syllable, expressed as a kind of breath sound, faintly continuing the previous vowel
anusvāra	*ṃ*	Occurs as a nasal sound before a hard consonant, sounding like the 'm' in the word 'sum'

Consonants

If vowels are viewed as the life principle of the Sanskrit language, consonants are its body: the 'stuff' that makes up language and gives it form. Consonants can be divided into two types: generic consonants, and an assortment of semivowels, sibilants and an aspirate. Like the vowels, each type of consonant is classified according to where the sound is produced (i.e. gutteral, palatal, etc.). Where an 'h' follows a consonant this represents an *aspirated sound*, in which the consonant is pronounced with a noticeable emission of breath. In fact, the 'th' and 'ph' sounds as they are commonly pronounced in English are not found in Sanskrit, although the 'ph' sound can be found in modern Indian languages influenced by non-indigenous languages such as Farsi. Thus the famous Āyurvedic medicament *triphala* is pronounced 'tri-pah-la' in Sanskrit and 'tri-fah-la' in the Farsi-influenced Hindi.

Generic consonants

Guttural	*k*	'k' as in 'kite'	kh (aspirated)	*g*	'g' as in 'gum'	gh (aspirated)	*ṅ*	'ng' as in 'finger'
Palatal	*c*	'c' as in 'chair'	ch (aspirated)	*j*	'j' as in 'jar'	jh (aspirated)	*ñ*	'ni' as in 'onion'
Cerebral	*ṭ*	't' as in 'tea'	ṭh (aspirated)	*ḍ*	'd' as in 'day'	ḍh (aspirated)	*ṇ*	'n' as in 'fund'
Dental	*t*	As in first sound of 'thirty'	th (aspirated)	*d*	As in the first sound in 'thus'	dh (aspirated)	*n*	'n' as in name
Labial	*p*	'p' as in 'punch'	ph (aspirated)	*b*	'b' as in 'butter'	bh (aspirated)	*m*	'm' as in 'mother'

Semivowels

Palatal	*y*	'y' as in 'young'
Cerebral	*r*	'r' as in 'real'
Dental	*l*	'l' as in 'laugh'
Labial	*v*	'v' as in 'vast', but without pressing the upper teeth hard against the lower lip

Sibilants

Palatal	*ś*	'sh' as in 'shut'
Cerebral	*ṣ*	'sh' as above, but with the tip of the tongue touching the hard palate
Labial	*s*	's' as in 'sip'

Aspirates

h	'h' as in 'harmony'

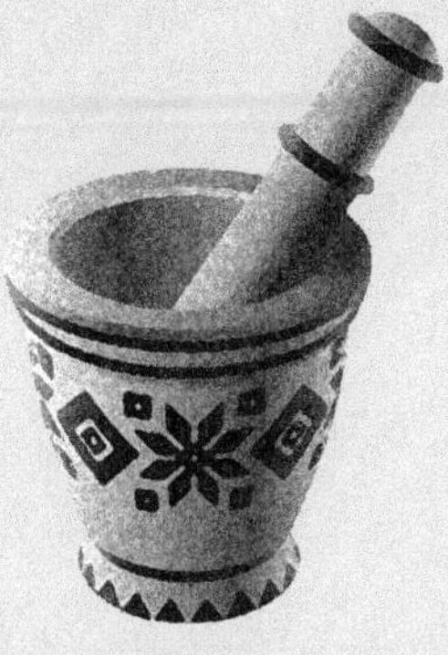

PART 1

THEORY AND PRACTICE OF ĀYURVEDA

PART 1

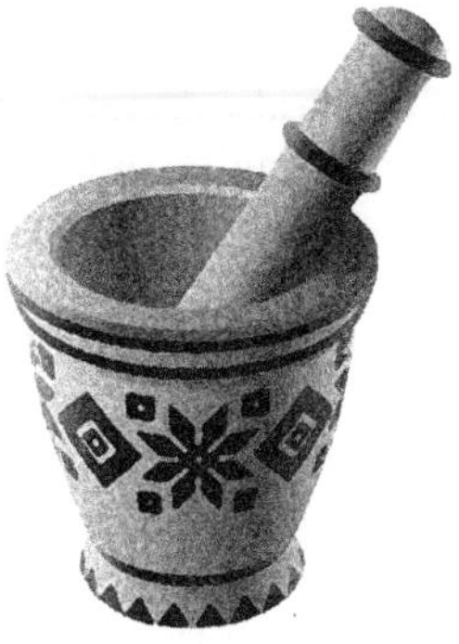

Chapter 1

FOUNDATION

OBJECTIVES

- To understand the anthropological and philosophical origins of Āyurveda.
- To understand the bioenergetic and spiritual models underlying the system of Āyurveda.

1.1 ORIGIN OF ĀYURVEDA

According to tradition, the teachings of Āyurveda were recollected by Brahmā, the Lord of Creation, as he awoke to begin the task of creating the universe that we inhabit now. This idea suggests that Āyurveda transcends the period of this universe, stretching beyond the concept of time itself, having no beginning and no end. Brahmā taught this knowledge to Dakṣa Prajāpati (the protector of all beings), whom in turn taught it to the Aśvinī Kumāras (the twin holy physicians), who in turn taught it to Indra (King of the Gods). When disease and illness began to trouble humanity the great ***ṛṣis*** ('sages') of the world assembled in the Himalayan mountains, seeking to learn Āyurveda from Lord Indra. Among these sages one named Bharadvāja volunteered and made the journey to Indra's court on Mount Kailash,[1] where he undertook the study of Āyurveda. In a few short quatrains Lord Indra expounded the entire teaching of Āyurveda, and the profound nature of this unfolded like a lotus in the illuminated mind of the accomplished sage. After he had heard and understood this teaching Bharadvāja returned to establish the first school of Āyurveda, and revealed this knowledge to the assembled sages. These sages in turn taught this knowledge to their own disciples, and one named Punarvasu Ātreya held a competition to see which student best understood ***kāya cikitsā***, or the practice of internal medicine. Among his students the treatise of Agniveśa was judged best, celebrated by all who heard it, and thus the ***Agniveśa saṃhitā*** became the authoritative text on internal medicine. Although this text is no longer available it exists in a revised and edited version compiled by the physician Caraka, whose ***Caraka saṃhitā***, with the later additions of Dṛḍhabalā, is now considered the most authentic and authoritative text on the subject. A contemporary of Ātreya was Kasiraja Divodāsa Dhanvantari, the sage who revealed the art and science of surgery, or ***śalya cikitsa***, to his student Suśruta (whose name means to 'listen sweetly').[2] Suśruta compiled Divodāsa's teachings into a text, which along with the later revisions of the renowned Buddhist scholar Nāgārjuna, forms the ***Suśruta saṃhitā***, the primary Āyurvedic text on the theory and practice of surgery. Another important early text is the ***Kāśyapa saṃhitā***, which is concerned with the theory and practice of paediatric and obstetric disease (***kaumārabhṛtya***). Unfortunately only portions of this text have survived the millennia, and the remainder of the original texts on each of the separate specialities of Āyurveda are either hidden, have been damaged over time, or have been completely lost. Fortunately both the ***Caraka*** and ***Suśruta saṃhitās*** are broad enough in scope that they describe almost the entire system of Āyurveda.[3]

The ***Caraka saṃhitā*** states that the term 'Āyurveda' is derived from two words, ***āyus*** and ***veda***. Many Āyurvedic commentators define ***āyus*** as 'life', but ***Caraka*** expands upon this definition, telling us that ***āyus*** is the '. . . combination of the body, sense organs, mind and soul', the factor (***dhāri***) responsible for preventing decay and death, which sustains (***jīvita***) the body over time (***nityaga***), and guides the process of rebirth (***anubandha***). The second part of the word is ***veda*** and can be translated as 'knowledge' or 'science', but more specifically suggests a deeply profound knowledge that emanates from a divine source, and hence Āyurveda is known as the 'divine science of life'.

As a ***śāstra*** ('teaching') of the ***Vedas***, Āyurveda is allied with the four principle Vedas of ancient India, which similarly issued forth from Lord Brahmā at the time of Creation. The Vedas include the ***Ṛg veda***, ***Yajur veda***, ***Sāma veda*** and the ***Atharva veda***, and are considered by Hindus to be a sacred knowledge, an eternal and unending truth called the ***sanātana dharma***. The Vedas can be organised in a few different ways, including into six ***āñgas*** ('limbs') or six ***darśanas*** ('perceptions'). Among the six ***darśanas*** the theoretical structure of Āyurveda draws primarily from the ***Nyāya***, ***Vaiśeṣika*** and ***Sāñkhya darśanas***. Both the ***Nyāya*** and ***Vaiśeṣika darśanas*** are concerned with logic, analysis and distinction, whereas the ***Sāñkhya darśana*** is a kind of ontology that describes the emanation of the universe from a divine source (see Ch. 2). To a lesser extent Āyurveda also draws upon the other three ***darśanas***, including ***Mīmāṃsā*** (knowledge and 'interpretation' of Vedic rituals and rites), ***Yoga*** ('union', spiritual discipline) and ***Vedānta*** ('esotericism'). Although the teachings of the Vedas are at the theoretical core of Āyurveda, the practice of medicine in India has also been influenced by the later spiritual traditions of India, especially during the Buddhist period (c. 600 BCE–700 CE). (*Note.* BCE = before common era; CE = common era.) During this time several famous centres of medical learning evolved that taught an apparently advanced knowledge of surgery and other specialties, such as the ***Takṣaśilā*** university in what is now modern-day Afghanistan. One of the more interesting historical accounts of ancient Āyurvedic practices comes to us from the ***Vinaya piṭaka*** of the Pāli Canon, which recounts the tales of the famed physician Jīvaka Komārabhacca.

Both the ***Caraka*** and ***Suśruta saṃhitās*** are highly technical texts, and many subsequent Āyurvedic scholars felt the need to contribute to the storehouse of Āyurvedic literature, to make it easier to understand, to simplify and arrange the material in a more accessible way. Among these Āyurvedic scholars was Vāgbhaṭa (c. 600 CE), author of the ***Aṣṭāñga Sangraha*** and the

Box 1.1 *Jīvaka Komārabhacca*

Jīvaka was a famous Āyurvedic physician during the 6th century BCE, and personal physician to the Buddha. His life began under very humble circumstances, when he was found lying in a trash heap, having been abandoned by a prostitute. He was discovered by chance by a prince who found him still 'living' (***jīva***), named him Jīvaka, and raised him as a son. At a young age Jīvaka travelled to Takṣaśilā to study medicine. As part of their final examinations the teacher asked his students to search through the forest and find one thing that could not be used as a medicine. As the students made their way back from their search, each one of them had found something that had no use as a medicine. After waiting an exceptionally long time Jīvaka finally returned to his teacher, crestfallen and empty handed. He had found no substance which could not, in some way, be used as a medicine. To his surprise the teacher congratulated Jīvaka and gave him his blessing as a physician. The rest of the students were berated: only Jīvaka had truly understood the heart of Āyurveda.

Aṣṭāñga Hṛdaya, who created these texts for those of us of 'weaker intellect'. The ***Aṣṭāñga Hṛdaya*** is his most succinct compilation of the teachings of both Caraka and Suśruta. Together, the teachings of Caraka, Suśruta and Vāgbhaṭa form the ***bṛhat trayī***, the 'greater triad' of surviving texts that are the heart of Āyurvedic literature. Standing beside these is the ***laghu trayī***, or lesser triad, composed of comparatively later texts including the ***Mādhava nidānam*** (c. 700 CE), ***Śāraṅgadhara saṃhitā*** (c. 1300 CE) and the ***Bhāvaprakāśa*** (c. 1300 CE). Besides these texts, however, there are many more that are highly respected among Āyurvedic physicians, including the ***Cakradatta*** (c. 1100 CE) and the ***Bhaiṣajyaratnāvalī*** (c. 1700 CE). Due to the hard work of modern Āyurvedic scholars such as Dr K. R. Srikanthamurthy and Dr P. V. Sharma, many of these works are now available as English translations.

Given that the ***Aṣṭāñga Hṛdaya*** is eminently suitable to those of us suffering from an intellectual deficit I have chosen it as my primary inspiration, as well as additional materials from other texts listed in the bibliography, and teachings that have been communicated to me personally. Translated into English, the ***Aṣṭāñga Hṛdaya*** literally means the 'heart' (***hṛdaya***) of the 'eight limbs' (***aṣṭ*** + ***āñga***) of Āyurveda, which are the eight specialties originally revealed by Bharadvāja. These ***āñgas*** or ***cikitsā*** ('treatments') are:

1. ***Kāya cikitsā***: general internal medicine
2. ***Bāla cikitsā***: treatment of infants and children
3. ***Graha cikitsā***: treatment of spiritual possession and medical astrology
4. ***Ūrdhvāñga cikitsā***: treatment of the eyes, ears, nose and throat
5. ***Śalya cikitsā***: treatment requiring the use of a knife, i.e. surgery
6. ***Damṣṭrā cikitsā***: treatment of animal inflicted wounds, poisoning, i.e. toxicology
7. ***Jarā cikitsā***: treatment of ageing; i.e. ***rasāyana*** ('rejuvenative') therapies
8. ***Vṛṣa cikitsā***: treatment of impotence and sterility, i.e. ***vajīkaraṇa*** ('aphrodisiac') therapies.

Vāgbhaṭa tells us in the second verse of the ***Aṣṭāñga Hṛdaya*** that '. . . persons desirous of long life which is the means for achieving ***dharma*** ('duty'), ***artha*** ('wealth') and ***sukha*** ('satisfaction') should repose utmost faith in the teachings of Āyurveda'. I humbly invite the reader to consider this present text not the word of the ***ācaryās*** ('wise teachers') but as a condensed and hopefully useful guide for practitioners and lay persons alike. Any interpolations, inaccuracies or mistakes are my own and are not reflective of the vast storehouse of wisdom that is Āyurveda.

1.2 PHILOSOPHICAL ORIENTATION OF ĀYURVEDA

It seems to be an inherent aspect of human nature to recognise the basic duality that pervades life. The ancient Chinese describe the dynamics of yin and yang, Judeo-Christian culture teaches the concepts of good and evil, and Jungian psychoanalysis organises the psyche in terms of anima and animus. Even the binary function of the computer on which I am writing this text is an example of this intrinsic duality. Āyurveda, too, recognises this duality, although its characteristics are unique. According to ***Vedānta***, the last and most profound of the Vedic ***darśanas***, what we call reality is really a self-developed illusion called ***māyā***, created and perpetuated by the ignorance of the ego. It is this conditioned existence that fragments an experience of ***brahman***, the 'vast expanse' of the Whole, which is unattributed and unknowable. The attainment and integration of ***brahman*** into our consciousness is the ***mokṣa***, or liberation from this world of illusion, where suffering ceases and one merges with the Totality. The ego with its ignorance, aversion and attachments clings to this fragmented world, inventing semantical, personal, cultural and social realities that blind us to our true nature, that we are God:

> ***Pūrṇam adaḥ pūrṇam idam pūrṇāt pūrṇam udacyate***
> ***pūrṇasya pūrṇam ādāya pūrṇam evāvaśiṣyate***
>
> 'That is the Whole. This too is the Whole.
> The Whole comes out of the Whole.
> Taking the Whole from the Whole,
> The Whole itself remains.'
>
> -***Isa Upaniṣad***, invocation

There is perhaps no other hymn in the Vedic literature that so clearly defines the orientation of holism and holistic medicine. It is a realisation that transcends the knowledge we gain from our corporeal existence, where the fragmentation of knowledge ceases to obscure true understanding, where we arrive at a knowing that is complete, and yet cannot be described:

> ***Avijñātaṃ, vijānatāṃ, vijñātam, avijānatām***
>
> 'It is not understood by those who understand it,
> It is understood by those who don't understand it.'
> -***Kena Upaniṣad***, 2:3

Within a human being this pervasive and yet unrealised state of totality is called the ***jīvātmān***, and it is this that is the 'seed' or spark of life. From the accumulated ***karma*** ('actions') of repeated births, through the ignorance and desires of the ***ahaṃkāra*** ('ego'), each of us have bound up our true nature with tremendous ***saṃskāras*** – actions whose fruits have yet to be realised. It is our reaction to these fruits, either by luxuriating in or by being repulsed by them, that generates further ***karma***, binding us to ***saṃsāra***, the wheel of life and death. Thus the path that leads us from ***dukha*** ('suffering') to ***sukha*** ('happiness') lies between the push and pull of life. It is a paradoxical state, to be remote yet fully engaged, remaining as the Chinese Taoists say, as '. . . an uncarved piece of wood'. Freed from desire, ignorance and hatred, ***karma*** never has a chance to develop, and that which comes to fruit is allowed to ripen, without inducing a conditioned response. In this state of being the aspirant is freed from birth, and '. . . sees how all things pass away', entering into the abode of ***nirvāṇa***.[4]

1.3 THE *Pañca kośa*: THE FIVE SHEATHS OF BEING

According to the ***Taittirīya Upaniṣad*** a corporeal being is born with five sheaths (***pañca kośa***) that are organised into three bodies (***śarira***). The ***sthūla śarira*** or 'gross body' is definitive of physical being and is the corporeal manifestation of all the other ***śarira***: the gross yet highly organised manifestation of matter. It is also called the ***annamaya kośa***, or 'food sheath', and is discarded upon death. Progressing inwards, we come next to the ***sūkṣma śarira***, or 'subtle body', which comprises three ***kośas*** or 'sheaths':

1. The ***prāṇāmaya kośa***, comprising the five 'winds' or ***prāṇas*** (***prāṇa***, ***apāna***, ***udāna***, ***vyāna*** and ***samāna***) which provide the impetus and energy for all actions in the body (see 2.9 The ***subdoṣas***: subdivisions within each ***doṣa***). The five ***prāṇas*** are the vital force that underlies the function of the five ***karma indriyās*** ('organs of action'), i.e. the mouth, hands, limbs, eliminative organs and genitalia.
2. The ***manomaya kośa***, comprising the five ***jñāna indriyās*** ('organs of knowledge'), i.e. the nose, ears, eyes, skin and tongue. When these five senses are activated by the ***citta***,[5] or innate consciousness, they form the ***manas***, or 'lower mind'.
3. The ***vijñānamaya kośa***, comprising the ***ahaṃkāra*** ('ego') and ***buddhi*** ('intellect', or higher mind).[6]

The ***sūkṣma śarira*** is equivalent to the astral body of Western occultism, where the body exists in an energetic form but nonetheless retains aspects of individuality. It is a subtle realm experienced by most people in trance states, dreams and visions. As the ***sūkṣma śarira*** contains the five senses (***jñāna indriyās***) and the five organs of action (***karma indriyās***) with which we receive sensory information and act upon it, all corporeal activities are first manifest within this realm. It is within this subtle arena that everything we think or feel becomes manifest. Whether or not this manifestation occurs on a corporeal level is dependent upon the strength and clarity of a given thought or emotion. In the physical realm manifestation occurs relatively slowly, and because of this one

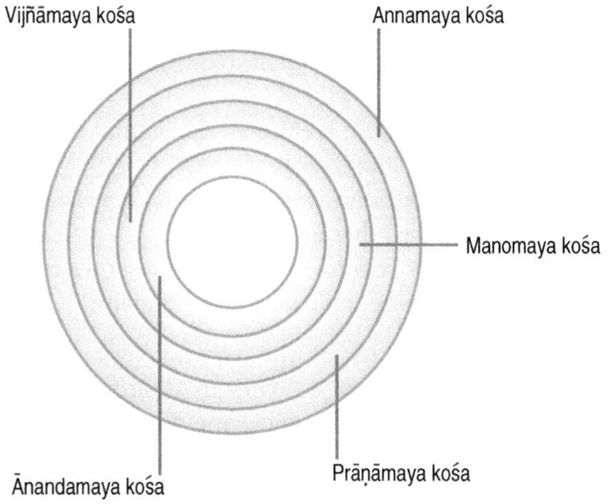

Figure 1.1 The ***pañca kośa***.

thought or feeling may be countered by another. This is why, if we want to obtain a result on a physical level, we must purify our intent and develop clarity about what it is we want. This is one of the purposes behind the use of ***mantra***, which through the repetition of special sounds organises consciousness in the ***sūkṣma śarira*** around a single purpose or vibrational quality. The ***sūkṣma śarira*** is also the realm within which the ***cakras*** exist, and through the conscious and directed flow of ***prāṇa*** ('vital force') through the energetic channel that connects them (i.e. the ***suṣumnā nāḍī***), we can awaken the spiritual energy in these energy centres. Many extrasensory abilities such as clairvoyance or the influence and guidance of other beings, such as channelling, occur within the ***sūkṣma śarira***.

The final body is the ***kāraṇa śarira*** ('causal origin'), also known as the ***ānandamaya kośa***, or 'bliss sheath'. This is perhaps the most appropriate place for us to designate the soul, the interface between the lower and higher aspects of our being. It is the most subtle state of being, beyond the push and pull of the ego (***ahaṃkāra***), resting in pure knowledge (***jñāna***), acting as the impetus for the development of the increasingly grosser forms of a living being.

The ***jīvātman***, the individuated aspect of ***brahman***, interfaces with these five sheaths to provide life, and in association with ***karma***, is bound to them, to ***saṃsāra***, the never-ending cycle of birth, death and rebirth. As beings evolve spiritually, consciously progressing inwards towards the attainment of ***mokṣa*** ('liberation'), they may find themselves partially existing within these subtle realms, developing certain spiritual powers called ***siddhis***, such as clairaudience, clairsentience or clairvoyance. It is even possible to be reborn within the heavenly realms of the ***sūkṣma śarira***, although this temptation is considered to be a serious pitfall in spiritual development. The ***sūkṣma śarira*** is the realm in which the ***devas*** ('heavenly beings') and ***asuras*** ('demons') are said to exist, enjoying the power and pleasure of the astral realms, living as immortals, or rather, as beings with extraordinary longevity and subtle powers. It was for this reason that the Tibetan *Bardo Thodol* ('Book of the Dead') was written, as a set of instructions to guide the dead past the enticing, yet illusory astral realms and onward to the greater realization of ***brahman*** (in Tibetan, 'dzogchen'). The beings that are said to exist within these subtle realms maintain different levels of awareness, some focused entirely on their own pleasures and desires, and others with a more noble intent, working towards their further development and for the benefit of all living beings. Fully realized beings, however, understand that any state of being is still a state in which ***karma*** and its fruit can be generated and thus know that they are subject to the unyielding power of impermanence and decay.

So far we have learned that ***prakṛti*** represents the created world, synonymous with the concept of ***māyā***, or self-created illusion. Although Āyurveda is the study of ***prakṛti***, it is a path of knowledge that is designed to explain phenomena within the veil of ***māyā***, a path through which we gain insight into its illusory nature. Āyurveda does not deny the importance of physicality, but advocates a specific methodology that facilitates the realization that ***prakṛti*** is ***puruṣa***. Thus, the correct study of Āyurveda and the practice of ***dharma*** will automatically lead us to the path of ***brahman***.[7]

1.4 THE *cakra* SYSTEM, *kundalinī* AND *aṣṭāñga* YOGA

Another system that provides a context for the practice of Āyurveda is the ***cakra*** system. This system, like the ***pañca kośa*** theory, describes the fundamental aspects of being, but also allows for a specific understanding of spiritual development and its concomitant effects upon the body, mind and emotions. The ***cakra*** system represents the dynamic structure of the subtle body, the etheric octave of the physical body. The term ***cakra*** means 'wheel,' and the seven major ***cakras*** are hierarchically arranged energy vortices within the subtle body:

1. ***Mūlādhāra cakra***: the 'root' ***cakra***
2. ***Svādhiṣṭhāna cakra***: the 'sex' ***cakra***
3. ***Maṇipūra cakra***: the 'digestive' ***cakra***
4. ***Anāhata cakra***: the 'heart' ***cakra***
5. ***Viśuddha cakra***: the 'throat' ***cakra***
6. ***Ājñā cakra***: the 'third-eye' ***cakra***
7. ***Sahasrāra cakra***: the 'crown' ***cakra***.

Each ***cakra*** represents certain energetic, mental and physical qualities, and from a spiritual perspective, certain life challenges and spiritual attainments.[8] These seven energy vortices are connected by the ***suṣumnā nāḍī***, the central axis or channel (***nāḍī***) of the body, like beads on a string. The ***suṣumnā nāḍī*** originates in the ***kānda***, or 'bulb', and rises upwards through the body and each ***cakra***, terminating at a region that corresponds with the crown of the head. The ***kānda*** represents a mass of potential energy within the lowest energetic levels of the physical body, thought by many to correspond with the sacral plexus. Although the impetus of this spiritual energy is to rise upwards through the ***suṣumnā nāḍī***, its movement is held in check by the continuous flow of ***prāṇa*** ('vital force') within two lesser channels that flow on either side of the ***suṣumnā nāḍī***, called the ***idā*** and ***pingalā nāḍīs***:

- The ***idā nāḍī***, or 'channel of comfort', represents the preserving aspects of the physical body and the feminine aspects of consiousness. It begins on the left side of the ***kānda***, rises up the back of the body, over the back of the head to the ***ājñā cakra***, or 'third eye', drops down and terminates in the left nostril.
- The ***pingalā nāḍī***, also known as the 'tawny current', represents the activating aspects of the physical body, as well as the masculine aspects of consciousness. It originates on the right side of the ***kānda***, rising upwards over the back of the right side of the head to the ***ājñā cakra***, drops down and terminates in the right nostril.

For most humans the ***idā*** and ***pingalā nāḍīs*** are the main pathways of energetic flow in the body, representing the duality of life and death, and the duality of consciousness. As ***prāṇa*** flows through them, the ***nāḍīs*** activate the dualistic and potentially negative aspects of each ***cakra***. When the flow of ***prāṇa*** is disrupted or blocked in these areas the result could be a variety of physical, emotional or mental problems that represent elemental qualities of the disturbed ***cakra***. To this extent, treatment can be given to improve energetic flow within the ***idā*** and ***pingalā nāḍīs*** to restore health, but in the spiritual tradition of ***hatha yoga***, the aspirant seeks to resolve all pain and suffering by directing ***prāṇa*** into the ***suṣumnā nāḍī***, the central channel. When ***prāṇa*** is directed into the ***suṣumnā nāḍī*** it awakens ***kundalinī***, the 'serpent power' of the Transcendent. ***Kundalinī*** is the potential mass of psychospiritual energy of the body, the capacity for spiritual transformation. It is the active, feminine aspect of the Divine called ***śakti*** that remains tightly coiled in the lowest aspect of the etheric body in spiritually unevolved beings.

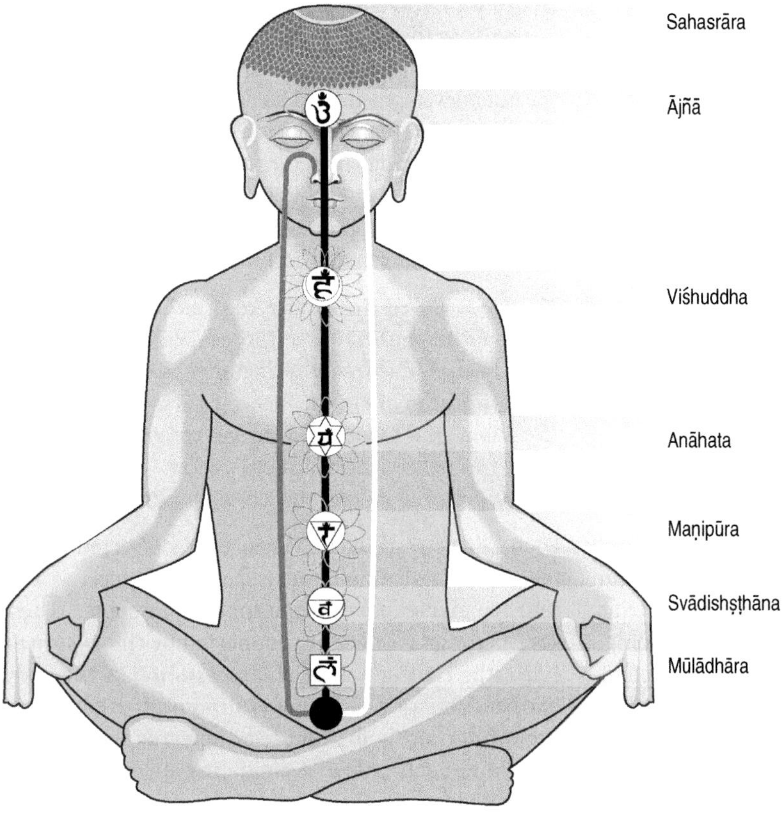

Figure 1.2 The ***cakra*** system.

Although there are a great many paths to spiritual liberation in India, most advocate a methodology that is more or less based upon ***aṣṭāñga yoga***, the 'eight' (***aṣṭ***) 'limbs' (***āñga***) of 'spiritual union' (***yoga***). ***Aṣṭāñga yoga*** is a highly specific set of guidelines that are traditionally considered to be the safest method to awaken ***kundalinī***, and can be practiced by anyone of any faith or spiritual practice. The eight limbs of ***aṣṭāñga yoga*** are:

1. ***Yama***: moral observance; skillful thoughts, works and actions directed externally
2. ***Niyama***: self-restraint; skillful thoughts, works and actions directed internally
3. ***Āsana***: posture; physical training
4. ***Prāṇayama***: breath control; breathing exercises
5. ***Pratyāhāra***: sensory inhibition; restraint of the senses
6. ***Dhāraṇā***: concentration; the ability to direct the mind
7. ***Dhyāna***: meditation; the ability to commune with that which we seek to understand
8. ***Samādhi***: ecstasy; complete integration.

The first five limbs of ***aṣṭāñga yoga*** are taken to make up ***hatha yoga***, and the latter three relate to the practice of ***rāja yoga***. The term ***hatha*** is derived from two words: '***ha***' meaning 'darkness' and '***tha***' which means 'light'. Thus ***hatha yoga*** is the path that seeks to unite the primordial aspects of the sun and the moon, the archetype of male and female, ***puruṣa*** and ***prakṛti***. ***Hatha***, however, also means 'forceful', referring to the practice of self-discipline and the effort it takes to rouse oneself to the calling of spiritual development. The goal of ***hatha yoga*** is the formation of a 'yogic body' (***yoga deha***), a body that is free from disease and the limitations of an ordinary human body, purified and cleansed for ***rāja yoga***.

While many confuse ***hatha yoga*** with the practice of ***āsana***, ***hatha yoga*** has a much broader outlook than the series of physical exercises it is often thought to be in the West. Ultimately the ***āsanas*** only serve to relax the body, making it able to withstand long periods of meditation. According to Patañjali, the author of the ***Yoga sūtra***, the only physical position (***āsana***) that it is important to cultivate is one that is 'stable' and 'pleasurable' (***sthirasukhamāsanam***), allowing for complete physical relaxation and mental clarity. Absolute proficiency in all the different ***āsanas*** is not considered necessary by most Indian spiritual traditions.

Rāja yoga, or the 'royal' ***yoga***, comprises the last three elements of ***aṣṭāñga yoga***, representing the teachings of ***Vedānta*** and the conscious direction of the mind towards spiritual liberation. Such an approach may combine an emphasis upon breathing techniques (***prāṇayama***), ***mantra*** and devotional exercises (***bhakti***). Other methods such as ***dhyāna*** ('meditation') are practised to facilitate a conscious understanding of the nature of self, where subject and object become one (***samādhi***).

Although ***aṣṭāñga yoga*** provides a clear path to divine knowledge, the actual practice involves a great deal of subtlety and aspirants are encouraged to seek instruction from experienced practitioners. The release of ***kundalinī*** is not a thing to play with, and without preparation the premature release of ***kundalinī*** is said to result in a variety of conditions, including inexplicable illness, erratic behaviours, anxiety, psychosis and memory loss. For those who are interested in researching ***kundalinī*** perhaps the best place to begin is with the works of Gopi Krishna, who, in his book ***Kundalini***: *The Evolutionary Energy in Man*, lucidly describes his experience with the awakening of the 'serpent power':

> 'Suddenly, with a roar like that of a waterfall, I felt a stream of liquid light entering my brain through the spinal cord. Entirely unprepared for such a development, I was completely taken by surprise; but regaining self-control instantaneously, I remained sitting in the same posture, keeping my mind on the point of concentration. The illumination grew brighter and brighter, the roaring loader, I experienced a rocking sensation and then felt myself slipping out of my body, entirely enveloped in a halo of light.'
>
> (Krishna 1971)

The awakening of ***kundalinī*** is the event that underlies the great revelations of all spiritual traditions, when the creative energy (***śakti***) of the individual unites with the ultimate awareness of the One (***śiva***). Through consistent spiritual practice ***kundalinī*** can be awakened from her dormant state, and like a snake-charmer we patiently entice this spiritual awakening to liberate us from the world of ***saṃsāra***. As ***kundalinī*** is called, she awakens each ***cakra*** to its purist potential, providing deep and truly profound insights into the nature of being.

ENDNOTES

1 Either literally, perhaps to a sage-King of the Himalayan tribes-people; or through meditation and revelation, Mount Kailash representing the pinnacle of human consciousness and divine revelation. In his role as King of the Gods, Indra represents the natural order which preserves life, harmony and goodness – in this sense, Āyurveda is an inherent principle of living in harmony with this natural order, i.e. *vis medicatrix naturae*.

2 The ***Suśruta saṃhitā*** reveres Divodāsa as Dhanvantari, an incarnation of Viṣṇu and the God of Āyurveda. By some accounts Divodāsa receives this knowledge directly from Indra, whereas in others he receieves it from Bharadvāja.

3 So far the debate as to the true age of the ***Caraka*** and ***Suśruta saṃhitās*** is unresolved. European indologists have dated the original authorship of these texts anywhere from the time of the Buddha (c. 600 BCE) to around 200 CE. In contrast, indologists from the sub-continent contend that the knowledge contained in these texts is much earlier, preserved over time by an ancient oral tradition. As the original authors, P. V. Sharma dates Atreya and Divodāsa to before 1000 BCE, while the ***Caraka saṃhitā*** itself was compiled some time between the 3rd and 2nd century BCE, and the ***Suśruta saṃhitā*** by about the 2nd century CE (Sharma 1992, 1999)

4 ***Anguttura-Nikāya*** VI:55, Pali Canon; ***nirvāṇa***, lit. 'extinction,' from the root ***nir*** ('to cease'), and ***vā*** ('to move').

5 The term ***citta*** is derived from the Sanskrit root of '***cit***' meaning to be 'aware.'

6 Within the ***vijñānmaya kośa*** the ***ahaṃkāra*** and ***buddhi*** compete for our attention, and together generate 'mundane knowledge' (***vijñāna***), as opposed to the higher aspects of knowledge, called ***jñāna***, which is the preserve of the ***buddhi*** and not influenced by the instability of the ***ahaṃkāra.***

7 It is not my intention to suggest that anyone need accept the religio-philosophical tenets of Hinduism to practice Āyurveda. Today in modern India people from every kind of faith study and practice Āyurveda. There is, however, a spiritual component to Āyurveda that cannot be denied: it is fundamental and cannot be separated out without seriously damaging the integrity of the system. Thus the reader is invited to adapt the study of Āyurveda to his or her own personal or religious philosophy. A purely existential or materialistic view of life, however, is incompatible with the principles of Āyurveda.

8 The ***Mūlādhāra cakra*** relates to the element of earth and the psychology of fear and instinct; the ***Svādhiṣṭhāna cakra*** relates to the element of water and the psychology of sensuality and desire; the ***Maṇipūra cakra*** relates to the element of fire and the psychology of anger and will; the ***Anāhata cakra*** relates to the element of wind and the psychology of compassion and love; the ***Viśuddha cakra*** relates to the element of pervasiveness and the psychology of insight and wisdom; the ***Ājñā cakra*** relates to the element of pure consciousness (***buddhi***) and the cessation of duality; the ***Sahasrāra cakra*** represents ***nirvāṇa*** ('the ceasing of all movement') and ***mokṣa*** ('the final liberation').

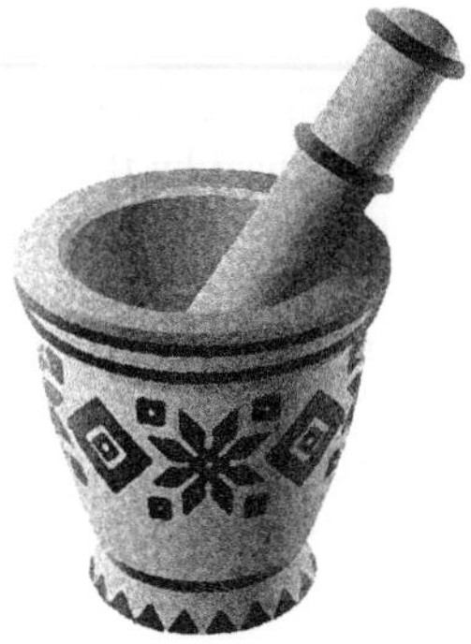

Chapter 2

THEORY

OBJECTIVES

- To review the philosophy of the ***Sāṅkhya darśana*** and its influence upon Āyurveda.
- To understand the framework and application of qualitative differences in Āyurveda.
- To introduce and detail the humoral system of Āyurvedic medicine.

2.1 THE *Sāṅkhya darśana*

An important component underlying the theoretical basis of Āyurveda is the ***Sāṅkhya darśana***, an ancient Vedic system of ontology that enumerates several distinct categories (***tattva***) of existence. This manifestation of increasingly grosser forms of existence begins with the evolution of ***prakṛti*** from ***puruṣa***. ***Puruṣa*** represents the latent force of nature, unexpressed and unknowable, synonymous with ***brahman*** and the ***atma*** ('great soul') described in the literature of ***Vedānta***. Emanating from ***puruṣa*** is ***prakṛti***, the principle of 'nature' and the infinite diversity of creation. Although ***prakṛti*** represents the totality of the universe it also represents the dualistic nature of existence, the separation of subject and object, and the subsequent delineation of dualistic attributes such as individuality and gender. Before creation there is only ***puruṣa***, an endless and timeless void of pure potentiality, but as desire (***taṇhā***) arises in ***puruṣa***, ***prakṛti*** is formed. This act of desire initiates the cycle of creation, emanating but divided from the totality of ***puruṣa***. The two principles of ***prakṛti*** and ***puruṣa*** are represented graphically as the sexual union of the goddess Śakti and the god Śiva, respectively. Śiva is portrayed as a corpse, lying supine, and Śakti sits astride him and copulates, taking the latent energy of Śiva and transforming it into the active energy of ***prakṛti***.

According to the ***Sāṅkhya darśana***, from the desire of ***prakṛti*** arises ***mahat***, the 'cosmic intelligence' and the knowledge of the transcendent Self that is within all. In this sense ***mahat*** most closely represents the Western concept of 'God', the total experience of the living universe, not as an individual being but as an omnipresence from which all natural laws emanate. Arising from ***mahat*** is ***ahaṃkāra***, the principle that fragments the unity of God into an individual sense of self. ***Ahaṃkāra*** is in many ways similar to the psychological concept of the ego, as a force that separates each of us into an individualised and incomplete experience of the Whole. When this principle of ***ahaṃkāra*** is at work in our consciousness, we each think that we are unique people. More closer to the truth is that only the conditions of the individual existence are different, not the function of ***ahaṃkāra***. It is the sense of 'me' that is ***ahaṃkāra***, the same sense of 'me-ness' that is possessed by each individual being. ***Ahaṃkāra*** resonates within the entire spectrum of individualised existence, from a purely aesthetic or abstract sense of self, to physiological activities such as the immune system that function to maintain that 'self-ness'.

From ***ahaṃkāra*** issues three primordial qualities, the ***mahaguṇas***, called ***sattva***, ***rajas*** and ***tamas***. In one sense, the ***mahaguṇas*** represent qualitative differences within the entire spectrum of individualised existence. ***Sattva*** can be thought of as the essence of creation, the quality of perception, clarity, equanimity and light. ***Rajas*** is the energy of creation, the quality of movement, change, transformation and colour. ***Tamas*** is the physical constitution of the created universe, the quality of cohesion, stasis, inertia and darkness. In regard to perceptual distinctions, ***sattva*** is also the principle of subjectivity, and from ***sattva*** arises the mind (***manas***), the five ***jñāna indriyās*** ('sense organs', i.e. ears, eyes, nose, mouth and skin), and the five ***karma indriyās*** ('organs of action', i.e. mouth, hands, limbs, genitalia and eliminative organs). ***Sattva*** thus embodies the essence of experience, the living subjective knowledge obtained from the objective experience. In contrast, ***tamas*** represents the object, the inanimate gross matter of the universe, devoid of sentience, and the confusion of subject with object. ***Tamas*** gives rise to pure physicality, such as the house that needs to be repaired and renovated, and the body (***annamaya kośa***, 'food sheath') that is released upon death. The emotional intensity with which we react to ***tamasic*** experiences is one example of just how powerfully subject becomes enmeshed with object, giving rise to ***dukha*** ('dissatisfaction'). Existing between ***sattva*** and ***tamas*** is ***rajas***, which acts as the catalyst that binds subject with object, connecting the subjectivity of mind and sense with the physical universe.

From ***tamas*** arises the five ***tanmātrās***, the subtle aspects of the material universe perceived by the five ***jñāna indriyās***. The five ***tanmātrās*** are ***śabda*** ('sound'), ***sparśa*** ('touch'), ***rūpa*** ('sight'), ***rasa*** ('taste') and ***gandhā*** ('smell'). From each of these subtle elemental aspects arises the ***pañca mahābhūtas*** ('elements'). These five elements are the basic principles of the universe and as such are the primary components of the human body. They are:

1. ***Pṛthvī***: earth, or the principle of inertia
2. ***Ap***: water, or the principle of cohesion
3. ***Tejas***: fire, or the principle of radiance
4. ***Vāyu***: wind, or the principle of vibration
5. ***Ākāśa***: ether, or the principle of pervasiveness.

It is incorrect to consider the ***mahābhūtas*** as 'elements' in the scientific sense of the word, as they are contained in varying proportions within the most minute subatomic phenomena. They are principles that provide the impetus for the creation of grosser materials, but are still to some extent a philosophical concept, in much the same way that the most subtle aspects of quantum theory remain unproven.

Each of the ***mahābhūtas*** forms different tissues of the body. As the principle of pervasiveness ***ākāśa*** relates to all hollow or empty places in the body, such as the orifices, channels and pores, as well as the ears that perceive the ***tanmatra*** of ***śabda*** ('sound'), and the different sounds that the body produces (e.g. during vocalisation, respiration, myocardial activity, nervous system activity etc.). From ***vāyu*** arises the skin, which perceives the ***tanmatra*** of ***sparśa*** ('touch'), and relates to the activities of the respiratory system. From ***tejas*** arises the eyes, which perceives the ***tanmatra*** of ***rūpa*** ('sight'), and is responsible for activities such as digestion and perception. From ***ap*** arises the tongue, which perceives the ***tanmatra*** of ***rasa*** ('taste'), and is responsible for fluid metabolism in the body, and to bind the tissues together. From ***pṛthvī*** arises the nose, which perceives ***tanmatra*** of ***gandhā*** ('smell'), and along with ***ap*** is responsible for the physical constitution of the body.

2.2 THE *guṇas*

The evolution of the ***mahābhūtas*** gives rise to the distinction of qualitative differences that can be objectively determined. In other words, one ***mahābhūta***

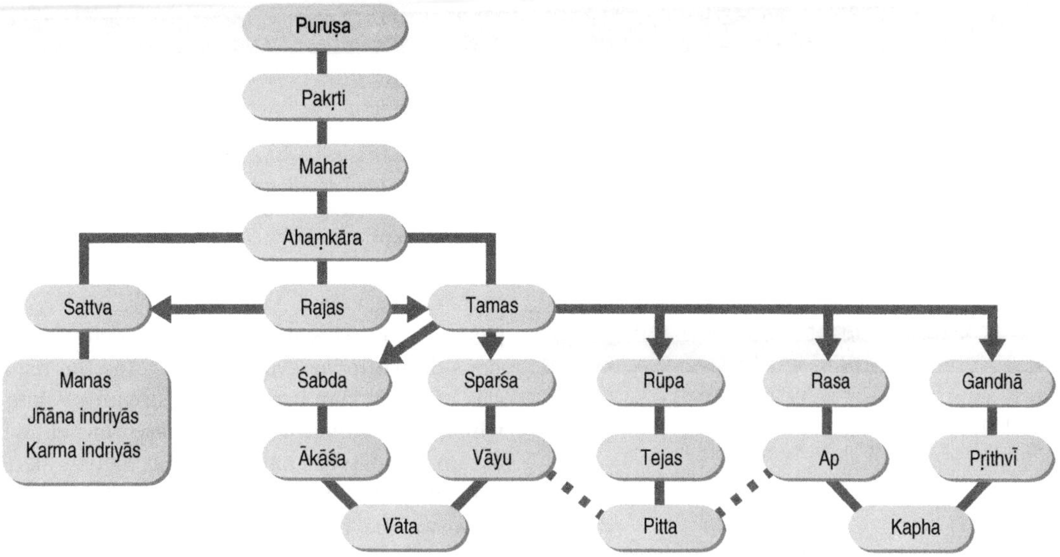

Figure 2.1 The ***sāṅkhya darśana.***

will display certain qualities that differentiate it from another ***mahābhūta***. It should be clear to the reader that individual ***mahābhūtas*** are impossible to perceive, and admixtures thereof perhaps too complex to quantify. While the ***mahābhūtas*** and thus the totality of corporeal existence cannot be perceived objectively, their presence can be inferred by the manifestation of certain qualities. To facilitate an understanding between the differences of the ***mahābhūtas***, Āyurvedic medicine maintains a list of qualities called the ***gurvādi*** ('ten pairs of opposite') ***guṇas*** ('qualities'), shown in Table 2.1.

Each of the ***gurvādi guṇas*** is associated with a particular ***mahābhūta***, and its opposite quality will be manifest in a ***mahābhūta*** that has an opposing action or effect. For example, the ***mahābhūta*** of ***pṛthvī*** ('earth') is associated with the quality of ***guru*** ('heavy'); the opposing quality of ***laghu*** ('light') is associated with the ***mahābhūta*** of ***vāyu*** ('wind'). Thus to some extent ***pṛthvī*** and ***vāyu*** have opposing forms and actions. Each pair of opposites is only one specific dimension in an interaction, however, with each subsequent pair representing a contrasting dimension. By recognising several different dimensions of interaction the result is a multidimensional model that explains the complexity of interactions that occur between the ***mahābhūtas***. Thus while ***pṛthvī*** ('earth') displays the quality of ***guru*** ('heavy'), it is also considered to be ***rūkṣa*** ('dry'). ***Vāyu*** ('wind') displays the opposite quality of ***laghu*** ('light'), but is also ***rūkṣa*** ('dry'). The relationship between ***pṛthvī*** and ***vāyu*** is therefore complex, displaying both similar and opposing qualities. Table 2.2 demonstrates the relationship of the ***gurvādi guṇas*** with the ***mahābhūtas***.

While all ten pairs of opposite qualities are generally considered in Āyurveda, for the purposes of diagnosis and treatment they are usually whittled down to three dominant dimensions of interaction that in large part guide the manifestation of all subsequent qualities, called the ***upakarmas*** (Table 2.3). As we

TABLE 2.1 The *gurvādi guṇas*: ten pairs of opposite qualities.

Guru ('heavy')	***Laghu*** ('light')
Manda ('slow')	***Tikṣṇa*** ('fast')
Śita ('cold')	***Uṣṇa*** ('hot')
Snigdha ('greasy')	***Rūkṣa*** ('dry')
Ślakṣna ('smooth')	***Khara*** ('rough')
Sāñdra ('solid')	***Drava*** ('fluid')
Mṛdu ('soft')	***Kaṭhiṇa*** ('hard')
Sthira ('stability')	***Cala*** ('movement')
Sūkṣma ('subtle')	***Sthūla*** ('obvious')
Viśada ('friction')	***Picchila*** ('slimy')

TABLE 2.2 Relationship between the *mahābhūtas*, *tanmātrās* and *guṇas*.

Mahābhūtas	*Tanmātrās*	*Guṇas*
Pṛthvī ('earth')	***Gandhā*** ('smell')	***Guru, manda, sthira, kaṭhiṇa, sthūla, sāñdra***
Ap ('water')	***Rasa*** ('taste')	***Śita, snigdha, mṛdu, guru, drava, manda***
Tejas ('fire')	***Rūpa*** ('sight')	***Uṣṇa, laghu, tikṣṇa, drava***
Vāyu ('air')	***Sparśa*** ('touch')	***Laghu, rūkṣa, cala, viśada, khara, sūkṣma***
Ākāśa ('pervasiveness')	***Śabda*** ('sound')	***Sūkṣma, viśada***

TABLE 2.3 The *upakarmas*.

Guru ('heavy')	***Laghu*** ('light')
Śita ('cold')	***Uṣṇa*** ('hot')
Snigdha ('greasy')	***Rūkṣa*** ('dry')

will see, these ***upakarmas*** form the basis of the six ***śamana karmas*** used in Āyurvedic therapeutics (see Ch. 11).

2.3 THE *tridoṣa* THEORY

When the ancient seers of Āyurveda contemplated the human body they must have had a sense of its incredible intricacy. An advanced knowledge of human anatomy described in the ***Suśruta saṃhitā***, combined with keen observations on the nature of being that is the hallmark of Indian spirituality, provided for an exceedingly lucid physiological model in Āyurvedic medicine. This model, however, is based on the notion that the human body is a holographic representation of the macrocosm. Āyurveda teaches that within our being, and within our bodies, exist all the clues and data we need to understand the universe: ***tvat tvam asi*** ('thou art that') commands the sage of the ***Upaniṣads***. We are, after all, as astronomers tell us, children of the stars.

With this insight into the complexity of our origin the sage understands that the knowledge of the body is never complete, a truth that is painfully obvious to anyone who tries to keep abreast of the myriad developments and contradictory opinions of medical science. The ancient seers knew well this merry-go-round of shifting phenomena and perceptions, identifying it as a property of ***saṃsāra***. According to this understanding ***saṃsāra*** represents the inexorable law of change, that no subject or object ever remains completely static. This means that the definitive conclusions drawn today eventually become the redundancies of tomorrow because the stream of data upon which these conclusions were based has changed. To use an analogy, the nature of objectivity is akin to the ancient light of the stars that fills the heavens at night: what we see now, objectively, has already become something else. On a physical level our response to any experience is affected by the slight delay it takes for our nervous system to receive and process the sensory information and output an appropriate response. Although for the most part imperceptible, this time lag means that our response is conditioned by the past, rather than what is actually happening in the moment.

Unlike a completely objective science, Āyurveda is orientated to help the practitioner understand the nature of ***saṃsāra***. To do this the Āyurvedic practitioner implements an approach that arises from principles that are based on the spiritual teachings of the ***Vedas***, as well as the experiences of the Self-realised sages that have passed beyond the edges of human consciousness. According to tradition, the principles of Āyurveda are emanations of an unchanging and eternal truth that reside in ***mahat***. In contrast, modern science is based upon the systematic observation, experimentation and analysis of ***saṃsāra***. The limits of human perception, including the technology that expands that awareness, are unconsciously guided by the principle of ***ahaṃkāra***. ***Ahaṃkāra*** represents the act of naming, identification and discrimination. It creates a vocabulary, a semantic description of a conditioned reality that lulls the scientist into believing in the idea of objectivity, that the individuated self can somehow observe the machinations of ***saṃsāra*** without that perception itself being affected. The ancient sages of Āyurveda did not seek to understand the minutiae of the human body nor pretended to have an objective perspective, but instead focused their attention on discovering the principles behind physiological activities. Thus when encountering a disease the Āyurvedic practitioner can largely ignore the complexity of pathological definitions and seek to understand the *principle* of the disease, thereby to develop a corresponding *principle* of treatment.

Having arisen from the ***mahābhūtas*** the human body can be seen to exhibit three principles of function, called ***vāta***, ***pitta*** and ***kapha***:

- ***Pṛthvī*** ('earth') and ***ap*** ('water') form ***kapha***
- ***Tejas*** ('fire'), and to a lesser extent ***ap*** ('water') and ***vāyu*** ('wind') form ***pitta***
- ***Vāyu*** ('wind') and ***ākāśa*** ('pervasiveness') form ***vāta***.

These three principles of function are called ***doṣas*** because they are subject to influences from both within and without. The term ***doṣa*** literally means 'blemish' because it is the increase, decrease and disturbance of one, two or all three of the ***doṣas*** that are responsible for all pathological changes in the body. Each ***doṣa*** has a specific ***pramāṇa*** ('quantity'), ***guṇa*** ('quality') and ***karma*** ('action') in the body. In an undisturbed state their function is said to be ***avikṛta*** ('normal'), the result of which is ***arogya*** (the 'absence of disease'). Foods, habits and environmental factors that are contrary to the qualities of a particular ***doṣa*** bring about its decrease, while foods, habits and environmental factors that are similar to a particular ***doṣa*** bring about its increase. Both of these states of increase (***vṛddhi***) and decrease (***kṣaya***) are considered abnormal (***vikṛta***), but it is increase that causes major disturbances, while decrease typically causes only minor disturbances.

The three ***doṣas*** are traditionally correlated with three types of eliminatory products: ***vāta*** is synonymous with 'wind' (i.e. flatulence), ***pitta*** with 'bile', and ***kapha*** with 'phlegm'. Although the descriptors of 'wind', 'bile', and 'phlegm' do not describe the complete activities of the ***doṣas***, they provide a convenient way to understand the implications of their manifestation when in a disturbed state.

Vāta doṣa

Vāta comes from the ***Sanskrit*** root word '***va***', referring to the qualities of movement and enthusiasm, and is the catalyst for all functions in the body to the extent that without its involvement ***pitta*** and ***kapha*** are said to be lame. The ***Caraka saṃhitā*** states that ***vāta*** is the grossest manifestation of the divine 'wind', and is responsible for the function of the entire body (***tantra yantra dhara***) and the originator of every kind of physiological action or anatomical structure (***ceṣtā pravartaka***). ***Vāta*** promotes and regulates the activities of the mind, carrying the perceptions of sensory cognition (***jñāna indriyās***) to the effector organs (***karma indriyās***) for a response. As the wind or 'flatus' that expels the faeces, ***vāta*** also promotes the expulsion of all wastes from the body, as well as the ejaculation of semen and the birthing of a baby. The activity of ***vāyu*** is present in conception, drawing the sperm and ovum together, guiding embryonic development. Given the important role that ***vāta*** plays it is perhaps no surprise that when it is retained or blocked in the body it becomes a major pathogenic influence.

As you may recall, ***vāta*** comprises the ***mahābhūtas*** of ***ākāśa*** and ***vāyu***. When ***vāta*** is disturbed the pervasive nature of ***ākāśa*** and the catabolic activity of ***vāyu*** represent widespread degenerative changes in the body, characterised by a lightness (***laghu***) and dryness (***rūkṣa***) of the tissues, which in turn promotes roughness (***khara***) and friction (***viśada***) in the body. ***Vāta*** is also ***śita*** ('cold') in nature although only because ***vāta*** assumes either ***śita*** ('cold') or ***uṣṇa*** ('hot') ***guṇas*** when exposed to their presence. Although ***vāyu*** and ***ākāśa*** are neutral in temperament the physical body is dominant in ***pṛthvī*** ('earth') and ***ap*** ('water'). Together, ***pṛthvī*** and ***ap*** create a cooling, solidifying influence, and thus ***vāta*** assumes a cold temperament in the body.

- The primary qualities of ***vāta*** are ***laghu*** ('light'), ***śita*** ('cold'), ***rūkṣa*** ('dry'), ***cala*** ('movement'), ***viśada*** ('friction'), ***khara*** ('rough'), and ***sūkṣma*** ('subtle').

Pitta doṣa

The function of ***pitta*** in the body is to provide heat due to the predominance of ***tejas*** in its composition, represented by the catabolic or 'cooking' action of digestion. This notion of cooking the ingested food, however, also extends to the concept of metabolism, and thus ***pitta*** is associated with metabolically active organs such as the liver, skin and blood. The term

pitta is derived from the root word ***tapas***, which means 'to heat' or 'glow'. ***Pitta*** also contains an aspect of ***ap*** in its constitution and thus to some extent displays ***snigdha*** ('greasy') and ***drava*** ('fluid') properties, characterised by the greasy, flowing and 'mobile' (***sara***) nature of bile, blood and sweat. ***Pitta*** is also ***laghu*** ('light') and ***tikṣṇa*** ('sharp') in nature, characterised by the catabolic action of ***tejas*** and ***vāyu*** that act together to combust solid substances into pure expressible energy.

- The primary qualities of ***pitta*** are ***laghu*** ('light'), ***uṣṇa*** ('hot'), ***snigdha*** ('greasy'), ***tikṣṇa*** ('sharp'), ***sara*** ('movement'), and ***drava*** ('fluid').

Kapha doṣa

In many ways ***kapha*** is opposite in nature to ***pitta***, attending to the structural functions of the body, lubricating, moisturising, nourishing and providing support. Comprising ***pṛthvī*** and ***ap***, ***kapha*** most strongly relates to the physical structure of the body, and is thus ***sthira*** ('solid'), ***guru*** ('heavy'), and ***sthūla*** ('gross') in nature. The term ***kapha*** is derived from the root word ***śliṣ***, which means 'to embrace', referring to the ***snigdha*** ('greasy') and ***picchila*** ('slimy') qualities that in combination with solidity and substance bind tissues together. These greasy and slippery properties of ***kapha*** also describe the nature and function of the generative organs, the creation of new life, as well as the lactating breast that can nourish another being.

- The primary qualities of ***kapha*** are ***guru*** ('heavy'), ***śita*** ('cold'), ***snigdha*** ('greasy'), ***sthira*** ('stable'), ***mṛdu*** ('softening'), and ***picchila*** ('slimy').

2.4 *Sthāna*: RESIDENCE OF THE *doṣas*

Despite the reality that each ***doṣa*** is involved in physiological processes all over the body, each also maintains a primary 'seat' of influence, or ***sthāna***. To some extent this idea is related to the often used transliteration of the ***doṣas***; i.e. wind, bile and phlegm. As the ***doṣa*** of wind, ***vāta*** is located in the ***antra*** ('colon') and ***basti*** ('bladder'), governing the regions of the body from the umbilicus downwards. As the ***doṣa*** of bile, ***pitta*** is located in organs such as the ***āmāśaya*** ('stomach'), ***yakrit*** ('liver') and ***plīhan*** ('spleen'), governing the area between the umbilicus and the diaphragm. As the ***doṣa*** of phlegm, ***kapha*** is located primarily in ***phuphusa*** ('lungs') and ***hṛdaya*** ('heart'), governing the areas from the diaphragm upwards.

2.5 *Kāla*: TIMING OF THE *doṣas*

Kāla ('time') relates to the influence of the ***doṣas*** in a variety of natural cycles: over a period of time such as in a day or a lifetime, or in specific processes, such as in digestion or disease. In every situation the Āyurvedic practitioner attempts to understand the state of the ***doṣas***. Generally speaking, ***kapha*** is dominant after sunrise and sunset, at the beginning stages of digestion (in the mouth and stomach), during childhood (***bālya***) and in the congestive, prodromal stage of disease. ***Pitta*** is dominant at midday and midnight, in the middle portion of digestion (in the lower fundus of the stomach and small intestine), during mid-life (***madhya***), and in the inflammatory or acute stage of disease. ***Vāta*** is dominant in the hours before dawn and sunset, in the latter part of digestion (in the colon), in the latter stages of life (***jīrṇa***), and in the chronic and degenerative stages of disease.

2.6 *Tridoṣa lakṣaṇas*: SYMPTOMOLOGY OF THE *doṣas*

The knowledge of which physical symptoms are associated with a particular ***doṣa*** or group of ***doṣas*** is the first step by which an Āyurvedic practitioner gathers clinical information, formulates a diagnosis and implements a principle of treatment. Thus certain symptoms are generally correlated with the effects of a particular ***doṣa***, based on the qualities that ***doṣa*** tends to exhibit. Thus the ***uṣṇa***, ***tikṣṇa*** and ***drava*** qualities of ***pitta*** suggest conditions such as burning sensations and diarrhoea; the ***manda***, ***snigdha*** and ***śita*** qualities of ***kapha*** suggest catarrhal conditions and lethargy; and the ***rūkṣa***, ***laghu*** and ***śita*** properties of the ***vāta*** suggest wasting and degenerative processes. In actual practice, however, each type of disease is further classified according to the ***doṣas***, even though a particular disease may be generally correlated with a particular ***doṣa***. Thus while a symptom such as diarrhoea is a manifestation of the ***uṣṇa*** and

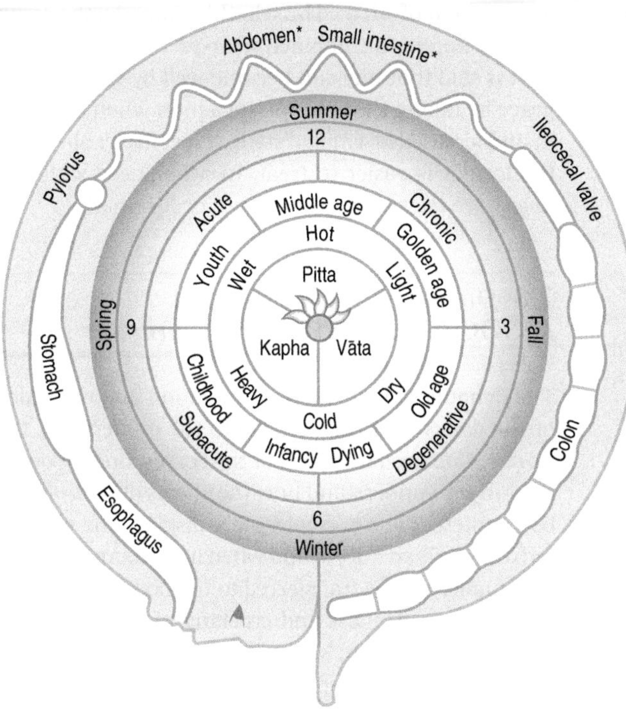

Figure 2.2 The tridoṣic wheel of life.

drava qualities of ***pitta***, an Āyurvedic practitioner will ascertain whether secondary characteristics suggest that the origin of the disease is other than ***pitta***. Thus in ***paittika*** variants of diarrhoea the patient will complain of burning sensations, thirst and a high fever, indicative of the ***uṣṇa*** properties of ***pitta***. If the patient discharges much mucus and complains of coldness and lethargy, then the diarrhoea might be classified as ***kapha***, indicated by the ***śita***, ***manda*** and ***snigdha*** properties of the symptomology. If the patient experiences frequent motions but only evacuates a relatively small volume, with much pain and flatulence, then the diarrhoea might be classified as ***vāta***, indicated by the ***rūkṣa***, ***cala***, and ***śita*** properties of the secondary symptoms. Thus a treatment regimen would be created to address the underlying cause of the condition, as well as address the primary symptomology.

The following are descriptions of ***vāta***, ***pitta*** and ***kapha*** in normalcy, as well as in a state of 'increase' (***vṛddhi***) and 'deficiency' (***kaśāya***). Generally speaking, the practitioner takes note of the increased state of a given ***doṣa***, not the deficiency, because it is an increased state of the ***doṣas*** which is responsible for causing disease.

Vāta lakṣaṇas

Vāta in normalcy protects the body by being the primary catalyst for all actions within it. ***Vāta*** bestows enthusiasm and desire, inspiration and expiration, all activities of body, mind, sense and speech, sexual function and the initiation of the urge and expulsion of wastes. When in an increased state, ***vāta*** produces emaciation and cachexia, a desire for hot food and drinks, a fear of cold, tremors and spasm, abdominal distension, constipation, weakness, fatigue, distortion of sensory function, excessive talking, giddiness, confusion, irreverence, fear, anxiety, nervousness, and black, blue, orange or clear discolorations of the skin, eyes, urine and faeces. When ***vāta*** is in a decreased state there is general bodily dysfunction, loss of sensation and consciousness and the general characteristics of a ***kapha*** increase.

Pitta lakṣaṇas

Pitta in a normal state attends to digestion and processing of wastes, appetite and thirst, complexion, eyesight, intelligence, courage and bravery, and suppleness of body tissues. When increased, ***pitta***

promotes excessive appetite and thirst, burning sensations, diarrhoea, anger, and yellow, red or green discolorations of the skin, eyes, urine and faeces. If ***pitta*** is in a decreased state the digestion will be poor, the skin will lose its lustre, and the patient will complain of the general symptoms of an increase in ***vāta*** and ***kapha***.

Kapha lakṣaṇas

The function of ***kapha*** in the body is to provide stability, structure, lubrication, endurance and strength. In an increased state, ***kapha*** results in a slow and sluggish digestion, excessive salivation, abundant phlegm and catarrh, lassitude, a desire for sleep, heaviness, coldness, obesity, dyspnoea, cough, sneezing, itching, and whitish, pink or clear discolorations of the skin, eyes, urine and feces. If ***kapha*** is decreased within the body there will be dizziness, emaciation, looseness and friction in the joints, palpitations, dry mucosa and the general symptoms of ***vāta*** increase.

For clarification, Table 2.4 describes the basic characteristics and the increased (***vṛddhi***) symptoms of each ***doṣa***, as well as the effect of the ***doṣas*** upon the mind (discussed in more detail in Ch. 3). Where signs and symptoms include more than one ***doṣa*** this is taken to be a mixed condition (i.e. ***vāta-pitta***, ***vāta-kapha***, ***kapha-pitta***, ***vāta-kapha-pitta***).

2.7 *Caya* and *kopa*: INCREASE AND VITIATION OF THE *doṣas*

Āyurveda differentiates between a ***doṣa*** in an 'increased' state (***caya***) and in a ***doṣa*** in a 'vitiated' state (***kopa***). Generally, when a ***doṣa*** is in an increased state (***caya***, ***vṛddhi***) its effects are usually limited to the physiological activities and the ***sthāna*** it governs, with clearly definable signs and symptoms that relate only to that ***doṣa***. When in a vitiated (***kopa***) state, however, the affected ***doṣa*** can begin to affect the other ***doṣas***, resulting in a condition which is more complex, often with contradictory features, presenting greater difficulties in treatment. An example is haemorrhoids secondary to constipation, which may be the result of an increase in ***vāta***, eventually worsening to bleeding anal fissures because of the subsequent involvement of ***pitta***. Thus, in this example, the result of ***vāta kopa*** is a combined ***vāta-pitta*** condition.

It is said that one can become well by grace or disgrace by taking the appropriate action when a ***doṣa*** is in an increased or vitiated state, respectively: obviously the former is easier to treat. In a balanced state the ***doṣas*** are referred to as ***avikṛta***, or 'normal'.

2.8 *Doṣagati*: THE *doṣas* IN ASSOCIATION WITH THE *guṇas*

The dynamics of the increase, vitiation and normalcy of the ***doṣas*** is directly related to the influence of the ***guṇas***. One need only look at the corresponding opposite ***guṇa*** to understand how the effects of a ***guṇa*** can be countered. For example, ***vāta*** displays the characteristic of ***rūkṣa*** ('dry'), and when in an increased state this quality will be transferred to the body, with symptoms such as dryness and cracking of the heels. The use of a medication, such as ***taila*** (sesame oil), that displays the corresponding opposite quality of ***snigdha*** ('greasy') would thus be applied to alleviate ***rūkṣa*** and return ***vāta*** to normalcy. If ***vāta*** is in a vitiated state, however, and promotes the increase of ***pitta***, this could manifest as bleeding cracks on the heels. Thus the principle quality of ***snigdha*** would need to be combined with the quality of ***śita*** to relieve the additional symptoms of heat, using perhaps coconut oil or ***ghṛta*** (clarified butter), which have both 'cooling' (***śita***) and 'greasy' (***snigdha***) properties.

Uṣṇa ('hot') and ***śita*** ('cold') are the primary ***guṇas*** that drive the increase, vitiation and pacification of the ***doṣas***:

- The qualities of ***vāta*** (i.e. ***rūkṣa***, ***laghu***, ***khara***, ***viśada***, ***cala***) in association with ***uṣṇa*** results in the 'increase' (***caya***) of ***vāta***. These same qualities (i.e. ***rūkṣa***, ***laghu***, ***khara***, ***viśada***, ***cala***) in association with ***śita*** brings about the 'vitiation' (***kopa***) of ***vāta***. Qualities that are opposite in nature to ***vāta*** (i.e. ***snigdha***, ***guru***, ***manda***, ***picchila***, ***sthira***) in association with ***uṣṇa*** bring about its return to normalcy (***samya vāta***).
- The qualities of ***pitta*** (i.e. ***tikṣṇa***, ***laghu***, ***drava***, ***sara***) in association with ***śita*** results in the 'increase' (***caya***) of ***pitta***. These same qualities (i.e. ***tikṣṇa***, ***laghu***, ***drava***, ***sara***) in association with ***uṣṇa*** bring about the 'vitiation' (***kopa***) of ***pitta***.

TABLE 2.4 *Tridoṣa lakṣaṇas* : signs and symptoms of the *doṣas*.

Doṣa	*Guṇa*	Colour (*varna*)	Digestion (*agni*)	Symptoms of increase (*vṛddhi*)	Waste products (*malas*)	Mind and mental function (*manas*)
Vāta	***Rūkṣa, laghu, śita, khara, viśada, cala***	Black, blue, brown, orange, clear	Irregular, sensitive digestion; colic and bloating; astringent taste in mouth	Debilitating pain; loss of function; irregularities, abnormalities, deformities; fragility, wasting; dryness, stiffness, friction, brittleness, spasm, tremor; strong aversion to cold; symptoms worse with cold or dry weather; symptoms worse in early morning and late afternoon	**Faeces:** small amount, constipation, dry, painful and rough evacuation; dark brown to black in colour **urine:** decreased volume, increased frequency; tenesmus; without colour or dark orange to brown; frothy or very greasy **sweat:** minimal volume, even with exertion **mucus:** diminished secretion; dry, stringy, difficult to expectorate	Primarily auditory **balanced:** enthusiastic, motivated, joyful, artistic **imbalanced:** scattered, unsteadiness of mind, poor concentration, restless, anxious, insecure, fearful, lonely, depressed (bipolar), insomnia, delusional; fear of cold
Pitta	***Uṣṇa, laghu, snigdha, tikṣṇa, sara***	Red, yellow, green	Strong, quick digestion; acid reflux, loose motions; bitter taste in mouth	Burning pain, burning sensations; fever, thirst, inflammation, ulceration, purulence; haemorrhage, foul smell; strong aversion to heat; symptoms worse with hot weather; symptoms worse at mid-day and in mid-night	**Faeces:** moderate volume, increased frequency; watery, quick expulsion; burning sensation; yellow, green or reddish discolorations, with blood **urine:** moderate volume, increased frequency; burning sensation; yellow to green in colour, blood **sweat:** profuse without exertion, malodorous **mucus:** moderate secretion; yellowish to green, blood	Primarily visual **balanced:** courageous, intelligent, disciplined **imbalanced:** impatient, judgmental, driven, controlling, angry, violent, fanaticism, insomnia, hallucinatory; aversion to heat
Kapha	***Guru, snigdha, picchila, śita, sthūla, sāñdra, manda***	Clear, white	Slow, dull digestion; epigastric heaviness, catarrh; sweet taste in mouth	Dull aching pain; lethargy, catarrh; itching, hypertrophy, oedema, obesity, cysts, tumours; mild aversion to cold; symptoms worse with cold and wet weather; symptoms worse in mid-morning and mid-evening	**Faeces:** large volume, decreased frequency; solid, heavy, slow evacuation; rectal itching; whitish discoloration with mucus **urine:** increased volume, decreased frequency; mucus, turbid, calculi; clear or white in colour **sweat:** profuse only with exertion; sweet odour **mucus:** copious secretion; easy expectoration; clear to white in colour	Primarily kinesthetic **balanced:** compassionate, generous, nurturing **imbalanced:** slowness, dullness, apathy, attachment, sentimentality, worry, greediness, grief, depression (unipolar); desire for hot, aversion to cold

Qualities that are opposite in nature to **pitta** (i.e. **manda**, **guru**, **sāñdra**, **sthira**) in association with **śita** bring about its return to normalcy (**samya pitta**).

- The qualities of **kapha** (i.e. **snigdha**, **guru**, **sthira**, **manda**, **picchila**) in association with **śita** results in the 'increase' (**caya**) of **kapha**. These same qualities (i.e. **snigdha**, **guru**, **sthira**, **manda**, **picchila**) in association with **uṣṇa** bring about the 'vitiation' (**kopa**) of **kapha**. The opposite qualities (i.e. **rūkṣa**, **laghu**, **cala**, **tikṣṇa**, **viśada**, **khara**) in association with **uṣṇa** bring about its return to normalcy (**samya kapha**).

2.9 THE SUB-*doṣas*: SUBDIVISIONS WITHIN EACH *doṣa*

In order to differentiate the specific actions of each **doṣa** they are in turn divided into five sub-**doṣas** each. While the sub-**doṣas** of **vāta** (i.e. the five **prāṇas** of the **prāṇāmaya kośa**) have long been identified in Āyurveda and allied disciplines such as **hatha yoga**, the approach of dividing **pitta** and **kapha** into five subcomponents appears to be a relatively new innovation, first appearing in the work of Vāgbhaṭa (c. 600 CE). The approach of delineating five subcomponents for each **doṣa** is not integral to understanding the basic theory of Āyurveda, but it does provide the practitioner with a greater realm of subtly to work within, sometimes providing for specific therapies that can affect a particular aspect of the **doṣas**. By studying the sub-**doṣas** we can see how the specific activities of **tri-doṣa** begin to interact with specific elements of physiological function, leaving the emphasis of *principle* and entering into the realm of *specificity*.

2.10 SUB-*doṣas* OF *vāta*

- ***Prāṇa vāyu***
- ***Udāna vāyu***
- ***Samāna vāyu***
- ***Apāna vāyu***
- ***Vyāna vāyu***.

The sub-**doṣas** of **vāta** are the five **vāyus**, or 'winds' of the body, but should not be confused with the **vāyu** of the **mahābhūtas**.

Prāṇa vāyu

Prāṇa vāyu is the first and most important of the five **vāyus**, and ultimately all of the other **vāyus** are really just permutations of **prāṇa**. **Prāṇa** initiates and controls all binary functions in the body, such as inhalation and exhalation, contraction and expansion, and stimulation and relaxation. **Prāṇa** animates the cells of the body as the vital force, entering into the body and into the **hṛdaya** ('heart'), moving upwards to the brain, activating the **indriyās** ('senses'), **citta** ('mind') and **buddhi** ('intellect'). Specifically, **prāṇa** attends to the maintenance of cardiopulmonary activity, governs ingestion, chewing and swallowing, and initiates expectoration, sneezing and belching. **Prāṇa** is the bridge between the physical and astral bodies and, when death occurs, **prāṇa** leaves the body. Symptoms of a disturbance to the function of **prāṇa** include anxiety, central nervous system dysfunction and accumulated toxins. **Prāṇa** may be restored to normalcy by the practice of **prāṇayama**, good nutrition and adequate rest.

Udāna vāyu

Udāna vāyu is derived from the root word '**ud**' meaning 'upward', and thus represents the upward moving energy of the body, located in the chest. **Udāna** is in many respects similar to **prāṇa**, but is considered to be lighter (**laghu**) in nature, and acts as the complement of **prāṇa**. Thus **udāna** governs exhalation, removing carbon dioxide from the alveoli, whereas **prāṇa** governs inhalation and the absorption of oxygen. **Udāna** governs speech, controls the tongue, initiates effort, promotes enthusiasm, and together with **prāṇa**, governs memory. As the upward moving force **udāna** initiates growth, such as the development of a child learning to walk, or as the force that raises consciousness to new levels. **Udāna** lifts the intent of our aspirations and desires to the heavens above. Upon death **udāna** compels consciousness to leave the body and enter the astral realms, and guided by **karma**, propels the soul to its next manifestation. Disorders of **udāna** include suffocation, hyperventilation, hiccoughs, choking, sleep apnoea, emphysema, hoarseness and **kundalinī** disorders. And, because **udāna** and **prāṇa** are similar, a dysfunction of one will most likely be simultaneous with a dysfunction of the other. Measures to balance **udāna** include mindfulness of breath meditation (***anapānasati bhavana***) and the practice of ***prāṇayama***.

Samāna vāyu

Samāna vāyu is located in the ***āmashaya***, and initiates the function of ***pācaka***, the aspect of ***pitta*** that attends to digestion. ***Samāna*** promotes thirst, hunger and satiety, facilitates the separation of waste from nutrient, and assists in assimilation. The movement of ***samāna*** within the body is sideways, descriptive of the movement of chyme through the gastrointestinal tract. ***Samāna*** assesses or 'measures' the metabolic needs of the body and guides the process of anabolism and catabolism. ***Samāna*** is said to display a radiant quality, and when functioning correctly, displays that quality within the mind and body. Disorders of ***samāna vāyu*** include most problems of digestion, including gastric reflux, hiatus hernia, dyspepsia, biliousness, diarrhoea, constipation and diverticulitis. Measures to correct ***samāna*** include following an appropriate diet (see Ch. 7), and the use of ***dīpanapācana*** ('digestive stimulant') remedies such as ***Yavānī*** (*Trachyspermum ammi*) and ***Śūṇṭhī*** (*Zingiber officinalis*) to enkindle digestion.

Apāna vāyu

Apāna vāyu is located in the sacral plexus, primarily the ***vasti*** ('bladder') and ***antra*** ('colon'), governing the function of the pelvic organs. The movement of ***apāna*** is downward, controlling the activities of ***prāṇa*** and ***udāna*** by creating a negative pressure in the chest. ***Apāna*** is said to arise with the first breath after birth, in which ***prāṇa*** becomes rooted in the body to sustain life. ***Apāna*** is the root of all other ***vāyus*** in the body and controls their function, just as a young child flying a kite measures how much string to let out in order for the kite to fly. To use another analogy of the traditional Indian family, ***prāṇa*** is like the husband coming in and going out, providing the material sustenance, whereas ***apāna*** is the wife, rooted in the home, coordinating all of its activities. Despite the social importance given to the head of the family, however, the household and the health of the family rest with the mother. Thus, if there is a problem with ***apāna vāyu*** this dysfunction will eventually affect all the other ***vāyus*** in the body. ***Apāna*** governs the excretion of wastes, menstruation and ejaculation, facilitates the meeting of the ovum and sperm during conception, and is responsible for the expulsion of fetus during labour. ***Apāna*** governs gross motor functions, like walking, jumping and running. In the psycho-spiritual realm ***apāna*** guides the process of manifestation, moving potentiality downward into actuality. As the downward moving force ***apāna*** contains ***kundalinī***, placing limits upon the evolution of consciousness, and in this respect is opposite to ***udāna***. Disorders of ***apāna vāyu*** include miscarriage, premature ejaculation, flatulence, retained urine, urinary incontinence, dysmenorrhoea, uterine prolapse, prolapse of the colon, ectopic pregnancy, haemorrhoids and infertility. Steps that can be taken to correct the flow of ***apāna vāyu*** include the use of 'grounding' herbs such as ***Gokṣura*** root (*Tribulus terrestris*), as well as purgatives (***virecana***) such as ***Viḍaṅga*** (*Embelia ribes*) and ***Trivṛt*** (*Operculina turpethum*) and enema (***vasti***) therapy to direct ***apāna vāyu*** downwards. ***Apāna*** influences the other ***vāyus*** to such a degree that they may be treated in an

Box 2.1 *Prāṇayāma* and digestion

Prāṇayāma is a breath-control technique that modulates the nature and duration of breathing, emphasising aspects of inhalation, exhalation, and the pauses that exist between them. As we inhale ***prāṇa*** is brought into the body, where it descends and meets with ***apāna vayu***. During exhalation ***apāna*** rises to meet with ***prāṇa***. Holding the breath after inhalation moves ***prāṇa*** towards ***apāna***, and holding the breath after exhalation moves ***apāna*** towards ***prāṇa***. The activities of ***prāṇa*** and ***apāna***, in turn, impact upon the function of ***āgni***, the flame of digestion and metabolism that resides between them. During inhalation ***prāṇa*** activates ***āgni*** causing it to rise upwards, burning the ingested food. Upon exhalation ***āgni*** is drawn downwards, transferring the waste products of digestion downwards to ***apāna vayu*** to be eliminated. Thus an exhalation that is twice as long as the inhalation ensures that waste products are properly eliminated. When ***apāna vayu*** is excessive it limits the capacity of ***prāṇa*** to enter into the body, and thus the general practice of lengthening the exhalation in relation to the inhalation is a useful approach to rid the body of wastes and optimise health. This technique is used only for the duration of ***prāṇayāma*** and should not replace normal, relaxed diaphragmatic breathing at other times.

indirect fashion by giving direct treatment to ***apāna***. By strengthening the mother, the whole family is likewise strengthened.

Vyāna vāyu

Vyāna vāyu is rooted in the ***hṛdaya*** ('heart') but circulates through the body as spiral currents, moving like a wheel. ***Vyāna*** governs circulatory function, distributing oxygen, nutrients and heat throughout the body. On a more subtle level ***vyāna*** also circulates emotions and feelings in the body, and thus unresolved emotional issues may locate themselves in certain areas within the body and affect the function and flow of ***vyāna*** in these areas. ***Vyāna*** also provides the impetus for gross motor function, discharging the nervous impulse and stimulating the flow of secretions, including the movement of lymph. Disorders of ***vyāna*** include cyanosis, poor circulation, cold intolerance and problems with coordination. Measures to correct the flow of ***vyāna*** involve regular exercise, a healthy emotional life, and the moderate use of stimulants such as ***Śūṇṭhī*** (*Zingiber officinalis*) and ***Guggulu*** (*Commiphora mukul*).

2.11 SUB-*doṣas* OF *pitta*

- ***Pācaka pitta***
- ***Ranjaka pitta***
- ***Sādhaka pitta***
- ***Ālocaka pitta***
- ***Bhrājaka pitta***.

Pācaka pitta

Pācaka pitta is synonymous with the ***jaṭharāgni*** (i.e. ***agni***), the fire of digestion located in the stomach and small intestine. The function of ***pācaka*** is to digest the ingested food, and guide the manifestation of all subsequent forms of ***pitta***. ***Pācaka*** discriminates what substances to secrete during the process of digestion and the guides the enzymatic breakdown of nutrients. The influence of ***pācaka*** extends from the lower fundus of the stomach to the ileocaecal valve and is concentrated between the villi of the small intestine, its actions increasing in subtlety as it extends its influence from the jejunum to the ileum. The function of ***pācaka pitta*** is completely dependent upon the status of ***prāṇa***, and deficient ***prāṇa*** results in poor digestion. Symptoms of weak ***pācaka*** include anorexia, flatulence, bloating, constipation, malabsorption, chronic fatigue and arthritis. Symptoms of excess ***pācaka pitta*** include gastric and duodenal ulcers, diarrhoea, and dysentery.

Ranjaka pitta

Ranjaka pitta is located primarily in the liver, gall bladder, spleen and red bone marrow. It is identified by the colour red, travels in the bloodstream as haemoglobin and is manifested as the intrinsic factor required for the absorption of vitamin B_{12}. ***Ranjaka*** initiates haemopoiesis in the red bone marrow and stimulates erythropoietin secretion by the kidneys. ***Ranjaka*** assists in the emulsification of fats, forms the stool and gives it shape and colour. ***Ranjaka*** is connected to enthusiasm, will and desire, and a lack of these qualities indicates its deficiency. ***Ranjaka*** also relates to the colour of skin, and thus yellow or red discolorations can indicate a derangement of ***ranjaka***.

Sādhaka pitta

Sādhaka pitta is located in the ***hṛdaya*** ('heart'), the seat of the mind and emotions, and by extension can also be said to function in the brain. Along with ***prāṇa***, ***sādhaka*** governs intellect (***buddhi***), comprehension, recognition and sensory perception. It is thought by some to maintain the function of the hypothalamus, the part of the brain that is directly responsible for maintaining homeostasis in the body. ***Sādhaka*** is also synonymous with awareness, the capacity for reasoning, the ability to concentrate, and the strength of courage. ***Sādhaka*** helps to discriminate between illusion and reality, and is the fiery messenger within each of us that awakens higher consciousness. ***Sādhaka*** also maintains individual consciousness and relates to the ego-identification with the body (***ahaṃkāra***). In its higher manifestation ***sādhaka*** is an evolutionary force, whereas in its lower manifestation it maintains the illusions, delusions and hallucinations of the ego. It is thought that by meditating upon the flame of a ***ghṛta*** candle ***sādhaka*** can be stabilised, and with the practice ***mantra*** can elevate spiritual consciousness.

Box 2.2 Meditation on light

Gazing upon the flame of a ghee candle is considered to be a helpful way to strengthen the eyes and purify the consciousness. The light of a ghee candle is unique, closely resembling the golden rays of the sun as it rises. This exercise is performed for a few minutes each day prior to meditation, at dawn and at dusk, just until the eyes begin to water. A visual imprint will be left on the retina, and this imprint is made the object of meditation to awaken new levels of spiritual consciousness. A ghee lamp can be made by pouring a small portion of melted ghee into a small, heat resistant vessel, and placing a small piece of wick into the centre of the vessel.

Ālocaka pitta

Ālocaka pitta is located in the eye and governs its function, giving it its transparency and lustre. ***Ālocaka*** is responsible for the expansion and contraction of the pupil, and is present in the rods and cones of the retina that provide for the perception of colour, shading and detail. ***Ālocaka*** is also located in the occipital regions of the brain, transforming inverted images right side up and processing the visual experience. ***Ālocaka*** relates to the ***ājñā cakra*** as the mystical connection between the mind and vision, expressed by the axiom 'the eyes are the doorway to the soul'. A deficiency of ***ālocaka*** can manifest as poor eyesight, which can be corrected through vision exercises and gazing upon the flame of a ***ghṛta*** candle, as well as in the consumption of nutrients such as carotenoids, flavonoids and vitamin A that are required in order for ***ālocaka*** to function properly. An eyewash prepared from a filtered, cold infusion of ***Triphala*** is particularly beneficial to nourish and protect the eyes.

Bhrājaka pitta

Bhrājaka pitta governs the function, lustre and complexion of the skin, lying between the dermis and underlying muscle. ***Bhrājaka*** interfaces with the subtle aspects of the body that are accessed by the stimulation of certain pressure points (***marmas***). ***Bhrājaka*** relates to the sensation of touch, and absorbs and digests topical applications such as fomentations, salves, medicated oils, liniments, and ointments. A deficiency of ***bhrājaka*** is indicated by not learning from tactile input, such as burning or cutting oneself on a frequent basis. The aggravation of ***bhrājaka*** is indicated by most acute, exquisitely sensitive inflammatory skin reactions.

2.12 SUB-*Doṣas* OF *Kapha*

- ***Avalambaka kapha***
- ***Kledaka kapha***
- ***Bodhaka kapha***
- ***Tarpaka kapha***
- ***Śleṣaka kapha***.

Avalambaka kapha

Avalambaka kapha is the primary form of ***kapha*** in the body, located in the chest, within the pleura of the lungs (***phuphphusa***) and the pericardium of the heart (***hṛdaya***), but also in the ileosacral joint (***trika***). ***Avalambaka*** most closely represents the status of the ***ap mahābhūta*** in the body, lubricating, nourishing and binding the body together. In the lungs ***avalambaka*** lubricates the bronchial passages and alveoli, ensuring the proper functioning of lung tissue. In the heart ***avalambaka*** supports and protects the heart in the chest. ***Avalambaka*** also anchors the cilia of the respiratory tract to the basement membrane and acts with ***samāna vāyu*** to move foreign substances out of the body.

With the expansion of the diaphragm the secretion of ***avalambaka*** is initiated. Within the spinal column ***avalambaka*** maintains the stability of the spinal cord, acting as the 'soil' that holds and nourishes its roots (i.e. the sacral plexus). ***Avalambaka kapha*** also represents the unfolding of love within the heart. A deficiency of ***avalambaka*** relates to compromised cardiopulmonary function, with a dry hacking cough, pallor and wasting. Excessive ***avalambaka*** relates to an increase in phlegm and a productive cough, poor digestion, and lassitude.

Kledaka kapha

Kledaka kapha is another important form of ***kapha*** in the body, found in the mucus secretions of the gastrointestinal tract, protecting the underlying tissues of the stomach from the ***uṣṇa*** and ***tikṣṇa*** nature of digestion (i.e. HCl, digestive enzymes). The activity of ***kledaka*** also relates to the moistening and liquefaction of the ingested food, the lubrication of the faeces and the initiation of satiety. As well as lubricating and nourishing the digestive tract, ***kledaka*** relates to the function of all mucus membranes, including those of the urinary and reproductive tracts, integral in the generation of seminal fluids and vaginal secretions. ***Kledaka*** maintains the body's electrolyte balance and regulates the pH balance of the interstitium, blood, urine and sweat. With a deficiency of ***kledaka*** there will be dryness, which gives rise to irritation and ulceration. Traditional treatments to restore ***kledaka*** include fresh coconut juice, mineral-rich preparations such as lightly salted meat and vegetable broths, as well as demulcent herbs such as ***Yaṣṭimadhu*** root (*Glycyrrhiza glabra*) and ***Balā*** root (*Sida cordifolia*). Excessive amounts of ***kledaka*** impair digestion and create catarrhal conditions.

Bodhaka kapha

Bodhaka kapha is present in the mouth as the salivary secretions, assisting ***udāna*** in the function of the tongue and with ***kledaka*** in the first stage of digestion. ***Bodhaka*** specifically relates to the function of taste, needed to distinguish the six different ***rasas*** (see Ch. 6). A deficiency of ***bodhaka*** relates to a loss of taste sensation and a dry mouth, whereas excess ***bodhaka*** relates to excessive salivary secretion. Sweet and salty tasting foods nourish ***bodhaka*** but when consumed to excess can promote its dysfunction, thickening the secretions, making them more slimy (***picchila***) and greasy (***snigdha***). Bitter and astringent tasting foods inhibit the secretion of ***bodhaka*** whereas sour and pungent tasting foods tend to stimulate the secretion of ***bodhaka***.

Box 2.3 *Svastha*: signs and symptoms of good health

Among the many contributors to Āyurvedic medicine the name Bhadanta Nāgārjuna is significant. Nāgārjuna was a reputed Buddhist scholar and author of several Āyurvedic texts, including the Uttaratantra, which is a supplement to the ***Suśruta Saṃhitā*** that deals with the preparation of medicinal remedies. In another medical and alchemical treatise written by Nāgārjuna, called the ***Rasa Vaiśeṣika***, he lists 15 signs and symptoms of good health. These qualities described by Nāgārjuna indicate the perfect balance of the three doṣas:

1. Good appetite
2. No noticeable signs or symptoms of the digestive process (e.g. eructation, distension, pain, gurgling, etc.)
3. Two bowel movements per day, one in the morning and one in the evening
4. Normal urination
5. No belching or flatulence
6. Proper functioning of the ***ghrāṇa*** (nose), as a ***jñāna indriya*** (cognitive organ)
7. Proper functioning of the ***jihvā*** (tongue), as a ***jñāna indriya*** (cognitive organ)
8. Proper functioning of the ***cakṣu*** (eyes), as a ***jñāna indriya*** (cognitive organ)
9. Proper functioning of the ***tvak*** (skin), as a ***jñāna indriya*** (cognitive organ)
10. Proper functioning of the ***śrotra*** (ears), as a ***jñāna indriya*** (cognitive organ)
11. Peace of mind, free of concern from the physical body
12. Strength of body
13. Clear complexion, strong aura
14. Sleeping without difficulty
15. Arising easily with renewed energy in the early morning.

Tarpaka kapha

Tarpaka kapha is located in the head as ***soma***, the 'nectar' (***amṛta***) that exudes from the brain and neural tissues to protect and nourish the senses (***indriyās***). ***Tarpaka*** thus promotes memory and guides the process of laying down new neural pathways in the brain, recording the sensory experiences analysed by ***sādhaka pitta***. The activity of ***tarpaka*** can be found in tissues such as the myelin sheath, the meninges of the brain, and the cerebrospinal fluid that circulates around and protects the brain and spinal cord. ***Tarpaka*** is also present in lacrimal secretions and the vitreous body of the eye, as well as in the perilymph and otolithic membrane of the inner ear. The function of ***tarpaka*** is to slow neural activity, induce relaxation, and promote contentment and emotional stability. In states of deep sleep ***tarpaka*** becomes active, representing the awakening of the ***sākṣi***, the 'witness' of consciousness. ***Tarpaka*** is the link between deep sleep and meditation, and from the clarity of ***tarpaka*** it is said that one can see the past, present and future simultaneously. A deficiency of ***tarpaka*** includes dryness of the eye, vestibular problems, chronic insomnia, memory loss and diseases such as multiple sclerosis. Excess ***tarpaka*** can manifest as hydrocephalous, a tumour of the pineal gland, glaucoma, blockage of the tear duct, and excessive cerumen (ear wax).

Śleṣaka kapha

Śleṣaka kapha is situated in diarthroses (freely moveable joints) as synovial fluid, preventing the degeneration of the articular surfaces of the bones. ***Śleṣaka*** binds the joints together, and so also includes parts of the function of ligaments and cartilage. ***Śleṣaka*** also brings emotional support, a sense of mental stability and flexibility, and can be depleted by overwork, excessive responsibilities and chronic stress, resulting in dry, popping joints.

PART 1

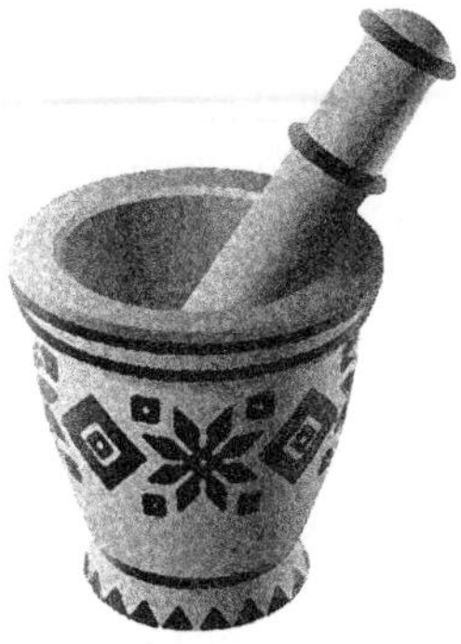

Chapter 3

CONSTITUTION AND CONSCIOUSNESS

OBJECTIVES

- To understand the concept and applicability of the physical constitution in Āyurveda.
- To understand the concept and applicability of the mental constitution in Āyurveda.
- To understand the concept of mind and consciousness from an Āyurvedic perspective.

3.1 *Prakṛti*: THE CONSTITUTION

When the ***śukra*** ('semen') meets the ***aṇḍāṇu*** ('ovum') in the fallopian tube to form the embryo, they each carry with them a similar combination and dominance of the ***doṣas*** present in the father and mother at the time of conception. The result of this union, as well as the time and season of conception, the food and habits of the mother during gestation, and the karmic influences of the being to be born, forms the ***prakṛti***, or constitutional nature of the embryo. Every person has a ***prakṛti***, which can be of seven types:

- ***Vāta***
- ***Pitta***
- ***Kapha***
- ***Vāta-kapha***
- ***Vāta-pitta***
- ***Pitta-kapha***
- ***Vāta-pitta-kapha***.

Because everyone is composed of all three ***doṣas*** these constitutional types are only indicative of the predominance of one, two or all three of the ***doṣas*** (called ***eka***, ***saṃsarga*** and ***sammiśra/sannipāta***, respectively). The activities of the ***doṣas*** in the ***prakṛti*** represent the normal activities of the body and are not necessarily reflective of any kind of diseased state (i.e. ***vikṛti***). Thus, ***prakṛti*** does not relate to treatment inasmuch as its knowledge assists with daily, preventative measures to optimise health. To some extent ***prakṛti*** can also assist in the formulation of a prognosis and in the individualisation of a treatment regimen. In some cases a patient will be seen to display a disease that is identical with their ***prakṛti***, but not necessarily.

In a state of disease the ***prakṛti*** can be very difficult to identify correctly because, like an onion, the

prakṛti is hidden within layers of the disease symptomology. Most Āyurvedic physicians will admit that it can be very difficult to determine one's own or someone else's ***prakṛti***, and thus it is generally recommended that treatment be provided on the basis that the human body has only one ***prakṛti***, predominant in ***pṛthvī*** and ***ap***. Treatment is thus directed to the specific signs and symptoms of the ***vikṛti*** ('disease'), rather than the ***prakṛti***. Learned Āyurvedic physicians suggest that it takes years of experience to accurately ascertain ***prakṛti***, although in certain cases, especially in ***eka prakṛtis***, it is possible to identify it correctly without too much effort.

Considering that ***doṣa*** means 'blemish', anyone who exhibits a particular ***doṣa*** or combination of the ***doṣas*** in their ***prakṛti*** will have a tendency when in a relative state of normalcy to exhibit minor symptoms native to those ***doṣa***(s). Although the ***prakṛti*** is a kind of blueprint for our development, the influence of the ***doṣas*** changes as each of us ages, and as a result the ***prakṛti*** may or may not be relevant to the maintenance of health. Some practitioners feel that it is even possible to change or modify one's ***prakṛti***, whereas others suggest that this is impossible. The concept of ***prakṛti*** resonates within ***jyotiṣ***, an ancient form of Vedic sidereal astrology that links ***prakṛti*** with the natal chart, or the position of the planets at birth. While this natal influence plays a significant role upon one's development, this chart is always in juxtaposition with the transit chart, the current position of the planets relative to the natal arrangement. Although insightful, the natal chart is not as significant in the assessment of the current status as is the transit chart. Corresponding with the transit chart is the concept is ***vikṛti***, or the 'disease tendency', which may or may not be similar to the ***prakṛti***. For example, Āyurveda recognises that an individual with a ***kapha prakṛti*** could have a ***vāttika*** disorder, such as anxiety. It is thus important to distinguish ***prakṛti*** from the disease state, or ***vikṛti***. Just by using treatments to balance ***prakṛti*** the treatment of a disease may not be effective.

Within Āyurvedic circles, especially in the context of the theories of rebirth and ***karma***, there is a tendency to rate each ***prakṛti*** in a hierarchical fashion. One opinion is that the ***eka prakṛtis*** are the most favourable (i.e. ***kapha***, ***pitta***, ***vāta***), followed next by ***saṃsarga prakṛtis*** (i.e. ***kapha-pitta***, ***kapha-vāta***, and ***pitta-vāta***), and then ***sannipāta prakṛtis*** (i.e. ***vāta-pitta-kapha***). Another perspective suggests that the ***sammiśra prakṛtis*** (i.e. all three ***doṣas*** in perfect balance) is the best ***prakṛti***, followed by the ***saṃsarga prakṛtis***, and then the ***eka prakṛtis***. Generally, ***kapha*** is considered to be the best ***prakṛti*** because the natural tendency towards disease is less, and a greater resistance and strength are displayed. ***Pitta*** is next, with a moderate resistance to disease. ***Vāta*** is considered to be the weakest ***eka prakṛti*** because it is the strongest ***doṣa***, and thus a ***vāttika prakṛti*** will display a greater tendency towards weakness and disease. ***Saṃsarga prakṛtis*** indicate that two ***doṣas*** are equally dominant, with ***kapha-pitta prakṛtis*** being the best in this category, followed by ***kapha-vāta*** and then by ***pitta-vāta***. The final category of ***prakṛti*** represents an equal dominance of all three ***doṣas***, and can be of two types. A ***sammiśra prakṛti*** represents all three ***doṣas*** is a state of perfect equilibrium, whereas a ***sannipāta prakṛti*** represents a constitution in which all three ***doṣas*** are imbalanced. The former ***prakṛti*** could thus be considered the best ***prakṛti*** and the latter the worst. Very often it is the state of mind and spiritual development that determines how a ***tridoṣaja prakṛti*** will manifest: if pure of mind, focused and disciplined, the ***sammiśra prakṛti*** will have few problems or obstacles to health. If confused, distracted, and undisciplined then the ***sannipāta prakṛti*** will be miserable. Thus in a ***sannipāta prakṛti*** the spiritual responsibility is much greater, but the reward is equally great. It is a calling, however, that only a few individuals will be able to answer.

The following are descriptions of each ***prakṛti***. This can be a somewhat speculative process as these types and especially the dual and tri-***doṣa prakṛtis*** are not as well defined in the ancient texts as one might wish. The process to determine the characteristics of each ***doṣa*** should largely be determined by assessing and comparing the various ***guṇas*** of the ***doṣas***, and relating this to observed physiological characteristics that are native to the person and do not represent pathological changes. Thus for most people the qualities of the ***prakṛti*** will be clearly evident during childhood and youth, when most people are healthy, but may become obscured with age and disease.

Kapha

Guru ('heavy'), ***snigdha*** ('greasy'), ***śita*** ('cold'), ***mṛdu*** ('soft'), ***sthira*** ('stable') and ***picchila*** ('slimy'). A general tendency to gain weight, with a heavy, sthenic build. The shoulders are broad and the torso, legs and arms are thick and large; in women the hips are broad and breasts are full. The musculature is well-developed but usually hidden by a layer of fat, hiding any angularities of the skeleton. The feet are large and thick. Facial features are broad and full, and generally well proportioned. The skin is soft and smooth, and the hair is generally smooth, thick and greasy. The orifices (eyes, nose, ears, mouth, rectum, uretha, vagina) are moist and well-lubricated. There is a tendency to lethargy or inactivity, although once motivated the energy released can be very powerful, with great endurance and a steady pace. A ***kapha prakṛti*** might suffer from minor congestive conditions, such as respiratory and gastrointestinal catarrh. They may display a mild aversion to cold and prefer warmer climates, but if they are physically active they can withstand even very cold weather quite easily.

Pitta

Uṣṇa ('hot'), ***tikṣṇa*** ('sharp'), ***snigdha*** ('greasy'), ***laghu*** ('light'), ***drava*** ('fluid'), ***sara*** ('movement'). Strong metabolism, strong digestion, and a general tendency to mild inflammatory states. Physically, the body is of average build, lighter than that of ***kapha***, with a well-developed musculature but generally less fat. The features are more angular than those of ***kapha***, and facial features are thinner, sharper and longer. The skin is often quite ruddy and there is a general tendency to excessive heat. Warm temperatures and hot climates are poorly tolerated. A tendency to excessive hepatic and gastrointestinal secretions, loose bowel movements, and more frequent urination. Generally more sensitive to sensory stimuli than ***kapha***, especially with light, heat and sound. Physically active, movements are co-ordinated, quick and efficient, sometimes aggressive, with determination and purpose.

Vāta

Laghu ('light'), ***śita*** ('cold'), ***rūkṣa*** ('dry'), ***cala*** ('movement'), ***viśada*** ('friction'), ***khara*** ('rough'), ***sūkṣma*** ('subtle'). A general tendency to being underweight and asthenic, with dry rough skin, small wiry muscles and irregular proportions. The bony prominences of the skeleton and the veins are easily observed due to a deficiency in the overlying muscular and fat layers. ***Vātaja prakṛtis*** will usually display a strong aversion to cold, with irregular or poor peripheral circulation. A tendency to more or less constant movement, often confused or peripheral to the situation at hand, including twitching, tapping, bouncing, picking and shaking. The joints often pop and crack, and the muscles have a tendency to go into spasm. ***Vāta*** is the most sensitive of the ***prakṛtis*** to sensory stimuli, with poor powers of recuperation and endurance. Digestive powers are typically weak or erratic, with a general tendency to constipation.

Saṃsarga and *sannipāta prakṛtis*

Prakṛtis that are either ***saṃsarga*** (two ***doṣas***) or ***sannipāta*** (three ***doṣas***) will display some of the ***guṇas*** of the involved ***doṣas***, although because some of these qualities are opposite in nature they may be poorly manifested. Generally speaking one ***doṣa*** will tend to dominate a ***sannipāta*** or ***saṃsarga prakṛti***, but the influence of the sub-dominant ***doṣa(s)*** will affect the overall manifestation.

Pitta-kapha prakṛtis will generally display a sthenic build and a layer of fat as in ***kapha prakṛti***, but there will be a tendency to a ruddier complexion and more physical activity that a pure ***kapha***. Warm, humid weather also adversely affects this ***prakṛti***.

Vāta-kapha prakṛtis will often display a lighter build and proportionally longer limbs, or are shorter and smaller, than a pure ***kapha***. There is generally more sensitivity to coldness than in any of the other ***doṣas***, and a similar tendency to mucus congestion and digestive weakness as ***kapha***. As there is less overt moisture in the body any congestive problems tend to worsen under the influence of dryness.

Vāta-pitta prakṛti is in many respects similar to ***vāta***, but generally with a stronger and more compact build, with somewhat larger muscles. There is a great deal of movement associated with this ***prakṛti***, combining a curious combination of determination and confusion. There is a general sensitivity to sensory stimuli such as light, heat, sound and dryness. Digestive secretions tend to be concentrated and intense, but are often irregular.

The ***sannipāta prakṛti*** is the most difficult to ascertain due to the expression of contradictory qualities present in all three ***doṣas***. A ***sannipāta prakṛti*** may be reactive to any change in diet, lifestyle or the environment, especially extreme changes. The result of this reactivity is minor conditions that change or alternate in nature, which have a greater tendency to manifest as ***vikṛti*** ('disease'). Generally speaking, a ***sannipāta prakṛti*** will tend to display signs of a ***vāta-pitta*** or ***vāta-kapha prakṛti***. Thus, the approach taken to balance the ***doṣas*** will be directed to ***vāta*** first, and then ***pitta*** or ***kapha***.

3.2 *Manas prakṛti*: THE CONSTITUTIONAL INFLUENCE UPON MIND

Apart from the symptoms that relate to physiology and disease, each ***prakṛti*** also influences mental and emotional characteristics. In most cases the features of the ***manas prakṛti*** are congruent with the physical ***prakṛti***, but sometimes they are not. In some cases the ***manas prakṛti*** represents an evolutionary change in the psychosomatic consciousness of a person, such as a person who has a ***vātaja prakṛti*** developing a more ***kaphaja*** mind, or vice versa. Over time the body will progressively express these mental qualities in a physical way, although inherent characteristics of the ***prakṛti*** may never be lost completely. To determine the nature of the various ***manas prakṛtis***, each type is identified according to the ***guṇas*** associated with each ***doṣa*** or combination of ***doṣas***.

Kapha manas

Guru ('heavy'), ***śita*** ('cold'), ***snigdha*** ('greasy'), ***sthira*** ('stable'), ***mṛdu*** ('soft') and ***picchila*** ('slimy'). A general tendency to mental lethargy and difficulty with abstract thinking. Minor difficulties in trying to follow conversations, especially when people are talking quickly. Generally easy-going and happy, good memory, they do not like to 'stir things up'. Benevolent, generous, and mothering, but with a tendency to become attached to people, places and things. Some difficulty controlling cravings to foods or pleasurable experiences, but not to the point of injury or harm. Kinesthetically orientated, speaks from physical, practical experiences. Grounded, earthy wisdom. A tendency to despondency, even depression, in cold, cloudy, wet weather. Dreams tend to be kinesthetic, joyful, and peaceful, and are associated with objects such as water, snow, the moon and flowers.

Pitta manas

Laghu ('light'), ***uṣṇa*** ('hot'), ***snigdha*** ('greasy'), ***tikṣṇa*** ('sharp'), ***sara*** ('moving') and ***drava*** ('fluid'). Generally charismatic, ambitious, courageous and extroverted. Usually passionate, dynamic and sometimes argumentative, a tendency to impatience and irritability, and in some cases can be aggressive or violent. Enjoys spicy foods, loud debates and is strongly interested in the opposite sex. Often insightful and perceptive, with a fluid, subtle intelligence that can provide clarity. Good critical thinking skills but a tendency to negative criticism and judgment. Self-disciplined and focused, sometimes obsessed, egotistical or proud. Generally sceptical and rational-minded. Speaks from theoretical knowledge, technique, logic or law. Dreams tend to be highly visual, vivid and emotional, sometimes with anger and violence, and are associated with objects such as the sun, fire and blood.

Vāta manas

Laghu ('light'), ***śita*** ('cold'), ***rūkṣa*** ('dry'), ***cala*** ('moving'), ***viśada*** ('friction), ***khara*** ('rough') and ***sūkṣma*** ('subtle'). Quick thinkers and quick learners, fond of theory and philosophy, sometimes with a poor memory or concentration. Generally enthusiastic at the outset of an enterprise, but have difficulty sustaining or following through. Often jumps to conclusions too quickly, or has unrealistic expectations. Ungrounded and irrational, sometimes paranoid and delusional. Pestering, obsessed, talkative, spiteful, angry and unreasonable. More affected by extra-sensory phenomena than the other ***doṣas***, and has difficulty relating to a commonly held reality. Generally more psychic and more creative than the other ***prakṛtis***. Often speaks from fantasy or from extrasensory experiences. May suffer from poor self-esteem, insecurity and loneliness and faithlessness. Generally fearful and anxious, and often appears distracted and confused. Unconventional, controversial, sometimes distorted or even perverted. Dreams tend to be highly auditory or visual, with feelings of despair and loneliness, and are associated with objects such as the wind and sky, and activities such as flying or moving quickly.

Saṃsarga and *sannipāta manas prakṛtis*

A pitta-kapha manas prakṛti will generally display similar properties to a ***kapha manas prakṛti***, but is more dynamic, passionate and ambitious. Although there is a tendency to be fairly conservative at the outset, once properly motivated and enthused a ***pitta-kapha manas prakṛti*** can be an instrument for significant social change. Quite often these are the most superficial and materially focused of the ***manas prakṛtis***, and as a result they are often quite successful but may lack any kind of spiritual perspective. The highly sensual nature of ***pitta-kapha*** may cause this type to be mildly addicted to various substances and activities, and have difficulty seeing the point in giving them up.

Vāta-kapha manas prakṛtis will generally display a strong sensitivity to other people, and are generally humble, considerate, shy and compassionate. They are often quite creative, highly imaginative and artistic, and are strongly inspired by the natural world. They tend to lack motivation and drive, however, and because they tend to have poor self-esteem, are negatively affected by criticism. ***Vāta-kapha manas prakṛtis*** tend to be something of a chameleon, and often have difficulty making a stand or confronting somebody on an important issue. In many cases this type will end up feeling unfulfilled in life, despite their inherent creativity.

Vāta-pitta manas prakṛtis are a volatile mix of ***vāyu*** and ***tejas***, and thus this ***prakṛti*** often suffers from mental volatility, sometimes expressing excessive confidence, even arrogance, but when criticised falls back into patterns of self-doubt and confusion. They are quite often highly reactive, explosive, and argumentative and often require a great deal of patience on the part of others. There are quite often brilliant thinkers, highly intelligent and very creative, and if they can find a loving and maternal environment in which to work, can be highly effective and very successful.

The ***sannipāta prakṛti*** is a combination of all three ***doṣas***, and thus the range of mental and emotional behaviours can vary to a great degree. Generally they will tend to display signs of a ***vāta-pitta*** or ***vāta-kapha prakṛti***. Thus, the approach taken to balance the ***doṣas*** will be directed to ***vāta*** first, and then ***pitta*** and ***kapha***.

3.3 *Triguṇa manas*: THE QUALITIES OF THE MIND

In Chapter 2 the basic components of the ***Sāṅkhya darśana*** were introduced, and specifically, the arising of the ***triguṇas*** of ***sattva***, ***rajas*** and ***tamas***. To recall this teaching, ***sattva*** is the principle of harmony, purity and light, ***rajas*** is the quality of conflict, movement and colour, and ***tamas*** is the quality of cohesion, stasis and darkness. Collectively, the ***triguṇas*** are the qualities that represent all phenomena.

Although we can apply ***tridoṣa*** to the mind and emotions, it is difficult to anticipate the wide variety of potential behaviours within each ***manas prakṛti*** from this alone. Āyurveda deepens this approach by ascertaining which of the ***triguṇas*** guide the consciousness of a particular ***manas prakṛti***. Thus we can use the ***triguṇa*** theory to describe more or less spiritually evolved forms of each ***prakṛti***.

When we speak of the mind and emotions, however, it is important to make the distinction between ***guṇa*** and ***doṣa***. In fact there is only one ***guṇa*** of the mind and it is ***sattva***. ***Rajas*** and ***tamas*** exist as ***doṣas*** of the mind that become vitiated and cloud the equilibrium and clarity of our true ***sattvic*** nature. Thus the pure mind that is directed to self-realisation is ***sattvic*** in nature, and the thoughts and emotions that swirl through it and disrupt this quest are ***rajasic*** and ***tamasic***. Spiritual evolution is the process by which we develop our ***sattvic*** or ***buddha*** nature, moving closer to the purity and absolute brilliance of the One. Thus, when we assess the mental state of a patient, for example, we are also trying to understand these elements of spiritual evolution.

Sattva

Sattvic individuals respond well to spiritual, vibrational or subtle therapies in the treatment of physical and psychological complaints. Techniques include self-inquiry, prayer, rituals, meditation, breathing exercises, ***mantra***, minerals and gems.

Rajas

Rajasic individuals respond well to natural, but more overt healing therapies such as self-discipline, dietary changes, nutritional supplementation, physical manipulation, music and colour therapies, and herbal and homeopathic treatment.

Tamas

Tamasic individuals display a poor compliance with holistic therapies, dietary or lifestyle recommendations, and have difficulty understanding the body other than how it functions as a kind of machine. More often than not, such individuals will turn to more invasive therapies such as pharmaceuticals and surgery for treatment.

In addition to the ***triguṇa*** model the ***Suśruta saṃhitā*** describes another model that breaks down the ***triguṇas*** into 16 archetypes. The first seven archetypes relate to ***sattva***, the second six are ***rajasic***, and the last three relate to ***tamas***. Each archetype within a ***sattvic***, ***rajasic*** or ***tamasic*** group is also arranged in a hierarchical fashion, the first being the most ***sattvic*** and the last being the most ***tamasic***.

Sattvic archetypes

1. ***Brahmā*** ('supreme deity'): pious, honest, compassionate, wise, charitable, hospitable, free of desire, hatred and ignorance, speaks from the heart, excellent memory
2. ***Māhendra*** ('king of the gods'): courageous, ready for action, charismatic, beneficent, protector of ***dharma***, ***artha*** and ***kama***, servant of the Earth
3. ***Varuṇa*** ('god of the waters'): courageous, capable, desires/achieves cleanliness, love of water, easily pleased but easily angered
4. ***Kaubera*** ('god of wealth'): charitable, tolerant, prosperous, enjoys comfort, surrounded by family and friends, intense anger and joy
5. ***Gāndharva*** ('celestial being'): artistic, musical, studious, enjoyment of fragrances and costume, pleasure-seeking
6. ***Yāmya*** ('god of death'): determined, efficient, impartial, fearless, free of passion, firm
7. ***Ṛṣi*** ('sage'): free of desire, meditative, disciplined, celibate, philosophical, habitually engaging in penance and fasting.

Rajasic archetypes

1. ***Asura*** ('demonic'): misguided, courageous, wealthy, unrestrained, jealous, charismatic, angry, selfish, self-aggrandising, reflective only after acting
2. ***Sarpa*** ('snake-like'): harsh, rough, angry, courageous, critical, capable, fickle, deceitful, causes dissension
3. ***Śākuna*** ('bird-like'): greedy, intolerant, restless, fearful
4. ***Rākṣasa*** ('impish'): prejudiced, angry, fearsome, irritable, jealous, critical, paranoid, lazy
5. ***Paiṣāca*** ('fiendish'): glutinous, rude, undisciplined, obsessed with sex, unclean, adventurous
6. ***Preta*** ('ghostly'): greedy, uncooperative, lazy, unhappy, unfulfilled, weak.

Tamasic archetypes

1. ***Paśu*** ('beast-like'): rude, boorish, weak intellect, secretive, obsessed with sex, uncooperative
2. ***Mātsya*** ('fish-like'): fearful, restless, foolish, obsessed with food, quarrelsome, idiotic
3. ***Vanaspati*** ('plant-like'): sedentary, oblivious, unconscious, removed from the pursuit of ***dharma***, ***artha*** and ***kama***.

3.4 *Manas*: THE MIND

There was a great deal of speculation in the philosophical teachings of ancient India as to the nature of the mind. There was a profound understanding that the mind and all that it embodies has an ethereal quality. We are apparently born with a mind and develop an identity with it, and carry it with us until it is lost upon death. But what is mind? How is it defined? Can you point to it? How can you define, by any means, what the mind is, when the mind itself is involved in the explanation? 'I think, therefore I am', wrote Descartes, but the Vedic sages might have asked: 'you think, but what is thought?' Inquiring into the nature of mind and its origination has been the preoccupation of Indian philosophy for millennia.

Where is your mind? Is it contained within the brain as modern science tells us? You watch a child playing in the playground, you see a bird sitting in a tree. Where is your mind? Is it in your head? Is it in your eyes? Or is your mind with the child, with the bird?

To understand your mind requires that you study it. At this moment please focus on your mind, finding that part of you that is thinking and chase it down. Take hold of it and look it squarely in the eye. Where is it? It disappeared! Where did it go? But like a flash it is back, thinking about how you couldn't find it.

To understand the mind requires that we witness it. Let go of your mind, see it as a river flowing in front of you. See how it moves, how the rapids and eddies swirl, how the river carries all kinds of debris in its waters, flowing past you endlessly. This is called ***sākṣi bhavana*** in the Vedic tradition, 'bearing witness' to the mind, and is a form of meditation.

According to science, a thought is said to result from a pattern of stimulation generated by many parts of the nervous system, determined and coloured by the limbic system, thalamus and reticular activating system as being pleasurable or painful, and given discrete characteristics by the cerebral cortex. A thought is a singular event in nervous function, a combined activity of the various aspects of the brain, integrating and analysing sensory information from all parts of the body into one definable 'eureka' of nervous function. Consciousness is one thought connected to another to form a continuous stream of thoughts. As David Frawley describes in his book *Ayurveda and the Mind: The Healing of Consciousness*, however, when brought under the lens of meditation, consciousness is like a pointillist painting, each thought working together to form an impression of experience, but not reality itself. Consciousness is like a movie, a series of snapshots flashed rapidly onto a screen, giving us the impression of continuity, but not the entire experience. We miss out on a great deal of information, and thus consciousness is a distortion, an incomplete knowing of the infinite nature of experience.

This view of consciousness is also illustrated by the writings of the Greek philosopher Zeno of Elea (c. 490 BCE). In his paradox entitled *The Dichotomy*, Zeno describes a runner in a race who must travel a given distance (d) in a given amount of time. Zeno suggests in this paradox that before the runner can finish the race, he must travel half the distance ($d/2$). And in order to travel half the distance, the runner must travel one-quarter the distance ($d/4$), and so on, over an infinite number of points ordered in the sequence $d/2$, $d/4$, $d/8$, etc. Because this sequence goes on forever, it therefore appears that the runner will never finish the race. Zeno's theory, however, is in direct contrast to the experience of the wildly cheering crowds who perceive the runner finishing the race. So who is right?

Measurement is an act of division, of separating the whole into a system of units. As Zeno illustrated in his paradox, there are an infinite number of points, both in time and space, that need to be crossed during the race. Although the crowd sees the runner finish the race, they do not perceive the infinite nature of time and space that has been crossed. Thus the observation of the runner finishing the race is not the complete experience, but a mental construct based upon incomplete data. This illustrates how our experience, or that which we interpret as being reality, is in fact only a small part of what is actually happening.

3.5 *Citta*: CONSCIOUSNESS

The underlying aspect of consciousness in Āyurvedic thought is called the ***citta***, the total potential field of conditioned consciousness. It is the repository of all aspects of conditioned existence, and records these influences upon itself. It includes the presence of subliminal activators called ***saṃskāras***, the psychic imprints that underlie our mental and emotional traits, derived from our experience over many lifetimes. These psychic imprints propel consciousness into action, regardless of whether the imprint is unconscious or conscious, internal or external, desirable or undesirable.

At the heart of this concept is the idea that it is these ***saṃskāras*** that bind us to the wheel of ***saṃsāra***. The chain of cause and effect that defines the existence of ***saṃsāra*** is called ***pratityasamutpāda*** (***pratitya*** 'dependent,' ***samutpāda***, 'origination'), first enunciated by Gotama Buddha soon after he had attained ***nirvāṇa***. The Buddha indicated that these ***saṃskāras*** exist and are created because of ***avidyā***, or 'ignorance', that what we hold to be reality is in fact a misconception that ultimately leads to ***dukha*** ('unhappiness').

According to the ***yogic*** tradition there are two forms of ***saṃskāras***; namely, those that promote the direction of consciousness externally and generate further ***saṃskāras***, called ***vyutthana*** ('waking consciousness'), and those that stem the flow of consciousness and thereby prevent the generation of further ***saṃskāras***, called ***nirodha*** ('conscious restriction'). ***Nirodha*** is said to be synonymous with the attainment of ***samādhi*** ('perfect concentration'), the highest limb of ***aṣṭāñga yoga***, an absorptive state in which subject and object become one.

Schematically, the ***yogic*** tradition indicates that the ***citta*** consists of the ***ahaṃkāra***, the ***manas*** and the ***buddhi***. The ***ahaṃkāra*** is for the most part considered synonymous with the Western concept of the ego, or that part of consciousness that retains a sense of individuality, that responds to perceptions, feelings and thoughts and thereby initiates a variety of activities. According to the Āyurvedic perspective the ***ahaṃkāra*** is the process of self-identification, an inner 'becoming' that associates and builds up a consciousness of itself from external relationships. This ***ahaṃkāra*** is said to arise because of a failure of our innate intelligence (***buddhi***), whose correct orientation directs us to our true Self, that we are Brahman. When the ***buddhi*** fails to perceive this it will mistake the body for the Self, and the limits of human sensory perception (and scientific instrumentation) for the whole of reality. The ***buddhi*** then becomes a tool of the ***ahaṃkāra***, which uses this intelligence to rationalise its existence, creating a mental illusion of reality. This tool is the ***manas***, or 'lower' mind, which concerns itself with the organisation of information received from the five senses. For this reason ***manas*** is often referred to as the 'sixth' sense, and with the five senses (***jñāna indriyās***) forms the sixfold base (***āyatana***) described in the Buddhist concept called ***pratityasamutpāda*** ('dependent origination'). According to the schemata of ***pratityasamutpāda***, the sixfold base undergoes 'contact' (***sparśa***) with corporeal phenomena (i.e. the ***tanmatras*** and ***pancabūthas***). This, in turn, gives rise to 'sensory impressions' (***vedanā***), 'desire' (***tṛṣṇā***), 'attachment' (***upādāna***), and then finally, 'becoming' (***bhava***). According to the Buddha this process of becoming (i.e. the ***ahaṃkāra***) provides the impetus for birth, which ultimately results in ageing, disease and death (***jarāmarana***), and thus ***dukha*** ('unhappiness').

If anything, the ***manas*** can be said to be driven by the senses, and can experience an endless number of mental formations as a result, all of which ultimately lead back to the same cycle of desire, attachment and becoming. In the ***yogic*** tradition the most direct method to uproot the activities of the ***manas*** is called ***pratyāhāra***, the fifth limb of ***aṣṭāñga yoga***. ***Pratyāhāra*** involves the withdrawal of the senses and the redirection of consciousness internally. The mind withdraws from the sensuous experience and redirects its focus to the nature of perceiving, to the nature of becoming. As the ***yogic*** text the ***Gorakṣa-paddhati*** states:

> 'Knowing that whatever he hears, be it pleasant or unpleasant, it is Self, and the ***yogi*** withdraws.'
> 'Knowing that whatever scent he smells with his nose, it is Self, and the ***yogi*** withdraws.'
> 'Knowing that whatever he sees with the eyes, be it pure or impure, it is Self, and the ***yogi*** withdraws.'
> 'Knowing that whatever he senses with his skin, tangible or intangible, it is Self, and the ***yogi*** withdraws.'
> 'Knowing that whatever he tastes with the tongue, be it salty or not, it is Self, and the ***yogi*** withdraws.'
>
> (Feurstein 1997)

The purification of the ***manas***, however, can also involve other methods, perhaps less radical than complete ***pratyāhāra***. Among these are the practice ***yama*** ('morality') and ***niyama*** ('self discipline'), and the three components of the traditional Indian ideal of the ***caturvarga***: ***dharma*** ('duty'), ***artha*** ('wealth'), ***kama*** ('pleasure').[9] Although these practices do not uproot the influence of the ***manas*** they create an inner equilibrium within the mind that allows for concentration and mental clarity.

Unlike ***manas***, the ***buddhi*** is pure awareness, or that which directly perceives. When directed by the ***ahaṃkāra*** the ***buddhi*** is really involved only in sensory perception, which results in ***manas***. When the ***buddhi*** has been purified from these limits, however, it is able to perceive directly the true nature of reality and becomes freed from the cloud of ***avidyā***, or ignorance, generated by the ***ahaṃkāra***. Hence, those who have attained this degree of perception are called ***buddha***, an 'awakened one'.

ENDNOTE

9 The fourth component of the ***caturvarga*** is ***mokṣa*** ('liberation').

PART 1

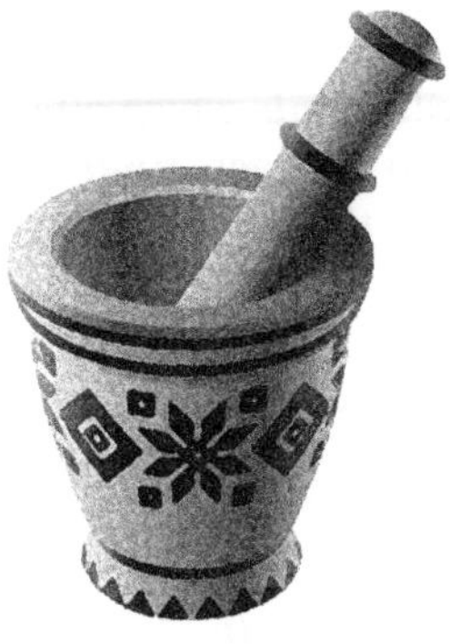

Chapter 4

THE PHYSICAL BODY

OBJECTIVES

- To understand the concept of digestion.
- To understand the concept of tissue development and metabolism.
- To understand the concept of vitality.
- To understand the concept of wastes and toxins.
- To understand the flow of energy, nutrients and tissues elements in the bioenergetic channels of the body.

4.1 *Agni*: THE FIRE OF DIGESTION AND METABOLISM

Agni is the fire within each of us that attends to digestion and metabolism, and in its higher form, represents vitality, perception and discrimination. It is characterised by the qualities of ***uṣṇa*** ('hot'), ***tikṣṇa*** ('sharp') and ***laghu*** ('light'), and in many ways resembles ***pitta***. It is incorrect, however, to assume that they are one and the same. ***Agni*** is the pure and cleansing fire of the body, whereas ***pitta***, as a ***doṣa***, ultimately represents the qualities of ***agni*** in a disturbed state.

Agni is located in the ***āmāśaya*** ('stomach and small intestine') as the ***jaṭharāgni***. Here the ***jaṭharāgni*** attends to separating the food into its subtle essence (***sūkṣma rasa***, which feeds the mind), its gross nutrient portion (***rasa***, which feeds the body) and waste (***kiṭṭa***, further separated into ***purīṣa*** and ***mūtra***, or faeces and urine, respectively). Beyond its role as the ***jaṭharāgni***, there are several different manifestations of ***agni*** in the body, each having a different name that relates to distinct metabolic processes. From the activity of post-synaptic enzymes that break down neurotransmitters, to ATP generation in the mitochondria, all metabolic processes are subsets of the ***jaṭharāgni*** of the ***āmāśaya***. Hence, when digestion is weak, metabolic activity suffers, energy levels diminish and waste products begin to accumulate in the body.

The negative effects of each ***doṣa*** results in a specific disturbance of ***jaṭharāgni***:

- In ***vāttika*** conditions the ***jaṭharāgni*** is ***viṣamāgni***, digestion that is erratic and irregular.
- In ***paittika*** conditions the ***jaṭharāgni*** is ***tikṣṇāgni***, extremely intense, with a burning sensation and thirst.

- In ***kaphaja*** conditions the ***jaṭharāgni*** is ***mañdāgni*** (also called ***agnimāndya***), characterised by sluggishness, with heaviness of the abdomen and lassitude.

In the absence of ***doṣa*** increase or vitiation, the ***jaṭharāgni*** is ***samyāgni***: correct, proper and normal.

Agni interacts with three different kinds of alimentary tract (***koṣṭha***), influenced by the predominance of a particular ***doṣa*** during gestation. ***Vāta*** is responsible for a ***krūra*** or hard bowel, producing dry, rough faeces that are difficult to evacuate. ***Pitta*** is responsible for a ***mṛdu*** or soft bowel, producing semi-solid or liquid faeces. ***Kapha*** is responsible for a ***madhya*** or medium bowel, which generally produces bowel movements that are neither too hard nor too soft. The nature of the bowel can be tested by introducing certain foods, such as ***ghṛta***, jaggery, milk or hot water. If these substances have a laxative effect, the bowel is stated to be ***mṛdu***; if they have a mild laxative effect, the bowel is stated to be ***madhya***; if they have no laxative effect, the bowel is stated to be ***krūra***.

It is important to remember that Āyurveda considers the partaking of food to be a ***yāga***, or 'sacrifice'. In the Hindu tradition, and in most spiritual traditions across the world, prayers are usually offered in the form of a sacrificial fire. A candle is lit, incense is burned, or certain herbs or foods are placed on a fire, and as these substances burn they release their smoky fragrance up to heaven, acting as a kind of vehicle for our prayers, hopes and dreams. ***Agni*** represents this sacrificial fire within us, and when we consume food our digestion becomes a spiritual catalyst. The act of eating therefore is a kind of spiritual ritual, where proper digestion depends upon eating in a conscious and mindful fashion. Thus meal times for the most part should be quiet, without distractions such as talking, television and books, with proper attention paid to eating slowly and chewing the food.

Besides the ***jaṭharāgni*** there are two additional kinds of ***agni*** or, rather, subsets of the ***jaṭharāgni***, that attend to the body's various metabolic activities:

1. ***Bhūtāgnis***: the types of ***agni*** which are responsible for the assimilation and metabolism of the five ***mahābhūtas***. Each of the ***bhūtāgnis*** (i.e. ***pārthiva***, ***āpya***, ***āgneya***, ***vāyavya*** and ***ākāśīya***) works on its respective elemental component (vis. ***pṛthvī***, ***ap***, ***tejas***, ***vāyu*** and ***ākāśa***) that form corporeality.
2. ***Dhātvāgnis***: ***dhātu***-specific ***agnis*** which attend to the particular function of each ***dhātu*** or support system (discussed in the next section).

4.2 *Sapta dhātus*: THE SEVEN SUPPORTS

As the ***tridoṣa*** theory is used to explain the principle of *function* in the human body, the ***sapta dhātus***, or 'seven supports', is used to describe the principle of *structure*. The ***sapta dhātus*** model is another aid for the practitioner to discover the specific actions of ***tridoṣa*** and understand their function within a structural model. Just as anatomy cannot be seriously studied without an understanding of physiology, any study of the ***dhātus*** must take ***tridoṣa*** into account. The seven ***dhātus*** and their most commonly translated definitions follow:

1. ***Rasa***: plasma
2. ***Rakta***: blood
3. ***Māṃsa***: muscle
4. ***Medas***: fat
5. ***Asthi***: bone
6. ***Majjā***: marrow
7. ***Śukra*** (men), ***ārtava*** (women): semen, menstrual blood.

The ***sapta dhātus*** is a model that describes the basic principles of structure, and does not literally represent the specific activities of their respective translated terms. For example, ***rakta*** does not represent the 'blood' inasmuch as it represents the 'blood essence'. All tissues and organs in the body arise from the combined effects of ***vāta***, ***pitta*** and ***kapha*** and are composed of all seven ***dhātus*** in varying proportions. Thus the blood will contain all the ***dhātus***, but arises principally from ***rakta***. It would be difficult to develop a general principle from an in-depth scientific analysis of blood because it has a multitude of functions and aspects. The term ***rakta*** is used to describe the essential nature of the 'blood', to understand its overall function within the human body. The following are descriptions of each of the ***dhātus***:

Rasa dhātu

When food is consumed it undergoes preliminary digestion in the ***āmāśaya*** under the influence of the

jaṭharāgni, separated into ***kiṭṭa*** ('waste'), ***āhāra rasa*** ('gross nutrient') and ***sūkṣma rasa*** ('subtle nutrient'). ***Āhāra rasa*** is that which enters into and nourishes the entire ***dhātu*** system, and is converted into the first ***dhātu***, i.e. ***rasa dhātu***, under the influence of a ***dhātu***-specific subset of the ***jaṭharāgni*** called the ***dhātvāgni***.

Rasa literally means 'taste', and in this sense, ***rasa dhātu*** is the essential nutrient quality of the food consumed. As it is created, ***rasa*** is directed to the ***hṛdaya*** ('heart') where it undergoes distribution throughout the body by the actions of ***vyāna vāyu***. ***Rasa*** is responsible for the nourishment of all the tissues of the body, circulating as a fluid that bathes the cells with vitality. One can think of ***rasa*** as the internal manifestation of the primordial ocean from which all life arose, as the amniotic and interstitial fluid that supports growth and maintains proper development. A secondary manifestation of ***rasa*** are endometrial fluids that support gestation and breast milk (***stanya***).

Rasa dhātu displays a strong resemblance to the qualities of ***kapha***, and in mental terms relates to feelings of purity, compassion and happiness. When functioning optimally ***rasa*** is an important component of vitality. If food is consumed that 'increases' (***caya***, ***vṛddhi***) ***kapha***, however, or if the ***jaṭharāgni*** is impaired, ***rasa dhātu*** will become vitiated and display the symptoms of ***kapha*** increase such as an increase of phlegm and catarrh. The symptoms of decreased (***kaśāya***) ***rasa dhātu*** are dryness, fatigue, emaciation, impotency, infertility and an increased sensitivity to sonic vibrations, all of which correspond to an increase of ***vāta***.

Rakta dhātu

Rasa dhātu is then converted by the ***dhātvāgni*** into ***rakta dhātu***, which is the 'blood essence'. Its primary function, along with ***rasa***, is the maintenance and nutrition of all bodily tissues, and is more closely associated with ***pitta***. ***Rakta dhātu*** gives rise to the haematopoietic system, including the liver and spleen, and connective tissue generally through its transformation into ***māṃsa dhātu***. More than any other of the ***dhātus***, ***rakta*** (blood) is an organ unto itself, and represents a phase of physiological function before it solidifies into specific tissues. As a result ***rakta*** is sometimes seen to function as a fourth ***doṣa*** and when vitiated produces diseases that are particular to it. In health ***rakta dhātu*** provides for a clear complexion and a deep passion for all living things.

Rakta dhātu is thought to generate the skin, seven separate and distinct layers (i.e. ***avabhāsini***, ***lohita***, ***śveta***, ***tāmra***, ***vedini***, ***rohiṇi***, ***māmsadhara***), in much the same way as cooking milk generates a layer of scum. Thus, skin disorders are seen as a manifestation of impurities within the blood. An increase in ***rakta dhātu***, either inherited from a vitiated ***rasa dhātu*** or by direct influence, can manifest as skin diseases, hepatomegaly, splenomegaly, hepatitis, jaundice, abscess with infection and inflammation, arthritis, gout, haemorrhages of the mouth, nose or anus (i.e. ***rakta pitta***), and a reddish discoloration of the eyes, skin and urine. A decrease of ***rakta dhātu***, transferred by a deficiency of ***rasa dhātu*** or other factors, manifests as a desire for sour and warming foods, anaemia, hypotension, dryness of the body, and a weak pulse.

Māṃsa dhātu

Rakta dhātu is then converted into ***māṃsa dhātu*** by the ***dhātvāgni***, which gives rise to all connective tissues excluding blood and bone. ***Māṃsa*** means 'flesh' and is responsible for enveloping and covering the bones, including tissues such as the muscles, tendons, ligaments, arteries, veins, lymphatic tissue and certain types of endocrine gland. In health ***māṃsa dhātu*** provides for a strong musculature and physical endurance, and contributes to feelings of charisma and courageousness. An increase in ***māṃsa dhātu*** can manifest as lymphadenitis, lymphadenopathy, goitre, malignant tumours, fibroids, abscesses and a general increase in body weight and musculature. A decrease in ***māṃsa dhātu*** is understood by signs and symptoms such as emaciation, fatigue, a lack of coordination, and muscular atrophy.

Medas dhātu

Māṃsa dhātu is converted into ***medas dhātu*** by the ***dhātvāgni***, and can be thought of as the principle of 'fat' tissue. The primary function of ***medas*** in the body is the protection of delicate organs (e.g. the kidneys) and tissues (e.g. the myelin that surrounds neurons), as well as lubrication and the storage of energy. In health ***medas dhātu*** provides for a melodious voice, a sense of joyfulness and a playful, humorous nature. An increase in ***medas dhātu*** may manifest as fatigue, shortness of breath, and sagging of breasts, buttocks and abdomen. A decrease in ***medas dhātu*** may manifest as nervous irritability, weak eyesight, dryness, joint weakness and emaciation.

Asthi dhātu

Asthi dhātu is the conversion of ***medas*** by the ***dhātvāgni***, and is the principle of all 'bone' tissue in the body. The primary function of ***asthi*** is the physical structure and shape of the body. In health ***asthi dhātu*** provides for a flexible nature, self-assurance, confidence, mental stability and a hard-working nature. An increase in ***asthi dhātu*** can manifest as the overgrowth of bone tissue such as bone spurs, bone cancer and metabolic diseases such as gigantism and acromegaly. A decrease of ***asthi dhātu*** can manifest as osteoporosis, brittle bones, splitting or cracking finger nails, alopecia and tooth decay.

Majjā dhātu

Majjā dhātu is the transformation of ***asthi*** by the ***dhātvāgni***, and is the principle of 'marrow,' or that which 'fills the bones'. ***Majjā*** is considered to generate the nervous system in the sense that it 'fills' the spinal column and cranium. Thus ***majjā*** can be thought of as the neural pathways along which electrical impulses flow, but should not be confused with the impulses themselves, which are governed by ***vāta***. In health ***majjā dhātu*** provides for a sensitive and receptive mind, a good memory and a compassionate nature. An increase of ***majjā*** usually manifests in ***kapha*** conditions, such as heaviness, lassitude, hypertrophy, and swelling of joints, and can manifest as obstinate ulcerous conditions. A decrease of ***majjā*** may manifest as a sensation of weakness or lightness in the bones, joint pain, rheumatism, giddiness and blindness.

Śukra/Ārtava dhātu

Majjā is converted by the ***dhātvāgni*** into the final ***dhātu*** of ***śukra*** in men, and ***ārtava*** in women. ***Śukra*** is responsible for the generation of semen within a male, while ***ārtava*** is the menstrual blood that usually indicates ovulation. Technically speaking the menstrual blood is not a ***dhātu*** but a kind of eliminatory product that indicates the health of the numerous ***aṇḍāṇu*** or 'ova' contained in the ovaries. In health ***śukra*** and ***ārtava dhātus*** provide for self-love, attractiveness and indicate the vitality of the person. In men, an increase of ***śukra*** can result in insatiable sexual urges, seminal calculi, odorous perspiration, greasy skin, greasy hair and acne. A decrease of ***śukra*** may result in impotency, premature ejaculation, prostatitis and urethritis. In women, a metabolic increase of ***ārtava*** (i.e. ***aṇḍāṇu***) can result in excessive sexual desire, a consistently short oestrus cycle, odorous perspiration, greasy skin, greasy hair and acne. A decrease of ***ārtava*** (i.e. ***aṇḍāṇu***) can result in frigidity, amenorrhoea, infertility, leucorrhoea, dysmenorrhoea, and menstrual blood that is pellet-like and malodorous. ***Śukra*** and ***ārtava*** also generate the ***ojas***, the final refinement of ***āhāra rasa*** by the body, which is discussed in the next section.

Dhātu transformation

Besides the process of ***dhātu*** transformation alluded to earlier, there are two other ways by which ***āhāra rasa*** circulates within the ***dhātus***. While the process of ***dhātu*** transformation previously described is much like the process by which cow's milk is transformed into ***dadhi*** (curd), which is then churned into butter and buttermilk, and then the butter finally made into ***ghṛta*** (clarified butter), the other two processes are somewhat different. The first analogy of cow's milk being transformed into ***ghṛta*** describes how an imbalance within ***āhāra rasa*** can affect each ***dhātu*** in succession, because the nature of what is being transformed is passed on through to the next ***dhātu***. The obvious deficiency of this analogy, however, is that it does not describe how metabolic wastes (***kiṭṭa***) are eliminated from the ***dhātus***. The second analogy is that the ***dhātus*** are nourished as if ***āhāra rasa*** is scattered on the ground as differing kinds of seed, with each ***dhātu*** as a different kind of bird that feeds on these seeds, selecting the ones most appropriate for its nourishment: what the birds leave behind is ***kiṭṭa***. This second analogy describes how an imbalance within ***āhāra rasa*** can affect one ***dhātu*** but not another, because it is a process of selectivity. The third method by which the ***dhātus*** are nourished is like the irrigation of a paddy (rice) field, with each paddy being irrigated by specific channels that draw water from the same main channel

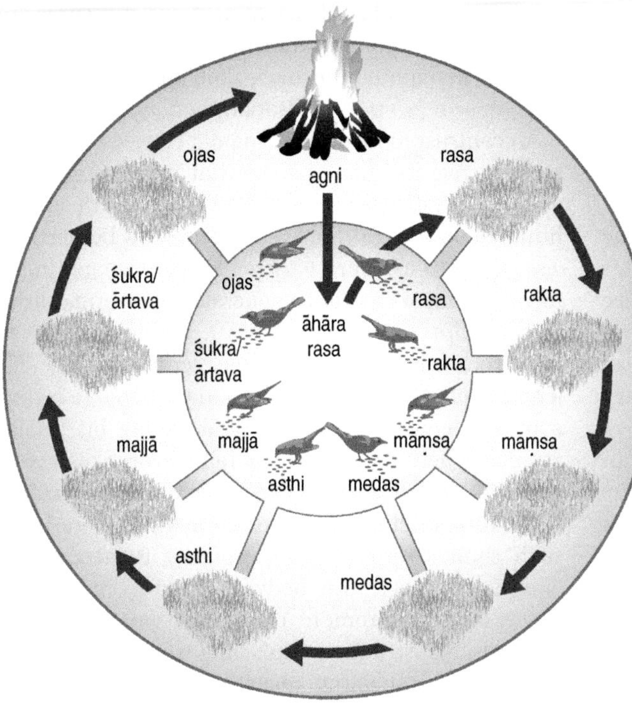

Figure 4.1 Transformation (*black arrows*), selectivity (*birds*) and irrigation (*paddy fields*) in ***dhātu*** metabolism.

that carries ***āhāra rasa***. This last analogy very much resembles the physiology of blood flow, from arteries to capillaries to the interstitium and then to the veins. Although these three models of ***dhātu*** metabolism may seem contradictory, all three processes of transformation (***kṣīradadhi***), selectivity (***khalekapota***) and irrigation (***kedārikulyā***) describe the complexity of ***dhātu*** metabolism, and occur simultaneously. In the case of ***kṣīradadhi*** (transformation), it is stated that after the food is digested it is present in the body as ***rasa*** for about 5 days, and then for 5 days for each successive ***dhatu*** until ***śukra*** and ***ārtava*** are formed. From this, ***ojas*** is directly nourished.

4.3 *Ojas*: THE VITAL ESSENCE

Ojas is the vital essence of the body, a subtle force that incessantly works to keep the body, mind and senses continuously refreshed. Āyurveda describes two types of ***ojas***: ***para ojas*** and ***apara ojas***:

- ***Para ojas***: also called the ***aṣṭā bindu*** ('eight drops'), located in the heart, representing the ***tejas*** of vitality and remaining constant in the body until death. Thus, ***para ojas*** is ***jiva***, the life force that separates the animate from the inanimate.
- ***Apara ojas***: also called ***ardhanjali*** ('one handful'), found in a continual state of flux, derived directly from the ***dhātus***, circulating throughout the body in the maintenance of health. In this text all subsequent references to the term '***ojas***' refer to ***apara ojas***.

Just as ***prāṇa*** represents the unblemished functions of ***vāta***, and ***agni*** represents ***pitta*** in an undisturbed state, ***ojas*** most closely resembles ***kapha***. Thus, those with a ***kapha prakṛti*** typically display an abundance of ***ojas***, providing for all the beneficial attributes of this ***prakṛti*** such as longevity, forbearance, generosity and strength. According to the ancient Vedic ***agnīṣomiya*** principle, ***ojas*** (***soma***) is the feminine counterpart to the masculine ***agni***, representing 'lunar' characteristics such as the ability to nurture, support, shelter and pacify. In contrast, ***agni*** represents solar, masculine characteristics such as the ability to consume, destroy, expose and invigorate.

As described earlier, ***ojas*** is the refinement of ***śukra*** and ***ārtava***, the final essence of the ***dhātus***. The process of ***dhātu*** transformation is dependent upon the health of the individual ***dhātus***, the channels (***srotāṃsi***) that carry them throughout the body (see 4.6 ***Srotāṃsi***: the channels of the body), and most importantly, the entire spectrum of ***agni***, from the processes of gastric digestion to the progressively subtle and discriminative efforts of tissue metabolism. Through the activities of ***agni***, ***ojas*** accumulates, supporting and nourishing the whole body, refreshing the senses and empowering the heart. Just as ***ojas*** is dependent upon ***agni***, however, so does ***ojas*** sacrifice itself to nourish ***agni***. ***Ojas*** 'gives' itself to ***agni***, providing the digestive tract and all subsequent tissues of the body the energy needed for proper function. Thus, ***ojas*** both feeds on and is fed to the ***dhātus***.

The principle function of any kind of therapy in Āyurvedic medicine is based upon understanding the dynamics of the ***dhātu*** cycle in individual patients. It explains why after any kind of ***śodhana*** ('purificatory') therapy in which the ***dhātus*** are purified a corresponding ***rasāyana*** ('rejuvenative') treatment is begun to rebuild the status of ***ojas***. This nourishment of ***ojas*** in turn nourishes ***agni*** and the ***dhātus***, and as a result provides for good health and longevity.

The status of ***ojas*** can be assessed by the lustre of the eyes, the strength of limbs, and the function of the mind and senses. The greatest concentration of ***ojas*** is found in the reproductive tissue, which is to say, the needs of reproductive function are served first in a hierarchical fashion among the various physiological systems. In normalcy ***ojas*** is for the most part distributed equally all over the body, whereas in acute disease or trauma the flow of ***ojas*** is blocked, and in chronic disease the flow of ***ojas*** gradually becomes deficient.

In the sexual act ***ojas*** concentrates in the reproductive organs to create life (***jiva***), but it is in the creation of this life principle that a 'little death' (in French, la petite mort) is brought to ***ojas***. In men the continual depletion of semen results in the loss of ***ojas***, and hence, a weakening of physiological function. In light of this and for several other reasons excessive sexual activity is discouraged in Āyurvedic medicine, and guidelines are provided for appropriate sexual activity in accordance with the seasons (see Ch. 5). Among some ***tantrik*** practices, however, a sexually active man suppresses the ejaculation of semen during copulation, and by utilising various techniques, attempts to use this energy to awaken ***kundalinī***. As a man ages the dynamic and masculine aspects of his fertility slowly decline, allowing the more feminine aspects of his nature to awaken. Thus, as men age, measures are usually taken to supplement the declining male essence, to maintain his masculine nature (see 11.13 ***Vajīkaraṇa karma***: virilisation therapy).

In contrast to men, the dynamic between ***ojas*** and reproductive function is somewhat more complex in women. Physiologically a woman is born with several hundred oocytes (***aṇḍāṇu***) that represent her fertility 'essence', just as semen (***śukra***) does for a man. Unlike men, who must constantly generate new sperm cells to produce ***ojas***, a woman draws a limitless supply of ***ojas*** from her ovaries until after menopause. The difference between a woman and a man therefore is that a man is constantly at risk of depleting his sexual essence, whereas a woman contains a large reserve of potential sexual energy. Thus, while men are counselled to restrict excessive sexual activity there is no such similar restriction for women. To access this energy, however, the body maintains regulatory processes that promote ovulation, which in turn results in menstruation. Thus, in a woman experiencing a normal healthy menstrual cycle all of her potential energy is available to her, whereas when menstruation is dysregulated the status of ***ojas*** weakens. Thus, time-honoured strategies that seek to maintain the menstrual cycle (e.g. ***ārtavajanana***, 'emmenagogues') help to make ***ojas*** available to the woman, even though they may not specifically nourish ***ojas***.

As a woman ages the number of oocytes becomes diminished and, as hormone levels drop off with menopause, a fire begins to awaken. This fire burns away aspects of her feminine essence, and she begins to take on more of the attributes of a man. Most women experience these symptoms as an intense flushing, which is sometimes quite uncomfortable. Although the flushing is probably a compensatory mechanism to liberate hormones such as oestrogen that are stored in fat, it also an alchemical process by which the fires of ***agni*** are stoked to convert the feminine essence into the dynamic aspects of spiritual awakening. As a woman loses the ability to create life, there is a physiological transition that directs a need to confront death, and thus menopause can be a time of great learning. On a physiological level treatment is directed to support the declining feminine essence by using herbal therapies that are similarly used to keep a man sexually potent. These herbs are specifically chosen for their ability to nourish ***ojas***, and lack the ***uṣṇa*** ('heating') properties of similar herbs used in men, e.g. ***Śatāvarī*** (*Asparagus racemosus*) (see 11.13 to ***Vajīkaraṇa karma***: virilisation therapy).

The importance of ***prāṇa*** cannot be overemphasised when it comes to the issue of ***ojas***. Life is dependent upon the air we breathe, and by the use of breath control methods like ***prāṇayama***, ***ojas*** can be increased and its circulation corrected. Without adequate ***prāṇa***, or in cases where the air we breathe is contaminated by pollutants (e.g. exhaust, recycled air, fine particulates, microbes), ***ojas*** undergoes decline. According to Caraka, those that wish to preserve ***ojas*** should:

> '. . . avoid unhappiness . . . (and take) diets and drugs which are conducive to the heart, ***ojas*** and channels of circulation . . . Tranquility and wisdom should be followed meticulously for this purpose.'
>
> (Sharma & Dash 1985)

4.4 *Malas*: BODILY WASTES

The term ***mala*** generally refers to any kind of impurity of the mind or body, but in Āyurvedic medicine usually refers to any 'waste' produced by the body. The ***malas*** are an important concept in Āyurveda, as health is absolutely dependent upon the proper formation and excretion of wastes. The improper formation and impaired excretion of waste products is considered to be an important factor in the development of disease. Thus the ***doṣas***, as 'wind', 'bile' and 'phlegm', also represent a kind of impaired eliminatory product.

The ***malas*** are said to be of two kinds: those that are ***sthūla*** or 'gross', and those that are ***sūkṣma***, or 'subtle'. The ***sthūla malas*** are ***purīṣa*** ('faeces'), ***sveda*** ('sweat') and ***mūtra*** ('urine'), collectively referred to as the ***trimalas*** ('three wastes'). The ***sūkṣma malas*** ('subtle wastes') comprise the remaining waste produced by the body.

Purīṣa ('faeces') is derived from the refinement of ***āhāra rasa*** during the digestion of food and the resultant formation of ***kiṭṭa*** ('waste', lit. 'that which must be eliminated'). When exposed to the ***uṣṇa*** ('hot') and ***tikṣṇa*** ('sharp') properties of ***agni***, ***kiṭṭa*** is formed into solid lumps that are referred to as ***purīṣa***. During the intense heat of digestion volatile substances are released from the ***kiṭṭa*** and are said to give rise to flatus, or ***vāta***. Although the regular elimination of ***purīṣa*** is considered to be of the utmost importance in Āyurveda, it is said that in cachexia (***rājyakśma***) the faeces should be protected. In such conditions (e.g. tuberculosis) the tissues of the body are being eliminated to excess, and by preventing the elimination of ***purīṣa***, the patient retains some of the strength lost by the ***dhātus***. ***Mūtra*** is formed in the same way as ***purīṣa***, but represents the liquid portion of indigestible products and bodily wastes.

The ***sūkṣma*** *or* subtle ***malas*** are formed as each ***dhātu*** metabolizes the ***sara*** ('essence') of the previous ***dhātu***. The following list details the waste products formed by each ***dhātu*** by the ***dhātvāgni***:

1. ***Rasa***: ***kapha doṣa***, as mucoid secretions
2. ***Rakta***: ***pitta doṣa***, as bilious secretions
3. ***Māṃsa***: impurities and wastes associated with the ***jñāna indriyās*** (i.e. nose, mouth, eyes, skin, and ears)
4. ***Medas***: ***sveda*** (perspiration)
5. ***Asthi***: ***nakha*** (nails), ***keśa*** (head hair) and ***loma*** (body hair)
6. ***Majjā***: ***akśi*** (greasy secretions of the eyes), ***tvak vit*** (sebaceous secretions), and ***purīṣa sneha*** (greasiness of the faeces)
7. ***Śukra/aṇḍāṇu***: none.

The state of a specific ***dhātu*** can be understood by the qualities of its excretion. If a given ***dhātu*** is producing excessive amounts of the waste product associated with it, then one needs to differentiate between the causes. If for example cerumen, a waste product of the ears and a ***mala*** of ***māṃsa***, is being produced in excess, then one needs to look at the state of ***māṃsa*** and the tissues it generates to understand the cause. ***Māṃsa*** generates muscle: is the patient thin and weak? If so, then there may be a problem with the ***māṃsa dhātvāgni*** such that the essence of the previous ***dhātu*** is being transformed into waste instead of healthy ***māṃsa***. Is the patient well built, with a good musculature? Then perhaps the cause is based in an excessive intake of dietary articles that specifically strengthen ***māṃsa***, i.e. meat and animal products. Similarly, in cases of excessive perspiration, is the cause too much fat (***medas***) or improper ***dhātu*** metabolism? Such an understanding of the ***dhātus*** enables the practitioner to refine the treatment strategy.

4.5 *Āma*: TOXINS AND WASTES

The status of ***agni*** is the focal point for diagnosis and treatment in Āyurveda. Its deficiency or impairment is the cause for the creation of ***āma***, which literally interpreted means 'undigested food stuff'. In a broader context, however, ***āma*** is the impairment of one's ability to derive nourishment from life, be it physical, emotional, mental or spiritual. A correctly functioning ***agni*** confers a harmonious benefit to the whole organism, with proper discrimination of the body, mind and senses.

As the by-product of poor digestion ***āma*** is opposite in nature to ***agni***, displaying qualities such ***guru*** ('heavy'), ***śita*** ('cold'), ***snigdha*** ('greasy'), ***picchila*** ('slimy'), and ***manda*** ('slow'). All qualities of ***āma*** are essentially identical to ***kapha***. The difference between ***āma*** and ***kapha***, however, is that instead of acting as a counterbalance to the activities of ***vāta***, ***āma*** accumulates in the ***srotāṃsi*** ('channels') and blocks the flow of ***vāta***. The labile nature of ***vāta*** causes it to move backwards when encountering this obstruction, reversing its flow in the body and thereby producing dysregulation and disease.

When ***agni*** is weak ***āma*** is formed instead of ***ojas***, and as a result, ***ojas*** gradually becomes deficient. And, because ***ojas*** feeds ***agni***, a deficiency of ***ojas*** results in a further diminution of ***agni***. In the dichotomy between ***ojas*** and ***agni***, ***āma*** represents an entropic tendency in the ***dhātu*** cycle. It is the accumulation of ***āma*** over many years that eventually robs ***ojas*** and ***agni*** of much of their power, facilitating the processes of degeneration, decay and death.

Although the qualities of ***āma*** are similar to ***kapha***, ***āma*** can associate with any of the ***doṣas***. In such a state a ***doṣa*** is said to be ***sāma***, or 'with ***āma***'. In the absence of ***āma*** a ***doṣa*** is said to be ***nirāma***, or 'without ***āma***'. The first treatment of any condition in Āyurvedic medicine is the elimination of ***āma*** and enhancement of ***agni***. If the condition persists beyond the use of these measures, a specific treatment is administered to the vitiated ***doṣa***(***s***). Table 4.1 describes the differences between ***sāma*** and ***nirāma*** conditions.

Intestinal permeability syndrome

To put a modern slant on the concept of ***āma***, let us examine the issue of intestinal permeability, or 'leaky-

TABLE 4.1 *Sāma* and *nirāma* conditions.

***Sāma* conditions**	***Nirāma* conditions**
Circulatory congestion, feeling of coldness	Circulation normal
Loss of strength	Normal strength
Lethargy and lassitude after eating	Energised and revitalised after eating
Poor appetite	Good appetite
Indigestion	Good digestion
Constipation	At least two bowel movements daily
Sinking stools with mucus congestion	Normal stools
Increased urination	Normal urination
Joint swelling and inflammation	Absence of joint swelling and inflammation
Headache	No headache
Thick tongue coating	Clear or thin white coating
Orbital oedema, eyes appear dull, poor vision	Eyes bright, shining, good vision
The above conditions made worse with cold and damp weather or climates, and worse at night	Health unaffected by changes in weather or climate

gut syndrome'. Succinctly put, intestinal permeability describes a process by which some agent or combination of agents initiates an inflammatory response in the digestive tract. Persistent gastrointestinal inflammation eventually disrupts the integrity of the mucosal lining of the gut, and tiny perforations allow for molecules larger than usual to pass across this barrier. These molecules can be derived from the diet, or may be in the form of microorganisms such as bacteria and fungi that naturally inhabit our digestive tract. In response to this infiltration, an immune response is initiated and the body begins to manufacture specific antibodies to these antigens. Unfortunately, many human tissues have antigenic sites almost identical to those substances that pass across a permeable intestinal wall. These antibodies then circulate throughout the body and bind with endogenous (self) antigens to initiate an inflammatory response.

Āyurveda describes a condition analogous to intestinal permeability, in which a deficiency of ***agni*** promotes the formation of ***āma***. ***Āma*** then enters into the ***dhātu*** cycle and begins to localise in areas such as the joints, or in already weakened or susceptible areas. Once ***āma*** is firmly wedged in these locations the ***doṣas*** become vitiated: first ***kapha***, with an increase in congestion; followed by ***pitta***, which sets up a cycle of inflammation; and then ***vāta***, which promotes degenerative changes. Thus the basic dynamics of intestinal permeability syndrome were identified several millennia ago in India as being an important causative factor in the development of disease, even if the pathogenic mechanisms described are somewhat different.

4.6 *Srotāṃsi*: THE CHANNELS OF THE BODY

The body contains several channels through which the ***doṣas***, ***dhātus*** and ***malas*** are transported, called ***srotāṃsi*** (sing. ***srota***). The impaired movement or obstruction of the ***doṣas***, ***dhātus*** or ***malas*** through a ***srota*** is called ***srotorodha***. ***Srotorodha*** interrupts proper tissue metabolism, causing the regurgitation of the ***doṣas***, ***dhātus*** and ***malas***, and the local formation of ***āma***. ***Āma*** then moves into the other ***srotāṃsi*** and circulates through the body, promoting systemic congestion.

A ***srota*** is either ***bāhya*** (an 'external' channel) or ***abhyañtra*** (an 'internal' channel). The ***bāhya srotāṃsi*** include the two nostrils, the two ears, the two eyes, the mouth, the urethra and the rectum. Females have two additional ***bāhya srotāṃsi***: the two lactiferous glands of the breasts (***stanyavaha srotāṃsi***), and the cervix (***ārtavaha srota***). There are 13 ***abhyañtra srotāṃsi***, each of which relates to specific organs, and are increased and vitiated by specific factors. The 13 ***abhyañtra srotāṃsi*** are listed as follows:

1. *Prāṇavaha srotāṃsi*

Function: provides the medium through which ***prāṇa*** flows, obtained on a corporeal level by the respiratory and gastrointestinal systems, and through the ***sūkṣma sarira***.
Governing ***doṣa***: ***vāta***.
Organs: correlates to cardiac function, the respiratory system and the activities of the digestive tract. In this sense, ***prāṇa*** is obtained from three sources:

(i) from the atmosphere, in which ***prāṇa*** is obtained by the cyclical nature of breathing, which in turn regulates the rhythm of the heart
(ii) from food, which contains smaller amounts of ***prāṇa*** that supply energy to the tissues of the body
(iii) from the subtle realm (***sūkṣma sarira***), where extrinsic ***prāṇa*** is absorbed from the universe, and especially from the sun.

The term ***hṛdaya*** ('heart') correlates to the general functions of the brain, and thus ***prāṇa*** has an important regulatory function in nervous tissue.
Cause of vitiation: consumptive diseases; suppression of natural urges; seasonal, environmental, lifestyle and dietary patterns that have a 'drying' (***rūkṣa***) nature; exertion and exercise while hungry.
Symptoms of vitiation: hyperventilation, shortness of breath, shallow breathing, asthma, hiatus hernia.

2. *Ambuvaha srotāṃsi*

Function: water metabolism; responsible for the hydration of bodily tissues and the production of urine.
Governing ***doṣa***: ***kapha***.
Organs: pancreas, palate.
Cause of vitiation: exposure to heat, indigestion, alcoholic drinks, eating excessively drying food, insufficient water intake.

Symptoms of vitiation: dryness of the oral mucosa, tongue and throat, lack of appetite, excessive thirst, diabetes, pancreatitis.

3. *Annavaha srotāṃsi*

Function: nutrient assimilation, transports assimilated nutrients to the ***dhātus***.
Governing ***doṣa***: ***pitta***.
Organs: stomach, duodenum.
Cause of vitiation: overeating, unwholesome foods, ***agnimāndya*** ('poor digestion').
Symptoms of vitiation: poor appetite, indigestion, malabsorption, anorexia, vomiting, dry tongue, dry lips.

4. *Rasavaha srotāṃsi*

Function: carries ***rasa*** throughout the body.
Governing ***doṣa***: ***kapha***.
Organs: heart, arteries, lymphatic tissue.
Cause of vitiation: excessive intake of ***guru***, ***śita*** or ***snigdha*** dietary articles (e.g. dairy, flour products); ***agnimāndya*** ('poor digestion').
Symptoms of vitiation: poor appetite, decrease in taste sensation, indigestion, malabsorption, anorexia, vomiting, abdominal heaviness, lethargy, fever, malaise, fainting, oedema, lymphatic congestion, frequent upper respiratory infections, anaemia, impotence/infertility, asthenia, premature ageing.

5. *Raktavaha srotāṃsi*

Function: carries ***rakta*** throughout the body.
Governing ***doṣa***: ***pitta***.
Organs: liver, spleen, red bone marrow, skin.
Cause of vitiation: consuming foods that are excessively ***uṣṇa***, ***snigdha*** or ***tikṣṇa*** in nature (e.g. alcohol, chilies, pork); toxins; excessive exposure to heat and the sun.
Symptoms of vitiation: skin disorders (e.g. psoriasis, eczema, herpes, erysipelas), menorrhagia, haemorrhage, rectal bleeding, hepatomegaly, splenomegaly.

6. *Māṃsavaha srotāṃsi*

Function: carries ***māṃsa*** throughout the body.
Governing ***doṣa***: ***kapha***.
Organs: tendons, muscles, ligaments, fascia, basement membrane of the dermis.
Cause of vitiation: sleeping after eating, eating excessive amounts of food, especially with ***guru*** and ***snigdha*** qualities (e.g. dairy, flour products, fatty meat).
Symptoms of vitiation: myoma, uvulitis, tonsilitis, epiglotitis, goitre, cervical adenitis, boils, non-malignant growths.

7. *Medovaha srotāṃsi*

Function: transports ***medas*** throughout the body.
Governing ***doṣa***: ***kapha***.
Organs: adipose tissue, kidneys, glandular tissue, serosal tissue of the viscera.
Cause of vitiation: lack of exercise, sleeping during the day, sleeping after eating, eating to excess (especially sweets), eating excessive amount of foods with a ***guru*** and ***snigdha*** quality; excessive alcohol consumption.
Symptoms of vitiation: benign cysts, obesity, atherosclerosis, dysuria, diabetes.

8. *Asthivaha srotāṃsi*

Function: carries ***asthi*** throughout the body.
Governing ***doṣa***: ***vāta***.
Organs: skeletal system, especially the sacrum and neck.
Cause of vitiation: excessive exercise, malnutrition, lack of sleep, ***vāta***-provoking foods and activities.
Symptoms of vitiation: osteoarthritis, osteoporosis, alopecia, dental caries, abnormal nail growth.

9. *Majjāvaha srotāṃsi*

Function: carries ***majjā*** throughout the body.
Governing ***doṣa***: ***vāta-kapha***.
Organs: nervous system, marrow.
Cause of vitiation: broken bones, compression (tight shoes and clothing), eating incompatible foods (e.g. fish and dairy).
Symptoms of vitiation: rheumatism, vertigo, fainting, memory loss, paralysis, tremors.

10. *Śukravaha srotāṃsi*

Function: carries ***śukra*** and ***aṇḍāṇu*** throughout the body, concentrates ***ojas*** in the reproductive organs during sexual activity.
Governing ***doṣa***: ***kapha***.
Organs: reproductive tissue.

Cause of vitiation: excessive sexual intercourse, suppression of ejaculation, suppression of sexual activities, excessive sexual stimulation without release, sexual activity concurrent with the need to urinate or defecate.
Symptoms of vitiation: spermatorrhoea, nocturnal emission, benign prostatic hyperplasia, amenorrhoea, leucorrhoea, dysmenorrhoea, uterine fibroids, infertility, miscarriage.

11. *Mūtravaha srotāṃsi*

Function: carries urine to elimination.
Governing ***doṣa***: ***vāta-kapha***.
Organs: urinary bladder and kidneys.
Cause of vitiation: overeating, suppression of the urge to urinate, sexual activity or the consumption of foods and beverages concurrent with the urge to urinate.
Symptoms of vitiation: frequency, tenesmus, calculi, pain upon voiding.

12. *Purīṣavaha srotāṃsi*

Function: carries faeces to elimination.
Governing ***doṣa***: ***vāta***.
Organs: colon and rectum.
Cause of vitiation: suppression of the urge to defecate, overeating, ignoring satiety, ***agnimāndya***.
Symptoms of vitiation: constipation, diarrhoea, irritable bowel syndrome, colitis.

13. *Svedavaha srotāṃsi*

Function: carries sweat to elimination.
Governing ***doṣa***: ***pitta***.
Organs: sudoriferous glands, hair follicles.
Cause of vitiation: excessive exercise, excessive exposure to heat, anger, fear, grief.
Symptoms of vitiation: absence of or excessive perspiration, dry skin, calloused skin, hypersensitive skin, horripilations (goose bumps), hives, burning sensations in skin.

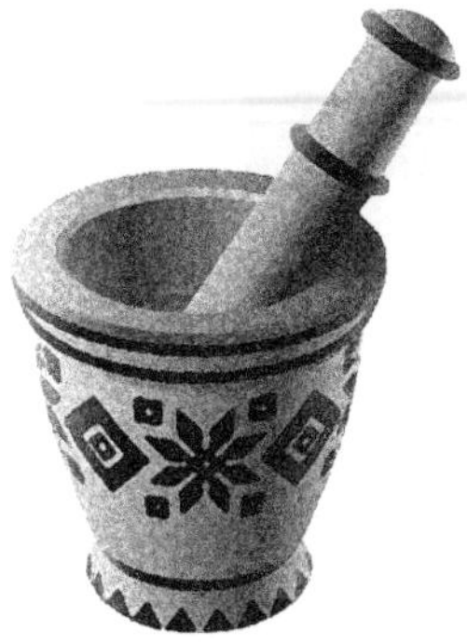

Chapter 5

ĀYURVEDIC LIVING

OBJECTIVES

- To review the components of the daily regimen prescribed by Āyurveda.
- To review the concept of morality and conduct in Āyurveda.
- To review the components of the seasonal regimen prescribed by Āyurveda.

5.1 *Dinācaryā*, *sadvṛtta* AND *ṛtucaryā*

Most systems of medicine admit that it is not enough to understand the cause and treatment of disease, that there must also be a method by which one can prevent it. Āyurvedic medicine maintains an awareness of these factors by examining the dynamic quality of each season, and similarly, the differing influences within each 24-hour period. Thus ***dinācaryā*** and ***ṛtucaryā*** are 'daily' (***dina***) and 'seasonal' (***ṛtu***) 'regimens' (***caryā***) to align dietary and lifestyle patterns with these influences. Extending beyond an assessment of environmental factors, it is also important to know how our behaviour and conduct causes the generation and ripening of karmic fruits, and as such it is useful to know which behaviours are conducive to 'spiritual progress' (***sadvṛtta***) and those that are not.

5.2 *Dinācaryā*: THE DAILY REGIMEN

Dinācaryā is the daily regimen described in Āyurveda, taking into account the dynamic quality of each day. At any given point during the day or night a particular ***doṣa*** is said to exert an influence, and thus the potential for an imbalance to occur in these periods must be moderated by a regimen that takes this into consideration. The cycles of the three ***doṣas*** in each day are shown in Table 5.1.

It is important to take note of the gradual transition between the different ***doṣas*** and the respective time of day each governs. Thus as morning wears on the influence of ***vāta*** will gradually diminish as ***kapha*** becomes dominant. Similarly, as the evening gets closer to midnight ***kapha*** gradually declines as the influence of ***pitta*** gradually increases. Thus there will

TABLE 5.1 ***Doṣa*** **influence and times of the day.**

Doṣa	Period of day	Approximate time of day
Vāta	Early morning, before and just after sunrise	3 a.m.–7 a.m.
Kapha	After sunrise to the end of morning	7 a.m.–11 a.m.
Pitta	Late morning to mid-afternoon	11a.m.–3 p.m.
Vāta	Mid afternoon to early evening	3 p.m.–7 p.m.
Kapha	Early evening to late evening	7 p.m.–11 p.m.
Pitta	Late evening to early morning	11 p.m.–3 a.m.

be times of the day and night when two ***doṣas*** are equally active, but only until the ascending ***doṣa*** becomes dominant.

Brāhmamuhūrta

The morning routine is especially important in Āyurvedic medicine, and much time was traditionally spent, even as it is today in modern India, on following specific morning regimens. It is said that one should arise early in the morning, before sunrise in the period of time called the ***brāhmamuhūrta***. This period of time, roughly between the hours of 3 and 7 a.m., is considered best for receiving ***brahman***, or 'divine knowledge'. As such it is a time of great spiritual influence, best for study and meditation. One of the functions of sleep is to relax the sense organs, thereby allowing for the free circulation of ***ojas*** to nourish the entire body. During the process of sleep we are able to experience the lifting of the veil of the ego (***ahaṃkāra***), where for a brief time we no longer create an identity based on the conditioned interpretation of sensory experience. The mind becomes unshackled, free from having to make sense of sensory experience, and interfaces with elements of the ***sūkṣma*** and ***kāraṇa śarīras***. In this state we can experience deep spiritual lessons through dream imagery and visions, which are lifted from the unconscious to consciousness by the functions of ***vāta***. Thus by awakening during the ***brāhmamuhūrta*** we naturally invoke ***vāta*** to catalyse unconscious spiritual revelations for use in our daily life, in much the same way that ***vāta*** appears to lift the sun from the edge of darkness to illuminate the day.

Box 5.1 Reclaiming dreams

Although every person enters into visionary states during sleep it is sometimes difficult to remember them. We might awaken with the thread of the dream upon our lips, but begin to lose it as we rouse ourselves and get on with our day. One way to recall these visionary states is to keep a journal at the bedside and upon wakening, spend about 5 minutes writing in a stream-of-consciousness fashion, writing down the first words that come into your head. At first these writings may not make much sense, but with consistent practice the spiritual intent of your nocturnal meanderings will become clearer, and you will begin recalling your dreams more clearly. Our dreams can even be a kind oracle, answering all kinds of questions, both spiritual and mundane. Sometimes visualisation can facilitate this process. Just before falling asleep create a mental image, such as standing before the sacred oracle at Delphi, at an ancient Confucian or Hindu temple, in an alpine meadow or any other sacred place. In this place humbly ask the residing forces to enlighten you with the answers you seek. Remember to receive these visions with an open mind, and do not be disturbed if the dream content is strange: over time you will come to know the meaning and significance of these dreams.

Apart from being a time of spiritual awakening the ***brāhmamuhūrta*** is also the time when we can take advantage of the ascending influence of ***vāta*** to cleanse our bodies of the accumulated ***kapha*** of sleep. Simple problems of lethargy, fatigue, mucus accumulation, liver and bowel congestion, headaches and other symptoms of a ***kapha*** increase are easily brought under control by waking up early. By and large the habit in the West of 'sleeping in' is an artifact of our artificial living environment. As anyone knows who has gone camping in the wilderness, the world awakes much earlier than we might otherwise be accustomed to. Simple techniques such as sleeping with one's head in an easterly direction in front of an uncurtained window will naturally re-orientate us to the Earth's circadian cycles. Persons exempt from waking up during the ***brāhmamuhūrta*** include diseased persons, the elderly, pregnant and lactating women, and young children.

Evacuation of wastes

After arising from bed one should attend to the purity of the body. In a state of health the evacuation of urine and faeces should occur without effort or treatment. If evacuation does not occur shortly after awakening, however, or there is a history of constipation, one or two glasses of warm water can be an efficient stimulant to peristalsis. In some cases in which constipation is the only complaint a stronger stimulant may be used. Among these are:

- ***Triphala*** 'powder' (***cūrṇa***), consisting of equal parts ***Harītakī*** fruit (*Terminalia chebula*), ***Āmalakī*** (*Phyllanthus emblica*) and ***Bibhītaka*** (*Terminalia belerica*). Approximately one large teaspoon (2–3 g) can be mixed in a small glass of water and left to steep overnight. First thing the next morning the glass is stirred again and left to settle once more, and then all the liquid is drunk, leaving the herbal residue behind at the bottom of the glass. Prepared as a cold infusion ***Triphala*** has a mild effect upon the bowels and helps to strengthen digestion and cleanse the ***dhātus***. For a stronger effect ***Triphala*** can be taken directly as tablets or powder drunk with water in a dosage between 1 and 3 g. When taken before bed ***Triphala*** has a mild aperient activity, whereas when taken first thing in the morning the effect is more laxative.
- If ***Triphala*** is insufficient to promote a bowel movement ensure more general changes to the diet, emphasising a diet high in leafy green vegetables, fibres such as flax, hemp or oat bran, and a probiotic supplement (e.g. acidophilus and bifidus). If the bowel movements tend to be quite hard and dry then the strategy should be to lubricate the intestines by increasing the amount of fat in the diet, and to take herbs such as ***Śuṇṭhī*** (*Zingiber officinalis*), ***Pippalī*** (*Piper longum*) and ***Hiṅgu*** (*Ferula foetida*) that enkindle ***agni*** and ensure proper digestion.
- If dietary measures fail to promote normal bowel movements then herbs that have a more laxative activity can be taken short term; for example ***Trivṛt*** (*Operculina turpethum*), Cascara bark (*Rhamnus purshiana*), or Da huang root (*Rheum palmatum*). The use of such laxatives is indicated only with simple constipation, and not in active inflammation or chronic indigestion.
- Enema (***vasti***) therapy may also be indicated in chronic constipation, but should be avoided on a regular basis as it will tend to promote rebound constipation. Please refer to Chapter 11 for more information on ***vasti*** therapy.

Cleaning the mouth

Cleaning the oral cavity is an important component of hygiene in Āyurveda, and involves cleaning the teeth (***dañtadhavana***), the tongue (***jihvānirlekhana***) and the use of gargles (***gaṇḍūṣa***). The teeth are cleaned with bitter, astringent and pungent tasting herbs, which traditionally took the form of twigs that were chewed, and then the frayed end used to gently brush the teeth. Today such chewing sticks are used all over the world instead of the abrasive plastic bristles of a modern toothbrush and saccharin-sweet toothpastes. It is stated that brushing the teeth specifically with bitter, astringent and pungent tasting herbs helps to cleanse the accumulation of ***kapha*** from the upper digestive tract and stimulate ***agni***. Typical herbs used in India to clean the mouth include the chewed twigs of ***Pippala*** (*Ficus religiosa*), ***Nimba*** (*Azadirachta indica*), ***Arjuna*** (*Terminalia arjuna*) and ***Karañja*** (*Pongamia pinnata*). Western equivalents such as Barberry root (*Berberis vulgaris*), Bayberry bark (*Myrica cerifera*), Prickly Ash (*Zanthoxylum americanum*) and Oak bark (Quercus spp.) can also be used, ground into a very fine powder and gently massaged into the teeth and gums as a dentifrice.[10] Contraindications for using very powerful ***kapha*** 'reducing' (***hara***) herbs for cleaning the mouth include fever, nausea, vomiting, EENT diseases and ***vāttika*** diseases of the head (e.g. trigeminal neuralgia). Herbs may also be chosen, however, for their utility to treat such diseases (e.g. by using ***vātāhara*** herbs such as ***Yaṣṭimadhu*** root (*Glycyrrhiza glabra*) and ***Balā*** root (*Sida cordifolia*) in trigeminal neuralgia).

One commonly used technique in Āyurveda to cleanse the tongue that is now making inroads into modern oral hygiene is that of the tongue scraper. Usually made out of a thin strip of gold or stainless steel, tongue scrapers are used to cleanse the tongue of the mucus coating found upon arising in the morning. While cleansing the tongue of some of the rather nasty oral bacteria that can accumulate in our mouths, Āyurvedic physicians believe that this procedure is specifically useful because it stimulates a reflex activity in the gastrointestinal tract, promoting good digestion and healthy elimination.

Gaṇḍūṣa or 'gargling' is performed after cleaning the teeth and tongue. Gargling with warm water is said to alleviate ***kapha***, and promote digestion and the elimination of ***āma***. Although water is most commonly used in cases of hoarseness or sore throat a variety of preparations can be used, including Indian herbs such as the fresh juice of ***Brāhmī*** (*Bacopa monniera*) or a decoction of ***Bibhītaka*** fruit (*Terminalia belerica*). Western herbs such as Sage (*Salvia officinalis*) and Purple Coneflower (*Echinacea angustifolia*) can also be helpful, used as an infusion or as diluted tinctures (2.5 mL per 50 mL of water as a rinse). For dryness of the pharynx, mouth and lips gargling with ***ghṛta***, coconut or sesame oil can be helpful.

Cleansing the eyes

Cleansing of the eyes is another facet of the traditional morning regimen, typically with collyriums (***añjana***) such as ***Sauvīrañjana***, which is prepared from the ore of antimony sulphide. This preparation is painted as a thick line on the lower eyelids, directly under the lashes, and is said to enhance vision and prevent eye disease.[11] A simple alternative to ***Sauvīrañjana*** is to collect the carbon from a wick burning in the oils of sesame, castor and ***ghṛta***: this can be done by placing a clean plate over the flame to collect the carbon as the candle burns. Both this preparation and ***Sauvīrañjana*** can also be applied at night, before bed.

Another commonly used preparation to cleanse and strengthen the eyes is ***Triphala***, as either an eyewash or as a medicated oil. To prepare a sterile eyewash a small amount of the ***cūrṇa*** is covered in about eight times the volume of hot water, steeped for 5–10 minutes and then strained through a piece of clean linen. When cool, the filtered infusion can be used to rinse the eye with the use of an eye cup. Alternatively, ***Triphala ghṛta*** can be applied, prepared by decocting one part ***Triphala*** in four parts ***ghṛta*** and 16 parts water until all of the water has evaporated. The resultant oil is then strained through fine linen, bottled and stored in a cool and dry location – to enhance shelf life a little vitamin E oil can be added as an antioxidant. A few drops are instilled in each eye before bed in conditions such as dry eye, glaucoma and diabetic retinopathy.

Non-indian alternatives used with an Āyurvedic rationale include a weak solution (3% v/v) of tinctures of Barberry root (*Berberis vulgaris*), Eyebright herb (*Euphrasia officinalis*), Rue (*Galega officinalis*) or Goldenrod herb (*Solidago* spp.), two to three drops instilled in each eye. Similar to ***Triphala***, these Western herbs can also be prepared as an infusion for an eye wash.

Another exceedingly beneficial collyrium is breast milk, which many mothers will observe to be the single best thing to treat almost any eye disorder in their infant, as well as in older children and adults. Human breast milk has the benefit of being both isotonic and demulcent, is rich in antimicrobial immunoglobulins, and is particularly helpful in soothing inflammation and dryness. Breast milk is a very important component in many traditional Āyurvedic ophthalmological preparations. As an alternative to breast milk fresh goat's milk is often used, especially in Āyurvedic ophthalmological preparations sold commercially.

Cleansing the nose, throat and lungs

In a state of health any accumulation of phlegm in the nose, throat or lungs should be relatively easy to expectorate, facilitated by the ***picchila*** and ***snigdha*** nature of ***kapha***, which governs these areas. When ***kapha*** becomes vitiated, however, or with the appearance of ***āma***, the respiratory secretions can become thick, heavy and congested, but are still more or less easy to expectorate. With an increase in ***vāta*** there is a drying and crusting of phlegm with breathing obstruction, and with ***pitta*** the phlegm is blood-streaked and the mucous membranes are sore. Although these symptoms can be a component of disease (***vikṛti***), in a mild form they are also manifestations of ***prakṛti*** as well as relatively minor disturbances to health, and thus a variety of daily regimens, many of them similar to the ***ṣatkarmas*** of ***hatha yoga***, are utilised to prevent and treat them.

Among these techiniques is ***nasya*** ('errhine'), a technique that can be utilised for cleansing the nostrils, nasal cavity, sinuses and nasopharynx. One of the most commonly used preparations for ***nasya*** is ***Aṇu taila***, a medicated herbal sesame oil, two to three drops (that which drips from the index finger) instilled deep into each nostril and inhaled. ***Aṇu taila*** is particularly effective in chronic sinusitis, but even plain unrefined sesame can be of benefit. The general nature of sesame oil is ***tikṣṇa*** ('sharp'), and upon administration it promotes a sensation of mild irritation that causes the liquifaction of ***kapha***, which is then subsequently expectorated. This type of ***nasya*** can be performed by most people, but is contraindicated in acute conditions of the nasopharynx, such as in a cold, fever or flu. Other useful ***nasya*** preparations include ***ghṛta*** medicated with ***Brāhmī*** herb (*Bacopa monniera*) or ***Vacā*** rhizome (*Acorus calamus*), both of which are particularly helpful to improve memory and concentration.

Another way to cleanse the nasopharynx is ***neti*** or 'nasal irrigation', which involves the use of a small pot (i.e. a ***neti*** pot) to administer a room temperature isotonic aqueous solution into the nasal passages, sinuses and nasopharynx via the nostrils. The best place to perform ***neti*** is over a bathroom sink in front of a mirror so you can observe the process. An isotonic solution can be prepared by dissolving a little sea salt in purified water, which, given the capacity of most ***neti*** pots, is about 1.25 mL of salt per 125 mL of water. The spout of the ***neti*** pot is inserted into the right nostril, the forehead gently tilted forwards and the chin upwards to the right so that the left nostril is below that of the right. The water is poured into the right nostril and will travel through the nasopharynx and exit through the left nostril into the sink. Care should be taken not to bend the head too far forward so that the nose is below the chin, as the water will not easily exit the nose this way. Performed properly no water will escape into the throat, and it is even possible to talk while performing ***neti***. Once complete the procedure is repeated by refilling the ***neti*** pot and repeating the same procedure with the other nostril. Following ***neti*** there may be a small amount of water remaining in the nasopharynx, which is normal. To remove any remaining water the hands are placed on the hips and a series of rapid, short and diaphragmatic exhalations (i.e. ***kapālabhāti***) are forced through the nostrils to remove any remaining water, gently tilting the body sideways to the right and then the left. ***Neti*** is a particularly helpful technique to treat hyposecretory states of the mucosa, to treat chronic stuffiness and sinus congestion, and to prevent respiratory allergies and sensitivities. As an alternative to water a weak infusion or decoction of various herbs such as ***Vāsaka***

Box 5.2 Nostril dominance

If you observe the passage of air through your nose as you breath you might notice that one nostril flows much more easily than the other. This is referred to as *nostril dominance*, a concept that has been a facet of ***hatha yoga*** for centuries. The dominance of a given nostril at any given time indicates which ***nāḍī*** is dominant. According to ***hatha yoga*** the functions of the body are manifest in the coordinated functions of the ***ida*** and ***pingalā naḍis***. The subtle energetic channel called the ***ida nāḍī*** terminates in the left nostril, and its counterpart the ***pingalā nāḍī*** terminates in the right nostril. The ***ida nāḍī*** represents the rest and restorative system of the body, and is associated with mental characteristics such as intuition, imagination, fantasy and subjectivity. When the ***ida nāḍī*** becomes dominant the body becomes quiet and relaxed. In contrast, the ***pingalā nāḍī*** is associated with activity and expenditure systems of the body, represents mental characteristics such as study, analysis and discrimination, and under its influence the body is hungry and is impelled to move. In most people, the dominant nostril alternates about every 90 to 120 minutes. In cases where natural, circadian cycles are ignored, there may be some fluctuation in this model. If one nostril is dominant for more than a few hours, however, this is an indication of a state of imbalance, and if this continues for more than 24 hours it may be a premonitory symptom of some kind of illness. Becoming aware of which nostril is dominant can also guide one's activities throughout the day. Activities such as working and eating are best performed when the right nostril is dominant, while activities such as relaxation and creative pursuits are best performed when the left nostril is dominant. Although our daily schedules may not be able to conform to the natural cycles of nostril dominance, there are things we can do to change which nostril is dominant at any given moment. If the left nostril is dominant just before eating or if you are having a difficult time concentrating, go out for a walk to activate the right nostril. Lying down on the left side of the body for a few minutes will also activate the right nostril, and conversely, lying down on one's right side will activate the left.

leaf (*Adhatoda vasica*) or Eyebright herb (*Euphrasia officinalis*) can be used in irritation and inflammation. In certain conditions of extreme debility and where ***āma*** has been removed, milk decoctions of nourishing herbs such as ***Aśvagandhā*** root (*Withania somnifera*), ***Balā*** root (*Sida cordifolia*) or ***Śatāvarī*** root (*Asparagus racemosus*) can also be used in ***neti***. ***Neti*** is generally contraindicated when the nasal passages are blocked, however, which will promote the retention of the liquid used: in such cases ***nasya*** is a better choice.

Another helpful technique to clear the lungs and respiratory passage is ***prāṇayama***, a unique form of breath control that is orientated towards controlling the nature and flow of ***prāṇa*** in the body. ***Prāṇayama*** is an esoteric practice of ***hatha yoga*** that is based on the belief that by controlling breath one gains conscious control over ***prāṇa***, the innate intelligence of the body. Although ***prāṇayama*** is a part of the ***hatha yoga*** tradition, it has since been integrated with Āyurvedic practices and is used as an important therapeutic tool that extends beyond the treatment of respiratory disorders. There are a variety of methods in ***prāṇayama***, including ***ujjayi***, ***śitali***, ***kabalābhati*** and ***bhastrika***, most of which require the instruction of a properly trained teacher. Among the easiest and safest techniques is ***nāḍī śodhana***, or 'alternate nostril breathing', which, technically speaking, is a preparatory technique for the more advanced techniques of ***prāṇayama***. ***Nāḍī śodhana*** is performed by alternating the inhalation and exhalation through one nostril while simultaneously blocking the other nostril. In the most common form of ***nāḍī śodhana*** the right hand is used: the index and middle fingers are placed in the middle of the brow (i.e. the ***ājñā cakra*** or 'third eye'), and the thumb and ring fingers are used to block the nostrils. First the thumb closes the right nostril by pressing it against the septum and an inhalation is taken through the left nostril. The ring finger of the right hand then blocks the left nostril and the thumb is released, and exhalation is performed through the right nostril. Without changing the position of the fingers the right nostril is then used to inhale while blocking the left nostril, and then the right nostril is blocked with the thumb and exhalation is performed by the left nostril. Altogether this counts as one cycle, and typically at least six cycles are performed after which the practitioner breathes normally for several seconds, and then initiates another round of cycles. In total there should be at least three rounds or 18 cycles. ***Nāḍī śodhana*** is typically performed while sitting cross-legged on the floor, with a straight back and relaxed shoulders, but can also be performed while sitting normally in a chair with a straight back.

The inhalation of smoke, called ***dhūma***, is also suggested by many Āyurvedic sources to be particularly helpful to cleanse the accumulated ***kapha*** from the respiratory tract. The smoke is inhaled through the nose with the help of a paper funnel: the pointed end inserted in the nostril and the open end over the burning ember; the inhaled smoke is exhaled through the mouth. A typical smoking preparation can be made by taking a pinch each of the powders of ***Haridrā*** rhizome (*Curcuma longa*), ***Marica*** fruit (*Piper nigrum*), and ***Yaṣṭi madhu*** root (*Glycyrrhiza glabra*), mixing them with a small quantity of ***ghṛta***, and heating them in a hot pan or on hot coals. Other potentially helpful Western herbs include Mullein (*Verbascum thapsus*) and Coltsfoot (*Tussilago farfara*), prepared in much the same way, or smoked in small amounts as a kind of cigarette (but inhaled through the nose, not the mouth). ***Dhūma*** is rarely utilised more than two to three times per week, and no more than one to two inhalations in each nostril per session. ***Dhūma*** is contraindicated in active inflammation of the nasopharynx and in dry, hyposecretive mucosa. As an alternative to ***dhūma*** the use of ***kapha***-reducing essential oils can be used, such as cedar, pine, spruce, rosemary, basil, frankincense, myrrh, eucalyptus, cajeput, camphor, ginger and clove, all of which can be used with humidifiers while sleeping and during the day, or for use in sauna and steam bath.

Stimulating digestion

The ancient custom of chewing ***betel*** (***pān***) finds its place in the daily routines recommended by Āyurveda. ***Betel*** nut (*Areca catechu*) is an important digestive stimulant with weak narcotic properties that gives the person who chews it a mild euphoria. ***Betel*** also has sialogogue properties, which not only assists in digestion but helps to maintain an oral pH that is conducive to good dental health. Another especially useful herb for this purpose is Toothache flower (*Spilanthes acmella*), which contains high levels of isobutylamides, the same class of chemical constituent as in ***Tuṃburū*** (*Zanthoxylum elatum*) and Purple Coneflower (*Echinacea angustifolia*) that provides for their characteristic 'tingling' sensation and sialogogue properties.

Other helpful digestive stimulants include aromatics such as ***Elā*** seeds (*Elettaria cardamomum*), ***Vacā*** rhizome (*Acorus calamus*), and ***Mustaka*** root (*Cyperus rotundus*), and bitter stimulants such as ***Nimba*** leaf (*Azadirachta indica*), ***Bhṛṅgarāja*** leaf (*Eclipta alba*) and ***Guḍūcī*** stem (*Tinospora cordifolia*).

Exercise

After attending to the purification of internal wastes and the stimulation of digestion, some form of exercise (***vyāyāma***) is indicated, usually to the capacity of 'one-half one's strength'. This is understood to mean that daily exercise should be performed to the point of perspiration of the face, axilla and limbs, with an accompanying sensation of dryness in the mouth. ***Vyāyāma*** is best implemented in winter and spring, whereas in the seasons of summer and autumn exercise should be performed to a milder degree. Although the different ***āsanas*** that make up ***hatha yoga*** come to mind for most people when thinking about Indian forms of exercise (e.g. ***sūrya namaskar***, or 'sun salutation'), wrestling and martial arts such as ***kālarippayattu*** and its East Asian equivalents (e.g. karate, ju sitsu, tae kwon do etc.) were traditionally considered to be very helpful, especially in younger people. Any form of exercise, however, that puts a repetitive strain on a specific part of the body, such as jogging, is not recommended.

Massage

After exercise ***abhyaṅga*** ('oleation') is utilised next, lightly massaging various oils over the entire body, paying particular attention to the head, ears, large joints and feet. The most commonly used oil is unrefined sesame oil (***taila***) but any number of pure or medicated oils can be used (see Ch. 7). Whereas a large amount of oil is used in ***pūrva karma*** (see Ch. 11), only a small amount of oil is used as part of ***dinācaryā*** – enough to coat the body but not enough to leave a greasy film. Used in larger amounts, however, ***abhyaṅga*** is particularly suitable for ***vāttika*** diseases but should be avoided in ***āma*** or ***kapha*** conditions. Oil in particular is a good solvent for much of the dirt and grime that accumulates on the body, and can be washed off during bathing. ***Paittika*** conditions benefit from the use of cooling oils such as coconut and ***ghṛta***, especially so if they have been medicated with ***pittahara*** medicaments or essential oils. ***Kapha*** conditions benefit from a dry massage, using herbal powders (*udavartana*) such as ***Triphala*** and ***Śūṇṭhī*** rhizome (*Zingiber officinalis*), raw silk gloves (***gharṣana***), or skin brushing with a brush or loofah (see Ch. 11). Such dry massage techniques are particularly helpful to reduce ***kapha***, fat and cellulite, and stimulate the lymphatic system. Such methods are typically applied to the peripheral parts of the body first, beginning with the feet and legs, and then the arms and back, and then lastly the torso and chest, to essentially move lymph to the heart where it is mixed with the blood and then directed to the liver and kidneys for elimination.

Bathing

Bathing (***snāna***) with warm water follows exercise and massage, and may be done with the addition of fragrant herbs or essential oils chosen on the basis of the ***prakṛti*** or the symptoms of disease (i.e. ***vikṛti***). For ***vāttika*** conditions herbs and essential oils can be chosen on the basis of their ability to reduce ***vāta***. Among these are epsom salts, and the 'oatmeal sock' method by which an old sock or linen bag is filled with oatmeal, tied off, and allowed to steep in a hot bath for 10–15 minutes. When the water is cool enough to bathe, the sock or bag is then squeezed out and sponged onto the skin, releasing its milky white 'juice' to soothe dry, irritated and inflamed skin. Useful essential oils to reduce ***vāta*** include chamomile, lavender, geranium, neroli, vetivert, rosemary, lemon balm, basil, sweet marjoram, bergamot, hyssop, lemon, clary sage, myrrh, frankincense, sandalwood, aniseed, cinnamon, eucalyptus and camphor. For ***paittika*** conditions only mildly warm water or even cool water should be used, along with cooling and pacifying herbs such as ***Candana*** wood (*Santalum album*) or ***Uśīra*** root (*Vetiveria zizanioides*) prepared as a decoction, as well as the oatmeal sock method described above. Useful essential oils to reduce ***pitta*** include chamomile, lavender, rose, gardenia, honeysuckle, ylang-ylang, vetivert, jasmine and sandalwood. For ***kapha*** conditions the use of warm water is similarly advised as in ***vāta*** to reduce coldness, but rather than a sitting bath a shower or steam bath should be used in preference due to their comparatively energising and stimulating properties. Helpful herbs to reduce ***kapha*** include ***Śūṇṭhī*** rhizome (*Zingiber officinalis*) and

Pippalī fruit (*Piper longum*), as well as essential oils such as cedar, pine, rosemary, basil, frankincense, myrrh, eucalyptus, cajeput, camphor, ginger and clove.

To remove dirt and excess oil Āyurveda recommends the application of herbal and bean powders to the moistened skin, rather than the detergents found in soap that strip the skin of its natural, protective oils and destroy the delicate bacterial ecology of the skin. Such powders include ***caṇa*** (garbanzo, chick pea) and ***mudga*** (green gram) that have absorbent and gently abrasive properties that remove dirt, oil and grime. For additional activities they can be blended with moistening and soothing herbs such as ground oatmeal or seaweed, or with astringing herbs such as any of the pond lilies or lotus flower roots (e.g. *Nelumbo, Nymphaea*), which have long been used by women all over the world to make the skin beautiful. In a similar vein, Āyurvedic medicine recommends the usage of herbal hair rinses to clean the hair, rather than the harsh detergents and chemicals found in commercial shampoos and conditioners. Like skin soap, the regular usage of shampoo strips the hair of its natural oils and nutrients, which are then replaced by the synthetic versions found in conditioners. Most people find that when they stop using such hair care products their hair becomes greasy and unmanageable. This response is more likely related to the fact that the hair follicles have become induced to secreting large amounts of oil to replace that which has been stripped away by shampoo. Technically speaking, the word 'shampoo' is a Hindi word referring to a vigorous head massage (***campū***), which correctly stimulates the hair follicles and distributes the natural oils throughout the hair. Such head massaging techniques are used in conjunction with herbal hair rinses that remove any excess oils and grime, but do not strip the hair completely. Examples of traditional Indian herbs that can be prepared as an infusion or decoction and then applied to the hair when cool are ***Japā*** flower (*Hibiscus rosa sinensis*), ***Śatapatrī*** flower (*Rosa* spp.), and ***Āmalakī*** fruit (*Phyllanthus emblica*). Herbs that are valued in Western herbal medicine include Rosemary leaf (*Rosmarinus officinalis*), Horsetail herb (*Equisteum arvense*), and Nettle leaf (*Urtica dioica*). Although it may take several weeks, the regular usage of head massage and herbal hair rinses instead of shampoos and conditioners will eventually normalise the secretion of the natural oils in the hair. Women in India are particularly noted for their beautiful thick hair, and up until very recently, only ever used hair rinses to clean and strengthen their hair, as well as cooling nourishing oils such as coconut that are applied to the head to keep it cool in hot weather.

Generally speaking only cool or room-temperature water should be used when bathing the head to avoid damage to the eyes and prevent hair loss. In particular, cold water is a useful treatment for acute psychological crises, such as mania, rage and other ***paittika*** mental manifestations, whereas warm water baths are best to pacify ***vāta*** and ***kapha***. Bathing with any kind of water is avoided in fever, influenza, pneumonia, indigestion, facial paralysis, diseases of the ears, eyes, nose and throat, and in persons who have just taken food.

Meditation

After exercise, massage and bathing the body is now supple and relaxed, and is best prepared for extended sitting for meditation, called ***bhavana*** or ***dhyāna***. Various meditative techniques exist, and not all are appropriate to each person. ***Vāttika prakṛtis*** will benefit from meditative techniques that involve much ritual, imagery, and visualisation. The quality of the ***vāttika*** mind is analogous to a team of wild horses, each pulling in opposite directions. Such meditative techniques provide an organised and structured environment to harness the lability of ***vāta***. ***Paittika prakṛtis*** will benefit from concentrated and disciplined meditative techniques such as mindfulness of breath or contemplating specific sense objects (i.e. smell, taste, sight, touch or hearing). The one-pointedness of such meditations purifies the mental fires of the ***paittika*** mind, clarifying intent and enhancing concentrative abilities. ***Kaphaja prakṛtis*** may want to emphasise devotional meditations such as meditating upon a deity (***bhakti yoga***), or perform more active forms of meditation such as walking meditation and ***karma yoga***. The use of more active forms of meditation helps to counter the relative stability, dullness and slowness of the ***kaphaja*** mind. None of these suggestions are static, however, and all of these techniques may be appropriate for all people at different stages of their lives, and in different situations.

Meditation is the process of understanding our various attachments, of freeing consciousness from a conditioned existence. It is the only technique that is mentioned in the ancient texts as being capable of bringing about the highest attainment of consciousness, with complete safety and total self-direction. Science has investigated some of the beneficial effects of meditation, such as the reduction of mental and physiological stress.

There are many different kinds of meditation: ultimately life itself is a kind of meditation and thus every activity a meditative exercise. The purpose of meditation is to be mindful, to be self-aware, to direct attention to our intent, thoughts and actions in every instance. For most this would be too difficult a task to do while living their everyday 'normal' life, and thus time is set aside on a daily basis to cultivate this state, to keep the flame of mindfulness alive so that it illumines our daily life. The benefit of regular morning meditation is to make us more mindful during the rest of the day. Some techniques require the repetition of a ***mantra***, or utilise visualisations – all this is unnecessary when the attention is directed inwards, to the nature of mind.

The simplest method of meditation is ***ānapānasati bhavana***, or mindfulness of breath meditation. The Vedic tradition states that breath, represented by the ***mantra*** 'so-ham', represents the division of consciousness. When we focus on the breath, when 'so' becomes 'ham', and 'ham' becomes 'so', we unite consciousness, and move beyond a state of duality.

Find a quiet location in your home where you will not be disturbed, turn off the lights, and draw the blinds or curtains. If you desire, light a small candle before you begin, and as you are lighting it imagine that this light represents the complete illumination of your consciousness. Assume a comfortable sitting posture on the floor, upon a folded blanket, or another firm surface. Ideally, sit in one of the three cross-legged yogic sitting postures, such as the ***padmāsana*** (1), the ***siddhāsana*** (2), or the ***sukhāsana*** (3) pose (see Fig. 5.1). Before attempting these postures you may want to stretch first, or practise a few simple yoga postures, stretching the arms, neck, torso, groin and legs.

If you have any difficulty with these sitting positions try placing a thin pillow under your buttocks. If you are still having some difficulty sit in a chair or on the edge of a bed. Try to keep your back reasonably straight, without being stiff or straining. Lay your hands in your lap, palm up, one palm resting upon the other, or place your palms over each knee. Close your eyes. As you breathe in focus your attention on the expansion and contraction of your abdomen. If your abdomen is not moving but your chest is, place your hands over your abdomen and try to bring your breath down to your abdomen. Once you have mastered this kind of breathing place your hands back in your lap or on your knees. Ensure that you are sitting up reasonably straight, almost as if each vertebra in your back were piled up one upon the other like a block tower, the spinal cord inside hanging vertical like a plumb line.

As you breathe in focus on the movement of the abdomen outwards, and as you exhale focus on the movement of the abdomen inwards. Keep your attention on the movement of your abdomen. Do not force or control your breath in any way – just breathe normally. Try not to follow the breath all the way down or all the way out: simply be aware of your breath. To help keep your focus on these movements mentally repeat to yourself 'rising, rising' as you breathe in, and 'falling, falling' as you breathe out.

An alternative method is to focus on the movement of air in and out of your nostrils. As you breathe in mentally repeat 'in, in' and as you breathe out mentally repeat 'out, out'. Feel the breath move in and out of your nose. If you are too congested to breathe easily through your nose bring your attention back to your abdomen.

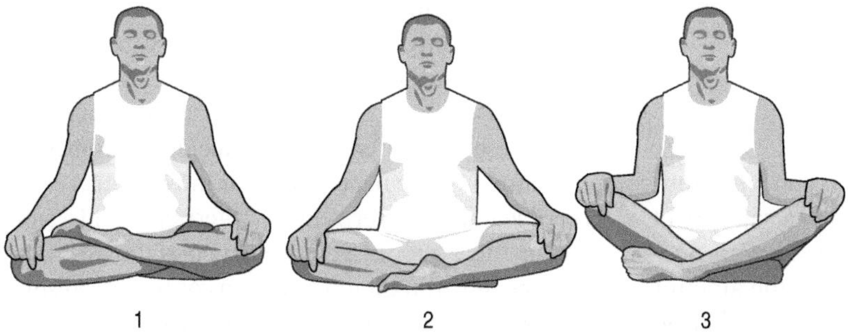

Figure 5.1 Meditative postures.

As you experiment with these different techniques during the first few minutes of meditation find which object of meditation is better for you, either the movement of your abdomen or the movement of air in and out of your nostrils. Once you have chosen a method, however, stick with it and do not alternate back and forth between the different methods.

As you focus on your breath, you may notice that thoughts or images enter into your consciousness. While meditating you may find yourself suddenly engaged in a long chain of thoughts, imagining some scenario, or seeing certain images. As you realise this try to bring your attention back to your breathing. Do not judge yourself, or the thoughts or images you experience: simply return back to the breath.

The task of mindfulness asks that you be aware of how your sensory experience colours and affects your consciousness. But rather than identify the purpose or intent of these sensations, the practice of meditation allows you to understand how fluid your day-to-day consciousness is. Meditation on the breath allows you to be an objective witness of your consciousness, rather than being a subjective participant. If thoughts come into your consciousness while meditating do not identify them or trace their source: mentally repeat 'thinking, thinking, thinking' until the thoughts dissipate into nothingness. Similarly, if you hear a noise do not try to determine the origin of the sound but simply identify its impact upon your consciousness by mentally repeating 'hearing, hearing, hearing'. If the noise generates a thought pattern repeat to yourself 'thinking, thinking, thinking'. If your body begins to hurt or you feel a tickling sensation somewhere do not give these sensations any credence while you are meditating: simply repeat to yourself 'feeling, feeling, feeling' until the sensation subsides.

Try to practice meditation for about 10–15 minutes each day, preferably during the ***brahmāmuhūrta***, in the morning hours just before sunrise. As you get used to the technique, try extending these periods of meditation to 20–40 minutes each day.

Eating

The partaking of food is the last of the morning routines, and for all meals is performed up to a capacity of one-half the stomach contents, consumed with one-quarter portion of water. This means that the amount of food to be consumed at any given meal should lead to satiation, to the appeasement of hunger, leaving some room in the stomach to accommodate gastric churning. In contrast, most people eat until they are 'stuffed', and think that symptoms experienced after eating, such as gastric fullness, difficulty breathing or moving, and the reflux of the ingested food into the oesophagus and mouth is for the most part normal. Most people are surprisingly unaware of this dynamic because for them it is not the need for food that drives its consumption, but rather, the 'taste' of food. If we recall from Chapter 2 it is the perception of taste (***rasa***) that gives rise of the ***mahābhūta*** of water (***ap***), which functions to create cohesiveness in the body but is also an energy that binds our perceptions to a lower order of reality. It is the function of water and the 'taste' of life that in turn binds us to ***saṃsāra***, which leads to dissatisfaction, unhappiness and pain. One important axiom I learned in my training is 'he who controls his tongue controls his life', indicating the pain and unhappiness that is generated when we eat in an unconscious fashion. Eating should be based upon fulfilling the needs of the stomach, not the tongue, which by its very nature is insatiable (as witnessed by that regretable second helping of pumpkin pie after the huge Thanksgiving turkey dinner . . .). According to the famed Āyurvedic scholar Nāgārjuna the process of digestion should be for the most part unnoticeable, and thus any problem experienced after eating should indicate that either the quantity of food was too much (or too little), that the ***agni*** is weak, or that the food chosen is simply inappropriate (***asātmya***). Āyurveda also recommends that small amounts of water be consumed with the meal to assist in digestion and to lubricate the food, but not in large gulps to 'wash it down'. It is said that water taken before meals or consumed in large amounts with the meal will inhibit digestion. Generally speaking, eating should be undertaken only when the stomach is completely empty, indicated by the absence of any taste and odour of the previous meal upon eructation (i.e. burping).

The remaining portion of the day is used to discharge one's duties, following the guidelines outlined in the next section (i.e. ***sadvṛtta***, 'good conduct'). Generally speaking, Āyurvedic medicine recommends a maximum of three meals a day for most people, eating larger meals in the morning and afternoon, and a small meal in the evening. The modern practice of eating many meals throughout the day to control blood sugar is ill-advised, and can usually be remedied by eating a larger, higher protein breakfast. In many cases people may find that when they eat higher-density nutrients such as proteins and fats they will eat less, and may be able to eat as few as two meals a day, a model followed by many traditional peoples across the world. Evening meals should always be taken before sunset, and bedtime should occur within the ***kapha*** dominant period (i.e. between 7 and 11 p.m.) to take advantage of the natural somnolence that this time of day produces. Staying up beyond 11 p.m. tends to activate ***pitta*** and fires of the mind, resulting in 'hunger', movement, and insufficient sleep, and when resorted to on a chronic basis, a commensurate loss of ***ojas***.

For more detailed information of dietary and lifestyle patterns for each ***doṣa*** please consult Appendix 2.

5.3 *Sadvṛtta*: GOOD CONDUCT

Āyurveda is not solely concerned with the health of the body but equally emphasises factors such as morality and proper conduct. Traditional Indian philosophy suggests that the body is but a vehicle for spiritual development and is of itself unimportant. Rather, it is the proper care and maintenance of the body and the prevention of disease that is important, for this liberates us from the discomfort, pain and sadness that might cloud our minds and inhibit spiritual development.

Most people in the West are familiar with the Ten Commandments as revealed to Moses and recounted in the Talmud. Āyurveda, too, advocates a similar system of ten 'sins', the first three relating to 'infractions of the body' (***kāyakarma***), the next four to 'infractions of speech' (***vācīkarma***), and the last three to 'infractions of the mind' (***manokarma***). Far from being a collection of simple morals to be followed blindly, this scheme is based upon an understanding of the mechanics of ***karma***, of how one skilful or unskillful action necessarily creates an equally charged reaction, and how this effect can be either productive or unproductive. The fruition of these ***karmic*** seeds can manifest at any given point in our long cycle of rebirth, when the necessary factors for their development are present. Thus, following such a scheme does not necessarily yield any immediate reward except to remove obstructions to further spiritual progress. The components of these 'ten sins' are as follows:

Kāyakarma (infractions of body)

1. ***Hiṃsā*** (violence): to cause injury or perpetrate violence on another sentient being is considered to be the foremost violation of good conduct, whether it leads to fatality or injury. In cases where the intent to cause harm is absent the gravity of the violation is considerably less. Sometimes our unintentional acts of violence are part of the fruition of another's unwholesome ***karma***.
2. ***Steyā*** (stealing): taking that which has been claimed by another, as well as claiming credit for works that are not of one's own creation.
3. ***Anyathākāma*** (improper sexual activities): traditionally this has referred to unlawful sexual conduct, e.g. sex with minors, sex with deceit (i.e. affairs), sex with teachers or students and sex with ***brahmacaryās*** (those who have given up normal human relations for a spiritual goal). ***Anyathākāma*** also refers to any sensual pleasure that is indulgent and does not serve health or the development of one's spiritual consciousness, such as a craving, fetishes, attachment, addiction and bad habit, in relation to food, sexuality or any other lifestyle activity.

Vācīkarma (infractions of speech)

4. ***Anrita vacana*** (falsehood): lying, mistruths, half-truths.
5. ***Paiśunya*** (slander): speech causing dissension, public attacks and criticism, breaching confidentiality.
6. ***Paruṣa*** (harsh speech): scolding, reviling, reproving with angry words, insult, sarcasm, negative criticism.
7. ***Saṃbhinna ālāpa*** (idle speech): mindless speech, blathering or talking just to make noise. Traditionally ***saṃbhinna ālāpa*** referred to the actions of one's self, but can also be seen as referring to the influence of the modern media. Television, cinema, the print media, radio and various forms of 'entertainment' such as video games are designed to be consumed mindlessly, without any 'digesting'. These influences can become lodged in the mind as a kind of mental toxin: ***āma*** that impairs the fire of consciousness. While many of these activities are enjoyable they should be closely monitored because they tend to create a blunted consciousness.

Manokarma (infractions of mind)

8. ***Vyāpāda*** (ill will): resentment, malice, anger, spite, animosity.
9. ***Abhidyā*** (jealousy): coveting another's possessions, relationships or powers; bearing ill-will towards another's success; rivalry, bad sportsmanship.
10. ***Dṛgviparyayā*** (improper interpretation): deliberate misunderstanding of another's actions; not listening to intuition; misinterpretation of information or knowledge; faithlessness, finding fault, necessarily taking an adversarial position, scepticism, closed mindedness.

The philosophy expressed in Vāgbhaṭa's ***Aṣṭāñga Hṛdaya*** is that all human activities should be directed towards the happiness of all sentient beings. While Vāgbhaṭa was expressing what is perhaps a characteristically Buddhist sentiment, it is a consistent theme in all Vedic sources, representing the compassion of the Divine Mother and the love she has for all her children. As an emanation of this divine energy (***śakti***) the ancient texts of Āyurveda counsel us to be honest, fair and balanced in our relations with others. Family and friends should be treated with the utmost respect and beneficence, and cordial and even helpful relations with rivals and competitors should be maintained. The poor and unfortunate, those suffering from disease and the circumstances of life, deserve every possible effort to alleviate that pain and suffering. We should all cultivate a pleasing and friendly countenance and avail ourselves to be of service. This means becoming adaptable and mutable to new circumstances and people, looking for integration rather than contrast. It does not mean that one should extinguish one's identity, but rather, place less value upon transitory emotions and thoughts that lead to feelings of alienation and suspicion. Āyurveda also mentions the quality of adoration, which in its modern context, refers to the validation and celebration of each person's unique talents and characteristics, including oneself.

An equally important theme in Indian spirituality was an understanding of how to develop one's 'personal power'. Archetypally this is the realm of initiation, the ego-driven individual transformed into the great ***yogin***, Lord Śiva besmeared with ash sitting on his tiger skin, perhaps equally represented by the Norse God Odin who sacrifices himself to obtain the magical power of the runes. In this realm we undergo a dramatic, sometimes painful transmutation, where our consiousness and everything we hold to be true is literally broken into pieces and we recognise the nature of duality (***dvaita***). The understanding of our dual nature is the first step on the path to the unification of opposites (***advaita***). Ultimately the will becomes one with Śiva, the source of All, the god Odin sacrificing himself to become Himself (i.e. ***svayambhu***, 'Self-become'). In this process of developing personal power Āyurveda thus acknowledges the cultivation of ***siddhis*** ('talents', 'powers') that can aid in the practice of medicine, and many of these form the highly specialised techniques of ***anumāna***, or inference and intuition in diagnosis (see Ch. 10). As a primary form of gaining knowledge and power all Āyurvedic physicians are instructed to direct their attention to the control of the mind and senses. Āyurveda states that the body is a sacred temple, and the senses are its sentinels: just as a beautiful temple or church is maintained and sustained by its residents, so will the proper correlation of sense and sense-object lead to a healthy body and mind.

5.4 *Ṛtucaryā*: SEASONAL REGIMEN

The influence of the solar cycle, or the time it takes for the earth to complete one orbit around the sun, can be divided into two equal periods, called ***dakṣiṇāyana*** and ***uttarāyaṇa***. The ***dakṣiṇāyana*** period begins with the summer solstice, the beginning of the decline of the sun's influence in the northern (***uttarā***) hemisphere and its increasing dominance in the southern (***dakṣiṇā***) hemisphere. During the ***dakṣiṇāyana***, especially in temperate areas such as North America and Europe, the lunar cooling influence of the moon begins to dominate, the sun and warm weather are gradually obscured by cloud and the environment becomes wet (***snigdha***), cold (***śita***), and windy (***cala***). Although marked by a brief period of fruition at the end of summer, the vital energy of the planet during the ***dakṣiṇāyana*** descends back into the earth to wait out the cycle of winter. If we remember that the human body is composed primarily of ***pṛthvī*** and ***ap*** we can see how the quality of these climactic influences (i.e. ***śita***, ***snigdha***, ***cala***) vitiates the basic characteristic of the human body, weakening ***agni*** and facilitating the production of ***āma***. In contrast, the

uttarāyaṇa period begins with the winter solstice, the time when the light of the sun begins to rise from its lowest point in the sky in the northern hemisphere to its highest. The powerful influence of the sun during this period gradually begins to dominate, and its progressively warming (***uṣṇa***) and drying (***rūkṣa***) qualities thin the congested properties of ***pṛthvī*** and ***ap***. Thus the period of time marked by ***uttarāyaṇa*** generally exerts a stimulating and tonic effect on the human body, enhancing ***agni*** and the elimination of ***āma***. In most of India and in tropical regions the beneficial attributes of the ***dakṣiṇāyana*** and ***uttarāyaṇa*** are reversed because the sun's influence is considerably greater in regions closer to the equator, and during the ***uttarāyaṇa*** the excessive heat of the sun depletes the qualities of ***pṛthvī*** and ***ap***. In contrast, the ***dakṣiṇāyana*** marks the period of the monsoons and cool weather, all of which provide relief from the depleting intensity of the sun. This variance in the effects of seasonal changes is perhaps why in the Vedic system of astrology called ***jyotiṣ*** the sun is considered to be a potentially malefic (harmful) influence in the chart, whereas in Western astrology the sun is generally considered to be a beneficial sign.

The ancient texts of Āyurveda describe six seasons, in contrast to the four generally recognised in the West. The seasons are identified as follows:

1. ***Hemañta***: early winter, mid-November to mid-January
2. ***Śirīṣa***: late winter, mid-January to mid-March
3. ***Vasanta***: spring, mid-March to mid-May
4. ***Griṣma***: summer, mid-May to mid-July
5. ***Varṣa***: monsoon, mid-July to mid-September
6. ***Śarat***: autumn, mid-September to mid-November.

While the above scheme takes into account the seasonal patterns of India it does not reflect the seasonal changes seen in temperate regions such as North America and Europe. Most notably, temperate regions display only four major seasons, they lack monsoons, and do not experience the season of ***śarat***, which in India is an intensely hot and humid period of weather that is experienced shortly after the monsoon. While this specific sequence might not be found in temperate regions, some regions will experience extended periods of hot, humid weather, typically during the height of summer (***griṣma***). This hot, wet weather aggravates ***pitta***, and thus measures are taken at this time to control ***pitta***,which are essentially the same as described for ***griṣma***. The seasons for most temperate regions are as follows:

1. ***Hemañta***: early winter, mid-November to mid-January
2. ***Śirīṣa***: late winter, mid-January to mid-March
3. ***Vasanta***: spring, mid-March to mid-June
4. ***Griṣma***, ***Śarat***: summer, mid-June to mid-September
5. ***Varṣa***: autumn, mid-September to mid-November.

Please note that this scheme does not take into account the entire scope of climatic variations found in temperate regions, nor yearly variations such as El Niño, and must be interpreted accordingly.

5.5 *Hemañta* AND *śirīṣa ṛtucaryā*: WINTER REGIMEN

It is during ***hemañta*** that the health potential is at its greatest due to the extrinsic cold of winter that contains the expansive nature of ***agni*** within the body. Thus the ***jaṭharāgni*** becomes concentrated and digestive capacity becomes strong to such an extent that if precautions are not taken its catabolic qualities will extend to the digestion of the body itself. Thus, generally speaking, a ***vātāhara*** routine is implemented at this time, using foods and therapies that are ***guru*** ('heavy') and ***snigdha*** ('moistening') in quality. Warm oil massages, especially those medicated with ***vātāhara*** herbs like ***Aśvagandhā*** root (*Withania somnifera*) and ***Balā*** root (*Sida cordifolia*), are used upon waking and before bed. Exercise is also an important and vital component of the winter regimen to ensure proper digestion and circulation of blood, and regular sexual activity and physical intimacy are recommended. Meals throughout the day should consist of warm soupy meat dishes and vegetable broths, high quality fats, moistening grains such as wheat, rye and brown rice, baked and steamed root vegetables, and if available, lightly steamed above-ground vegetables. Warming herbs and spices such as ginger, garlic, shallots, oregano, rosemary, basil, mustard, black pepper, cinnamon and cardamom can be used during this period. Although the variety of foods is limited, a number of foods can be eaten at this time that at other times might causes problems: any food that is cold, dry or raw, however, is usually avoided in winter. Modest amounts of naturally fermented beverages such as wine or dark beer may be consumed with meals in winter to assist in the digestion of the heavier, fatty foods consumed at this time, and to prevent the accumulation of ***kapha***. Wool, silk, heavy cotton, leather, fur and feathers are appropriate fabrics and materials for both wearing and sleeping under. Footwear and hats should always be worn, even inside if necessary. Fresh air is highly recommended during winter because of the excessive time usually spent indoors, as well as for the opportunity to exercise and stay active. In ***vāttika prakṛtis***, however, exposure to very cold weather should be avoided, and instead, time can be spent sitting beside a warm fire or in a heated room in front of a sunny window. The regimen for ***śirīṣa*** resembles ***hemañta*** in many respects, but should be adhered to even more rigorously, as the influences of deep winter are much stronger. Typically, there will be more ***rūkṣa*** ('dryness') and ***śita*** ('cold') qualities as winter wears on, especially in places that have a long winter.

5.6 *Vasanta ṛtucaryā*: SPRING REGIMEN

The cold weather of winter coupled with the ***guru*** ('heavy') and ***snigdha*** ('moistening') qualities of a ***vātāhara*** regimen causes an increase in ***kapha*** (see 2.7 Caya and kopa: increase and vitiation of the doṣas). With the increasing influence of the sun and the warm weather of ***vasanta*** (spring) this natural increase of ***kapha*** undergoes vitiation. This process is mirrored in the natural environment, when the snow that has accumulated in the mountains over winter begins to melt and flood the streams and rivers with water. Similarly, the ***guru*** ('heavy'), ***śita*** ('cold'), and ***snigdha*** ('wet') properties of ***kapha*** that accumulated over winter begin to 'melt' and flood the body, impairing ***agni*** and giving rise to such congestive conditions as a colds, flu, and hayfever. Thus, just as a landowner clears the dry streams and creek beds of debris in preparation for the spring run-off, so too should the eliminative faculties of the body be prepared at this time. The traditional practice in many cultures of a spring cleanse is an example of such a measure, best implemented just before the season has changed from winter to spring. ***Vamana***, or vomiting therapy, is usually considered to be the most effective technique (see Ch. 11), but the application of nasal medications (***nasya***, ***neti***), the consumption of simple and easily digestible foods, vigorous exercise, sauna and dry massage are also useful. A course of ***kaphahara*** herbs such as ***Śūṇṭhī*** rhizome (*Zingiber officinalis*), ***Pippalī*** fruit (*Piper longum*), and ***Dāruharidrā*** root (*Berberis aristata*) taken with honey would add to the effectiveness of such a cleanse, as would a period of vegetable juice fasting. In terms of diet, light and easily digestible grains such as barley, rice, millet, amaranth and quinoa are emphasised, along with leafy green vegetables and shoots, legumes, and stimulating herbs and spices such as pepper, ginger, mustard and fenugreek. Meat with a light property such as goat, lamb, poultry and rabbit are also appropriate. Naturally fermented beverages are also recommended at this time, especially bitter aperitifs and digestives.

5.7 *Griṣma* AND *śarat ṛtucaryā*: SUMMER REGIMEN

With the moist heat of spring, ***pitta*** undergoes ***caya*** ('increase'), and this increase coupled with the heat of summer leads to the ***kopa*** ('vitiation') of ***pitta***. During summer the ***jaṭharāgni*** is dislodged from the ***āmāśaya*** ('stomach') by the extrinsic heat, which offers up no resistance to contain it within the body, as is the case in winter. Sunstroke, heatstroke, fever and diarrhoea are all common features of this event. If the weather becomes particularly hot and humid, this is the season of ***śarat***, when ***pitta*** is in its most vitiated state. Summer is also the season when the ***dakṣiṇāyana*** begins, evidenced by the blazing heat that begins the downward spiral of seasonal dissolution. ***Pitta*** generally has a catabolic effect on the body and if antagonised by hot weather, this continued and unchecked catabolism eventually leads to ***vāta caya***. Thus, to control ***pitta***, foods that are sweet, light, cooling and liquid should be consumed to preserve the moist structure of the body. Dairy products, if of good quality and if there is no underlying sensitivity, may be consumed in moderation. Large amounts of fermented dairy products such as cheese are to be avoided, however, but yogurt can be mixed with cool water, a little sugar and blended with fresh aromatic herbs such as mint, cilantro and rose petals as a refreshing drink. Milk decoctions can be especially helpful at this time, prepared by boiling milk and water with herbs such as cardamom and ginger, and sweeteners such as ***guḍa*** (jaggery). The bulk of the diet, however, should be composed of easily digestible grains such as basmati and jasmine rice, as well as lightly steamed and raw vegetables, some legumes such as mung and tofu, and fresh seasonal fruit. Meat, poultry and fish may also be taken, but in lesser quantities than in winter, and with fresh aromatic herbs such as cilantro, fennel, dill and basil to ensure proper digestion. Alcohol is strictly avoided in warm weather, however, as are foods with a distinctly pungent or sour taste. Some pungent tastes, however, such as those found in cardamom and ginger are said to be ***sattvic*** in nature, and can be used in moderation. Salty taste, which many Āyurvedic texts list as contraindicated, can be be a helpful strategy to reduce ***pitta***. In this regard, purified table salt (NaCl) should be avoided, emphasising salts rich in micronutrients such as rock salt (***saindhava***) and unrefined sea salt taken with sweet foods to restore the electrolyte balance of the body (***kledaka kapha***). During particularly hot and humid weather (***śarat***) foods that have an astringent and bitter taste to cool the body and reduce vitiations of ***pitta*** should be predominant in the diet. Lifestyle habits should include the avoidance of direct sunlight, mild physical exercise and limited sexual activity. Useful pursuits include residing near running water, sleeping outside under the moonlight, bathing in cool water, and decorating one's surroundings and body with fresh flowers and natural floral scents. Light oil massages may be indicated, with cooling oils such as coconut scented with floral fragrances.

5.8 *Varṣa ṛtucaryā*: AUTUMN REGIMEN

In autumn the weather changes from the heat and dryness of summer, and becomes cool (***śita***), windy (***cala***), and wet (***snigdha***). The result of this transition is that the already weakened digestive capacity undergoes further decline, and ***vāta***, which is already in an increased state, undergoes vitiation. Thus, during the autumn, seasonal and climatic factors conspire to make this the most difficult time to retain one's health, to 'hold on' to the energy of the earth as it sinks back down into itself to wait out winter. Blustery clouds of cold rain, wet snow and fog promote ***āma*** and impair circulation, and thus ***vāta sāma*** conditions such as inflammatory joint disease may be initiated or exacerbated at this time. In ancient India the rainy season of autumn was considered to be the worst time for travel and activity, and even homeless ***sannyāsins*** such as Buddhist monks would take up residence during this time. During autumn ***vātāhara*** regimens are typically employed, but must be tempered to inhibit the formation of ***āma***. Using the analogy of the plant, autumn is a time of rendering, of separating the animate from the inanimate, storing that which nourishes (in the roots) and discarding that which has outlived its usefulness (the leaves and aerial parts). Thus special purificatory measures such as ***vamana*** and ***virecana*** are traditionally implemented at this time, followed by ***vasti*** (see Ch. 11). While nourishing and greasy foods can be consumed, they should be complemented with sour, salty and pungent tastes to both pacify ***vāta*** and prevent ***āma***. Both animal and vegetable broths are useful at this time, as are baked, boiled and steamed root vegetables and squashes. Whole grains that impart a warming and lightening energy are helpful in autumn, such as as barley, rice, millet, amaranth and quinoa. Naturally fermented foods are especially helpful, such as pickled garlic, sauerkraut, miso and umeboshi, as well as spicy tasting wines, all of which help to pacify ***vāta***, enhance ***agni***, and break up the congestion of ***āma***.

Based on the dynamics of seasonal influence, Table 5.2 lists the effects of each season upon the ***doṣas***.

5.9 *Ṛtusandhi*: TRANSITIONAL PERIODS

There is a period of time each season, approximately 1 week before and after its commencement, when the new or previous season exerts its influence. During this time the body is particularly susceptible to disease and any new regimen must be implemented gradually to avoid negative effects. Āyurveda encourages us to understand the circadian rhythms of the natural environment, paying close attention to factors such as changing climate, bird migrations, and the growth patterns of local plants for clues as to the transition between the seasons.

5.10 CLIMATIC INFLUENCES

The specific influence of the climate and geography can also influence the ***doṣas***. Warm and dry climates such

TABLE 5.2 Seasonal influence of the ***doṣas***.

Season	*Doṣa*
Winter (***hemañta, śirīṣa***)	***Vātacaya, pittahara, kaphacaya***
Spring (***vasanta***)	***Vātāhara, pittacaya, kaphakopa***
Summer (***griṣma, śarat***)	***Vātāhara, pittakopa, kaphahara***
Autumn (***varṣa***)	***Vātakopa, pittahara, kaphacaya***

as desert regions increase ***vāta*** and ***pitta***, and decrease ***kapha*** and ***āma***. Cold and wet climates such as temperate rain forests increase ***vāta***, vitiate ***kapha*** and ***āma***, and decrease ***pitta***. Hot and wet climates increase ***kapha*** and ***āma***, vitiate ***pitta***, and decrease ***vāta***. Cold and dry climates vitiate ***vāta*** and decrease ***pitta***, ***kapha***, and ***āma***.

ENDNOTES

10 It is important to ensure that the powders are finely sieved as any extraneous fibres can abrade the gums and become lodged in the teeth.

11 There has been recent concern that a similar preparation called ***kohl*** contains high levels of lead and could be toxic. The use of ***Sauvīrañjana*** without proper supervision is not recommended.

PART 1

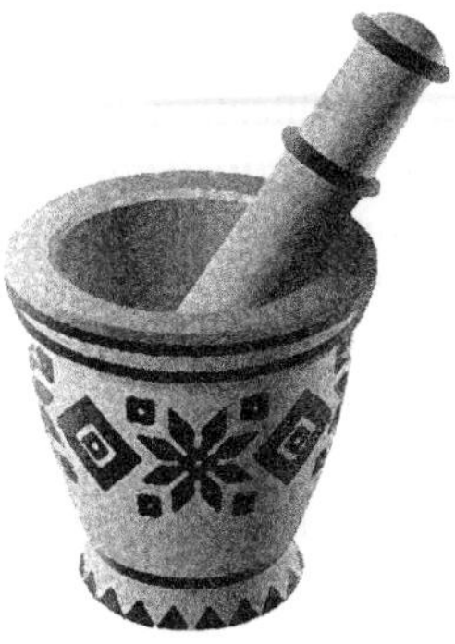

Chapter 6

PHARMACOLOGY AND PHARMACY

OBJECTIVES

- To understand the conceptual basis of Āyurvedic pharmacology.
- To understand the influence of the taste of a drug upon the body.
- To understand the influence of taste after digestion upon the body.
- To understand the influence of the energetic qualities of a drug upon the body.
- To understand the effect of a drug upon specific disorders and diseases.
- To understand the influence of inexplicable or spiritual qualities upon the activity of a drug.
- To review the basic components of Āyurvedic pharmacy.
- To review the concept of combining drugs with certain foods, condiments and liquids to modify their biological effects.

6.1 *Dravyguṇa*: DEFINITION, SCOPE AND BACKGROUND

Dravyguṇa is the limb of Āyurveda that concerns itself with the properties and actions (***guṇa***) of medicinal agents (***dravya***).[12] The first branch of ***dravyguṇa*** is ***nāmarūpavijñāna***, a 'system' (***vijñāna***) of mnemonics detailing the various synonyms that describe specific characteristics of a given medicament. These different 'names' (***nāma***) usually refer to 'morphological characteristics' (***rūpa***), but ***nāma*** might also refer to a medicinal use or another unique attribute. An example is the variance in synonyms of Turmeric rhizome (*Curcuma longa*), which includes ***Haridrā*** (referring to its natural 'yellow' dye), ***Varṇā*** (indicating its usefulness in disorders of 'complexion') and ***Niṣā*** (which explains that the root is best harvested at 'night'). The second branch of ***dravyguṇa*** concerns itself with explaining the 'properties' (***guṇa***) and 'actions' (***karma***) of medicaments, something that modern science might understand as pharmacology, and is known as ***guṇakarmavijñāna***. The ***guṇakarmas*** were introduced in Chapter 2 to illustrate the nature and function of the ***gurvādi guṇas*** in the human body. Building upon ***guṇakarmavijñāna***, the third branch of ***dravyguṇa*** is ***prayogavijñāna***, describing the therapeutic indications of specific medicines, as well as pharmacy. The fourth and last aspect of ***dravyguṇa*** is ***bheṣajakalpanā***, referring to the collection and storage of drugs and various methods of processing.

6.2 *Dravya* AND ITS CLASSIFICATION

A substance becomes a ***dravya*** only when its specific 'qualities' (***guṇa***) are taken into consideration, and thus a ***dravya*** is dependent upon the 'purpose' (***artha***) and 'rationale' (***yukti***) of its usage (Sharma 1976). When viewed as a singular phenomenon, a ***dravya*** has no inherent quality: it is the perceptive process, viz. the five senses and the mental impressions that are formed, which give rise to ***guṇa***. Āyurveda designates a ***dravya*** as strictly ***pañcabautika*** or 'formed of the elements', and is devoid of *atma* ('consciousness') and therefore insentient (Sharma 1976). Thus it is the conscious usage of a substance that makes a ***dravya***.

Dravyas are grouped in several ways depending upon the source within the extant literature of Āyurveda, but both Suśruta and Caraka group ***dravyas*** according to therapeutic action. Caraka enumerates 50 groups, each group containing 10 herbs named according to the general action of that group, such as 'analgesics' (***vedanāsthapāna***), 'diuretics' (***mūtravirecanīya***) and 'antihelminthics' (***kṛmighna***). Suśruta categorises each therapeutic group with the name of a notable representative of that group, an example being the ***pippalyādi*** group, the suffix ***'ādi'*** meaning 'etcetera', with the herb ***Pippalī*** (*Piper longum*) being representative. Suśruta also provides therapeutic indications for each of these groups, the ***dravyas*** within the ***pippalyādi*** group, for example, are indicated in ***vāta*** and ***kapha*** disorders, respiratory ailments, anorexia, poor digestion, flatulence and tumours.

Other methods of ***dravya*** classification include whether its activity 'decreases' (***doṣapraśamana***), 'increases' (***doṣapradūṣaṇa***) or 'balances' (***svasthahita***) a specific ***doṣa***, or whether the ***dravya*** can be used to 'pacify' an aggravated ***doṣa*** (***śamana***) or to expel an aggravated ***doṣa*** by means of 'purificatory' methods (***śodhana***), e.g. ***pañca karma***. ***Dravyas*** can also be classified according to the predominance of any one of the ***mahābhūtas***, illustrated in Table 6.1.

6.3 *Rasa*: THE SIX TASTES

The simplest method by which a ***dravya*** can be analysed is through the tongue (and oral cavity), by noticing the specific taste sensations called ***rasa***. In itself ***rasa*** does not provide any definite information but gives possible indications of a medicament's composition, character, property and pharmacological effect. ***Rasa*** also has several other meanings in Āyurveda, being another name for mercury (Hg), the expressed juice of a plant, and the product of digestion that circulates within the ***dhātus***.

There are six ***rasas*** in ***Āyurveda***, each generated by a specific combination of two different ***mahābhūtaṣ*** They are as follows:

TABLE 6.1 The *mahābhūta dravyas* (Sharma 1976).

Mahābhūta	*Jñāna indriyās*	*Rasa*	*Guṇas*	*Karma*
Pṛthvī	***Gandhā*** (smell)	***Madhura***, slightly ***kaśāya***	***Guru, khara kaṭhiṇa, manda, sthira, sāñdra, sthūla***	Condensing (anabolic), downward-moving (e.g. purgation)
Ap	***Rasa*** (taste)	***Madhura***, slightly ***kaśāya, lavaṇa***	***Snigdha, śita, manda, guru, drava, mṛdu, picchila***	Moistening, binding, oleation, pleasing
Tejas	***Rūpa*** (vision)	***Kaṭu***, slightly ***amla, lavaṇa***	***Uṣṇa, tikṣṇa, sūkṣma, laghu, viśada***	Metabolic, digesting, illuminating, tearing, upward movement (e.g. emesis)
Vāyu	***Sparśa*** (touch)	***Kaśāya***, slightly ***tikta***	***Sūkṣma, khara, śita, laghu, rūkṣa, viśada***	Drying, emaciating, roughening, mobility
Ākāśa	***Śabda*** (sound)	Unmanifest	***Ślakṣna, sūkṣma, mṛdu, viśada***	Softening, lightening, emptying

1. ***Madhura*** ('sweet'): composed of ***pṛthvī*** and ***ap***
2. ***Amla*** ('sour'): composed of ***ap*** and ***tejas***
3. ***Lavaṇa*** ('salty'): composed of ***pṛthvī*** and ***tejas***
4. ***Kaṭu*** ('pungent'): composed of ***tejas*** and ***vāyu***
5. ***Tikta*** ('bitter'): composed of ***ākāśa*** and ***vāyu***
6. ***Kaśāya*** ('astringent'): composed of ***pṛthvī*** and ***vāyu***.

Knowing that each ***rasa*** is composed of a particular combination of the ***mahābhūtas*** is a process of inference, taking into account the particular qualities that each taste exhibits. Every ***dravya*** contains all ***rasas*** because each thing contains a combination of all the ***mahābhūtas***. It is the predominance, however, of one and/or another ***mahābhūta*** in a given substance that explains ***rasa***. The ***rasas*** that are difficult to ascertain, or tasted secondarily, are called ***anurasas***. Typically, an ***anurasa*** adds to the overall activity of the ***dravya***, but is weaker than the primary ***rasa(s)***. The classification of ***rasa*** is not static, however, because changes that occur to the ***dravya*** over time, including processing and storage, may alter the original ***rasa***, e.g. an ethanol extract (tincture) will add ***kaṭu rasa*** to the overall ***rasa*** of the crude ***dravya***.

The characteristics and qualities of ***rasa*** are best understood in context with the ***guṇas***. A ***rasa*** does not have any inherent quality because it is the sense-object of the tongue. However, a ***guṇa*** can be detected by ***rasa*** because the ***guṇas*** are projected from the ***pañcabautik*** ('elemental') composition of the ***dravya*** itself. Using the ***upakarmas*** of ***uṣṇa-śita***, ***guru-laghu*** and ***rūkṣa-snigdha***, each ***rasa*** can be seen to exhibit a specific range of activities:

1. ***Madhura*** ('sweet') is ***snigdha*** ('greasy'), followed by ***śita*** ('cold') and then ***guru*** ('heavy')
2. ***Amla*** ('sour') is ***uṣṇa*** ('hot'), followed by ***snigdha*** ('greasy') and then ***laghu*** ('light')
3. ***Lavaṇa*** ('salty') is ***guru*** ('heavy'), followed by ***uṣṇa*** ('hot') and then ***snigdha*** ('greasy')
4. ***Kaṭu*** ('pungent') is ***uṣṇa*** ('hot'), followed by ***rūkṣa*** ('dry') and then ***laghu*** ('light')
5. ***Tikta*** ('bitter') is ***śita*** ('cold'), followed by ***rūkṣa*** ('dry') and then ***laghu*** ('light')
6. ***Kaśāya*** ('astringent') is ***rūkṣa*** ('dry'), followed by ***śita*** ('cold') and then ***guru*** ('heavy').

6.4 ACTION OF THE *rasas* UPON THE *doṣas*

Each ***rasa*** has a specific activity upon the ***doṣas***, ***dhātus*** and ***agni***.

Madhura rasa (sweet)

Dravyas or foods with a predominance of ***madhura rasa*** increase the qualities of ***guru*** and ***snigdha*** in the body due to the dominating influence of ***pṛthvī*** and ***ap mahābhūtas***. ***Madhura dravyas*** are often the first choice when treating ***pitta*** or ***vāta***, although ***vāttika*** conditions may require the inclusion of a ***dravya*** that contains ***uṣṇa*** to counterbalance the ***śita*** quality of ***madhura***, while in ***paittika*** conditions some degree of ***rūkṣa*** may be needed to counteract ***snigdha***. ***Madhura rasa*** is anabolic in nature, used to maintain growth and development, utilised in the general treatment of debility, ageing and reproductive deficiencies. It represents the essential quality of love, nourishment and sustenance, and has a harmonising, satiating and pleasing effect, helping to balance the effects of opposing ***rasas*** in formulations, e.g. Glycyrrhiza glabra. Although it is never completely avoided, ***madhura*** is contraindicated in ***kaphaja*** conditions such as cough, asthma, diabetes, obesity, fever and ***mañdāgni***. ***Madhura rasa*** is also said to promote obesity and parasitic infections (e.g. helminths, candidiasis). Examples of ***madhura dravyas*** include Indian herbs such as ***Balā*** (*Sida cordifolia*), ***Gokṣura*** (*Tribulus terrestris*), and ***Kūṣmāṇḍa*** (*Benincasa hispida*), Western herbs such as Marshmallow root (*Althaea officinalis*) and Slippery Elm bark (*Ulmus fulva*), as well as most grains, fruits and animal products.

Amla rasa (sour)

Dravyas or foods with a predominance of ***amla rasa*** increase the qualities of ***uṣṇa***, ***snigdha*** and ***laghu*** in the body due to the dominating influence of the ***ap*** and ***tejas mahābhūtas***. The qualities of ***amla*** resemble that of ***pitta***, and the catalysing, 'cooking' and churning activity of the gastrointestinal tract, related to the digestive acid and enzymes as well as the fermentative activities of probiotic bacteria. ***Amla***

is generally used in the treatment of ***mañdāgni***, digestive disorders and ***vāttika*** conditions, but is contraindicated in ***paittika*** disorders, including haemorrhage, gastrointestinal inflammation, jaundice or burning sensations. Although ***amla*** generally counters ***mañdāgni***, in some cases it may increase ***kapha*** because of the presence of ***ap*** in its composition, although only if used without skill or to excess. Examples of ***amla dravyas*** include Indian herbs such as ***Āmalakī*** fruit (*Phyllanthus emblica*) and ***Amlavetasa*** (*Garcinia pedunculata*), Western herbs such as Rosehips (*Rosa* spp.), and also Chinese herbs such as Shan za fruit (*Crataegus pinnatifida*) and Chen pi (*Citrus reticulata*), as well as fermented foods and beverages.

Lavaṇa rasa (salty)

Dravyas or foods with a predominance of ***lavaṇa rasa*** increase the qualities of ***uṣṇa***, ***snigdha*** and ***guru***[13] in the body due to the dominating influence of ***pṛthvī*** and ***tejas mahābhūtas***. In many respects ***lavaṇa*** relates to the dissolved minerals and electrolytes that conduct an electrical current throughout the body, and thus plays a key role in the activity ***vāta*** and the function of the nervous system. Due to the influence of ***tejas, lavaṇa rasa*** tends to increase ***pitta***, although certain kinds of ***lavaṇa dravyas*** such as ***saindhava*** are stated to posses a comparatively cooling activity and are helpful in ***paittika*** disorders such as diarrhoea or heat stroke. ***Lavaṇa*** tends to promote the mobilisation or liquefaction of ***kapha*** due to its ***uṣṇa*** and ***snigdha*** qualities, but can also promote congestive conditions such as oedema because of the ***guru*** quality of ***lavaṇa***, especially when taken in large amounts. Generally speaking, ***lavaṇa dravyas*** are used in the treatment of cough (to liquefy ***kapha***), to restore the electrolyte balance of the body (to decrease ***vāta***), and to enhance appetite (increase ***agni***). Contraindications for ***lavaṇa dravyas*** include hypertension, skin diseases, oedema, ascites, haemorrhage and gastrointestinal inflammation. Examples of ***lavaṇa dravyas*** include the various salts used in Āyurvedic medicine (e.g. ***saindhava***, ***sāmudra***, ***audbhida***, ***sauvarcala***, ***viḍa***), seaweeds, Western herbs such as Nettle leaf (*Urtica dioica*), foods such as celery, and ocean fish like mackerel.

Kaṭu rasa (pungent)

Dravyas or foods with a predominance of ***kaṭu rasa*** increase the qualities of ***uṣṇa*** and ***laghu*** in the body due to the dominating influence of ***vayu*** and ***tejas mahābhūtas***. ***Kaṭu rasa*** acts in opposition to the basic nature of ***kapha***, and is an important ***kaphahara rasa***. ***Laghu*** and ***uṣṇa guṇas*** are dominant in ***pitta***, however, and thus ***kaṭu rasa*** is avoided in ***paittika*** conditions. This same ***laghu*** nature of ***kaṭu*** will also act to increase ***vāta***, but if ***kaṭu*** is used in small amounts and counterbalanced with ***dravyas*** that are ***snigdha*** and ***guru*** (e.g. ***ghṛta***), it can be used in ***vāttika*** conditions to reduce ***śita***. When taken internally, ***kaṭu*** has a special property to promote the proper flow of energy in the body, harmonising the interior with the exterior parts of the body, and helps to direct the movement of the other ***rasas***. As a result, ***katu*** is often included in various formulations to ensure the absorption and movement of a remedy throughout the body, e.g. *Zingiber officinalis*. Externally, ***kaṭu*** is used to promote local blood flow. Generally speaking, ***kaṭu rasa*** is used in the treatment of ***mañdāgni***, dysentery, helminthiasis, colds and flu, asthma, cough, obesity, diabetes and certain skin diseases. ***Kaṭu rasa*** is contraindicated in gastrointestinal inflammation, haemorrhaging, burning sensations, reproductive deficiency and urine retention. Examples of ***kaṭu dravyas*** include Indian herbs such as ***Pippalī*** fruit (*Piper longum*) and ***Śūṇṭhī*** rhizome (*Zingiber officinalis*), Western herbs such as Cayenne fruit (*Capsicum minimum*), and spicy tasting foods such as tomatoes, peppers and garlic, as well as distilled alcohol.

Tikta rasa (bitter)

Dravyas or foods with a predominance of ***tikta rasa*** increase the qualities ***śita*** and ***rūkṣa*** in the body due to the dominating influence of ***vāyu*** and ***ākāśa mahābhūtas***. ***Tikta*** stimulates very specific regions of the tongue and soft palate that can initiate reflex eliminatory responses such as nausea and vomiting, and as such, ***tikta rasa*** is often used to enhance the eliminatory faculties of the body. Formulations to reduce ***pitta*** will often include ***madhura rasa*** to offset the ***laghu*** qualities of ***tikta***, whereas formulations to reduce ***kapha*** will benefit from adding ***kaṭu rasa*** to offset the ***śita*** nature of ***tikta***. While ***vāttika*** conditions may benefit from ***tikta rasa*** to assist in the removal of ***āma***, such formulations need to be balanced with ***rasas*** such as ***amla***, ***kaṭu*** and ***lavaṇa*** to avoid increasing ***vāta***. ***Tikta rasa*** is used in the general treatment of ***mañdāgni***, ***srotorodha*** (congestion of the ***srotāṃsi***), dysentery, helminthiasis, gastrointestinal inflammation, jaundice and diseases of the liver, skin diseases, fever, obesity, diabetes and excessive secretions. ***Tikta rasa*** is contraindicated in dryness, coldness, asthenia, debility and reproductive deficiency. Examples of ***tikta dravyas*** include Indian herbs such as ***Nimba*** leaf (*Azadirachta indica*) and ***Bhūnimba*** herb (*Andrographis paniculata*), Western herbs such as Gentian root (*Gentiana lutea*) and Goldenseal root (*Hydrastis canadensis*), and vegetables such as endive and bitter melon (karela).

Kaśāya rasa (astringent)

Dravyas or foods with a predominance of ***kaśāya rasa*** increase the qualities of ***rūkṣa***, ***śita*** and ***guru*** in the body due to the dominating influence of ***pṛthvī*** and ***vāyu mahābhūtas***. ***Kaśāya*** is used therapeutically to decrease the excessively ***snigdha*** properties of ***kapha***, and the ***uṣṇa*** and ***laghu*** properties of ***pitta***. Although ***guru***, ***kaśāya rasa*** is exceptionally ***rūkṣa*** in nature and will increase ***vāta***. Similar to ***kaṭu***, ***kaśāya*** has a systemic effect when taken internally, serving to tighten and toughen the tissues of the body by absorbing excess fluids and binding proteins together. ***Kaśāya rasa*** is used in the general treatment of diarrhoea, haemorrhage, wounds and respiratory catarrh, and is contraindicated in dryness, coldness, debility and ***mañdāgni***. Examples of ***kaśāya dravyas*** include Indian herbs such as ***Bibhītaka*** fruit (*Terminalia belerica*) and ***Kuṭaja*** (*Holarrhena antidysenterica*), Western herbs such as Alum root (*Heuchera cylindrica*) and Uva ursi leaf (*Arctostaphylos uva-ursi*), as well as astringing beverages such as black tea.

6.5 ACTION OF THE *rasas* UPON THE *dhātus*

The activity of the ***rasas*** upon the ***dhātus*** can be divided into either a 'nourishing' (***bṛmhaṇa***) or 'depleting' (***langhana***) activity. Broadly speaking, only ***madhura*** can be considered ***bṛmhaṇa*** due to its capacity to increase and nourish all the ***dhātus***. ***Amla*** and ***lavaṇa rasa*** could be considered ***bṛmhaṇa*** because of their stimulant effect upon the ***jaṭharāgni***, but they are not nourishing or vitalising, and even deplete ***śukra/aṇḍāṇu*** when used to excess. ***Lavaṇa rasa*** causes water retention and in excess promotes congestion, but this cannot be considered to be nourishing as such. ***Tikta***, ***kaṭu*** and ***kaśāya rasas*** all have a 'depleting' (***langhana***) effect on the body.

TABLE 6.2 ***Rasas*** in association with the ***mahābhūtas***, ***guṇas***, and ***doṣas***.

Rasa	*Mahābhūtas*	*Guṇas*	Effect on *Doṣas*
Madhura	***Pṛthvī*** (earth) ***ap*** (water)	***Guru*** (heavy), ***snigdha*** (greasy), ***śita*** (cold)	***Vātapittahara, kaphakopa***
Amla	***Ap*** (water) ***tejas*** (fire)	***Uṣṇa*** (hot), ***snigdha*** (greasy), ***laghu*** (light)	***Vātakaphahara, pittakopa***
Lavaṇa	***Pṛthvī***(earth) ***tejas*** (fire)	***Uṣṇa*** (hot), ***snigdha*** (greasy), ***guru*** (heavy)	***Vātapittahara, kaphakopa*** (int.) ***kaphahara*** (ext.)
Kaṭu	***Vāyu*** (wind) ***tejas*** (fire)	***Uṣṇa*** (hot), ***rūkṣa*** (dry), ***laghu*** (light)	***Kaphahara, pittakopa***
Tikta	***Vāyu*** (wind) ***ākāśa*** (pervasiveness)	***Śita*** (cold), ***rūkṣa*** (dry), ***laghu*** (light)	***Pittakaphahara, vātakopa***
Kaśāya	***Pṛthvī*** (earth) ***vāyu*** (wind)	***Rūkṣa*** (dry), ***śita*** (cold), ***guru*** (heavy)	***Pittakaphahara, vātakopa***

6.6 ACTION OF THE *rasas* UPON *agni*

Based upon the ancient Vedic concept of ***agnīṣomiya*** (***agni*** and ***soma***) Āyurveda classifies the ***rasas*** according to their ability to enhance the solar (***agni***) or lunar (***soma***, or ***ojas***) aspects of the body. Within the ***tridoṣa*** theory, ***agni*** relates to ***pitta***, ***kapha*** relates to ***soma*** (***ojas***), and ***vāta*** stands between them as the catalyst (***prāṇa***). Those ***rasas*** that contain ***agni*** are ***agneya***, while those that contain ***soma*** are ***saumya***. Tables 6.3 and 6.4 describe their differences and relative degrees of hot or cold.

The ***agneya rasas*** (***kaṭu***, ***amla*** and ***lavaṇa***) stimulate the appetite and promote digestion. Although ***tikta*** belongs to the ***saumya*** group it promotes digestion by clearing away ***kapha*** and ***āma***, and promotes the activity of ***samāna vāyu***. The ***guru*** and ***śita*** qualities of ***madhura*** and ***kaśāya*** have an adverse effect upon the ***jaṭharāgni***. Thus, while the most nourishing foods contain ***madhura rasa***, they may have a detrimental effect upon the ***jaṭharāgni***, or if the ***jaṭharāgni*** is already impaired, facilitate the production of ***āma***.

6.7 *Vipāka*: POST-DIGESTIVE EFFECT

Vipāka is a controversial subject in some respects because the process it claims to describe cannot be observed directly, but only inferred by observing its effect upon the body. ***Vipāka*** is the process whereby the ***rasa*** of the ingested ***dravya*** is modified by the differing activities of the digestive process. When a substance is ingested, digestion begins in the mouth with salivary secretion (***madhura*** and ***lavaṇa***), followed by the secretions of the stomach and small intestine (***amla***, ***katu***) and liver (***tikta***), and ending with bacterial fermentation (***amla***, ***kaṭu***) and water resorption (***kaśāya***) in the colon. Thus, ***vipāka*** describes in part where in the gastrointestinal tract the ***rasa*** of a given ***dravya*** will exert its activity, and how it might affect the state of the ***doṣas*** within their seats (see 2.4 ***Sthāna***: residence of the ***doṣas***).

TABLE 6.3 The *agneya rasas*.

Degree of *agni*	*Agneya rasas*
Hot in the third degree	***Kaṭu***
Hot in the second degree	***Amla***
Hot in the first degree	***Lavaṇa***

TABLE 6.4 The *saumya rasas*.

Degree of *soma*	*Saumya rasas*
Cold in the third degree	***Tikta***
Cold in the second degree	***Madhura***
Cold in the first degree	***Kaśāya***

The ***Suśruta*** and ***Caraka saṃhitās*** differ in some respects in describing ***vipāka***. According to Suśruta, ***vipāka*** is only of two types: ***guru*** or ***laghu***. Caraka, however, details three ***vipākas***: ***madhura***, ***amla*** and ***kaṭu***. One could rationalise that Suśruta's scheme is a classification according to the ***dhātus*** (anabolic versus catabolic), whereas Caraka's method is based on the three ***doṣas*** of ***kapha***, ***pitta*** and ***vāta*** (i.e. ***madhura***, ***amla*** and ***kaṭu***, respectively). This is understandable if we remember that Suśruta, as a surgeon, was concerned with anatomy, and Caraka, as a physician, was concerned with physiology. Both methods, however, can be understood in relation to ***tridoṣa***:

1. ***Vipāka*** according to Suśruta
   - ***guru vipāka*** will increase ***kapha*** and decrease ***pitta*** and ***vāta***
   - ***laghu vipāka*** will increase ***pitta*** and ***vāta***, but decrease ***kapha.***
2. ***Vipāka*** according to Caraka
   - ***madhura vipāka*** will increase ***kapha*** and decrease ***pitta***
   - ***amla vipāka*** will tend to aggravate ***pitta*** but pacify ***vāta***
   - ***kaṭu vipāka*** will increase ***vāta*** and decrease ***kapha***.

A ***guru vipāka*** is the result of ***madhura*** and ***lavaṇa rasas***, whereas a ***laghu vipāka*** is the result of the remaining four ***rasas***. A ***madhura vipāka*** is the result of ***madhura*** and ***lavaṇa rasas***, an ***amla vipāka*** is the result of ***amla rasa***, and ***kaṭu vipāka*** is the result of ***kaṭu***, ***tikta***, and ***kaśāya rasas***. While most ***dravyas*** adhere to this scheme, some do not. The ***rasa*** of **Bibhītaka** (*Terminalia belerica*), for example, is primarily ***kaśāya***, but the ***vipāka*** is ***madhura***. This type of exception exists for many of the more important ***dravyas*** used in Āyurvedic medicine.

The significant differences between ***rasa*** and ***vipāka*** relate to their effects: ***rasa*** has an immediate, localised effect on the gastrointestinal tract, whereas ***vipāka*** has a delayed, systemic effect on the organism. Thus ***vipāka*** can be seen to be an extension of the effect that the ***rasas*** have on the body, rather than existing as an entirely different process.

6.8 *Vīrya*: ENERGETIC QUALITIES

Vīrya is the specific potency by which a ***dravya*** acts, based primarily on whether it is ***śita*** or ***uṣṇa***. This concept borrows heavily from the ancient Vedic ***agnīsomīya*** principle, the primordial division of heat and cold, of light and darkness, and male and female. Although ***uṣṇa*** and ***śita*** are the primordial energetic attributes that drive all energetic changes in the body, in practice we can see that any number of qualities can be described to differentiate the energetic quality of one particular ***dravya*** from another. Thus a ***dravya*** with an ***uṣṇa*** and ***rūkṣa vīrya*** would be distguished from another that is similarly ***uṣṇa***, but is also ***guru***, ***snigdha***, ***laghu***, ***picchila*** etc. Most Āyurvedic texts describe these additional qualities separately under '***guṇa***,' but this is a needless sub-classification: in actual practice any and all of the ***gurvādi guṇas*** could be used to describe the different energetic possibilities of a ***dravya***, but most of these also require ***uṣṇa*** or ***śita*** to become manifest (i.e. they are all products of interactions between the ***agnīṣomiya*** principle). Table 6.5 lists the activity of the six primary energetic qualities (i.e. the ***upakarmas***), their effect upon the ***doṣas***, their general effect and their respective elemental combination(s).

As ***uṣṇa*** and ***śita*** are the primary energetic qualities, most ***dravyas*** will display either of them, usually with secondary attributes of the remaining ***upakarmas***, such as ***laghu*** or ***guru***, and ***snigdha*** or ***rūkṣa***. Sometimes a ***dravya*** will be neutral in temperament, however, which is to say, neither ***uṣṇa*** nor ***śita*** seem especially predominant. In this case, the secondary energetic attribute(s) would become the primary one(s).

In every respect ***vīrya*** supersedes the actions of ***rasa*** and ***vipāka***, although more often than not the relationship between them is congruent, even when considering non-Indian plants, as shown in Table 6.6.

There are, however, a number of contradictions to this rule of congruency so one cannot substitute theory for an intimate knowledge of the ***dravya*** in question. For example, although meat has a ***madhura rasa***, its ***vīrya*** is ***uṣṇa***: this explains the benefit of using meat to counter the ***rūkṣa***, ***laghu*** and ***śita*** qualities of ***vāta***. ***Āmalakī*** fruit (*Phyllanthus emblica*) has a definite ***amla rasa***, but its ***vīrya*** is ***śita***: thus as a cooling remedy ***Āmalakī*** is used to treat ***pitta***, and as a sour-tasting fruit it enhances digestion and normalises ***agni***. ***Harītakī*** fruit (*Terminalia chebula*) has a ***kaśāya rasa***, but its ***vīrya*** is ***uṣṇa***, drawing out and digesting ***āma***, while countering the ***śita vīrya*** of ***vāta***. The degree of exceptional characteristics that a given ***dravya*** displays is often proportionate to its usefulness, and such herbs that contain contradictory qualities are often a better choice in the treatment of complex disease states.

6.9 *Karma*: THERAPEUTIC ACTION

Karma refers to the specific therapeutic activity of a given ***dravya***, a concept that in many ways resembles that of Western herbal medicine. In fact, the entire terminology of therapeutic actions commonly used in Western herbal medicine such as 'stomachic', 'carminative', and 'purgative' may be used in Āyurveda without contradiction, because these too describe the observed effects of a ***dravya***. ***Karma*** literally means 'action', and the therapeutic activity of a given

TABLE 6.5 The composition and effect of *vīrya*.

Vīrya	Effect upon the *doṣas*	General effect	*Mahābhūtas*
uṣṇa	***Vātakaphahara, pittakopa***	***Svedana*** ('heating')	***Tejas***
śita	***Pittahara, vātakaphakopa***	***Stambhana*** ('cooling')	***Ap***
guru	***Vātāhara***	***Bṛmhaṇa*** ('nourishing')	***Pṛthvī, ap***
laghu	***Kaphahara***	***Langhana*** ('depleting')	***Tejas, vāyu***
snigdha	***Vātāhara***	***Snehana*** ('moistening')	***Ap***
rūkṣa	***Vātakopa, kaphahara***	***Rūkṣana*** ('drying')	***Vāyu, pṛthvī***

TABLE 6.6 Relationship of ***vīrya*** with ***rasa*** and ***vipāka***, with examples.

Rasa	*Vipāka*	*Vīrya*	Example
Madhura	***Guru***	***Śita***	Marshmallow root (*Althaea officinalis*), decreases ***pitta*** and ***vāta***
Lavaṇa	***Guru***	***Uṣṇa***	Kelp (*Fucus vesiculosis*), decreases ***vāta***
Amla	***Laghu***	***Uṣṇa***	Shan za fruit (*Crataegus pinnatifida*), decreases ***kapha*** and ***vāta***
Kaṭu	***Laghu***	***Uṣṇa***	Cayenne fruit (*Capsicum minimum*), decreases ***kapha***
Tikta	***Laghu***	***Śita***	Goldenseal root (*Hydrastis canadensis*), decreases ***pitta*** and ***kapha***
Kaśāya	***Laghu***	***Śita***	White Oak bark (*Quercus alba*), decreases ***kapha*** and ***pitta***

dravya is an effect (***karma***) based upon the collective activities of ***rasa***, ***vipāka*** and ***vīrya***.

Āyurvedic medicine describes 20 basic ***karmas***, each derived from the ***gurvādi guṇas***. Each of the ***gurvādi guṇas*** can be identified with a specific effect or activity (***karma***) in the body, and these actions form the basis for the observed effect of different medications and therapies. These effects are listed in Table 6.7.

While all the different ***karmas*** are recognised and form the basis of a therapeutic rationale, they are broadly separated based on the actions of ***tikṣṇa*** ('fast') and ***manda*** ('slow'). Thus any ***karma*** is of two basic types: ***śodhana*** ('purificatory') or ***śamana*** ('pacificatory'). ***Śodhana karmas*** are most commonly referred to as the ***pañca karmas***, used on an in-patient basis, and are ***vamana*** ('vomiting'), ***virecana***

TABLE 6.7 ***Gurvādi guṇas*** and their ***karmas*** ('actions').

Guṇa	*Karma*	Meaning
Guru	***Bṛmhaṇa***	To nourish, grow, expand
Laghu	***Laghu***	To lessen, reduce, diminish
Śita	***Stambhana***	To arrest, retain, make firm
Uṣṇa	***Svedana***	To inspire, perspire, make soft
Rūkṣa	***Śoṣana***	To dry, dehydrate, suck out
Snigdha	***Kledana***	To moisten, hydrate, anoint
Manda	***Śamana***	To appease, allay, suppress
Tikṣṇa	***Śodhana***	To counter, arouse, purify
Sthira	***Dhāraṇā***	To hold, preserve, sustain
Cala (sara)	***Preraṇa***	To release, expend, excite
Mṛdu	***Ślathana***	To slacken, loosen, weaken
Kaṭhiṇa	***Dṛḍhīkarana***	To strengthen, tighten, fortify
Viśada	***Kṣālana***	To strip away, remove, scrape
Picchila	***Lepana***	To plaster, anoint, soothe
Ślakṣna	***Ropaṇa***	To unite, anoint, sustain
Khara	***Lekhana***	To attenuate, scrape, diminish
Sūkṣma	***Vivaraṇa***	To expand, unfold, express
Sthūla	***Samvaraṇa***	To conceal, cover, suppress
Sāñdra	***Prasādana***	To render pure, pacify
Drava	***Vilodana***	To mix together, churn

('purgation'), ***vasti*** ('enema'), ***nasya*** ('errhine'), and ***rakta mokṣaṇa*** ('venesection') (see Ch. 11). ***Śamana*** therapies are treatments used on an out-patient basis, and include ***bṛmhaṇa*** ('nourishing'), ***langhana*** ('depleting'), ***svedana*** ('heating'), ***stambhana*** ('cooling'), ***rūkṣana*** ('drying'), and ***snehana*** ('moistening') (see Ch. 11). The five types of ***śodhana karmas*** and six types of ***śamana karmas*** form much of the therapeutic basis of Āyurvedic medicine. In addition to the ***karmas*** derived from the ***gurvādi guṇas***, however, texts such as the ***Śāraṅgadhara saṃhitā*** (c. 13th CE) mention other types of actions, some that describe a physiological response or activity, and others correlated to the alleviation of a particular symptom or disease. Following the work of scholars such as P. V. Sharma (1976), some of the many actions described in Āyurveda are listed as follows, described on the basis of which physiological system they tend to affect:

Digestion

- ***Dīpana***: ***dravyas*** that enkindle ***agni***, e.g. ***Guḍūcī*** vine (*Tinospora cordifolia*).
- ***Pācana***: ***dravyas*** that 'cook' or denature the food that has been consumed, e.g. ***Marica*** fruit (*Piper nigrum*).
  (Many ***dravyas*** in fact contain both the activities of ***dīpana*** and ***pācana***, e.g. ***Harītakī*** fruit (*Terminalia chebula*), and are called ***dīpanapācana***.)
- ***Anulomana***: ***dravyas*** that assist in digestion and promote normal bowel movement, e.g. ***Ajamodā*** fruit (*Trachyspermum roxiburghianum*).
- ***Āsyasravaṇa***: ***dravyas*** that promote the flow of saliva, e.g. ***Tuṁburū*** fruit (*Zanthoxylum alatum*).
- ***Vamana***: ***dravyas*** that promote emesis, e.g. ***Madanaphala*** fruit (*Randia dumetorum*).
- ***Chardinigrahaṇa***: ***dravyas*** that act as antiemetics, e.g. ***Śatapuṣpā*** fruit (*Foeniculum vulgare*).
- ***Bhedana***: ***dravyas*** that forcibly expel the contents of the bowel, e.g. ***Kaṭuka*** rhizome (*Picrorrhiza kurroa*).
- ***Recana***: ***dravyas*** that forcibly expel the contents of the bowel in liquid form, e.g. ***Trivṛt*** root (*Operculina turpethum*).
- ***Arśoghna***: ***dravyas*** that treat haemorrhoids, e.g. ***Harītakī*** fruit (*Terminalia chebula*).
- ***Śulapraśamana***: ***dravyas*** that act as intestinal antispasmodics, e.g. ***Śūṇṭhī*** rhizome (*Zingiber officinalis*).
- ***Purīṣasaṅgrahaṇa***: ***dravyas*** that act as intestinal astringents, e.g. ***Kuṭaja*** bark (*Holarrhena antidysenterica*).
- ***Kṛmighna***: ***dravyas*** that act as antihelminthics, e.g. ***Viḍaṅga*** fruit (*Embelia ribes*).

Circulatory system

- ***Hṛdaya***: ***dravyas*** that treat diseases of the heart, e.g. ***Arjuna*** bark (*Terminalia arjuna*).
- ***Śoṇitasthāpana***: ***dravyas*** that stop bleeding, e.g. ***Nāgakeśara*** flower (*Mesua ferrea*).
- ***Raktaprasādana***: ***dravyas*** that purify the blood, e.g. ***Mañjiṣṭhā*** root (*Rubia cordifolia*).

Respiratory system

- ***Kāsahara***: ***dravyas*** that act as antitussives or bronchial sedatives, e.g. ***Khakhasa*** immature capsule (*Papaver somniferum*).
- ***Svāsahara***: ***dravyas*** that alleviate bronchial constriction, e.g. ***Bibhītaka*** fruit (*Terminalia chebula*).
- ***Chedana***: ***dravyas*** that act as expectorants, e.g. ***Vāsaka*** leaf (*Adhatoda vasica*).
- ***Svarya***: ***dravyas*** that promote the voice, e.g. ***Guggulu*** resin (*Commiphora mukul*).
- ***Hikkānigrahaṇa***: treatments that stop hiccoughs, e.g. ***prāṇayama***.

Urinary system

- ***Mūtravirecana***: ***dravyas*** that act as diuretics, e.g. ***Gokṣura*** fruit (*Tribulus terrestris*).
- ***Mūtrasaṅgrahaṇa***: ***dravyas*** that act as urinary astringents, e.g. ***Jambū*** fruit (*Syzygium cumini*).
- ***Mūtraviśodhana***: ***dravyas*** that act as anti-infectives in the urinary tract, e.g. ***Candana*** wood (*Santalum album*).
- ***Aśmaribhedana***: ***dravyas*** that act to remove stones, e.g. ***Agnimañtha*** root (*Premna integrifolia*).
- ***Śothahara***: ***dravyas*** that relieve oedema, e.g. ***Bilva*** leaf (*Aegle marmelos*).

Nervous system, brain and sense organs

- ***Medhya***: ***dravyas*** that promote ***buddhi***, e.g. ***Maṇḍūkaparṇī*** leaf (*Centella asiatica*).

- ***Cakṣuṣya***: ***dravyas*** that enhance eyesight, e.g. ***Āmalakī*** fruit (*Phyllanthus emblica*).
- ***Nasya***: ***dravyas*** that restore the sense of smell, e.g. ***Kaṭphala*** bark (*Myrica nagi*).
- ***Madakārī***: ***dravyas*** that intoxicate, e.g. ***Pārasikayavānī*** root (*Hyocyamus niger*).
- ***Saṃjñāsthāpana***: ***dravyas*** used to restore consciousness, e.g. ***Vacā*** rhizome (*Acorus calamus*).
- ***Nidrājanana***: ***dravyas*** that promote sleep, e.g. ***Sarpagandhā*** root (*Rauwolfia serpentina*).
- ***Vedanāsthāpana***: ***dravyas*** that relieve pain, e.g. ***Guggulu*** resin (*Commiphora mukul*).
- ***Vyavāyi***: ***dravyas*** that act very quickly by spreading all over the body, e.g. ***Bhaṅgā*** flower (*Cannabis indica*).

Reproductive system

- ***Vajīkaraṇa***: ***dravyas*** that enhance fertility, e.g. ***Aśvagandhā*** root (*Withania somnifera*).
- ***Prajāsthāpana***: ***dravyas*** that prevent miscarriage, e.g. ***Śatāvarī*** root (*Asparagus racemosa*).
- ***Stanyajanana***: ***dravyas*** that promote milk production, e.g. ***Yavānī*** fruit (*Trachyspermum ammi*).
- ***Ārtavajanana***: ***dravyas*** that promote menstruation, e.g. ***Kumārī*** leaf juice (*Aloe vera*).

Skin

- ***Svedana***: treatments that promote sweating, e.g. steam bath.
- ***Snehana***: ***dravyas*** that smooth the skin, e.g. fat, oil.
- ***Rūkṣana***: ***dravyas*** that roughen the skin, e.g. ***Yava*** fruit (Barley).
- ***Varnya***: ***dravyas*** that promote complexion, e.g. ***Haridrā*** rhizome (*Curcuma longa*).
- ***Kaṇḍūghna***: ***dravyas*** that stop itching, e.g. ***Nimba*** leaf (*Azadirachta indica*).
- ***Kuṣṭhaghna***: ***dravyas*** that relieve skin diseases, e.g. ***Kuṣṭha*** root (*Saussurea lappa*).
- ***Romasañjanana***: ***dravyas*** that promote hair growth, e.g. ***Nirguṇḍī*** leaf (*Vitex negundo*).

Metabolism

- ***Jvaraghna***: ***dravyas*** that reduce fever, e.g. ***Kiratatika*** (*Swertia chiretta*).
- ***Dāhapraśamana***: ***dravyas*** that reduce heat and burning sensations, e.g. cool milk.
- ***Vidāhi***: ***dravyas*** that cause burning sensations, e.g. ***Vaṃśayava*** fruit (*Bambusa arundinacea*).
- ***Viṣaghna***: ***dravyas*** that alleviate poisons, e.g. ***Śiriṣa*** (*Albizzia lebbeck*).
- ***Sandhānīya***: ***dravyas*** that promote healing, e.g. ***Yaṣṭimadhu*** root (*Glycyrrhiza glabra*).
- ***Medohara***: ***dravyas*** that reduce fat, e.g. ***Guggulu*** resin (*Commiphora mukul*).
- ***Lekhana***: ***dravyas*** that dry up excessive moisture in the body, e.g. ***Yava*** fruit (Barley).
- ***Grāhī***: ***dravyas*** that dry up the excessive moisture in the body and are ***dīpanapācana***, e.g. ***Śyonāka*** root (*Oroxylum indicum*).
- ***Rasāyana***: ***dravyas*** that ward off old age and disease, e.g. ***Punarnavā*** root (*Boerhavia diffusa*).
- ***Balya***: ***dravyas*** that increase strength, e.g. ***Balā*** root (*Sida cordifolia*).
- ***Jīvanīya***: ***dravyas*** that energize the body, e.g. ***Jīvantī*** root (*Leptadenia reticulata*).

Srotāṃsi

- ***Pramāthi***: ***dravyas*** that remove the accumulated ***doṣas*** from the ***srotāṃsi***, e.g. ***Marica*** fruit (*Piper nigrum*).
- ***Abhiṣyandī***: ***dravyas*** that block the ***srotāṃsi*** because of their ***guru*** and ***picchila*** nature, causing heaviness and congestion, e.g. ***dadhi*** (yogurt, taken internally).
- ***Sūkṣma***: ***dravyas*** that enter into even the most minute channel of the body, e.g. ***Saindhava*** (rock salt).

Doṣas

- ***Vātāhara***, ***vātaghna***: ***dravyas*** that decrease ***vāta***.
- ***Vātakopa***: ***dravyas*** that increase ***vāta***.
- ***Pittahara***, ***pittaghna***: ***dravyas*** that decrease ***pitta***.
- ***Pittakopa***: ***dravyas*** that increase ***pitta***.
- ***Kaphahara***, ***kaphaghna***: ***dravyas*** that decrease ***kapha***.
- ***Kaphakopa***: ***dravyas*** that increase ***kapha***.
- ***Tridoṣahara***, ***tridoṣaghna***: ***dravyas*** that reduce all three ***doṣas***.

6.10 *Prabhāva*: SPIRITUAL POTENCY

Prabhāva refers to the activity of a ***dravya*** that cannot be rationalised within the conceptual framework of ***dravyguṇa***. Whereas ***rasa***, ***vipāka*** and ***vīrya*** are described as ***cintya*** ('explicable'), ***prabhāva*** is said to be ***acintya*** ('inexplicable'). A classic illustration of ***prabhāva*** can be found when we compare the herb ***Citraka*** (*Plumbago zeylanica*) with ***Dañtī*** (*Baliospermum montanum*). Both of these ***dravyas*** have the identical ***rasa***, ***vipāka*** and ***vīrya***, but the latter is a strong purgative while the former is not. Thus ***prabhāva*** describes how certain ***dravyas*** seem to display a specificity in action that cannot be matched by another herb which otherwise exhibits the same qualities. More often than not, ***prabhāva*** refers to the tropism of a ***dravya*** to a specific ailment, such as ***Arjuna*** (*Terminalia arjuna*) for diseases of the heart.

Prabhāva is also representative of the spiritual basis of Āyurvedic medicine. In regard to medicinal plants, ***prabhāva*** is the teacher (***guru***), the healing wisdom of the plant that cannot be rationalised but understood only through the experience of spiritual insight. This approach finds resonance in other herbal traditions, such as shamanism, where plants are not simply viewed as another kind of organism, but rather, as representatives or manifestations of powerful spiritual energies (e.g. the sacred and mysterious plant called ***Soma*** mentioned in the ***Ṛg veda***). Furthermore, ***prabhāva*** explains how a ***dravya*** can be used in such small amounts that its action cannot be explained by its biochemical constituents, as is the case with highly potentised alchemical preparations such as ***bhasmas***, or more recently, with the use of flower essences and homeopathic remedies.

Prabhāva also refers to techniques used in processing a ***dravya***, such as the addition of semi-precious and precious metals and gems, and the chanting of ***mantras*** for specific periods of time during different stages of processing. Although such techniques may seem alien and superstitious to the Western mind, they have their basis in science. Such traditional methods used in the processing of crude aconite, for example, resulted in a preparation that was assessed to be non-toxic, even at dosages eight times greater than the LD_{100} for the crude drug (Thorat & Dahanukar 1991).

6.11 *Bhaiṣajya vyākhyāna*: PRINCIPLES OF PHARMACY

It is rare that a ***dravya*** can be taken in its natural or raw state as a medicament without first preparing it in a certain fashion, to either remove impurities and toxins, or to make the medicament more bioavailable. The following techniques discuss the most commonly used procedures in Āyurvedic herbal pharmacy, but do not represent all the different techniques used in Āyurvedic medicine.

Pañca kaśāya: aqueous extracts

The ***pañca kaśāya*** are the 'five aqueous extracts', consisting of:

1. ***Svarasa***: expressed juice, prepared by taking the fresh plant, wrapping it in cloth and pounding and squeezing it to express the juice. If the fresh plant is not available, one may also take one part of the dried powder and mix it with twice the amount of water. This is allowed to sit overnight before being squeezed out through a cloth. ***Svarasa*** is considered to be the heaviest to digest and most potent of the ***pañca kaśāya***, and is typically dosed at a half a ***pala*** (12–24 mL), twice daily. Prepared as needed.
2. ***Kalka***: bolus, is prepared by grinding the ***dravya*** in a mortar and pestle and adding just enough water to make a paste. Honey and/or ***ghṛta*** are often added to the preparation. ***Kalka*** is typically dosed at one ***karṣa*** (12 g), twice daily. Prepared as needed.
3. ***Kvātha***: decoction, prepared by boiling one part (by weight) of the coarsely powdered ***dravya*** in 16 parts water (by volume) in a covered earthenware pot, over a medium-low heat until it is reduced to one quarter of its original volume. ***Kvātha*** is typically dosed at two ***palas*** (96 mL). Prepared as needed.
4. ***Hima***: cold infusion, prepared by allowing one part (by weight) of the coarsely ground ***dravya*** to infuse in eight parts (by volume) of water overnight. ***Hima*** is typically dosed at two ***palas*** (96 mL), twice daily. Prepared as needed.
5. ***Phāṇṭa***: warm infusion, prepared by infusing one part (by weight) of the coarsely ground powder

dravya in four parts (by volume) of hot water for 8–10 minutes. The resultant preparation is then filtered out through a cloth or sieve. ***Phāṇṭa*** is typically dosed at two ***palas*** (96 mL), twice daily. Prepared as needed.

Cūrṇa: powdered *dravya*

Cūrṇa refers to the finely powdered, finely sieved ***dravya***. ***Cūrṇa*** are typically dosed at one ***karṣa*** (12 g) twice daily, and administered with some combination of honey, ***ghṛta***, sugar or fried ***Hiṅgu*** (*Asafoetida ferula*). If taken with liquid such as water or milk, the liquid portion should be four times the volume of the ***cūrṇa***. Stored in a dark-coloured vessel, in a cool location, the shelf life of a freshly powdered ***cūrṇa*** is 6 months to a year.

Guggulu: resins

Guggulu are a class of medications that are prepared by macerating ***dravyas*** with the purified resin of ***Guggulu*** (*Commiphora mukul*). There are two ways to purify ***Guggulu***. In the first method, the resin is purified by first picking out adulterants by hand, breaking the resin into small pieces, bundling these pieces in a piece of cloth, and then boiling it in various fluids including cow urine, a decoction of ***Triphala***, or milk. When the resin is a soft mass it is taken out and spread over a wooden board that has been oiled with ***ghṛta*** or ***taila*** and any further adulterants are removed by hand. The resin is then fried in ***ghṛta*** and then ground into a powder in a mortar. The second method to prepare a ***guggulu*** is to steam or boil the bundled resin until it melts through the cloth into the fluid, leaving behind the adulterants. The fluid is then filtered and boiled again until all the water has evaporated and only the resin remains. This resin is collected, dried in the sun, and then pounded with ***ghṛta*** in a mortar until it has a waxy consistency. Once prepared according to either method, the resin is then mixed with various ***dravyas*** to create specific formulas. ***Guggulu*** are typically administered with warm water, honey, fresh plant juices or herbal decoctions, in doses of about three ***māṣas*** (3 g), twice daily. Stored in a dark-coloured vessel, in a cool location, the shelf life of a ***guggulu*** can be 2–3 years.

Guṭikā and *vaṭī*: pill

Guṭikā and ***vaṭī*** are prepared by either cooking and macerating the powdered ***dravya*** with an excipient such as jaggery, sugar or ***Guggulu*** (*Commiphora mukul* resin), or macerating it uncooked with a liquid or honey, and rolling it into pills when the desired consistency is achieved. ***Guṭikā*** and ***vaṭī*** are used according to the strength of the patient, based on the potency of the ***dravyas*** used, as well as the actual size of the pill itself. The dosage for ***guṭikā*** typically ranges between one and two ***guñja*** (125–250 mg), or from two to four ***māṣa*** (2–4 g), depending on the formulation, twice daily. Stored in a dark-coloured vessel, in a cool location, the shelf life of ***guṭikā*** and ***vaṭī*** can be 2–3 years.

Avaleha: confection

Avaleha is prepared by reducing a ***kvātha*** over a very low heat until all the water has evaporated, after which the resultant tarry residue is collected and mixed with ***ghṛta***, jaggery or honey. ***Avaleha*** is dosed at one ***pala*** (48 g) once to twice daily, with four times the volume of any such liquid that is appropriate. Many ***avaleha*** recipes are extremely complex in nature and this simple rendering does not account for the preparation of all ***avalehas***, and thus dosages may be different. Stored in a dark-coloured vessel, in a cool location, the shelf life of an ***avaleha*** can be 2–3 years.

Sneha: medicated fats and oils

Sneha are typically prepared by taking one part powderd ***dravya*** (by weight) to four parts fat or oil (by volume), to 16 parts water (by volume). This preparation is then brought to the boil and simmered over a low heat until all the water has evaporated. The resultant preparation is then cooled and strained through a fine cloth. Some ***sneha*** formulations use a different proportion of ***dravya*** to oil to water, and some use other liquids such as milk instead of water. The internal dosage for ***sneha*** typically ranges between one half and one ***karṣa*** (6–12 g), once to twice daily. Externally, ***sneha*** is used in large volumes, between one and four ***prasthas*** (768–3072 mL) per day. For ***nasya*** (nasal administration), the dosage ranges from two to ten ***bindus*** (drops), depending on the formula and the treatment. Stored in a dark-coloured vessel, in a cool location, the shelf life of ***taila*** (medicated sesame oils) can be 2–3 years, whereas ***ghṛta*** (medicated ghee) can actually increase in potency over decades if properly stored. Any stored fat should be free of a rancid or musty odour or flavour.

Āsava and *Ariṣṭa*: galenicals and fermented liquids

Āsava and ***ariṣṭa*** are two types of fermented medicinal preparation, the difference being the use of cold and boiled water, respectively. A typical ***āsava*** or ***ariṣṭa*** may consist of one part (by weight) of the dried herb mixed with 5 parts (by weight) of honey, 10 parts (by weight) of jaggery and 25 parts (by volume) of water. In the case of ***āsava*** the above ingredients are mixed together without heat, poured into an earthenware vessel, sealed well, wrapped in cloth, and buried in the ground for a period of about 1 month. ***Ariṣṭa*** are prepared in a similar manner, except that the ***dravya*** is boiled in the water first, and when cool, honey and jaggery are added later. Both ***āsava*** or ***ariṣṭa*** are typically dosed between one and two ***karśas*** (12–24 mL), twice daily. Stored in a dark coloured vessel, in a cool location, the shelf life of an ***āsava*** or ***ariṣṭa*** can be decades, in which it will increase in potency over time.

Vartti, netrabindu and *añjana*: collyriums and eye drops

Vartti are generally prepared by grinding the powders of the various ***dravyas*** in the formula with fluids such as water, milk, cow urine, and herbal decoctions to make a paste, which is later rolled into thin sticks about 2 cm in length, and then shade dried. For administration these are applied to the lower eyelid. ***Netrabindu*** is a filtered aqueous preparation of various ***dravyas*** that is instilled directly into the eye. ***Añjana*** is a powder or paste of various ***dravyas*** applied to the lower eyelid. Prepared as needed.

Kṣāras: alkalis

Kṣāras are alkaline remedies that are taken both internally and externally. The ***dravyas*** are burnt, reduced to an ash and allowed to cool. The ash is then mixed with six times the volume of water and then strained through a cloth, repeating the process until a clear liquid is obtained. The liquid is then heated until it has evaporated, leaving behind a solid white substance. This is then packed into air-tight bottles and administered with some kind of liquid, in doses ranging from one to two ***guñjas*** (125–250 mg), or from one to two ***māṣas*** (1–2 g), twice daily. Stored in a dark-coloured vessel, in a cool location, the shelf life of a ***kṣāra*** is indefinite.

Bhasmas: purified calcinations

Bhasmas are a kind of alchemical preparation, representing the purified, fully calcified ash of various substances including minerals, plants and animal products. Depending on the ***dravyas*** used, the first stage in preparing ***bhasmas*** is ***śodhana*** ('purification'). For example, a certain mineral is repeatedly heated and then immersed into various substances including ***taila***, buttermilk, cow urine, decoctions and fresh plant juices. When this process is deemed complete the ***dravya*** is powdered and formed into small cakes that are dried in the sun. In some cases the result of ***śodhana*** is sufficient to be used as a remedy, whereas other substances must continue on to the second stage of preparation of ***marana***, or 'killing', which more properly describes a ***bhasma***. According to traditional practices a pit of a specified diameter and depth is dug and half filled with dried cow dung, which is a combustible fuel. The purified, powdered ***dravyas*** are placed into a well-sealed crucible and put on top of the cow dung, and then covered with more cow dung until the pit is full. The pit is then set on fire and allowed to burn completely. After the crucible is allowed to cool, the seal is broken and the calcified ***dravyas*** are taken out, triturated with various substances, and then formed into cakes that are once again allowed to dry in the sun. These cakes are then subjected to this process again and again, sometimes 10, 100 or even 1000 times. The net result is a highly purified and complex preparation that is different from the ingredients that went into it, which results in a significantly different biological activity. Thus even potentially toxic minerals such as arsenic or mercury are used.[14] The preparation of ***bhasma*** is a highly technical process that can take several months or even years to complete, and requires special training. ***Bhasmas*** are considered to be the most potent of Āyurvedic remedies, used in small doses, typically between a half and four ***guñja*** (62.5–500 mg), mixed with various substances including honey, ***ghṛta*** and ***svarasas***. Stored in a dark-coloured vessel, in a cool location, the shelf life of a ***bhasma*** is indefinite.

6.12 *Anupāna*: VEHICLE

A special category of Āyurvedic pharmacy called ***anupāna*** relates to the usage of certain ***dravyas*** to assist in the metabolism of the medication, or to enhance its medicinal activity. ***Anupāna*** literally refers to drinking 'water' (***pana***) 'after' (***anu***) the medicament has been consumed, but in a broader context has come to mean any substance taken with or after the medicament. Commonly used ***anupāna*** include water, milk, honey, ***ghṛta***, sesame oil, jaggery, treacle, rice, ***saindhava***, meat broth and fresh plant juices. If a fat is used as an ***anupāna*** it is usually followed with a little warm water. Even the same ***dravya*** has different effects when it is combined with a different ***anupāna***. For example, the daily usage of ***Harītakī*** fruit (*Terminalia chebula*) as a ***malaśodhana*** ('alterative') and ***rasāyana*** ('rejuvenative') remedy and the choice of ***anupāna*** is affected by the season in which it is consumed. Thus ***Harītakī*** is traditionally taken every morning with salt during the monsoon (***varṣa***), with jaggery in autumn (***śarat***), with ***Śūṇṭhī*** rhizome (*Zingiber officinalis*) in the first half of winter (*Hemañta*) and ***Pippalī*** fruit (*Piper longum*) in the second half (***Śirīṣa***), with honey in the spring (***vasanta***), and with treacle during the summer (***griṣma***). In this way, the various ***anupāna*** modify the biological activities of ***Harītakī*** and make its usage more appropriate to the given season.

6.13 *Bhaiṣajya kāla*: DOSING STRATEGY

Compared to other medical systems Āyurvedic medicine maintains a relatively sophisticated dosing strategy, dependent upon a number of factors, including the disease being treated and the specific ***doṣas*** underlying the pathology. The following is a list of the methods used:

1. ***Abhakta***: prescribed dose is taken on an empty stomach; ***abhakta*** is the most potent of dosing strategies, generally reserved for ***kaphaja*** conditions or otherwise strong patients.
2. ***Prāgbhakta***: prescribed dose is taken before meals to correct ***apāna vāyu*** and to reduce ***medas*** (fat).
3. ***Madhyabakta***: prescribed dose is taken with meals, indicated in digestive disorders to correct ***samāna vāyu*** and ***paittika*** conditions.
4. ***Adhobakta***: prescribed dose is taken after meals, to exert a ***bṛṃhaṇa*** effect, in diseases of the upper body, and in disorders of ***vyāna*** and ***udāna vāyu***.
5. ***Samabhakta***: prescribed dose is taken mixed with food, indicated in paediatric and geriatric complaints, in patients suffering from poor appetite or weakness, in cases where there is an aversion to taking the medication, or where the disease has spread throughout the body.
6. ***Antarābhakta***: prescribed dose is taken after the midday meal, indicated in disorders of ***vyāna vāyu*** and in patients with otherwise good digestion.
7. ***Sāmudga***: prescribed dose is taken before and after a small meal, indicated in disorders of ***vāta***, such as tremor, spasm and convulsions.
8. ***Muhuḥ muhuḥ***: prescribed medication is taken frequently throughout the day, irrespective of meal time, in dyspnoea, vomiting, thirst and poisoning.
9. ***Sagrāsa***: prescribed dose is taken with the first morsel of a meal, used to enhance digestion with ***dīpana dravyas*** and when prescribing ***vajīkaraṇa dravyas***.
10. ***Grāsāntara***: prescribed medication is taken in divided doses between each morsel of food, during the evening meal, indicated in disorders of ***prāṇa vāyu*** and in diseases of the heart.
11. ***Niṣā***: prescribed dose is taken just before bedtime, in the treatment of EENT diseases, to exert a ***bṛṃhaṇa*** effect, and to promote a restful sleep (Sharma 1976).

ENDNOTES

12 The other limbs of Āyurveda include anatomy (***śarira***), physiology (***prakṛti vijñāna***) and pathology (***vikṛti vijñāna***).

13 Some texts classify ***lavaṇa*** as being ***laghu*** but this does not conform to my experience. Excessive salt (NaCl) intake causes oedema and promotes hypertension, both of which are ***kapha*** disorders and occur as the result of the ***guru*** properties of ***lavaṇa***. When applied topically, however, ***lavaṇa*** has ***uṣṇa*** and ***laghu*** properties and promotes the removal of ***kapha***.

14 A recent study published by Saper et al (JAMA 292(23): 2868–2873) found that some Āyurvedic products contain potentially toxic minerals such as lead, mercury and arsenic. Unfortunately this study does not discriminate between those products that intentionally contain these metals in significant

amounts, and those that appear to be adulterated and contain relatively small amounts. The vast majority of manufacturers in India follow good manufacturing practices (GMPs) and can ensure the safety and purity of their products – a very few companies, however, and especially those that produce very inexpensive products (i.e. 'knock-offs') that can be found in Indian grocery stores, may not follow the proper GMPs, and should be avoided. The fact that some Āyurvedic products intentionally contain heavy metals is a separate issue. Such products undergo extensive processing according to traditional methods, and the few published studies indicate that they are safe (see: Pattanaik et al 2003 Toxicology and free radicals scavenging property of Tamra Bhasma. *Indian Journal of Clinical Biochemistry* 18(2): 181–189; Chandra & Mandal 2000 Toxicological and pharmacological study of Navbal Rasayan – a metal based formulation. *Indian Journal of Pharmacology* 32:369-371). Nonetheless, it is understandable that practitioners in the West would be concerned about the ingestion of heavy metals, given a similar concern over these same metals in the food supply, vaccines and dental amalgams. I take the opinion that Āyurvedic protocols should rely on the safe, effective and natural therapies discussed in the most ancient of Āyurvedic practices. While potentially toxic purified mineral preparations may be effective, Western practitioners will require significantly more scientific evidence of their safety before they could ever be used in practice.

PART 1

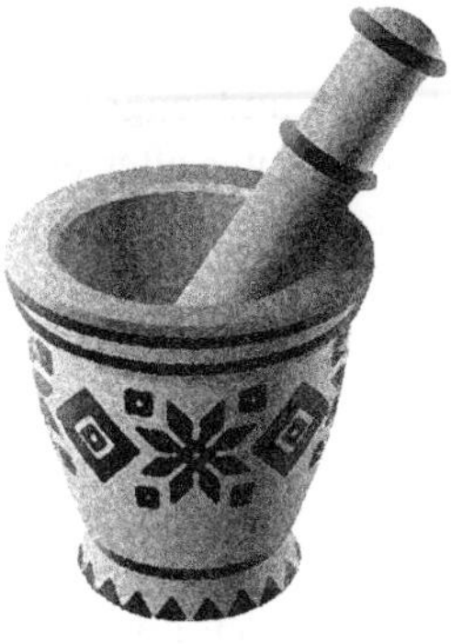

Chapter 7

FOOD AND DRINK

OBJECTIVES

- To understand and review the influence of specific dietary articles upon the humoral system of Āyurveda.

Many of the recommendations of ***dinācaryā*** and ***ṛtucaryā*** would be incomplete without the inclusion of a system of knowledge that guides the myriad choices available to us in our diet. Āyurveda divides the classification of diet in two basic categories, ***dravadravya vijñanīya*** ('knowledge of liquids') and ***annasvarūpa vijñanīya*** ('knowledge of food').

Despite the fact that more recent texts on Āyurveda suggest that there are certain dietary regimens that are best suited to the individual ***doṣas***, this is not a concept found in any traditional text on Āyurveda. Traditional Āyurvedic physicians recognise that there are certain foods that influence the individual ***doṣas***, and that a true understanding of diet comes from appreciating each individual dietary article, rather than memorising a list of dietary 'dos and don'ts'. Most of the foods mentioned in these ancient texts, however, are outside of India, and thus we are left to consider non-Indian foods from an Āyurvedic perspective. Beyond any regimen, all diets for all people should be healthy, diverse and wholesome, and attempt to reflect the season and the local ecology.

7.1 WATER

Of the liquids, water is considered to be the most important in Āyurveda. The biological activity of water is said to be different if it is hot, tepid or cold, and its qualities are dependent upon the location from which it is collected. It is fairly clear from the ancient texts that the utmost importance was attached to making sure the source of water was pure and uncontaminated.

In ancient India freshly collected rainwater was highly valued for health. It is said to be rejuvenating (***rasāyana***), strength promoting (***balya***), life giving (***jīvanīya***), promotes contentment (***sukha***), enhances the intellect (***medhya***), and alleviates all three ***doṣas***. In this industrial age, however, rain often contains the residue of airborne pollutants. These industrial pollutants are now dispersed widely across the entire surface of the earth, and although one may live in a pristine environment this does not mean that the rainwater is not contaminated.

According to Āyurveda the water from fast-flowing glacial rivers is considered to be the best substitute for rainwater; it is ***rasāyana*** ('rejuvenative'), and alleviates all three ***doṣas***. The water from slower flowing rivers and streams, which is murky and brown, contains algae and other plant material said to promote congestion, parasitic infection, circulatory disturbances, and aggravate all three ***doṣas***. The water from underground springs alleviates ***kapha***, promotes digestive function, and is ***hṛdaya*** ('cardiotonic'). The water collected from artesian wells stimulates digestion function, alleviates ***kapha***, and aggravates ***pitta***. Lake water can relieve the symptoms of excessive ***pitta***, whereas water taken from ponds and small pools aggravates ***vāta***. Water that has been collected and allowed to sit in a crystal vessel and exposed to the rays of the sun all day, and then exposed to the rays of the moon all night, is said to be ***rasāyana*** ('rejuvenative'), ***balya*** ('strength-promoting'), ***medhya*** ('intellect-promoting'), and alleviates all three ***doṣas***.

Water in excessive amounts is considered detrimental for persons suffering from ***agnimāndya*** (weak digestive function), and is thus consumed in lesser quantities in such situations. Clearly the modern practice of consuming eight glasses of water a day is not appropriate for every person. Small amounts of water on a frequent basis are better for hydration, whereas large amounts of water consumed all at once is ***mūtravirecana*** ('diuretic') and ***virecana*** ('purgative'). With regard to the seasons, water should be consumed in greater quantities in the summer, and less so in the other seasons, but as it is essential to life it is never prohibited completely. The best guide to water consumption is to rely on one's desire for it (e.g. thirst), and to watch for symptoms associated with dehydration such as dryness of the oral cavity, constipation, headache or low blood pressure. The consumption of water before eating inhibits digestive function, promotes weight loss and aggravates ***vāta***. Consuming water after meals promotes congestion, weight gain and aggravates ***kapha***. Drinking small amounts of water after every few mouthfuls with meals enhances digestive function and promotes the normalcy of the ***doṣas***.

Cold water relieves the effects of aggravated ***pitta*** and poison, inhibits digestion, and is useful for intoxication, exhaustion, fainting, fatigue, vertigo, thirst, heat and sunstroke. Cold water is contraindicated in constipation, flatulence, throat diseases, nascent fevers, rhinitis, upper respiratory tract infections, coughs, hiccoughs, chest pain, urinary tract disorders, cataracts, anorexia, anaemia, poor circulation and tumours. Cold water is not taken after ***snehapāna***, a therapy in which a large amount of oil is ingested orally (see 11.3 ***Pūrva karmas***: ***snehana***).

Warm water stimulates digestive function, soothes throat irritations, cleanses the urinary tract, relieves hiccoughs and dispels intestinal fermentation. It is particularly suitable for both ***vāttika*** and ***kaphaja*** conditions, and finds its best use in the nascent symptoms of an upper respiratory tract infection. Water that has been boiled to three quarters of its original volume is stated to alleviate ***vāta***; that which has been boiled to one half its original volume alleviates ***pitta***; and water that has been boiled to one quarter of its original volume is constipative and alleviates ***kapha***. This ability to modify the effect of boiled water is a useful factor to take into account when preparing decoctions (***kvātha***) for individuals. Hot water is contraindicated in physical and mental exhaustion, convulsions, bronchial asthma, hunger and haemorrhage. Boiled water that has been cooled is best for both ***kaphaja*** and ***paittika*** conditions, but if left overnight will aggravate all three ***doṣas***.

Water is an extremely important substance, and in many respects is the ultimate ***anupāna***, acting as a solvent and carrier for the medicinal substances it is mixed with. Depending upon its quality and source, water can energise and potentise a medication, or it can impinge or inhibit a medicinal effect. Water also appears to have the ability to record influences upon itself, and can be energised by succusion, meditation and prayer. To some extent these ideas are supported by scientific research, most notably in the work of physicist Louis Rey of Lausanne, Switzerland, who suggests that water has a kind of 'memory' of molecules that have been diluted away, demonstrated by a technique that measures thermoluminescence (Rey 2003).

7.2 DAIRY PRODUCTS

Milk is given much importance in Āyurveda, and the milk of different animals has distinct dietary and therapeutic applications. As in the West, cow's milk is by far the most commonly consumed milk in India, although for many people (especially in non-urban areas) milk is obtained fresh, unpasteurised and unprocessed. In constrast, the industrial product called milk in the Western world that is heavily promoted by government agencies, marketing boards and the dairy industry, is in many respects an entirely different substance to the health-giving food that cow's milk was considered to be in the ancient Āyurvedic texts. Herbicide and pesticide residues that act as carcinogens and endocrine disrupters, pathogenic bacteria, the presence of growth hormones, antibiotic residues and heavy metal contaminants like cadmium have all contributed to make industrial cow's milk an unfit product for regular consumption. At the least I recommend that cow's milk be as fresh as possible, preferably from a local supplier or one's own animals, unpasteurised and free from herbicides, pesticides, hormones and antibiotics.

Besides those factors mentioned above, there are two more factors to consider before consuming any kind of milk:

1. ***Sātmya***: the consideration of whether milk is an appropriate food for a particular person, based on cultural and racial differences. Most East Asian people, for example, do not produce the enzyme lactase needed to break down the milk sugars, and can experience severe intestinal cramping and bloating after dairy consumption. Other people regardless of race also exhibit allergies and sensitivities to cow's milk, in all likelihood because of its premature introduction into the diet as young children or infants.
2. ***Agni*** and ***āma***: the digestive capacity of one who wishes to consume milk must be taken into account. When digestion is weak, there is usually ***āma***. If milk is consumed in such a scenario, ***agni*** will continue to be impaired and the undigested milk will feed ***āma***.

Go dugdha ('cow's milk') is considered to be ***guru*** ('heavy') and ***snigdha*** ('greasy') in nature, ***śita*** ('cold') in action, ***rasāyana*** ('rejuvenative'), ***bṛmhaṇa*** ('nourishing'), ***stanyajanana*** ('galactagogue'), and ***bhedhana*** (mildly 'laxative'), alleviating ***vāta*** and ***pitta***. ***Go dugdha*** increases ***kapha*** and promotes ***srotorodha*** (***srota*** 'congestion') in ***āma*** conditions. The milk of a black cow is considered to be the most wholesome, whereas the milk of a white cow is stated to aggravate ***kapha***. Although all milk is best consumed fresh, if cow's milk must be pasteurised it is best decocted with ***kaṭu dravyas*** such as ***Śūṇṭhī*** rhizome (*Zingiber officinalis*), ***Elā*** seed (*Elettaria cardamomum*) and ***Tvak*** bark (*Cinnamomum zeylanicum*) and drunk warm.

Takra ('buttermilk') is the somewhat acidic liquid separated from butter during churning, considered to be ***śita*** in nature, ***dīpanapācana*** (enhances ***agni*** and 'cooks' ***āma***), and ***stambhana*** ('constipating'). It is useful in the treatment of throat irritation and inflammation, but like cow's milk is avoided in ***srotorodha***. ***Takra*** is especially useful in the treatment of and recovery from dysentery, often boiled with herbs such as ***Haridrā*** rhizome (*Curcuma longa*), ***Śūṇṭhī*** rhizome (*Zingiber officinalis*), and fresh curry leaves (*Bergera koenigii*).

Ajā dugdha ('goat's milk') is similar to cow's milk in many respects, but is ***laghu*** ('light') in nature, ***dīpana*** (enhances ***agni***), ***stambhana*** ('constipating'), and is particularly useful for cachexia, haemorrhoids, diarrhoea, menorrhagia and fever. In many areas of India ***ajā dugdha*** is the first choice when weaning children off breast milk. Like cow's milk, goat's milk should be consumed warm, and can be similarly decocted with ***kaṭu dravyas***. Due to their instinsic nature, goats cannot be intensively farmed like cows, require large pastures to browse in, and thus typically eat a broader range of foods than cows. Thus goat's milk is in every way superior to industrial cow's milk, and often contains a broader range of nutrients.

Avi dugdha ('sheep's milk') can also be thought of as an alternative to cow's milk. It is ***guru*** ('heavy') and ***snigdha*** ('greasy') in nature, and is considered to be almost identical to cow's milk, useful in ***paittika*** and ***vāttika*** conditions, dry hacking coughs, and alopecia.

Mahisi dugdha ('water buffalo milk') is excessively ***guru*** ('heavy'), ***snigdha*** ('greasy') and ***śita*** ('cold') in nature. It is most often used by the poorer classes in India instead of cow's milk, and imparts a similar flavour to goat's milk. Given its heavy and greasy properties ***mahisi dugdha*** is used therapeutically for a condition called ***bhasmika***, in which dietary articles pass through the patient very quickly and the hunger is insatiable. Water buffalo milk is also said to be ***stambhana*** ('constipating'), ***balya*** ('enhances strength'), and ***nidrājanana*** ('promotes sleep').

Navanīta is fresh butter churned from cow's milk, and is ***vajīkaraṇa*** ('aphrodisiac') and specific to ***vāttika*** and ***paittika*** complaints. ***Ghṛta*** or ***ghee*** is made by heating fresh unsalted butter over a low heat and rendering the pure butter oil from the milk solids, the latter of which are discarded. The ***rasa*** of ***ghṛta*** is ***madhura*** ('sweet'), its ***vīrya*** is ***śita*** ('cold'), and its primary ***guṇas*** are ***guru*** ('heavy') and ***snigdha*** ('greasy'). When applied topically ***ghṛta*** is anti-inflammatory and finds special utility in skin conditions such as eczema, rashes, ulcers, and herpetic lesions, especially when medicated with ***raktaprasādana*** ('blood-cleansing') ***dravyas***, e.g. ***Mahātikta ghṛta***. Medicated ***ghṛta*** preparations are also used in oleation therapies (***abhyaṅga***) for their ability to treat psychological disturbances (e.g. insanity, bipolar disorders) and other nervous system disorders (e.g. epilepsy, paralysis). ***Ghṛta*** is an important medicament used in the treatment of many ophthalmological disorders, and is often decocted with the formula ***Triphala*** for this purpose. Internally, ***ghṛta*** is used with other herbs as an ***anupāna*** and is ***yogavāhī***, meaning that it contains the ability to augment the effects of any medicinal agent combined with it. ***Ghṛta*** is especially suited to paediatrics and geriatrics, and is a ***rasāyana*** in ***paittika*** conditions. ***Ghṛta*** is considered a highly auspicious food within Hindu culture, and is used in many forms of ***pūja*** ('worship') ceremonies as an agent of purification. ***Ghṛta*** is often combined with honey for its nutritive effects, but never in equal quantities. Although it is a ***rasāyana*** and can help to improve digestive function, ***ghṛta*** can block the channels of the body (***srotorodha***) and promote the accumulation of ***āma*** if ***agni*** is weak. ***Ghṛta*** that has been aged in excess of 10 years is thought to be much stronger in its overall action than fresh ***ghṛta***, and has a ***kaṭu*** ('pungent') ***vipāka***, is ***pramāthi*** (decongests the ***srotāṃsi***), ***medhya*** ('intellect promoting') and alleviates all three ***doṣas***. It is a tradition among some Indians to bury well-sealed vessels that contain ***ghṛta*** that are to be dug up several years later and used by succeeding generations.

When cow's milk is allowed to ferment the resultant preparation is ***dadhi*** or curd (yoghurt). Although high in beneficial commensal bacteria (e.g. *Lactobacillus*, *Bifidus*), it is generally not recommended for daily consumption in Āyurveda. Generally speaking, ***dadhi*** promotes digestion, is constipative and strengthening. It is specific for diarrhoea and dysentery, anorexia, dysuria and in chronic fever where ***āma*** has been removed (***nirāma jvara***). ***Dadhi*** is thought to promote congestion (***kleda***) and burning sensations (***daha***), which can lead to fever, diseases of the blood, cold sores and other skin diseases. There are different varieties of ***dadhi***, however, each classified on the basis of the fermentation period. ***Dadhi*** that has been fermented for a short period of time is stated to have a ***madhura*** ('sweet') ***rasa***, and can be helpful to relieve ***vāta*** and ***pitta***, whereas ***dadhi*** that has been fermented for longer has a ***kaṭu*** ('pungent') ***rasa***, better used in ***kaphaja*** conditions. Āyurveda recommends that ***dadhi*** should be consumed by itself, or with honey or jaggery, and never in the evening. The watery portion of ***dadhi***, called ***mastu***, has all of the benefits of ***dadhi*** but none of its disadvantages and is an excellent food, containing the highest amounts of beneficial bacteria.

Panir is a cultured dairy product that very much resembles what in the West is called cottage cheese or kefir. ***Panir*** is ***guru*** ('heavy'), ***snigdha*** ('greasy') and mildly ***śita*** ('cold') in nature and is a good food in ***vāttika*** and ***paittika*** conditions only as long as ***agni*** is strong enough to digest it. ***Panir*** tends to promote ***kleda*** ('congestion'), and hence is an especially poor choice in ***kaphaja*** conditions. Most other kinds of cheese that are available in the West such as cheddar, montery jack and mozzarella are excessively ***guru*** ('heavy') and ***snigdha*** ('greasy') in quality, and are intolerable in anything except small amounts or in those people with a ***tikṣṇa agni***. Aged and hard cheeses such as parmensan, romano and feta have a ***kaṭu*** ('pungent') ***rasa*** and can be used in ***vātaja*** and ***kaphaja*** conditions in small amounts.

Even though many people within the last few generations in the West missed out on it, it is now clearly established that human milk should be the first food of any newborn. Therapeutically, the milk of lactating women alleviates ***vāta*** and ***pitta*** without aggravating ***kapha***, nourishes the ***dhātus***, and stimulates digestive function. Breast milk finds special therapeutic utility in diseases of the eye, such as conjunctivitis, and can be mixed with other herbal preparations for more serious ophthalmological conditions. Breast milk is also used in ***nasya*** for diseases of the head and in neurological disorders.

7.3 FRUIT

Most fruits generally aggravate ***kapha*** and relieve ***pitta*** because of their ***śita*** ('cold') and ***guru*** ('heavy') qualities, and depending upon the kind of fruit, may aggravate or pacify ***vāta***. Of all the fruits Āyurveda considers ***drākṣā*** ('grapes') to be among the best, but these of course must be organically produced or otherwise naturally grown, and I believe, also refers to eating the seeds along with them, which contain potent anti-oxidant compounds. The following list describes the actions of fruits upon the ***doṣas***:

Aggravates *vāta*

- Dried fruit, cranberries, sour and acid-tasting fruits, unripe fruit.

Pacifies *vāta*

- Most local and seasonal fruits, consumed individually and in small amounts, e.g. raspberry, strawberry, pear, blueberry, peach, grape, and apple.
- Cooked fruits such as baked apples, baked pears, and stewed fruit (e.g. prunes, raisins, etc.), prepared with ***ghṛta*** and ***dravyas*** such as ***Tvak*** bark (*Cinnamomum zeylanicum*) and ***Elā*** seed (*Elettaria cardamomum*).
- Any tropical fruit, e.g. mango, pomegranate, papaya, guava, litchi (lychee), melon, banana, etc.

Aggravates *pitta*

- Sour and acid-tasting fruits, including lemons, sour oranges; papaya or strawberry consumed to excess.

Pacifies *pitta*

- Most local and seasonal fruits can be eaten freely, such as raspberry, plum, pear, cranberry, grape, and apple; sweet citrus fruits can also be consumed in moderation.
- Most tropical fruits, e.g. mango, pomegranate, papaya, guava, litchi, melon, banana, etc.

Aggravates *kapha*

- Most fruits are generally avoided because of their excessive water content (***snigdha***) and cold (***śita***) nature.

Pacifies *kapha*

- Small amounts of dried fruit, cranberry, grapefruit, lemon, lime, and sour-tasting fruits.

7.4 VEGETABLES

Among all the different foods, vegetables stand out for their health-giving properties and their generally beneficial effects upon all three ***doṣas***. In this respect vegetables are closely allied with medicinal plants, some such as ***Śūṇṭhī*** (*Zingiber officinalis*) and ***Laśuna*** (*Allium sativum*) straddling the definition of food and medicine. Although all vegetables are generally beneficial each ***doṣa*** may require that these vegetables be prepared by a specific method.

The consumption of raw vegetables is generally not advised in Āyurvedic medicine due to their excessively ***śita*** ('cold') ***vīrya***, and are specifically contraindicated in ***vāttika*** and ***kaphaja*** conditions. To some extent the issue also relates to potentially pathogenic microorganisms that can be found on raw vegetables, especially in developing countries that often lack sufficient sanitation. In most cases raw vegetables should be avoided, and at the least should be lightly steamed or juiced, preferably with ***dravyas*** that have an ***uṣṇa*** ('hot') ***vīrya*** such as fresh ginger root, garlic and shallots. In contrast, ***paittika*** conditions may benefit from limited amounts of raw vegetables such as celery and carrot sticks to cool the body and reduce excess heat. Fried vegetables are only really indicated in ***vāttika*** conditions, and aggravate both ***pitta*** and ***kapha***, and can promote ***āma***. Most deep-fried foods are similarly congesting and even toxic considering their transfatty acid content – at the least, deep-frying should use heat-resistant oils such as ***ghṛta*** and coconut oil. The following lists the interaction between vegetables and the ***doṣas***:

Aggravates *vāta*

- Raw vegetables generally, mushrooms,[15] potatoes.

Pacifies *vāta*

- All cooked vegetables generally, but especially root vegetables and winter squashes, steamed, boiled, baked or stir-fried.

- Well-cooked onions and garlic.
- Cruciferous vegetables (broccoli, cabbage, etc.) are ***śita*** ('cold') and ***laghu*** ('light') in nature, and should be cooked with ginger or other herbs such as cumin, rosemary, and garlic, and consumed with fats such as butter, olive oil or ***ghṛta***.
- Seaweed, in soups and broths.
- Fermented vegetables, e.g. sauerkraut, pickles, umeboshi plum.

Aggravates *pitta*

- Onions, chilies, tomatoes, eggplant (aubergine), garlic, turnip, radish, avocado, watercress, seaweed, pickles.

Pacifies *pitta*

- Most vegetables, preferable steamed, juiced or raw, especially cooling vegetables such as leafy greens, cucumber, lettuce, dandelion, cilantro, sprouts and celery.

Aggravates *kapha*

- Raw vegetables, mushrooms.
- Fried vegetables.

Pacifies *kapha*

- All vegetables, steamed or baked.
- Bitter or pungent tasting leafy greens.
- Raw vegetables only with ***uṣṇa*** ('hot') ***dravyas*** such as cayenne and black pepper.
- Sprouted beans and seeds in moderation.
- Small amounts of fermented vegetables and unsweetened pickles.

7.5 GRAINS AND CEREALS

Most grains and cereals have a ***madhura*** ('sweet') ***rasa***, a ***guru*** ('heavy') and ***uṣṇa*** ('hot') ***vīrya***, and are mostly ***bṛmhaṇa*** ('nourishing') in action. Grains and cereals are thus generally considered to be most appropriate in ***vāttika*** conditions, although certain grains, such as rice, barley, quinoa or amaranth appear to be suitable to all three ***doṣas***.[16] Refined cereals such as white flour that have been stripped of their original nutrient content aggravate all three ***doṣas***, promote ***āma*** and should be avoided. Whole grain flour, although largely considered to be better than white flour, can still impair gastric motility and aggravate ***kapha***, weaken ***agni***, and facilitate the production of ***āma*** due its ***guru*** and ***picchila*** nature. Whole grain flours are also particularly susceptible to rancidity, due to the polyunsaturated fat content, and should be freshly ground and used as soon as possible. Generally speaking, it is best to consume boiled or naturally fermented grains, such as oatmeal and steamed rice, or homemade idli (fermented rice/urad bean cakes) and sourdough bread. It has become increasingly clear that a long-term diet rich in grains and cereals poses several potential health problems. Foods with a high glycaemic index can promote alterations in blood sugar, leading to hypoglycaemia, as well as induce a state of hyperinsulin secretion and insulin resistance, leading to diabetes and cardiovascular disease. Grains and cereals also contain a chemical called phytic acid that binds to certain minerals such as calcium and iron, and minimises their absorption in the digestive tract to promote nutrient deficiencies. Further, a diet rich in grains may also be abundant in compounds called lectins, which irritate and inflame the gut wall. Thus, in many cases, a grain-based diet is contraindicated in inflammatory bowel disorders, and in autoimmune conditions like ***āmavāta*** (rheumatoid arthritis) that are thought to have an enteropathogenic origin. Despite the fact that the modern Indian diet obviously relies upon grains and legumes to feed an enormous population, there is no indication in the extant Āyurvedic literature that a primarily grain-based or vegetarian diet should take preference over a more balanced diet: indeed, the Ā yurvedic texts recommended a wide assortment of foods, including meat, to maintain health.

The following list details the effects of grains and cereals upon the ***doṣas***:

Aggravates *vāta*

- Insufficiently cooked grains; grain foods with light (***laghu***) and dry (***rūkṣa***) properties such as granola, muesli, corn, millet, yeasted bread, popcorn, rice cakes, puffed grains, tortilla chips.

Pacifies *vāta*

- Boiled and fermented grains, including oats, rice, rice noodles, quinoa, amaranth, buckwheat, khuskhus (couscous), whole wheat pasta, whole wheat chapatti, corn flour tortilla, sourdough bread (lightly toasted).

Aggravates *pitta*

- None, except light or toasted grains consumed to excess (e.g. granola, muesli, corn, millet, bread, popcorn, rice cakes).

Pacifies *pitta*

- Boiled and toasted grains, including oats, rice, rice noodles, quinoa, amaranth, buckwheat, khuskhus, whole wheat pasta, whole wheat chapatti, corn flour tortilla, sourdough bread (lightly toasted).

Aggravates *kapha*

- Most grains, especially white rice, yeasted bread, pasta, wheat, rye and oats.

Pacifies *kapha*

- Boiled and fermented rice, quinoa, amaranth, millet, barley, corn; grain foods with light (***laghu***) and dry (***rūkṣa***) properties such as granola, muesli, corn, millet, popcorn, rice cakes, puffed grains, etc.

7.6 LEGUMES

Although legumes are an important non-animal source of protein, they typically display a ***rūkṣa*** ('dry'), ***laghu*** ('light') and ***śita*** ('cold') ***vīrya***, and hence most are contraindicated in ***vāttika*** conditions. Similar to grains and cereals, legumes have been shown to contain potentially toxic or health-damaging constituents, such as lectins, phytates and protease inhibitors. Thus legumes may promote nutrient deficiencies, which is in keeping with the Āyurvedic perspective, as well as inflame the intestinal wall, and thus are contraindicated in inflammatory bowel disease and autoimmune disorders. Like grains and cereals, most legumes are rich in carbohydrates, and should be avoided in hypoglycaemia and diabetes, or at least be consumed with fats and oils to lower the glycaemic index. Some legumes such as soy are now very common in our modern diet, often as a hidden ingredient in prepackaged foods and meat, and many people are allergic or have sensitivities to soy. As legumes will typically provoke ***vāta*** in most people, they should be soaked overnight, cooked with ginger and other ***uṣṇa*** ('hot') ***dravyas***, and eaten with fat such as ***ghṛta***. In countries like Japan, beans such as soy are rarely consumed without first being fermented, as in natto, miso and tempeh, which helps to deactivate some of the health-damaging constituents. Another frequent error that is made when preparing bean dishes such as ***dahl*** is using too great a volume of beans. According to traditional Indian cookery, ***dahl*** is a thin, watery broth made with beans and spices. In a given meal, the actual volume of beans consumed is actually fairly small. Many Westerners that emulate an Indian diet prepare far too large an amount needed for one meal, and mistakenly rely upon this as their primary source of protein, eschewing the benefits of egg or dairy in an otherwise vegetarian diet. The primary reason why most people in India exlusively rely upon legumes as their primary source of protein is because of extreme poverty, although some believe a vegetarian diet more beneficial to cultivate a ***sattvic*** state of mind.[17]

The following lists the effects of legumes upon the ***doṣas***:

Aggravates *vāta*

- All legumes, including soy, lentils, split peas, kidney, garbanzo, lima, pinto, navy, peanut.

Pacifies *vāta*

- There are no beans that truly pacify ***vāta***, but some legumes and legume products such as ***urad dhal*** (black gram), adzuki, mung, soft tofu, natto, and tempeh can be consumed in moderation if prepared with warming herbs and spices such as ginger, cumin, garlic, basil and oregano.

Aggravates *pitta*

- Peanut.

Pacifies *pitta*

- Most legumes are acceptable for ***pitta***, but because they have a ***laghu*** ('light') ***vīrya*** they should not be consumed to excess.

Aggravates *kapha*

- Peanut, ***urad dhal***.

Pacifies *kapha*

- Most legumes are useful for relieving ***kapha***, used in moderation.

7.7 NUTS AND SEEDS

Nuts and seeds are the most ***bṛmhaṇa*** ('nourishing') foods of the vegetable kingdom, and are an excellent source of dietary fat. Nuts and seeds are the fruit of the plant, the final ***dhātu*** produced, and are closest in quality to ***śukra/aṇḍāṇu*** (semen/ovum) in humans. Thus nuts and seeds directly nourish the reproductive organs, if taken in appropriate amounts. The ***vīrya*** of most nuts and seeds is ***guru*** ('heavy'), ***snigdha*** ('greasy') and ***uṣṇa*** ('hot'). Care should be taken to eat nuts and seeds as fresh as possible, as many will become rancid shortly after being hulled. Many nuts such as pistachio also contain high levels of fungal mycotoxins that result from improper storage and act as liver carcinogens. If taken in excessive amounts, nuts and seeds facilitate the production of ***āma*** and will aggravate ***kapha***. The following lists the effects of nuts and seeds on the ***doṣas***:

Aggravates *vāta*

- None, except in large amounts (i.e. more than a small handful), and improperly chewed.

Pacifies *vāta*

- Flax, hemp, sesame, pumpkin, walnut, cashew, sunflower, coconut, pecan, filbert, brazil, almond, etc.

Aggravates *pitta*

- Most nuts and seeds are generally avoided in ***paittika*** conditions because of their ***snigdha*** ('greasy') and ***uṣṇa*** ('hot') ***vīrya***.

Pacifies *pitta*

- Pumpkin seeds, coconut, almond, melon seeds.

Aggravates *kapha*

- Most nuts and seeds are generally avoided in ***kaphaja*** conditions because of their ***snigdha*** ('greasy') and ***guru*** ('heavy') ***vīrya***.

Pacifies *kapha*

- Pumpkin, melon seeds.

7.8 MEAT AND ANIMAL PRODUCTS

Of all the food groups, meat and animal products are the most ***bṛmhaṇa*** ('nourishing'), and are generally considered to have a ***guru*** ('heavy'), ***snigdha*** ('greasy') and ***uṣṇa*** ('hot') ***vīrya***. Meat and animal products generally pacify ***vāta***, but some can aggravate both ***pitta*** and ***kapha***.

Although India is renowned for its vegetarian culture, Āyurveda does not prohibit meat as a dietary article, and nor are the vast majority of people in India vegetarian, at least by choice. It is clear that traditional Āyurvedic medicine considered meat to be an excellent food to relieve deficiency (***langhana***) conditions. In the West, however, gross nutritional deficiency is rarely an issue, although many people feel much better when they consume good quality meat on a daily basis, especially if they live in cold, dry climates. In northern climes it is clear that animal products have always been an important staple to people that reside in these areas, and if living in such a climate, it is as well to follow these practices. It is important to remember, however, that meat carries with it a greater investment in the economy of cause and effect, when a sentient being is killed and eaten to nourish another. Above all, meat is a medicinal food, and should be consumed when needed, with respect and honour for the animal which has sacrificed its life to nourish your own. If such an approach were taken in the West, much of the objectionable and cruel practices of the meat industry would be replaced by those that preserve and honour the dignity of the animal. Further, industrially produced meat is typically deficient in key trace minerals, low in omega-3 fatty acids, high in saturated fat, and rife with antibiotic and hormone residues. Such meat and animal products should be avoided in all conditions in favour of those that are organically grown, pasture-raised and free-range.

The consumption of the different kinds of meat can be based upon the nature of the animal in relation to the ***doṣas***. Thus, timid animals such as rabbit and venison might be avoided in ***vāttika*** conditions but are used in ***kaphaja*** conditions because of their comparatively ***laghu*** ('light') and ***rūkṣa*** ('dry') ***vīrya***. Passive and sedentary animals such as beef and buffalo are contraindicated in ***kaphaja*** conditions, but are useful in ***vāttika*** conditions because of their ***sthira*** ('stable'), ***sāñdra*** ('solid') and ***madha*** ('slow') qualities. Red meat is generally avoided in ***paittika*** conditions, but is useful in ***vāttika*** conditions because of its comparatively ***uṣṇa*** ('hot') ***vīrya*** (indicated by the red colour of the meat). The ***uṣṇa*** property of lean red meat can be appropriate in ***kaphaja*** if the animals are not sedentary, such as venison, moose or elk. Goat meat and mutton are two of the few red meats that are tolerated in ***paittika*** conditions, are similarly helpful in ***vattaika*** conditions, and can even be used in ***kaphaja*** conditions in small amounts. Most fish is good for all three ***doṣas*** but tropical fish is said to have an ***uṣṇa*** ('hot') ***vīrya*** and is traditionally avoided in ***paittika*** conditions. Cold water fish, however, is unlikely to have this effect, although cold water fish with a high fat content is contraindicated in ***kaphaja*** conditions.

The following details the effects of the different kinds of meat upon the ***doṣas***:

Aggravates *vāta*

- No meat is contraindicated for ***vāta***, but some meats such as pork and beef can be difficult to digest, and should be consumed in small amounts and with herbs and spices that enhance digestion.
- As ***vāttika*** conditions speak of an extreme sensitivity to psychic stimuli, the act of killing an animal for food carries with it a downward moving, negative energy that can act in opposition to the nourishing qualities of the meat. In such conditions, the kind of meats should be chosen carefully, selecting only meat that has been cared for lovingly during its life and sacrificed humanely.

Pacifies *vāta*

- Almost all meats pacify ***vāta***, especially those cooked in soups and stews with ***kaṭu*** ('pungent') ***dravyas*** such as onion, shallots, garlic, ginger, etc. Acceptable animal products include eggs, poultry (especially duck and goose), wild fish, shellfish, wild game, beef, pork, goat, lamb, mutton, etc.

Aggravates *pitta*

- Pork, beef, tropical fish, shellfish.

Pacifies *pitta*

- Poultry (particularly the white meat), cold water fish (salmon, halibut, herring, etc.), fish roe, rabbit, goat, lamb, mutton.

Aggravates *kapha*

- Pork, beef, lamb, fish, shellfish.

Pacifies *kapha*

- Poultry, wild game, goat, rabbit.

7.9 FATS AND OILS

Fats and oils are an important food, medicament and vehicle (***anupāna***, see Ch. 6) in Āyurvedic medicine. Generally speaking, oils and fats are a primary treatment to ***vāta*** due to their generally moistening and warming nature. They are typically used to a lesser extent in ***paittika*** and ***kaphaja*** conditions, although some oils are an exception to this rule.

The most commonly used oil in Āyurvedic medicine is sesame oil (***taila***). ***Taila*** is the cold-pressed oil from raw ***tila*** ('sesame seed') and is the primary medium for the many medicated oils used in Āyurveda. ***Taila*** has a ***madhura*** ('sweet') ***rasa***, an ***uṣṇa*** ('hot') and ***guru*** ('heavy') ***vīrya***, and is ***bhedana*** ('aperient'), ***vajīkaraṇa*** ('aphrodisiac'), ***balya*** ('strength promoting'), ***varnya*** ('enhances complexion'), and pacifies ***vāta***. Taken internally in large amounts ***taila*** is ***vidāhi*** ('promotes burning sensations'), and can be used in the treatment of intestinal parasites (***kṛmighna***). Used topically ***taila*** is ***medhya*** ('intellect promoting'), ***romsañjanana*** ('promotes hair growth'), ***dīpana*** ('enhances ***agni***'), and ***balya*** ('counters fatigue').

Besides ***taila***, ***ghṛta*** is the next most commonly used oil, used in both cooking and as a medicine.

A number of other oils are also used, however, and the following is a list of common food oils used in both Āyurveda and in the West, and their effects upon the ***doṣas***. Needless to say, perhaps, but this list refers only to high-quality, fresh, cold-pressed 'extra-virgin' oils, and generally not to those that have been refined or rendered with the use of chemical solvents or heat:

1. Olive: decreases ***vāta***, increases ***pitta*** and ***kapha***
2. Coconut: decreases ***vāta*** and ***pitta***, increases ***kapha***
3. Sunflower: decreases ***vāta*** and ***pitta***, increases ***kapha***
4. Safflower: decreases ***vāta*** and ***pitta***, increases ***kapha***
5. Walnut: decreases ***vāta***, increases ***pitta*** and ***kapha***
6. Flax: decreases ***vāta*** and ***pitta***, increases ***kapha***
7. Hemp: decreases ***vāta*** and ***pitta***, increases ***kapha***
8. Castor: decreases ***vāta*** and ***kapha***, increases ***pitta***
9. Mustard: decreases ***vāta*** and ***kapha***, aggravates ***pitta***
10. Almond: decreases ***vāta*** and ***pitta***, aggravates ***kapha***
11. Canola: decreases ***vāta*** and ***pitta***, aggravates ***kapha***
12. Peanut: aggravates all three ***doṣas***
13. Fish: decreases ***vāta*** and ***pitta***, increases ***kapha***.

Although there is no mention of them in the Āyurvedic literature it is clearly wise to avoid both hydrogenated oils and trans-fatty acids, as the consumption of these fats has been shown to promote a wide range of diseases, including cancer and cardiovascular disease. This includes margarine, most oils added to packaged foods, blackened meat from high heat broiling, and any vegetable, fruit or seed oil sold in a clear container without refrigeration (monounsaturated fats such as olive oil are to some extent an exception to this rule). In a similar fashion, the fat of meat from animals raised in large industrial operations and fed only grain-based fodder is exceptionally unhealthy, much higher in saturated fat and concomitantly lower in essential omega-3 fatty acids than that found in pasture-raised, grass-fed animals.

7.10 SWEETENERS

There are many kinds of sweetener used in Āyurvedic medicine, mostly as ***anupāna***. Sweets are also very popular as a food and condiment in India, but this is not reflective of the perspectives found in ancient texts like the ***Caraka saṃhitā*** or ***Aṣṭāṅga Hṛdayam***. Intensely sweet foods such as cane sugar and honey are considered to be a kind of medicine in Āyurvedic medicine, with powerful healing properties. Used to excess, however, or simply to feed the impulses of the tongue, sweet foods are a kind of poison that aggravates all three ***doṣas***.

Madhu ('honey') is a highly valued sweetener in Āyurveda, and is considered to be ***rūkṣa*** ('dry'), ***uṣṇa*** ('hot') and somewhat ***guru*** ('heavy') in nature. ***Madhu*** is ***dīpanapācana*** ('enhances ***agni***' and 'cooks' ***āma***), ***grāhī*** ('checks excessive secretion'), ***śoṇitasthāpana*** ('antihaemorrhagic'), ***varnya*** ('enhances complexion'), ***medhya*** ('promotes intellect'), ***vajīkaraṇa*** ('aphrodisiac'), and alleviates ***kapha***. Taken internally ***madhu*** is used in the treatment of peptic and duodenal ulcer, bronchitis, asthma, hiccoughs, vomiting and diarrhoea. Externally, honey is used to heal bruises, soothe inflamed skin, resolve ulcers, unite broken bones and enhance the complexion. Like ***ghṛta***, ***madhu*** is ***yogavāhī***, enhancing the activity of the medicaments taken with it. ***Madhu*** may be used safely with ***ghṛta*** (but only in disproportionate quantities) for ***vāttika*** disorders, and as an ***anupāna*** for ***rasāyana*** ('rejuvenative') and ***vajīkaraṇa*** ('aphrodisiac') therapies. ***Madhu*** is a mild irritant to ***pitta***, which is offset if at least twice the amount of ***ghṛta*** is used in combination. Aged ***madhu*** has less of the nourishing, ***bṛmhaṇa*** qualities of fresh honey, but has a greater ability to alleviate ***kapha***.

Āyurveda prohibits the internal use of heated honey. This is because wild bees gather nectar indiscriminately from any kind of plant, regardless of whether the plant is toxic or not. Thus all honey contains a certain amount of toxins,[18] and because the nature of poison is ***uṣṇa***, when honey is heated the latent toxins become active. This is also why the internal consumption of ***madhu*** is avoided in hot weather.[19]

Guḍa, or jaggery (solidified cane sugar juice), is ***snigdha*** ('greasy'), ***śita*** ('cold') and ***guru*** ('heavy') in nature, and is by far the best sweetener and ***anupāna*** to use in ***paittika*** conditions. It may be used in ***vāttika*** conditions as well, as long as the ***dravya*** accompanying it has an ***uṣṇa*** ('hot') property, but should be avoided in ***kaphaja*** disorders, and can promote ***kṛmi*** ('intestinal parasites'). ***Guḍa*** is said to be ***bhedana*** ('aperient') and ***balya*** ('strength promoting'), and is used therapeutically in the treatment of ***dahi*** ('burning sensation') and ***tṛṣṇā*** ('thirst'). Aged ***guḍa***, however, is said to have a ***laghu*** nature, and is considered to be ***hṛdaya*** (cardiotonic) and nourishing. Refined ***guḍa***, which includes both white and 'brown' (caramelised) sugar, aggravates all three ***doṣas***, promotes ***kṛmi*** ('parasites'), and should be avoided. Molasses is ***guru*** ('heavy') and ***snigdha*** ('greasy') in nature, and is well suited to ***vāttika*** conditions. Maple syrup and other syrups derived from tree sap are similar in many respects to ***guḍa***, and may represent a better choice for people living in temperate climates when consumed in small amounts, as an ***anupāna***.

7.11 ALCOHOL, COFFEE AND TEA

Although the ancient texts of Āyurveda speak of the dangers of alcohol, much of what is written seems to indicate that alcohol has many benefits. All of these references to alcoholic beverages are to certain kinds of wine or beer that have been naturally fermented. Wine (***madya***) prepared from grapes, consumed in moderate amounts and taken with meals, is considered to be ***dīpana*** ('stimulant to digestion'). Beer (***surā***) prepared from rice is considered to be ***guru*** ('heavy') in nature, and ***balya*** ('strength-promoting'), ***stanyajanana*** ('galactagogue') and ***bṛmhaṇa*** ('nourishing') in action, useful in the treatment of oedema, haemorrhoids, abdominal bloating, malabsorption syndromes and dysuria. ***Yavasurā***, or beer prepared from barley (the dominant form of beer in the West), is said to be ***guru*** ('heavy') and ***rūkṣa*** ('dry') in nature, inhibits digestion, promotes bloating, and aggravates all three ***doṣas***.

Alcohol is generally avoided in ***paittika*** complaints because the nature of addiction involves a dysfunction of the discriminative faculties (i.e. ***pitta***), but also because alcohol is ***uṣṇa*** ('hot') in nature. Naturally fermented alcohol is predominant in ***madhura*** ('sweet') and ***amla*** ('sour') ***rasa***, and is ***uṣṇa*** ('hot'), ***laghu*** ('light'), and ***snigdha*** ('heavy') in quality, consumed with meals in small amounts to treat ***vāttika*** and ***kaphaja*** conditions. Distilled alcohol (e.g. scotch, bourbon, vodka) has a ***kaṭu*** ('pungent') ***rasa***, and is ***uṣṇa*** ('hot'), ***laghu*** ('light'), and ***rūkṣa*** ('dry') in quality, used to control ***kaphaja*** conditions and coldness in small amounts.

Neither coffee nor tea is mentioned in the ancient texts of Āyurveda, despite the fact that these are both exceptionally popular beverages in modern India, often consumed with large amounts of sugar, boiled milk and aromatic spices. Taken in small amounts and infrequently, neither of these beverages poses any prominent risk to health, although both ***vāttika*** and ***paittika*** conditions can be aggravated by their regular usage. In ***kaphaja*** conditions both coffee and tea may have some minimal benefit (taken without sugar), as the stimulatory effect of the methylxanthines counters the lethargic nature of ***kaphaja*** and enhances mental clarity. Unfortunately both coffee and tea inhibit digestive function when taken on a chronic basis. Taken before meals, coffee and tea effectively inhibit the appetite by enhancing the breakdown of glycogen into glucose, temporarily elevating blood sugar levels. If taken after meals, however, coffee and tea work to enhance stomach emptying, strongly induce gall bladder secretion and thus mass peristalsis, such that food is moved quickly through the gut without first having undergone adequate digestion. The methylxanthines in coffee and tea artificially induce a state of nervous excitation called the 'fight or flight' response, and in large doses can promote nervous irritability, anxiety and tachycardia. I generally find that most patients feel healthier and have more energy when they avoid coffee and tea, although discontinuing coffee can promote a few days of headaches from rebound vasodilation of the cerebral arteries.

7.12 SUMMARY OF DIETARY GUIDELINES AND ***tridoṣas***

The following tables summarise what foods will typically pacify (reduce) or aggravate (increase) the affected ***doṣa***. For specific dietary and lifestyle guidelines for each ***doṣa*** please consult Appendix 3.

TABLE 7.1 *Vāta doṣa.*

Pacifies ***vāta***	Aggravates ***vāta***
Oils and fats: animal fats (free-range), olive oil, coconut oil, ***ghṛta***, butter	Canola, refined oils, margarine, trans-fatty acids and hydrogenated fats
Cane sugar juice (in small amounts)	
Cooked fruits such as apple sauce, baked pears, stewed prunes, with spicy herbs (ginger, cinnamon, cardamom, clove)	Unripe fruit, raw fruit, dried fruit, cranberries, sour citrus
Steamed vegetables, baked vegetables, especially squash and root vegetables (except potatoes)	Raw vegetables, field mushrooms
Oats, basmati rice, quinoa, amaranth	Granola, corn, millet, rice cakes, manna bread, flour, pastries
Legumes (with spicy herbs and fat): natto, miso, tofu, adzuki, mung beans	Most legumes: soy, lentils, split peas, kidneys, garbanzo, pinto
Seeds and nuts (in small amounts): sesame, pumpkin, almond, brazil, pecan, coconut	Seeds or nuts in excess
Eggs, poultry, shellfish, beef, pork, goat, lamb, goat's cheese, whole dairy (in moderation, always warm, with spices)	No meat contraindicated

TABLE 7.2 *Pitta doṣa.*

Pacifies ***pitta***	Aggravates ***pitta***
Coconut oil, ***ghṛta***, cold-pressed vegetable oils, fish fats (in moderation)	Mustard, canola, refined oils, margarine, trans-fatty acids and hydrogenated fats
Cane sugar juice, jaggery, maple syrup (in moderation)	Honey, white sugar (to excess)
Raw fruits, especially in hot weather; raspberry, plum, pear, blueberry, grape, apple, melon	Sour and acidic fruits, including sour oranges, lemon, lime; papaya or strawberries to excess
Raw and steamed vegetables, broccoli, chard, celery, salad greens, cucumber, green beans, peas, cauliflower, cilantro, sprouted beans and seeds	Raw onion, chilies, tomatoes, eggplant (aubergine), peppers, daikon radish
Oats, basmati rice, quinoa, amaranth, khuskhus, whole wheat pasta, whole wheat chapatti, pumpernickel, manna bread	Refined flour products
Most legumes in moderation	Legumes to excess
Seeds and nuts: pumpkin, coconut, almond, melon, brazil, cashew, filbert	Seeds or nuts to excess
Eggs, poultry, cold-water fish, rabbit, game, goat, mutton	Pork, beef, tropical fish, shellfish, yogurt

TABLE 7.3 ***Kapha doṣa.***

Pacifies ***kapha***	Aggravates ***kapha***
Mustard oil	Most fats and oils; canola, refined oils, margarine, trans-fatty acids and hydrogenated fats
Honey	Sweet or sweetened foods
Dried fruit, apple, cranberry, grapefruit, lemon, lime, papaya	Raw vegetables in excess, field mushrooms
Raw vegetables (in moderation): sprouted beans and seeds, spicy salad greens; steamed vegetables	Flour products, white rice, yeasted flour products, pasta, wheat, rye, spelt
Brown rice, quinoa, amaranth, millet, kasha, barley, popped grains, granola, rice cakes	Peanuts, black gram
Most legumes, with spicy herbs	Most seeds and nuts
A few seeds: pumpkin, melon	Most animal products, fatty meats, especially to excess
Poultry, wild game, goat, fish, mutton	Dairy products

ENDNOTES

15 Āyurveda generally abhors the ingestion of fungi, which is typical of other fungiphobic cultures such as many of the First Nations of North America. In contrast, the experiences of fungiphilic cultures found in Europe and China have shown that fungi have many beneficial and medicinal effects. Most fungi are avoided in ***kaphaja*** or ***āma*** conditions, but some, such as Reishi, Maitake and Shitake, may be helpful in such states.

16 In regard to rice, the ancient Āyurvedic commentators preferred certain varieties over others, such as ***raktasāli*** (red rice) and ***ṣaṣtika*** (60 day rice). Further, these traditional rices did not undergo extensive milling and retained all or a portion of their inner husk, which is rich in bran and anti-oxidant compounds. Completely milled rice, and certainly parboiled rice, which unfortunately makes up a large part of the rice now consumed in India and the rest of the world, is a pale comparison of the health-giving food mentioned in Āyurveda.

17 Even now, vegetarianism in India is not a strict veganism: fresh and fermented unpasteurised dairy products are a major component of the vegetarian diet.

18 Honey manufactured from the nectar of several species of ***Rhodendron*** and other members of the Ericaceae contains grayanotoxins that can cause dose dependent symptoms of toxicity such as acute salivation, vomiting, paralysis, and hypertension (Lampe 1988 JAMA 259(13): 2009).

19 It is interesting to note that heated honey is used in traditional Chinese medicine, such as stir-frying it with Gan cao (*Glycyrrhiza uralensis*) to modify the activity of Licorice, to 'strengthen the middle', and enhance digestion. Despite the idea that heated honey is never taken internally, the ***Madanapala nighaṇṭu*** indicates that heated honey can be taken with water in diseases caused by ***āma***, presumably to enhance ***agni***.

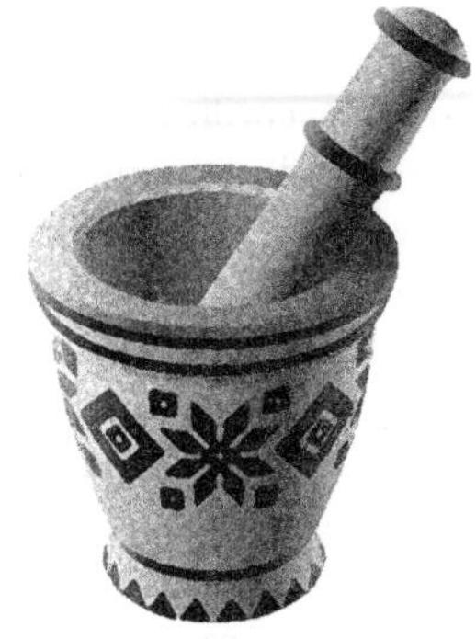

Chapter 8

PATHOLOGY AND DISEASE

OBJECTIVES

- To understand the concept of disease.
- To understand the causes of disease.
- To understand the manifestation of disease.

8.1 *Vikara*: DISEASE IN ĀYURVEDA

From an Āyurvedic perspective health is defined as the equilibrium between the ***doṣas***, ***dhātus*** and ***malas***. When there is a disruption to this equilibrium the result is ***vikara*** or 'disease'. ***Vikara*** can be seen to have several different synonyms, each of which details an aspect of disease, including:

1. ***Vyādhi***: 'pain', literally referring to the sensation of a pricking pain, but can be thought of as the experience of pain.
2. ***Pāpa***: 'evil' or 'sin', referring to the desires and ignorance of the ***ahaṃkāra*** ('ego') that perpetuates the illusion of individuality, of being separate from the Whole. Such an orientation creates a downward spiral into dissolution and promotes disease.
3. ***Āma***: 'undigested food', referring to toxins and waste products that impair metabolic activities.
4. ***Bādha***: 'trouble', referring to the hindrance and obstacles that disease brings to spiritual progress.
5. ***Dukha***: 'sorrow' or 'work', referring to the sadness and extra effort that disease brings.

The etymology of the modern English word 'disease' suggests that the 'ease' by which life is lived becomes hindered or blocked in some way. While disease can be at the least an inconvenience, it often strikes at the core of our being, challenging basic assumptions, attitudes and behaviours, and as such has profound lessons to teach, providing opportunities for an expanded awareness of life and death. Disease and dying are powerful teachers, and in this respect should be honoured, embraced and understood, and given our complete attention and concern.

Although Āyurvedic medicine considers the nature of ***vikara*** as being profound and important, others might argue that some disease is a meaningless, random event. In many cases it seems as though a disease is unrelated to factors of personal responsibility, such as influenza or the plague that appear to affect people indiscriminately. According to Āyurvedic medicine there is no disease that is a random event: it is solidly built on the foundation of previous actions, some of which may be beyond our ability to fully comprehend, especially if we insist upon finding a *single* causative factor. Thus, rather than simply attributing an epidemic to a viral or bacterial pathogen, Āyurvedic medicine always considers co-factors such as diet, lifestyle and the environment. Thus, in the case of epidemic disease an Āyurvedic physician would analyse individual factors such ***agni*** and ***ojas***, and then regard the time of season and the health of the surrounding ecology. Treatments would be given to control the disease in a symptomatic way, but ultimately the treatment is directed towards strengthening ***agni*** and nourishing ***ojas***, and making any modifications to the environment as seems necessary.

In the Western medical model, and even in the later teachings of Āyurveda, a great deal of emphasis is placed upon the differentiation of disease states. While this is a practical approach, it is a process that inevitably leads to the fragmentation of knowledge. To some extent this process is complete in Āyurvedic medicine, because as a classical science the number of basic diseases has not been added to for centuries. In contrast, the number of diseases described in modern medicine is ever-increasing, despite being hampered by a comparatively limited materia medica. Modern medicine has thus become increasingly specialised, such that it is rare nowadays to find a medical doctor who has skills in a variety of specialties, such as gastroenterology, obstetrics and infectious disease. In comparison, Āyurvedic physicians traditionally worked with all kinds of diseases, in both genders, with the young and old, and even treated domesticated animals such as horses and cows. Āyurvedic physicians profess to practice the 'knowledge' (***veda***) of 'life' (***āyus***), and thus specialise in understanding the manifestation of this life principle and the individual living bodies that arise from it. From an Āyurvedic perspective there are quite possibly as many diseases as there are people that experience them, because each state of illness arises from unique physical, emotional, mental and spiritual factors. These factors are then assessed according to relativistic theories such as ***tridoṣa*** and ***agniṣomiya*** (***agni*** and ***ojas***). The advantage that Āyurveda has over the fragmented science of pathology is that disease can be understood as a manifestation of relatively simple principles, regarding the body as a whole, and attempting to understand the flux manifested in the ***doṣas***. As the ***Aṣṭāñga Hṛdaya*** states, '. . . the physician who knows not the name of the disease, but recognises and understands the influence of the ***doṣas***, need never be embarrassed'.

8.2 *Pañcavidha kāraṇa*: THE FIVE CAUSES OF DISEASE

Āyurveda clearly states that all disease is made manifest through the increase and vitiation of the ***doṣas***. Generally speaking, there are five basic factors that affect the ***doṣas***:

1. ***Asātmyeñdriyārtha***: the improper correlation of sense objects (stimuli) with the ***jñāna indriyās*** ('sense organs')
2. ***Prajñaparādha***: crimes against wisdom
3. ***Kāla*** and ***deśa***: seasonal, climatic, ecological and geological factors
4. ***Karma***: the cause and effect relationship of thoughts and actions generated through the repetitive cycles of birth, life and death
5. ***Āma***: toxins and retained waste products, derived endogenously or exogenously.

8.3 *Asātmyeñdriyārtha*: SENSE AND SENSE OBJECTS IN DISEASE

As the first causes of disease, ***asātmyeñdriyārtha*** is divided into three separate categories relating to the use of one's senses.

Atiyoga

The first misuse of the senses is ***atiyoga***, in which one or more of the five senses (i.e. nose, tongue, eye, skin or ear) are over-used or over-stimulated:

Smell: to expose oneself to excessively heavy, sharp or pungent fragrances and perfumes.

Taste: to over-indulge while eating, or eating too much of one particular food item.

Sight: to stare excessively at a certain object, or at bright objects.
Touch: to expose oneself to extreme temperatures, or engage in excessive and indulgent forms of tactile stimuli on a chronic basis.
Hearing: to listen to loud or stimulating sounds.

Hīnāyoga

Hīnāyoga is the under-usage of the senses, something that is perhaps not all that common in our comparatively over-stimulated society. A good example would be a form of asceticism that deprives certain kinds of sensory experience, or chronically emphasising one kind of sensory experience over another. We have been given all five senses to use for our spiritual development and to ignore any one of them is to deprive ourselves of true spiritual growth. Remember that each of the ***pañcabhūtas*** are manifest in the ***tanmātrās***, and each of these stimulates a specific ***jñāna indriya***. It is only through understanding the subtle nature of sense that we gain true insight into the nature of reality. Examples of under-usage are:
Smell: the avoidance of otherwise pleasing fragrances or odours.
Taste: excessive fasting, or eating an unvaried diet.
Sight: to not move the eyes around, change one's focus or remain in darkness for long periods of time.
Touch: to avoid physical affection and touch.
Hearing: to avoid the sound of voices or music.

Mithyāyoga

Mithyāyoga is the distorted or unnatural usage of the senses, either the over-use or under-use for an end that is destructive to oneself or another being. In many respects the insatiable desires of the Western world for certain commodities deprives those that produce them from living complete and whole lives. One example might be our craving for sugar that results in vast tracks of monocultured sugar cane, produced with herbicides and pesticides that have replaced traditional crops in developing countries. The social repercussions of such desires change social and cultural patterns in these countries, where traditional sustainable values are discarded for the fragmentation of industrialisation. ***Mithyāyoga*** would also indicate the pleasure taken in harming or torturing another individual, or the pleasure taken in watching such acts (even in the form of the so-called 'horror movie'). Examples of distorted usage are:
Smell: to expose oneself to toxic, putrid and otherwise harmful odours.
Taste: to not follow appropriate dietary guidelines, to consume spoilt, foul or toxic foods.
Sight: to strain the eyes by focusing on tiny or distant objects, to watch lewd, horrifying and violent acts.
Touch: to touch broken and uneven surfaces or unclean objects, to cause physical pain.
Hearing: to listen to the sound of someone screaming or moaning in pain, to expose oneself to harsh and fearful sounds.

8.4 *Prajñaparādha*: CRIMES AGAINST WISDOM

The second cause of disease according to Āyurveda is ***prajñaparādha*** (lit. 'crimes against wisdom'). These are acts performed by a person with body, mind or speech whose comprehension, intelligence, intent or memory is deranged in some fashion. There are 12 aspects:

1. Forced expulsion or suppression of natural urges

Such activities generally upset the flow of ***vāta*** in the body and cause its vitiation. Āyurveda lists 13 bodily urges that should not be suppressed, as follows, which also describes the result of their suppression:

(a) Sleep: insomnia, exhaustion, headaches, depletes ***ojas***
(b) Crying: eye diseases, throat diseases, disrupts ***prāṇa***
(c) Sneezing: headache, trigeminal neuralgia, respiratory disorders
(d) Breathing: dyspnoea, cough, depletes ***ojas***
(e) Belching: cough, hiccough, dyspnoea, palpitations
(f) Yawning: tremors, numbness, convulsions, disrupts ***prāṇa***
(g) Vomiting: nausea, oedema, fever, skin diseases
(h) Eating: low appetite, malabsorption, hypoglycaemia, mental/emotional irritation
(i) Drinking: thirst, dehydration, constipation, fatigue, urinary disorders
(j) Urination: urinary disorders, lower backache, headache

(k) Ejaculation: prostatic hypertrophy, incontinence, insomnia, mental/emotional frustration
(l) Defecation: constipation, abdominal pain, bloating, dysuria, poor appetite, autotoxicity, spasm
(m) Flatulence: constipation, abdominal pain, bloating, dysuria, joint pain.

2. Indulgence in violence

This refers to, as well as overt physical violence, any harm wished upon another being, or actions by which we injure another being in any sense. When we take out our anger, rage or frustration on another being we generate unwholesome ***karma*** and perpetuate the cycle of violence. We should instead look to why it is we are experiencing these feelings and find appropriate ways to vent their expression, and find peaceful solutions to problems in which violence or aggression seems like the only answer.

3. Over-indulgence in sexual activity

This point refers specifically to men, who are considered to have a finite sexual capacity that fluctuates according to age and seasonal influences (see Ch. 4). It also refers, however, to excessive sexual activity to the extent that it becomes indulgent, interfering with ***dharma*** ('duties and obligations') and ***artha*** ('generation of wealth and abundance'). In ancient India sexuality was never viewed as inherently 'bad' or 'dirty' as it was in the West, but rather, as a natural and celebrated form of human expression. Some Āyurvedic texts such as the ***Aṣṭāñga Hṛdaya*** even contain rather 'steamy' passages that deal with sexuality, but later texts such as the ***Bhāvaprakāsa*** have a fairly rigid and patriarchal approach.[20] Although ***kama*** ('pleasure') is an essentially positive and worthy pursuit, like all indulgent acts sensuality and sexuality are thought to contain illusory elements that can blind us to deeper insights, and thus confuse our actions such that sexuality becomes an end in and of itself.

4. Postponement of healing a disease

When any disease manifests, Āyurveda considers this to be a clarion call from our higher self to attend to the maintenance of health and equilibrium. By not acknowledging illness or taking the appropriate measures to treat it, illness and disease worsen, and lead to an increasingly poor prognosis.

5. Inappropriate treatments

Āyurveda suggests that we should seek the most appropriate form of treatment for any imbalance or disease, one that seeks to resolve the fundamental issue rather than suppressing the symptoms. Many treatments employed by modern medicine are orientated towards symptom management instead of prevention and cure, and are thus regarded as a ***prajñaparādha*** ('crime against wisdom').

6. Disregard for modesty and customs

This point refers to appropriate and inappropriate behaviours in specific social contexts. Āyurveda counsels us to be respectful of majority opinions and practices, which creates trust and faith in our actions. Being mindful of social customs integrates us within the social dynamic and removes restrictions upon how others see us, allowing us to fulfil our ***dharma*** with the least hindrance. It also allows others to feel that they have space to be who they are, even if you are proposing change or reform.

7. Disrespect to the venerable and the aged

Āyurveda counsels us to show utmost respect and courtesy to those who have attained significant positions of (spiritual) influence, and honour our elders and seniors for their life experience and practical wisdom. This does not mean that one needs to sacrifice one's integrity, only create a space for the venerable that is open-minded, non-judgemental and respectful. Most traditional cultures revolve around the decisions and insights of their elders, whereas in our increasingly puerile society, elders and seniors are obsolete, sequestered away in senior centres and resorts far away from the children and adolescents who could best benefit from their grace, compassion and wisdom.

8. Travelling at improper times and in improper places

Āyurveda traditionally acknowledges certain times of the year that are considered to be bad times to travel, especially when the weather is poor. Travel during autumn (***varṣa***) was typically avoided, and even the wandering ***sannyasin*** ('religious ascetic') would temporarily take up residence in a village or a monastery until the weather improved. During ***varṣa***, ***vāta*** is already said to be in an increased state, and thus excessive movements such as travelling will compound the effects of this seasonal tendency and promote the vitiation of ***vāta***. Certain places such as burial grounds and cemeteries were traditionally considered to be dangerous places to be at certain times, such as during a full moon, or in the middle of the night.

9. Friendship with those who commit crimes against wisdom

Āyurveda suggests that by maintaining friendships with persons who have little or no moral character we expose ourselves to negative influences that may cause us to commit ***prajñaparādha***. Āyurveda states that these people do not need to be judged, reviled and rejected, but that we should maintain a certain distance that prevents us from coming under their direct influence.

10. Abandoning good habits

Indulgent attitudes such as 'just this once', are behaviours that, when taken alone, may seem harmless but provide precedents for repeated incident. Although these influences are often hidden until after the act has been committed, the effect of these habits begins to accumulate and promote imbalance, both in mind and body. Firmness and discipline of mind and body, as well as compassion for one's weakness, is the only way to address such behaviours. The satisfaction of maintaining this kind of integrity, despite the inconvenience that it can cause, allows for the continuous flow of spiritual energy.

11. Negative thoughts and emotions

Although it is difficult to inhibit negative thoughts altogether, Āyurveda suggests that we need to actively create feelings of love, compassion and charity to counter them, and direct these positive feelings towards ourselves and all other living beings. We might be inclined to think that our lives are difficult and unfair, but if we can find even just one thing to be thankful for we have the seed of how to change our lives. We see that true satisfaction comes when we turn inward, and at least feel that awesome power that sustains each of us, which truly loves us, and become grounded in this. We cease comparing ourselves to others, developing externalised criteria for happiness: we love ourselves so completely that it becomes a great romance, a profound love. This is the ***sattvic*** power of ***ahaṃkāra***, recognised by the Buddha in the ***Anguttara nikāya***, who, in his journey for enlightenment, found that 'in whatever quarter of heaven I searched, none could I find whom I loved as dearly as myself'. This great love affair is recognised as a facet of all living beings, and is thus honoured, respected and shared because it is good and leads to happiness. The heart is opened and we become a well-spring of our own divine beauty. Eventually this, too, is seen as a kind of subtle self-deception, however, and we know that even positive thoughts can cloud the intelligence. True wisdom is manifest only in the equanimity and freedom of ***buddhi*** ('pure awareness').

12. Over, under or perverted usage of the body, mind and speech

This point has been covered under ***sadvṛtta*** in Chapter 4. Āyurveda states that all thoughts, words and actions generate ***karma***, and at some point in the future these actions will come back to haunt us. If we are lucky, these bad events happen soon after the act has been perpetrated, and we see a cause and effect relationship and an immediate opportunity to remove an obstruction. If we are unlucky this ripening may manifest at some distant point in the future, even in another life, where a cause and effect relationship is difficult to perceive and may provoke an unskilful response.

8.5 *Pariṇāma*: SEASONAL AND CLIMATIC FACTORS IN DISEASE

The third cause of disease, called ***pariṇāma***, relates to periods (***kāla***) of seasonal and climatic changes and distortions. Like ***asātmyeñdriyārtha***, these factors can be understood to be of three types: ***atiyoga*** ('excess'), ***hīnāyoga*** ('deficient') and ***mithyāyoga*** ('distorted'). ***Atiyoga kāla*** relates to excessively hot weather or extended periods of rain, which can affect both ***pitta*** and ***vāta***. ***Hīnāyoga*** refers to excessively cold or dry weather, which affects ***kapha*** and ***vāta***. ***Mithyāyoga*** refers to unseasonable weather, particularly in the transitional periods between seasons (***ṛtusandhi***), and can aggravate any of the three ***doṣas***. ***Pariṇāma*** however also indicates an ecological perspective upon disease: that excess, deficiencies and distortions in the natural environment create disease in humans and other living creatures. This suggests that the human relationship with the natural environment should be respectfully maintained and cultivated.

8.6 *Karma* AND DISEASE

The fourth cause of disease is the ripening of unwholesome ***karmic*** fruits, which manifest only when the conditions are right for them to do so. In some respects it is a highly esoteric subject but one that cannot be avoided, especially when we confront the issue of disease. If disease is indeed a manifestation totally or in part due to ***karmic*** influences then the opportunity to see disease and death as a healing journey cannot be over-estimated. According to ***jyotiṣ***, or Vedic astrology, specific ***karmic*** influences can be seen in an astrological chart by the position of ***Śani*** ('Saturn'), ***Rāhu*** ('lunar north node') and ***Ketu*** ('lunar south node'). Specific regimens such as the repetition of ***mantra***, the performance of good works (***karma yoga***), asking a deity for assistance (***bhakti yoga***), the wearing of certain colours, precious metals and gem stones, and avoiding negative thoughts can all be utilised to negate the effects of unwholesome ***karma***, but nothing may stop its effects entirely.

8.7 *Āma* AND DISEASE

The fifth and final cause of disease is ***āma***, the metabolic and psychological residue that impairs the function of the body, mind and senses. By disrupting the flow of energy in the body, ***āma*** promotes the vitiation of ***vāta***, the ***doṣa*** most associated with the disease process. ***Āma*** is easily recognised by ***kaphaja*** symptoms such as lethargy, fatigue, a lack of enthusiasm, mucoid congestion, weak digestion, constipation, abdominal distension, orbital oedema, rectal itching and a thick coating on the tongue. ***Āma*** can associate with any ***doṣa***, especially in ***vāttika*** conditions, in which the patient becomes weak and thin while continuing to display what might be considered ***kaphaja*** symptoms. The concept of ***āma*** was introduced in Chapter 4, and is explored further in Chapters 9 and 10.

8.8 *Rogamārgas*: THE PATHWAYS OF DISEASE

Āyurveda recognises three pathways of disease (***rogamārgas***), or three distinct levels in which disease will manifest in the body. The first pathway of disease is the 'inner pathway' or ***añtarmārga***, consisting of the digestive and respiratory systems. Although it is called the 'inner pathway', it is actually the most superficial level that disease can manifest in, and is thus comparatively easy to treat. Examples of conditions that manifest on this level include vomiting, gastritis, abdominal bloating, constipation, diarrhoea, piles, coughing, dyspnoea and fever. Treatments typically consist of internal therapies such as ingestion, inhalation and enema.

The second pathway of disease is the ***bāhya rogayana***, or 'outer pathway', consisting of the circulatory, lymphatic and integumentary systems. The outer pathway of disease is a little more difficult to treat, as conditions within this pathway can be considered to be conditions of the inner pathway that have been driven deeper, from the gastric and respiratory mucosa into the blood, lymph and skin. Examples of conditions on this level include eczema, acne, boils, psoriasis, granuloma, warts, swollen lymph nodes, oedema and arterial disease. Treatments for the ***bāhya rogayana*** typically consist of internal therapies in combination with external therapies such as ***svedana*** ('diaphoresis').

The third pathway of disease is the ***madhyama rogamārga*** or 'middle pathway', consisting of deeper, harder to reach tissues such as the nervous and endocrine systems, the kidneys, heart, bones and muscles. It is the deepest level in which a disease can manifest, and also represents the most difficult kind of disease to treat. It is called the 'middle pathway' because it is sandwiched between the other two levels, making accessibility difficult. Examples of conditions on this level include paralysis, mental disorders, seizures, wasting, osteoporosis, rheumatoid arthritis, renal failure and heart disease. Typically, a combination of both internal and topical therapies will be required.

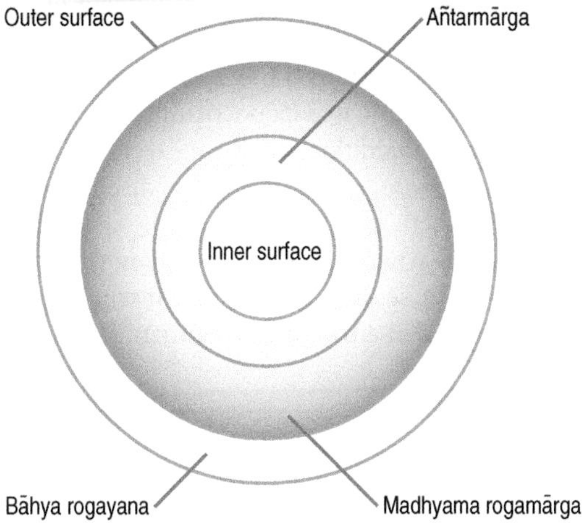

Figure 8.1 The rogamārgas.

8.9 *Vyādhyāvasthā*: THE PATHOGENESIS OF THE DISEASE

As we have learned in the previous sections, the ***doṣas*** are responsible for all negative changes in the body, not as causal agents per se, but as mediators of internal and external influences. In Chapter 2 we learned how to identify the ***doṣas*** according to their ***lakṣaṇas*** ('symptoms') and how they undergo ***caya*** ('increase') and ***kopa*** ('vitiation'). In truth, this process is only a simplified description of ***vyādhyāvasthā*** ('pathogenesis'), in which three separate categories are recognised:

1. ***Ṣatkriyākālas***: sixfold progression of ***doṣa*** increase, vitiation and disease manifestation
2. ***Vegavasthā*** and ***avegavasthā***: exacerbatory and remissive symptoms
3. ***Doṣapāka avasthā***: the digestion and removal of ***āma***.

Ṣatkriyākālas

The first classification of ***vyādhyāvasthā*** describes a sixfold process of pathogenesis, in which the ***doṣas*** go through progressive stages called the ***ṣatkriyākālas***:

1. ***Caya*** (**'accumulation'**): the ***doṣa***(***s***) undergo ***caya*** ('increase') in their ***sthānas*** (lit. 'seat' or 'location'): ***vāta*** in the ***antra*** ('colon') and ***vasti*** ('urinary bladder'); ***pitta*** in the ***āmāśaya*** ('stomach and duodenum') and ***yakrit*** ('liver'); and ***kapha*** in the ***hṛdaya*** ('heart') and ***phuphphusa*** ('lungs').
2. ***Prakopa*** (**'aggravation'**): the ***doṣa***(***s***) undergo further increase within their respective sites (***sthāna***) and begin to manifest as amorphous health issues, as a sense of physical uneasiness that is indiscernible but definitely noticeable.
3. ***Prasāra*** (**'migration'**): the increased ***doṣa***(***s***) now begin to migrate from their respective ***sthānas*** into other locations of the body, settling in weak areas of the body.
4. ***Sthānasaṃśraya*** (**'localisation'**): the ***doṣa***(***s***) now settle into weakened ***dhātus***, and begin to alter their function.
5. ***Vyakti*** (**'manifestation'**): the ***doṣa***(***s***) now begin to manifest discernible signs and symptoms, mostly in the acute stage. At this stage the disease can be classified, and the specific characteristic of the ***doṣas*** can be identified.
6. ***Bheda*** (**'fruition'**): the nature of the condition becomes chronic and the debilitating effects of the disease become manifest. The person afflicted with the disease becomes weakened and treatment becomes progressively more difficult.

Vegavasthā and *avegavasthā*

The second classification of ***vyādhyāvasthā*** is ***vegavasthā***, the stage 'during the attack' (acute symptoms), and ***avegavasthā***, the stage 'between the attack' (chronic or remissive symptoms). The knowledge of these states allows the practitioner to establish a clear line of treatment. During ***vegavasthā*** the treatment consists of balancing the ***doṣas*** (***śamana***), while during ***avegavasthā*** the treatment is focused on removing the cause of the disease (***śodhana***), strengthening digestion (***dīpanapācana***) or attending to rejuvenation (***rasāyana***).

Doṣapāka avasthā

The third classification of ***vyādhyāvasthā*** is ***doṣapāka avasthā***. The term ***paka*** means 'digestion', and it is at this stage that ***āma*** becomes separated from the ***doṣas*** and ***dhātus*** and is digested. The ***doṣas*** also begin to normalise and move to the ***koṣṭha*** (lit. 'digestive tract', but referring to all aspects of elimination).

Doṣapāka avasthā is noted by such symptoms as a normalisation of body temperature, lightness of the body, renewed sensory perception, increased strength and an improvement in mental and emotional clarity. Such symptoms indicate a good prognosis, and it is usually at this stage that therapies such as ***pañca karma*** are most favourable (see Ch. 11). Although they can bear some resemblance to one another, ***doṣapāka avasthā*** must be clearly separated from ***avegavasthā***, and vice versa.

8.10 *Dvividha roga*: THE TWO KINDS OF DISEASE

Āyurveda identifies two basic pathological processes: that which is a 'primary manifestation' (***svātantra***), and that which is a 'secondary manifestation' or a sequela (***paratantra***). ***Svātantra*** diseases are easily identified, and have specific causes and easily recognisable symptoms and signs. In contrast, ***paratantra*** diseases are opposite in nature and do not have specific causes, nor do they manifest in predictable or easily discernible ways. ***Paratantra*** diseases are the sequelae (secondary conditions) of ***svātantra*** diseases, and thus their treatment is dependent upon the removal of the primary condition. If during treatment, however, the sequelae of the primary disease remain unchanged, then specific treatment is also given to them. In cases where the signs and symptoms of the sequelae are worse than the primary disease, they are given preference in a treatment regimen.

ENDNOTE

20 Most historians agree that ancient India has fairly strong matriarchal roots, but in response to successive invasions by Arabs, Persians and Europeans during the medieval period India became an increasingly patriarchial society, in which women and sexuality became increasingly limited in their expression. India is only now reclaiming its heritage in this regard, such as the efforts made by the government in the state of Kerala to promote economic and societal prosperity by ensuring literacy among women.

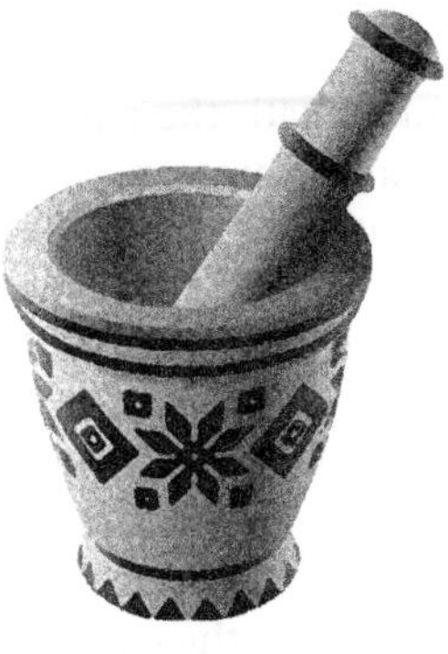

Chapter 9

CLINICAL METHODOLOGY AND CASE HISTORY

OBJECTIVES

- To review the clinical methodology of Āyurveda.
- To review case history techniques in Āyurveda.

9.1 *Nidāna*: CLINICAL ASSESSMENT

In Chapter 8 we learned that ***vikara*** ('disease') and its various synonyms are classified according to the concept of ***nidāna***, which means 'causes'. ***Nidāna*** is the model of aetiology and pathology in Āyurvedic medicine, and under this practice the signs and symptoms of a patient are classified according to specific criteria, assessed by a thorough examination of the case history (***daśavidha parīkṣā***), physical observation (***pratyakṣa***), and specialised assessment techniques (***aṣṭāsthāna parīkṣā***). Chapter 9 details the components of ***daśavidha parīkṣā***, or the 'ten methods of assessment' used to analyse the case history, whereas Chapter 10 details the ***aṣṭāsthāna parīkṣā***, eight specialised assessment techniques, including pulse and tongue diagnosis.

9.2 *Trividha parīkṣā*: THREE SOURCES OF KNOWLEDGE

Before we can even begin to study the patient, Caraka tells us that we must consider three basic sources of knowledge when gathering the evidence to support any kind of therapeutic regimen. These are ***āptopadeśa***, ***pratyakṣa*** and ***anumāna***.

Āptopadeśa

Āptopadeśa is derived from the term '***aptas***', referring to persons whose memory and comprehension are sound and complete. Specifically, Caraka tells us that ***āptopadeśa*** refers to wise teachings that help us understand the nature of health and disease, such as

Āyurveda. In context with ***nidāna*** however, ***āptopadeśa*** means 'interrogation', referring to questions asked of the patient, family and friends to determine the case history.

Pratyakṣa

Pratyakṣa means 'direct observation', or the use of one's own senses and mind to observe the patient. This includes techniques such as visual observation, auscultation, percussion, palpation and odour. When the patient complains of digestive disorders, for example, this may include observing the abdomen for distension, protuberances or discolorations, listening to the abdomen for borborygmi (intestinal gurgling), tapping the abdomen to determine the nature of the abdominal distension, gently pressing upon the different areas of the abdomen to determine the presence of any swellings or masses, and smelling the patient's breath.

Anumāna

Anumāna are factors in the patient's health that cannot be observed directly. For example, if a patient complains of a bad taste in their mouth this cannot be observed or experienced directly. Instead, an Āyurvedic physician must rely upon the 'case history' (***āptopadeśa***) by asking the patient questions, and by utilising specialised techniques of 'inference' (***anumāna***). For example, Caraka mentions that flies are more often attracted to a person who has a sweet taste in his or her mouth, which generally speaking denotes an increase of ***kapha***. Similarly, Caraka states that the determination of ***raktapitta***, a haemorrhagic disease caused by ***pitta***, can be tested by having a dog taste the blood – if the dog rejects the blood then the bleeding disease is inferred to be ***raktapitta***. Thus ***anumāna*** is any source of medical information that is arrived at purely through inferential means, no matter how simple, skilled or unique the techniques are. Although ***anumāna*** refers specifically to those techniques mentioned under ***aṣṭāsthāna parīkṣā*** (see Ch. 10), one could consider certain medical tests as a kind of ***anumāna*** since these tests do not describe the nature of a disease, only a temporary fragment or snapshot of the blood, urine, saliva, etc., and should be carefully interpreted in context with the patient's case history and physical signs and symptoms.

Caraka states that it is of the utmost importance to base any therapy upon these three aspects of knowledge, first beginning with one's own training and the case history of the patient (***āptopadeśa***), and then through direct observation (***pratyakṣa***) and then specialised diagnostic techniques (***anumāna***). When any one of these three aspects in data collection is ignored, or if one is overemphasised (as is often the case with blood tests, pulse diagnosis, etc.), Caraka states that the knowledge obtained is fallible. Fallibility in assessment leads an inaccurate diagnosis and ineffective or even harmful treatments.

9.3 CRITERIA FOR PHYSICIANS, PATIENTS AND TREATMENT LOCATION

Healing best occurs when the physician acts with wisdom, when the patient maintains the best mental state and actions conducive for healing, and when the environment is well-suited for healing to take place. Caraka states that the physician should be pure from both mental as well as physical defilements, possessing all the normal sense faculties as well as the necessary equipment to undertake clinical assessment. The physician should be an expert in the observation of life and its various manifestations, and should have studied the medical texts and committed them to memory. The physician should also have practical experience in the treatment of disease, and should display this skill in assessment as well as in the analysis of the condition and in the determination of the treatment. Physicians are also counselled by Caraka to be sympathetic and kind to all patients, and reside in a state of equanimity regardless of prognosis. This later point is particularly germane, especially with novice physicians, who have a tendency to take the progress of their patient somewhat personally.

The qualities of the patient are also important to consider, and in ancient texts such as the ***Aṣṭāṅga Hṛdaya*** and the ***Caraka Saṃhitā*** physicians are encouraged only to work with patients who listen to and practice the advice given to them. It is important that the patient has a strong will power and control over the senses, and is capable of accurately reporting the details of his or her health to the attending physician. The Āyurvedic texts state that the physician should reject patients who are ungrateful, rude and impolite, those who are sceptical or afraid of the treatment regimen, those who have no will power, or those patients that are constantly in a hurry and too busy to follow through with the recommendations. Although it is the duty of physicians to be compassionate, Āyurveda suggests that the physicians should not hesitate to distance themselves from bad patients, in order to protect their honour and the honour of the medicine.

According to Caraka the clinic or hospital should be designed by an architect trained in ***vastu śāstra***, the ancient science of Indian architecture. In many respects ***vastu śāstra*** bears some similarity to the better-known Chinese system of feng shui. According to ***vastu śāstra***, the building is viewed as a body composed of different energies that are represented by different deities. For example, the very centre of the house corresponds with Brahmā, the Lord of Creation, and is traditionally left empty (such as a courtyard) to invite Brahmā into the heart of the home. ***Vastu śāstra*** states that disease can occur in someone who lives in a house that was not built properly, and that the location or type of disease may indicate the afflicated part of the house.

The building should be strong and well-built in a location free from high winds, although it should be constructed in such a way that gentle winds can pass through it if desired, freshening the interior environment. The building should not be built in mountainous places (for lack of accessibility), and nor should it be located next to a bigger building (which brings misfortune upon it). Dusty locations, wet environments, or locations with foul or toxic smells should be rejected as building sites. The attendants that work in the clinic or hospital should be enthusiastic, skilled and compassionate. Caraka states that people well versed in music and poetry should also be encouraged to participate in the healing centre. Outside the building a herb and vegetable garden should supply medications and food for the clinic or hospital, and certain animals, such as a cow and her calf, and birds such as quail and partridge, should be kept by the facility for the benefit and enjoyment of the patients and faculty.

9.4 *Nidāna pañcakam*: THE FIVE METHODS OF INVESTIGATION

There are five methods by which an Āyurvedic physician gathers clinical information to formulate a diagnosis, called ***nidāna pañcakam***. They are:

1. ***Nidāna***: aetiology of the disease
2. ***Pūrvarūpa***: prodromal symptoms
3. ***Rūpa***: symptomology
4. ***Upashya*** and ***anupaśaya***: trial and error
5. ***Saṃprāpti***: pathology.

Nidāna

Nidāna as 'aetiology' refers to the causative factor of disease (***vikara***), the basic components of which have already been discussed in Chapter 8. Since the ***nidāna*** or cause of a specific disease may be the same for another disease, such as the consumption of unwholesome foods or lack of sleep, ***nidāna*** alone cannot provide enough information to diagnose a specific disease, and thus more information is required.

Pūrvarūpa

Pūrvarūpa are the premonitory symptoms, or generalised symptoms that appear before the appearance of a disease. In some cases these symptoms are non-specific, such as fatigue in ***jvara*** ('fever'), and do not indicate the involvement of a specific ***doṣa***. In other cases, however, the ***pūrvarūpas*** are highly specific. In the case of ***jvara*** for example, yawning is given as a ***pūrvarūpa*** of ***vātaja jvara***, burning sensations in the eyes for ***paittika jvara***, and a loss of appetite in ***kaphaja jvara***. The identification of specific ***pūrvarūpas*** may help in the early diagnosis of a disease, assisting in the efficacy of preventative treatments and in the differentiation of the syndrome from other conditions.

Rūpa

Rūpa are the signs and symptoms of ***doṣa*** vitiation that are characteristic of a particular syndrome or disease. In the earlier Vedic literature all disease is described as being one of two archetypal forms: ***takman*** (***jvara***), a disease of 'fever' and 'excess'; and

yakṣma (***kaśāya***), a disease of 'wasting' and 'deficiency'. In this respect ***takman*** represents the acute, immediate stage of disease, whereas ***yakṣma*** relates to the chronic, end-stage of disease. The comparatively later ***Caraka*** and ***Suśruta saṃhitās*** expand upon this simple dichotomy and enunciate several different diseases (or stages) that exist between them, and over the centuries the number of diseases gradually increased, finally culminating in the ***Mādhava nidānam*** (c. 7th century CE), a text that solely specialises in pathology. This approach of differentiating signs and symptoms into specific diseases appears obviously similar to modern pathology, but in actual fact diseases in Āyurveda are also arranged to illustrate the spectrum of different treatments within the ***takman*** and ***yakṣma*** dichotomy. In describing diseases such as ***jvara*** ('fever'), ***atisāra*** ('diarrhoea') and ***kasa*** ('cough') Āyurvedic medicine orientates the practitioner to a specific set of symptoms, as well as specific set of remedies that can be used to treat them, e.g. ***Guḍūcī*** (*Tinospora cordifolia*) for ***jvara***, ***Dāḍima*** (*Punica granatum*) for ***atisāra***, and ***Vāsaka*** (*Adhatoda vasica*) for ***kasa***, etc. While each disease category displays general characteristics it also contains potentially diverse manifestations based on the differing activities of the ***doṣas***, ***dhātus*** and ***malas***. Thus while ***jvara*** ('fever') is generally characterised by an increase in body temperature, secondary symptoms are based on the underlying manifestation of the ***doṣas***, identified by the ***guṇas*** each sign or symptom represents, for example:

- In ***vāttika jvara***, the ***rūpa*** is noted by qualities such as rapid temperature fluctuations (***cala***), dryness of the throat and lips (***rūkṣa***), insomnia (***śita***, ***laghu***), dehydration (***rūkṣa***, ***laghu***), headache (***śita***), constipation (***rūkṣa***), bloating (***laghu***, ***cala***), excessive yawning (***laghu***, ***cala***).
- In ***paittika jvara***, the ***rūpa*** is noted by qualities such as a very high and constant temperature (***uṣṇa***), diarrhoea (***sara***), insomnia (***uṣṇa***, ***laghu***), mucosal ulceration (***uṣṇa***, ***snigdha***), burning sensations (***uṣṇa***), and thirst (***uṣṇa***).
- In ***kaphaja jvara***, the ***rūpa*** is noted by qualities such as a feeling of coldness (***śita***), mild temperature increase (***śita***), lassitude (***guru***), stiffness (***śita***), nausea and vomiting (***śita***), horripilation (***śita***), mucus congestion (***snigdha***, ***śita***), rhinitis (***śita***, ***snigdha***), and a lack of appetite (***śita***, ***guru***).

As a result of understanding these subtypes of ***jvara*** we are inclined to use antifebrile herbs such as ***Guḍūcī*** (*Tinospora cordifolia*) in combination with herbs that are specific to the ***doṣa*** or ***doṣas*** manifest: for example, with ***Harītakī*** (*Terminalia chebula*) and ***saindhava*** in ***vātaja jvara***; with ***Uśīra*** (*Vettivera zizanioides*) and ***Candana*** (*Santalum album*) for ***paittika jvara***; and ***Kaṇṭakāri*** (*Solanum xanthocarpum*) and ***Śūṇṭhī*** (*Zingiber officinalis*) for ***kaphaja jvara***, etc. Thus each sign or symptom described as ***rūpa*** immediately announces its complement in nature, be it any influence, such as a herb, food, place, person, colour, ***mantra*** etc. What remains is for the Āyurvedic physician to understand, analyse and integrate these relationships. Even the most skilled Āyurvedic practitioner, however, may be unable to ascertain these relationships, and based on their best understanding will formulate a hypothesis, a method of trial and error called ***upaśaya*** and ***anupaśaya***.

Upaśaya and *anupaśaya*

The term ***upaśaya*** refers to the administration of treatments orientated to relieve the signs and symptoms of a given condition, and is of two types: ***viparīta upaśaya*** and ***viparītārthakāri upaśaya***. ***Viparīta upaśaya*** is the successful administration of medicaments that are opposite in nature to the condition being treated, essentially an allopathic effect ('opposite cures opposite'). For example, the Indian herb ***Pippalī*** fruit (***Piper longum***) displays qualities such as ***uṣṇa***, ***rūkṣa*** and ***laghu***, and these are used to counter the ***śita***, ***snigdha*** and ***guru*** nature of ***kaphaja*** diseases such as ***kasa*** ('cough'). Similarly, the ***rūkṣa*** and ***śita guṇas*** of ***Kuṭaja*** bark (*Holarrhena antidysenterica*) are used in ***paittika*** conditions such as ***atisāra*** ('diarrhoea'), and the ***uṣṇa*** and ***guru*** qualities of ***Aśvagandhā*** root (*Withania somnifera*) are used to counter ***vātaja*** diseases such as ***kaśāya*** ('consumption'). We could even consider the usage of drugs such as acetaminophen in the treatment of fever to be ***viparīta upaśaya***, although because acetaminophen only suppresses inflammation and does not resolve the underlying cause of the disease its usage could be considered a ***prajñaparādha*** ('crime against wisdom'), or ***vyādhi asātmya*** ('unwholesome').

The second classification of ***upaśaya***, called ***viparītārthakāri upaśaya***, is the administration of treatments that have qualities of a similar nature to the condition being treated but also bring relief. For example, an Āyurvedic physician might use the emetic herb **Madanaphala** (*Randia dumetorium*) in the treatment of vomiting, usually in doses well below those that could be considered to have a physiological effect. ***Viparītārthakāri upaśaya*** is an expression of the homeopathic axiom 'like cures like' coined by Samuel Hahnemann, an idea similarly found in almost every other traditional system of medicine, including those of ancient Mesopotamia and Egypt. Although Āyurvedic physicians are traditionally trained in some homeopathic treatments, in India, as well as in ancient Mesopotamia and Egypt, this class of treatment was more often a matter of religious and spiritual speculation and hence officiated by a class of skilled priests or spiritual intermediaries. With the evolution of a secular form of homeopathic medicine in the West, however, homeopathic principles in Āyurvedic medicine evolved into a separate system of 'Indian' or 'Āyurvedic' homeopathy, which is based on both Āyurvedic and modern homeopathic principles.

The opposite of ***upaśaya*** is ***anupaśaya***: treatments that promote a worsening of the signs and symptoms of a disease. ***Anupaśaya*** can be the result of treatments that are either similar or opposite to the qualities of the condition being treated. When ***anupaśaya*** occurs treatment is withdrawn immediately and a new approach is undertaken. It is important to distinguish ***anupaśaya*** from other clinical events, however, such as insufficient dosage, too high a dosage, and drug interactions.

Saṃprāpti

Saṃprāpti is the course by which a ***doṣa*** becomes vitiated and produces a specific disease. This is unlike ***vyadhavasthā*** described in Chapter 8, which is a more general model relating to the pathogenic influence of the ***doṣas***. ***Saṃprāpti*** is divided into five parts:

1. ***Sāṅkhya***: ***Sāṅkhya saṃprāpti*** is the enumeration of several distinct disease states, such as ***jvara*** (fever), ***chardi*** (vomiting) and ***kuṣṭha*** (skin disease), each with unique clinical features. In turn, each disease is then classified according to the ***doṣas***. ***Jvara*** for example, is classified into 25 categories, depending upon the state of the ***doṣas***, the duration of the condition, stress, injury, environmental influences, etc.
2. ***Vīkalpa***: ***Vīkalpa saṃprāpti*** is simply the recognition of the quality (***guṇa***) of a specific symptom and its correlation with a particular ***doṣa***. Thus the ***drava*** (liquid) alteration of the bowel movement in diarrhoea indicates ***pitta***, because ***drava*** is a ***guṇa*** of ***pitta***. Similarly, if the eyelids go into spasm, this is identified as excess movement (***cala***), and is correlated with ***vāta***.
3. ***Prādhānya***: ***Prādhānya saṃprāpti*** constitutes an analysis of which ***doṣa*** is the predominant ***doṣa*** in the pathology or pathologies, especially when a disease arises from the vitiation of two or more ***doṣas***.
4. ***Balā***: ***Balā saṃprāpti*** is an analysis of the strength of the disease, based on an assessment of the ***nidāna***, ***pūrvarūpas*** and ***rūpas***. If all three factors are clearly manifested then the disease is said to be severe, whereas if they are only partially manifested the disease would be classified as mild to moderate.
5. ***Kāla***: ***Kāla saṃprāpti*** is the analysis of biological, daily and seasonal influences that indicate the influence of the different ***doṣas*** in disease. In some cases it can be observed that a condition manifests only at a certain time of day. In ***kāsa*** (cough) for example, if the symptoms manifest only in the morning or the evening, then this would clearly be distinguished as a ***kaphaja kāsa***.

9.5 *Daśavidha parīkṣā*: TEN METHODS OF EXAMINATION

It is important that the practitioner gain a thorough knowledge of the patient's state prior to treatment, and Āyurvedic tradition suggests that case history taking should contain ten components, called ***daśavidha parīkṣā***:

1. ***Dūṣyam***: the state of the ***dhātus***
2. ***Kālam***: the staging or progression of the condition
3. ***Prakṛti***: the constitution of the patient
4. ***Vayaḥ***: the age of the patient
5. ***Balām***: the strength of the patient
6. ***Agni***: the digestive capacity of the patient
7. ***Sattva***: the mental and emotional state of the patient
8. ***Sātmya***: the lifestyle habits of the patient

9. ***Deśam***: the environment in which the patient lives
10. ***Āhāra***: the dietary habits of the patient.

9.6 *Dūṣyam*

For a disease to develop, there are three factors that must be present: a 'cause' or 'causes' (***nidāna***), the vitiation of the ***doṣas***, and the subsequent impact upon the ***dhātus***. A cause cannot act independently to initiate a disease, but does so only through the vitiation of the ***doṣ as***, which then act upon the ***dhātus*** to bring about their ***vṛddhi*** ('increase') and ***kaśāya*** ('decrease'). Each ***dhātu*** should thus be examined to determine its status, which will indicate which ***doṣas*** are involved in the illness:

Rasa

Vṛddhi: ***kapha lakṣaṇas***, e.g. of phlegm, mucus discharge.
Kaśāya: ***vāta lakṣaṇas***, e.g. dryness, fatigue, emaciation, impotency, infertility, increased sensitivity to sonic vibrations.

Rakta

Vṛddhi: ***pitta lakṣaṇas***, e.g. skin diseases, hepatomegaly, splenomegaly, hepatitis, jaundice, abscess with infection and inflammation, arthritis, gout, haemorrhages of the mouth, nose or anus (***rakta pitta***), reddish discoloration of the eyes, skin and urine.
Kaśāya: ***vātakapha lakṣaṇas***, e.g. desire for sour and warming foods, anaemia, hypotension, dryness of the body.

Māṃsa

Vṛddhi: ***kapha lakṣaṇas***, e.g. lymphadenitis, lymphadenopathy, goitre, malignant tumours, fibroids, abscesses, obesity.
Kaśāya: ***vāta lakṣaṇas***, e.g. emaciation, fatigue, a lack of coordination, muscular atrophy.

Medas

Vṛddhi: ***kapha lakṣaṇas***, e.g. fatigue, shortness of breath, sagging of breasts, buttocks and abdomen, obesity.
Kaśāya: ***vāta lakṣaṇas***, e.g. nervous irritability, weak eyesight, dryness, osteoarthritis, poor mineralisation, emaciation.

Asthi

Vṛddhi: ***kapha lakṣaṇas***, e.g. bone spurs, bone cancer, gigantism, acromegaly.
Kaśāya: ***vāta lakṣaṇas***, e.g. osteoporosis, brittle bones, splitting or cracking fingernails, alopecia, tooth decay.

Majjā

Vṛddhi: ***kapha lakṣaṇas***, e.g. heaviness, lassitude and hypertrophy, swelling of joints, muscular paralysis.
Kaśāya: ***vāta lakṣaṇas***, e.g. sensation of weakness or lightness in the bones, joint pain, rheumatism, vertigo, progressive blindness, loss of sensory function.

Śukra

Vṛddhi: ***kaphapitta lakṣaṇas***, e.g. insatiable sexual urges, seminal calculi, odorous perspiration, greasy skin, greasy hair, acne.
Kaśāya: ***vāta lakṣaṇas***, e.g. impotency, infertility, premature ejaculation, erectile dysfunction, chronic prostatitis, chronic urethritis.

Aṇḍāṇu

Vṛddhi: ***kaphapitta lakṣaṇas***, e.g. insatiable sexual urges, a consistently short oestrus cycle, odorous perspiration, greasy skin, greasy hair, acne.
Kaśāya: ***vāta lakṣaṇas***, e.g. frigidity, infertility, amenorrhoea, chronic leucorrhoea, premenstrual depression, menstrual blood which is pellet-like and malodorous, chronic menstrual pain.

9.7 *Kālam*

Kāla literally means 'time', and, in regard to the examination of the patient, refers to the progression or the staging of the condition or disease in relation to a therapeutic regimen. This is not to assess the progress of the condition in relation to biological rhythms or determine a prognosis as in ***kāla saṃprāpti***, so much as it is to understand the difference between the administration of a timely remedy (**kālaha**) and an untimely one (**akālah**). Even though a certain remedy could be helpful to the patient, it must be in accordance with the current signs and symptoms, but with the ultimate aim of re-establishing the balance between the **doṣas**, **dhātus** and **malas**. In the case of diarrhoea (**atisāra**), for example, remedies such as **Jātīphala** (*Myrsitica fragrans*) that are **stambhana** ('constipating', 'cooling') should not be used too soon. Instead the treatment should be directed to **agni** first with the use of **dīpanapācana** remedies. In another example, **kāla** could refer to the supplementation of iron and vitamin B complex in persons with a chronic bacterial infection. In this example, the vitamin–mineral combination could prove helpful to address an underlying nutritional deficiency, but should only be given after the infection has been completely resolved, as the bacteria can utilise these nutrients to assist in their own reproduction. Thus, **kāla** is the development of a treatment protocol based upon individual factors such as the staging or progression of the condition.

9.8 *Prakṛti*

The knowledge of the patient's **prakṛti** is helpful in determining their underlying strength (**balā**), in developing individualised preventative regimens, and in formulating a prognosis. In the latter case, a **vikṛti** that corresponds with the **prakṛti** is usually more difficult to treat.

The different **prakṛtis** are based upon the primary **guṇas** that they display. Tables 9.1–9.3 correlate the qualities of the **doṣas** with the physical characteristics that form the **prakṛti**.

9.9 *Vayaḥ*

Vayaḥ refers to the age of the patient and the life span. According to Caraka a variety of factors are involved in the determination of lifespan. These include the actions of previous lives as well as the actions of one's current life, such as the prevention of injury, the consumption of wholesome foods, the successful treatment of disease and the pursuit of

TABLE 9.1 ***Kapha prakṛti.***

Kapha guṇas	**Manifestations**
Guru	Heaviness and largeness of body; bones, veins and tendons well covered
Snigdha	Oiliness of body
Śita	Mild hunger and thirst, mild perspiration, dislikes cold
Mṛdu	Suppleness of tissues, pleasing appearance
Sthira	Slow in initiating activity, slow and deliberate movement; slow digestion
Picchila	Smoothly gliding joints, smoothness of skin, clarity of complexion

TABLE 9.2 ***Pitta prakṛti.***

Pitta guṇas	**Manifestations**
Uṣṇa	Intolerance of hot things, ruddy complexion, increased density of moles and freckles, thin hair
Tikṣṇa	Strong hunger and strong thirst, angular features
Snigdha	Moistness of body
Laghu	More muscular, less fat
Drava	Increased excretion of the *malas* (perspiration, faeces and urine)
Sara	Physically active, moves quickly

TABLE 9.3 ***Vāta prakṛti.***

Vāta guṇas	**Manifestations**
Laghu	Thinness of body; bones, tendons and veins prominent
Śita	Intolerance of cold, stiffness
Rūkṣa	Dryness and coarseness of skin and hair; dry faeces
Cala	Constantly moving, active, fidgety
Viśada	Cracking and popping of the joints
Sūkṣma	Instability in movement

spiritual happiness. In Āyurvedic terms, the life span is divided into three parts:

1. ***Bālya*** ('child' hood): Childhood encompasses the time from birth onwards until puberty (***vṛddhi***). During childhood it is said that ***kapha*** is the predominant ***doṣa***, indicated by the soft, fat and moist bodies of children, and the minor congestive conditions that often occur as the immune system develops. Psychologically, however, the dominant ***doṣa*** during childhood is ***vāta***, as children are highly suggestive, sensitive and attuned to both negative and positive influences in their environment.
2. ***Madhya*** ('middle' age): Middle age encompasses the time from puberty until the first stages of physical degeneration (***parihāni***) begin to manifest, by about the age of 60 or 70. The height of middle age occurs in the 3rd and 4th decades in which the body is full grown (***sampūrṇata***), and the person is at the height of their physical prowess, skill and mental aptitude. During this time ***pitta*** is the dominant ***doṣa*** both physically and psychologically, accounting for the ability to understand one's duties and responsibilities and project one's will in the world.
3. ***Jīrṇa*** ('old' age): Old age encompasses the period of time from the first stages of physical degeneration until death; that is from the 6th and 7th decades onwards. Physically, this time is marked by the influence of ***vāta***, indicated by the encroaching influences of cold, dry and light qualities that promote physical degeneration and a gradual decline in strength, memory, speech and courage. Psychologically this period of life most closely resembles that of ***kapha***, and many seniors can be seen to display ***kaphaja*** qualities such as compassion, sentimentality and generosity, although psychological factors are also affected by the increasing influence of ***vāta***, which in conjunction with ***kapha*** can promote psychological traits such as confusion, lethargy and dullness of mind.

Based on the concept of ***prakṛti***, ***kaphaja prakṛtis*** are stated to have the longest lifespan, followed by ***pittaja prakṛti***, and then ***vātaja prakṛti***, which typically has the shortest. Apart from ***prakṛti***, a variety of Āyurvedic texts provide a number of features that can be used to determine health and longevity. When a baby was born a number of factors were taken into consideration to determine potential longevity. According to Caraka there is a specific symmetry in babies that generally indicates a long life. The ears should be large and thick, with large lobes and a large tragus (the auricular cartilage anterior to the external meatus). The forehead should be broad and have three transverse lines, and the hair on the head should be soft, moist and thick. The nose should be straight and the nasal bone wide, the jaw should be broad and large, and the lips should be neither very thin nor very thick. The neck should be neither thin nor thick, and the chest should be broad. The arms and hands should be large and plump, and the nails of the hand should be firm, round, and slightly convex. The waist should be less than three-quarters the width of the chest. The buttocks should be round, firm and plump. The thighs should be round and plump, and taper downwards. The calves, ankles and feet should be rounded and soft, and be neither excessively thin nor too thick.

In adults, the ***Aṣṭāñga Hṛdaya*** indicates that the hair should be soft, the forehead high, and the ears should be thick and broad. The sclera of the eyes should be white, and demonstrate a clear demarcation between the iris and sclera, the eyes protected by thick eyelashes. The nose should have a slightly elevated tip, with a straight and full septum. The lips should be red and thick, the lower jaw and chin fully developed, the teeth large, thick, smooth and evenly placed, and the tongue pink, broad and thin. The neck should be short, thick and round, and the shoulders should be firm and muscular. The abdomen should be firm, even, and smooth, and the umbilicus with a right whorl. The nails should be pink, smooth, thick, convex and hard. The hands and feet should be large, the fingers long and separate. The vertebral column and joints should be large, but hidden by the surrounding tissues. The lustre of the skin should be slightly greasy and shining. Derivations from this ideal include the eight unsatisfactory body types (***nindita***), including ***aroṃa*** ('absence of body hair'), ***atiloma*** ('excess body hair'), ***atikṛṣṇa*** ('excessively dark skin'), ***atigaura*** ('excessively white skin'), ***atisthūla*** ('obesity'), ***atikṛśa*** ('asthenia'), ***atidīrgha*** ('excessively tall') and ***atihrasva*** ('excessively short').

9.10 *Balām*

The term ***balā*** refers to the strength of an individual, and is of three types. ***Sahajā balām*** is the innate strength of the individual, and corresponds to the ***para ojas***. Thus the strength that an individual is born with generally corresponds with the ***prakṛti***, with ***kaphaja prakṛti*** being the strongest, ***pittaja prakṛti*** being moderately strong, and ***vāttika prakṛti*** being the weakest. ***Yuktikṛtham*** is the 'acquired' strength of an individual, corresponding with ***apara ojas***. This corresponds with the 'dietary' (***āhāra***) and 'lifestyle habits' (***sātmya***) of the individual. ***Kālajam*** is the strength of an individual that is based upon the 'seasonal influence' (***ṛtucaryā***). The ideal manifestation of strength is a well-developed musculature with a good ability to carry heavy loads, and to walk up hills relatively easily.

Caraka states that there are three grades to ***balā***, listed as ***pravara***, ***madhya*** and ***avara balā***. ***Pravara balā*** is 'great strength', ***madhya balā*** is 'medium strength', and ***avara balā*** is 'poor strength'. The importance in distinguishing the strength of the individual is found in the varying strengths of medicines that could potentially be administered during treatment. If ***tikṣṇa dravyas*** are given to a weakened individual for example, the result could be harmful or even fatal. Weak persons are thus given ***mṛdu*** ('soft') and ***sukumāra*** ('mild') ***dravyas***. On the other hand, if such remedies were given to a strong person, there may be no change in the course of the disease, which may indicate the need for a stronger approach.

Caraka also mentions that the ***kāla saṃprāpti***, or the appearance of signs and symptoms, may sometimes obscure the true nature of the condition, and that this is a potential error the physician must guard against. Caraka states that strong individuals suffering from a severe disease may manifest only mild symptoms. Similarly, a weak patient suffering from a mild disease may manifest severe symptoms. If remedies that are weak or mild in nature are given to the strong patient suffering from a strong disease, Caraka states that the disease will eventually get worse. If strong remedies are used in a weak patient suffering from a mild disease, the patient will also get worse.

9.11 *Agni*

Caraka says that ***agni*** is the focal point of treatment, and the root of ***balā*** ('strength'), ***arogya*** ('health'), ***āyus*** ('longevity'), ***varna*** ('complexion'), ***sukha*** ('happiness'), ***ojas*** ('resistance to disease'), and ***tejas*** ('energy'). Thus, the digestive capacity of the patient should be ascertained. Generally speaking, the ***agni*** is assessed according to the influence of the ***doṣas*** ***Vāttika*** afflictions of ***agni*** are associated with a ***viṣamāgni***, or an irregular digestion. ***Paittika*** conditions are associated with a ***tikṣṇāgni***, or a digestion that is unusually strong and fast. ***Kaphaja*** conditions are associated with a ***mañdāgni***, or a digestion that is weak and slow (see 4.1 ***Agni***: the fire of digestion and metabolism).

9.12 *Sattva*

Sattva is an assessment of the patient's mental and emotional state. ***Sattva*** can be classified in two ways: by determining the general mental and emotional capacity, and by assessing the predominance of ***sattva***, ***rajas*** or ***tamas***. The strength of an individual's mental capacity is graded according to their ability to withstand mental, physical and emotional hardship. ***Pravaram*** is the ability to withstand a high degree of hardship, such that adverse conditions are faced with courage, grace and hope. ***Madhyamam*** is the ability of an individual to withstand hardship only when they have the love and support of others around them, and when they realise that they are not the only person in the world that is experiencing ***dukha*** ('sorrow'). Individuals classified as ***avaram*** have a difficult time gaining any strength from others, and have little ability to face hardship on their own. They are susceptible to fear and cannot tolerate any negative influences (such as media reports of tragedies) or the sight of physical injury.

Sattva is also an assessment of the patient's mental and emotional orientation, classified according to the predominance of ***sattva***, ***rajas***, or ***tamas***. Please review section 3.3 ***Triguṇa manas***: the qualities of the mind.

9.13 *Sātmya*

Sātmya means what is 'normal', or the 'habit' of the patient, referring specifically to their current lifestyle habits, generally in context with the disease being treated, as well as other factors such as the ***prakṛti*** and ***deśa***. Ultimately, it is an assessment of whether these habits are conducive to the successful treatment of the condition, and if these habits are congruent with the patient's ***prakṛti*** and ancestral background. In a rather obvious example, the consumption of devitalised and refined food in a patient suffering from a debilitating condition would be ***asātmya***, or incongruent with the needs of the patient. Similarly, the same person staying up late at night would also be ***asātmya***. Thus, encouraging the patient to eat an easily digestible diet of whole foods and making sure to get adequate sleep would be an example of recommendations that are ***sātmya***. In another example, the consumption of foods that have a ***guru*** and ***snigdha*** quality in a patient with a ***kaphaja prakṛti*** would also be ***asātmya***, as would a lifestyle that is luxurious and deficient in strenuous physical exercise.

Sātmya also refers to the need for the patient to consume an appropriate diet, with an emphasis towards those foods that are generally regarded as being high in quality. Traditionally speaking, some Āyurvedic commentators elevate certain dietary articles over others, such as ***rakta śāli*** (red rice) among grains, ***saindhava*** (rock salt) among salts, ***drākṣā*** (grapes) among fruits, ***jīvantaka*** tuber (*Leptadenia reticulata*) among vegetables, ***ghṛta*** (clarified butter) among fats, and ***ena māṃsa*** (venison) among meats. The emphasis in the patient's diet, however, should be to choose the healthiest local foods available, with an emphasis upon ***deśa***, or ancestral influences. Thus for people of Northern European descent the Indian red rice may not be the most appropriate and best food, and measures should be undertaken to implement the ancestral diet to as great a degree as possible. Within the confines of ***sātmya***, however, the emphasis should still be as varied as possible, and all six ***rasas*** should be present in the diet. This kind of diet is called ***pravaram***, or 'wholesome'. When only one or two ***rasas***, such as salt and sweet, are dominant in the diet, this is called ***avaram***, or 'unwholesome'.

9.14 *Deśam*

The term ***deśa*** means habitat, and in the context of examination refers to environmental factors in the patient's life. This includes the current residence of the patient, the place of birth, and the knowledge of what constitutes a polluted environment.

Generally speaking, a living environment is of three basic types:

1. ***Jāṅgala***: arid environments
2. ***Anūpa***: marshy environments
3. ***Sadhāraṇa***: temperate environments.

The ***doṣa*** that is predominant in a ***jāṅgala*** environment is ***vāta***. People who inhabit a ***jāṅgala*** environment are said to have coarse and hard bodies, but are strong and long-lived. A ***jāṅgala*** environment is said to produce few diseases, due to the ***laghu*** and ***rūkṣa*** qualities of this environment, which tends to inhibit the formation of ***āma***. The ***doṣa*** that is predominant in an ***anūpa*** environment is ***kapha***. People who inhabit an ***anūpa*** environment are said to have soft bodies, are more delicate, and have a shorter life span. An ***anūpa*** environment is said to produce many diseases, due to the ***snigdha*** and ***śita*** qualities of this environment, which tend to promote the formation of ***āma***. Inhabitants of a ***sadhāraṇa*** environment may experience both the qualities of ***jāṅgala*** and ***anūpa***, but experience them to a lesser degree. In a ***sadhāraṇa*** environment there is no ***doṣa*** that is particularly dominant, and thus the ***doṣas*** here are influenced more by dietary and lifestyle habits.

In examining ***deśa***, the place of birth should also be taken into account. The type of environment in which the patient gestated and was born in will always have an influence upon what kind of weather is preferred. A patient born in a warm tropical environment, for example, will tend to have a body that is adjusted to this kind of environment, even if this is not representative of their ancestral environment. If such a person were to move to a more northerly environment, he or she would experience the cold to a greater degree, but be more tolerant of warm weather than his or her peers born in a temperate environment. Over time, however, the body will begin to adapt to a new environment, especially if measures are taken to implement wholesome local diets and lifestyle regimens. Thus, a person born in a warm tropical environment and now living in a colder environment could ameliorate the influence to a certain degree by eating more warming foods and making sure to get plenty of exercise during winter. Conversely, a patient born in a more northerly, temperate environment would do well when visiting tropical countries to avoid the intense heat of the day and by eating foods that are cooling to the body.

Lastly, ***deśa*** refers to the general health of our local ecology. Caraka list features in air, water and land quality that can indicate polluted elements in our ecology. Polluted in this sense includes many elements, including those of natural origin as well as from human activity.

1. ***Air pollution***: foul and abnormal smells, smoke, haze, gases, alterations to the colour of the atmosphere, blowing sand or dust; the appearance of the sun and moon as coppery, reddish or white coloured; constant cloud; absence of wind, excessively high winds or constantly shifting winds; seasonal abnormalities; frequent meteorites and thunderbolts.
2. ***Water pollution***: foul or abnormal smell, taste, appearance or texture; a decline in the diversity and number of aquatic species; absence of birds.
3. ***Land pollution***: abnormalities in the natural smell, colour, taste and texture of the land; having a withered, dried or broken appearance; large tracts of land covered exclusively in weedy plants; an abundance of animal pests (rodents, mosquitoes, flies, cockroaches, etc.); behaviour of local animals that can be regarded as bewildered, painful and confused; behaviour of its human inhabitants that can be regarded as immoral, dishonest and impolite; noise pollution (sounding as if the 'country is seized by demons').

According to Caraka, these factors found in air, water and land pollution ultimately give rise to epidemic disease.

9.15 *Āhāra*

Āhāra is an analysis of the patient's current diet against what has been determined to be ***sātmya***, as well as the strength of digestion (***agni***). Rather than simply asking them what they eat, it is often more effective to have the patient record each food and beverage each day and the time it was consumed in a journal, as well as record any symptoms. The modern usage of techniques such as Coco's pulse test, which are said to help determine the presence of allergenic foods in the diet, can also be used by these patients to determine which foods are ***avaram*** ('unwholesome'). The patient should be taught to recognise and record even minor symptoms experienced after eating, such as an increase in catarrh, minor skin irritations or flatulence. Generally speaking, ***kaphaja*** afflictions to ***agni*** will be noted as symptoms and signs that appear during or just after eating while the food is still in the stomach; ***paittika*** symptoms and signs will noted within 3–4 hours after eating, while the food is transiting the small intestine; ***vātaja*** afflictions to ***agni*** tend to occur within 8–10 hours after eating, when the food is transiting the colon. When an individual is able to consume a large amount of food on a regular basis the person is said to have a good ***āhāra śakti*** (digestive power), whereas a person who cannot eat much without bloating or discomfort is said to have a poor ***āhāra śakti***.

PART 1

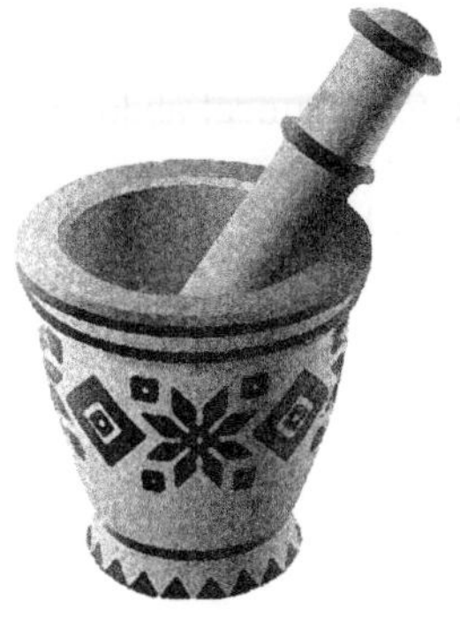

Chapter 10

CLINICAL EXAMINATION

OBJECTIVES

- To understand and discuss specialised clinical techniques in Āyurveda.

10.1 *Aṣṭāsthāna parikṣā*: THE EIGHT METHODS OF DIAGNOSIS

There are several methods of diagnosis (***parīkṣā***) in ***Āyurveda***, identified as ***aṣṭāsthāna parīkṣā***, consisting of eight (***aṣṭā***) seats (***sthāna***):

1. ***Akṛti parīkṣā***: observation of the build and general physical characteristics
2. ***Śabda parīkṣā***: examination of the voice
3. ***Dṛk parīkṣā***: examination of the eyes and eyesight
4. ***Sparśa parīkṣā***: palpation
5. ***Mūtra parīkṣā***: examination of urine
6. ***Purīṣa parīkṣā***: examination of faeces
7. ***Nāḍī parīkṣā***: examination of the pulse
8. ***Jihva parīkṣā***: examination of the tongue.

The purpose of diagnosis in Āyurvedic medicine is simply to collect data. Some of these techniques are a matter of 'direct perception' (***pratyakṣa***), such as ***akṛti*** and ***sparśa parīkṣā***, whereas others are a matter of 'inference' (***anumāna***), such as ***nāḍī parīkṣā***. It is always easier to base an overall diagnosis on something that can be directly perceived. Although inferential methods like ***nāḍī pariskṣā*** can offer deep insights, they are notoriously difficult to quantify and in many cases two practitioners can come to entirely different conclusions using the same methods. Ideally, the practitioner should base any diagnostic conclusions on three aspects: the 'case history' (***āptopadeśa***), 'direct observation' (***pratyakṣa***), and 'inference' (***anumāna***). Where a treatment is based on only one or two of these components, the treatment may not be appropriate.

10.2 *Akṛti parīkṣā*: THE OBSERVATION OF BUILD

The observation of a patient's overall physical structure is a useful means of understanding the general state of nutrition, eliminative functions and any obvious disease characteristics. It is important to add that all observations are relative to the racial heritage of each person. The observation of the patient's general characteristics should begin as soon as the patient enters the room, and may be noted down when convenient. The following are the basic characteristics to look for, understood in the context of ***tridoṣa*** (indicated by V, P or K):

1. ***Frame***: whether large (K); medium (P); small (V)
2. ***Musculature*** and ***adiposity***: overweight, well-distributed (K); well-muscled (P); asthenic, or overweight in upper body only (V)
3. ***Complexion***: pale and white (K); yellowish to red (P); translucent, greyish (V)
4. ***Face***: large eyes, thick eyelashes, thick eyebrows, large septum, rounded nose, thick lips (K); medium eyes, reddish sclera, thin eyelashes and eyebrows, sharp nose, ruddy face, acne on cheeks (P); smallish eyes, dark circles under eyes, dry skin, deviated septum (V)
5. ***Hair***: thick, wavy (K); thin, balding (P); dry, split ends (V)
6. ***Fingernails***: strong, thick, white (K); soft, pink, peeling, frequent hang-nails (P); brittle, ridged, variable shape (V).

Akṛti is a method of assessment that can potentially confuse the practitioner, because elements of the ***prakṛti*** may be taken to be the ***vikṛti***. As a general rule of thumb, look for features that appear to represent pathological changes as opposed to constitutional factors. Thus the patient's frame or facial structure may tell us little about the ***vikṛti***, but the skin, hair, fat distribution and complexion typically provide more immediate indications of a disease process. In severe wasting or obesity, however, the frame may indeed tell us about the pathology. Generally speaking, determine if the weight gain or weight loss is proportional to the skeletal structure. Thus true pathological wasting is noted by disproportionately large bony prominences, and true obesity by a fleshy structure on a comparatively small frame (e.g. small hands and feet) or regions of disproportionate adiposity (e.g. truncal-abdominal obesity).

Akṛti also involves observing how a patient moves their body, whether they are slow and lethargic (***kapha***), fast and determined (***pitta***), or confused and disorientated (***vāta***).

10.3 *Śabda parīkṣā*: VOICE DIAGNOSIS

The voice can indicate many things about a person's health, his or her resistance to disease, as well as mental, emotional and spiritual development. Generally speaking, voices that are melodious, deep, laughing, pleasing to the ear, like water flowing through a creek, are considered to be ***kapha*** in nature, expressing a harmonious mind and a tranquil emotional life. Immune function is typically strong although there may be a tendency towards cardiovascular stasis, diabetes, and emotions such as sentimentality and worry. Voices that are harsh, passionate, critical, loud and angry are considered to be ***pitta***, expressing a sharp mind and a florid emotional life. There may be ulcerous conditions, head injuries, and hepatic congestion. Voices that are weak, confused, subtle, and alternate between fast and slow are considered to be ***vāta***, expressing a disassociated mind and a chaotic emotional life. There may be exhaustion, constipation, chronic illness and anxiety.

10.4 *Dṛk parīkṣā*: EXAMINATION OF THE EYES

The examination of the eyes in Āyurvedic medicine is a somewhat less detailed process compared to specialised assessment techniques such as iridiagnosis, but many of the same principles can be employed. ***Dṛk parīkṣā*** is used to assess both eye function and what the eyes reveal about the rest of the body. The typical tools required when examining the eyes include a high-powered flashlight to illuminate the eye and at least a 5× hand lens to note its discrete features.

Each of the ***doṣas*** plays a key role in the function of the eyes. ***Kapha*** governs the supply of nutrients (***āhāra rasa***) to the eye, whereas ***pitta*** is involved in the metabolism and discharge of wastes into the venous system that drains the eye. ***Vāta*** plays a key role to ensure a balance between ***kapha*** and ***pitta*** in the eye, as well as the proper movement of the eye and the conduction of the visual images to the brain via the optic nerve. The vitiation of one, two or three of the ***doṣas*** in the eye are understood by correlating these signs and symptoms with the ***lakṣaṇas***, or clinical features of the ***doṣas*** (see: 2.6 ***Tridoṣa lakṣaṇas***: symptomology of the doṣas):

- ***Kaphaja*** afflictions to the eyes manifest as a sticky, white exudate, orbital swelling or oedema, itching, and whitish discolorations of the lens, iris, sclera or conjunctiva. The patient complains of whitish or clear spots that impair vision. The eyes seem to move lazily, have a gentle gaze, and open and close slowly. A dull frontal or sinus headache may accompany symptoms, with nausea and a weak appetite.
- ***Pittaja*** afflictions to the eyes manifest as a purulent, yellowish-green exudate, inflammation and burning sensations, photophobia, and yellowish, red or greenish discolorations of the lens, iris, sclera or conjunctiva. The patient complains of yellowish, red or greenish spots or streaks that impair vision, and may complain of hallucinations. The eyes are bright and moist, and stare with intensity. A sharp, burning headache pain over the eyes or temples may accompany symptoms, with loose motions, thirst and burning sensations.
- ***Vātaja*** afflictions to the eyes manifest as dryness and scratchiness of the eyes, impaired eye movement, ocular muscle spasm, rapid eye movement and twitching, squinting and fluttering of the eyelids. The eyes are lustreless and dull, may appear contracted within the eye-sockets, and may be surrounded by a purplish or bluish colour. The patient complains of dark-coloured spots that impair vision, or sporadic and intense flashes of light. A severe lancinating pain in the eyes and head may accompany symptoms, with anxiety, nervousness, constipation and other ***vattika*** symptoms.

As mentioned, ***dṛk parīkṣā*** can also be used to assess other regions of the body, based on the concept that each discrete region of the body is a holographic representation of the entire body (e.g. the ear, hand, tongue, foot, etc.). Using the Āyurvedic concept of the ***rogamārgas*** the structure of the iris can be divided into three basic concentric regions, each of which corresponds with the three pathways of disease: the ***añtarmārga*** (the inner), the ***madhyama rogamārga*** (the middle) and the ***bāhya rogayana*** (the outer) (see 8.8 ***Rogamārgas***: the pathways of disease). The areas just outside the pupil, but contained within the collarette (the 'wreath' that surrounds the pupil) indicates the status of the ***añtarmārga***, or inner pathway, comprising the digestive system and aspects of the respiratory system. The ***madhyama rogamārga***, or middle pathway, is found just outside the collarette and extends near to the edges of the iris, and comprises the central and peripheral nervous systems, the endocrine, renal and musculoskeletal systems, and the viscera such as heart, liver, spleen, pancreas and lungs. The ***bāhya rogayana***, or outer pathway, is contained in the periphery of the iris, comprising the lymphatic, circulatory and integumentary systems.

Another useful method to assess the iris is to divide the regions of the eye into three regions that represent the ***sthānas***, or seats of influence, of ***vāta***, ***pitta*** and ***kapha*** (see 2.4 ***Sthāna***: residence of the doṣas). If we examine the iris like the face of a clock, these three regions can be easily identified:

- In a clockwise direction, the regions roughly located between 9 and 11 o'clock, and 1 and 3 o'clock, represent the regions of the body contained within the ***kapha sthāna***, i.e. the head, neck, lungs, heart, etc.
- In a clockwise direction, the regions roughly located between 7 and 9 o'clock, and 3 and 5 o'clock, represent the regions of the body contained within the ***pitta sthāna***, i.e. the liver, gall bladder, stomach, pancreas, spleen, etc.
- In a clockwise direction, the regions roughly located between 5 o'clock and 7 o'clock, and at the top from 11 to 1 o'clock, represent the regions of the body contained within the ***vāta sthāna***, i.e. the pelvis, colon, kidneys, adrenals, reproductive organs, and the central nervous system, etc.

By noting features in these regions, such as the stromal density of the iris and pigmentation, and by correlating these to the symptomology of the ***doṣas*** (see 2.6 ***Tridoṣa lakṣaṇas***: symptomology of the doṣas), the iris may indicate a particular dysfunction in a specific region of the body. Stromal density of the iris is an important consideration in traditional iridiagnosis, and while the density of these fibres does not change over time, they may be an indication of constitutional defects in a particular region of the body. Impairments in stromal density are seen as an

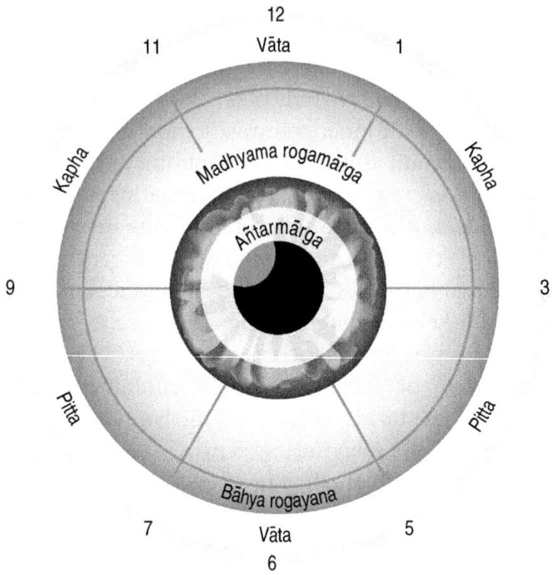

Figure 10.1 ***Tridoṣic*** eye assessment.

interruption in the fibres that make up the iris, giving rise to craters and cavities, referred to as lacunae, that are best seen by shining a bright light across the surface of the iris.

10.5 *Sparśa parīkṣā*: PALPATION

Palpation is an especially important diagnostic tool that is too often ignored by practitioners. In the Western herbal tradition, the eclectic physician John M. Scudder (1874) states in his text *Specific Diagnosis* that practitioners should acquaint themselves '. . . with the education of the blind, to see the range of this sense which in the majority has such imperfect development'. Such sentiments are reflective of Āyurvedic practices, in which the senses of the pracitioner become finely attuned through daily meditative practices. The sensation of touch arises from the influence of ***vāta***, the impetus and vehicle of thought and emotion. By developing the skill of palpation the practitioner has access to a body of knowledge that can guide the overall diagnosis and remove much guesswork from the diagnostic equation.

If performing a complete examination the patient should be asked to remove his or her clothes and lay supine on an examining table, covered with a sheet or light blanket. The practitioner may examine each area of the body separately, folding up the portion of the sheet that is covering the part of the body to be inspected. The examining room should be well lit, preferably with natural light, and warm enough for an unclothed patient. All of the body regions should be examined, paying close attention to the cervical region, the axila, the abdomen and the inguinal region.

There are five primary factors in ***sparśa***: moisture, temperature, texture, mobility and turgor, and sensitivity:

1. ***Moisture*** is assessed by distinguishing perspiration, oiliness and dryness. Moist skin would typically indicate ***kapha*** or ***pitta***, but this feature has to be assessed in context with other features, such as temperature and colour. Thus, in greasy and inflamed skin, such as acne, this would indicate a ***pitta*** or a combined ***pitta-kapha*** condition. If on the other hand the skin is moist but cool, this would suggest ***kapha***. In ***vāttika*** conditions there will be dryness, flakiness, roughness, discoloration, tenesmus, irregularities, a lack of symmetry and hardness. A patient who, for all intents and purposes, appears to be ***kapha*** but has dry skin, may in fact be hypothyroid, a combined ***vāta-kapha*** condition. Similarly, inflamed skin that is dry indicates a combined ***vāta-pitta*** condition.
2. ***Temperature*** is assessed with the back of the fingers, identifying the warmth or coolness of the skin, paying particular attention to any areas that appear red. ***Paittika*** conditions such as hyperthyroidism will be noticed as a generalised warmness as in a fever, and ***vāta-kapha*** conditions such as hypothyroidism will be noted as a generalised coolness. Focal areas that are warm or cool to the touch suggest local inflammation and a circulatory deficiency, respectively.
3. ***Texture*** is assessed by noting characteristics such as smoothness and roughness of the skin, but also the topography, such as areas that seem knotted, hard, pinched or fibrotic. Patients with a hypofunctioning thyroid will often manifest rough, dry skin, which is a ***vāta-kapha*** condition. Women who complain of cyclic breast pain may have fibrotic nodules that can be assessed in the breast tissue at certain times during the oestrous cycle. Nodules that appear slowly and do not change

with the oestrous cycle, however, may be dermoid cysts or a tumour, suggesting ***kapha*** or a combined ***kapha-pitta*** disorder. Similarly, subcutaneous cysts found elsewhere in either men, women or children are usually related to ***pitta*** and ***kapha***.

4. ***Mobility*** and ***turgor*** are assessed by lifting a fold of skin and noting the ease by which it moves (mobility) and the speed with which it returns to normal (turgor). In oedema (***kapha***) there will be decreased mobility, whereas in dehydration (***vāta***) there will be decreased turgor. With inflammation (***pitta***) there will be immobility.
5. ***Sensitivity*** is noted by how the patient responds to the practitioner's touch. Light touches and gentle rubbing tends to pacify ***vāta*** but aggravates ***pitta***. Medium to strong pressure tends to pacify ***pitta***, whereas this may or may not alleviate ***kapha***. Upward movements tend to alleviate ***kapha***, whereas downward motions tend to reduce ***pitta*** and ***vāta***.

10.6 *Mūtra parīkṣā*: EXAMINATION OF URINE

The assessment of the urine requires that the patient collect a small amount of urine at midstream, into a clean, clear plastic or glass vessel. Once voided, urine will oxidise very quickly and the original aromatic odour will degrade into one dominant in ammonia, and thus an assessment should be made as soon as possible after voiding. Stale urine that has not been refrigerated will often be much darker and cloudier than original due to the proliferation of bacteria. In Āyurvedic assessment there are five basic aspects to urine examination:

1. ***Colour*** and ***transparency***. In health, the urine should be a clear pale yellow colour, but under the influence of different foods, herbs, and supplements the colour may display some variability. Bright yellow, almost neon in colour, is often the result of vitamin B-complex supplementation. Pink or reddish urine that suggests blood but is translucent may be due to anthocyanins, a pigment found in red vegetables such as beets. Patients who subsist on diets high in protein may have a greenish urine due to the presence of a potassium salt of indole, formed by the putrefaction of protein in the intestine. Herbal laxatives such as ***Āragvadha*** fruit (*Cassia fistula*), Turkey Rhubarb root (*Rheum palatum*) or Cascara Sagrada bark (*Rhamnus purshiana*) contain anthraquinones that can colour the urine orange. Food coloring agents can colour the urine, such as methylene blue, present in some proprietary pills, which can colour the urine green. Drugs can also colour the urine, such as tetracyclines (yellow), phenindione (pink), rifampicin and phenazopyridine (red), and methyldopa and iron sorbitol (black).

   After ruling out the variety of exogenous agents that can colour the urine, the practitioner can then freely examine the urine. In dehydration (***vāta***) the urine will be an amber, dark yellow or orange colour, depending on the severity of the condition. Although small amounts of blood are undetectable, larger amounts can give the urine a smoky appearance. Bile pigments can give the urine a brownish colour with a green tint at the surface, and when shaken in a test tube will cause a yellow froth, indicating a ***paittika*** disorder. Urine that has been allowed to stand unrefrigerated may become darker than when first voided, due to the presence of pus or phosphates.

   Urine in ***kaphaja*** conditions will tend to be clear and pale, and if turbid, will have a slightly cloudy appearance suggesting the presence of calculi, mucus or semen. In ***paittika*** conditions the urine will tend to be yellow to red in colour. In ***vāttika*** conditions the colour of the urine can be variable, either clear or quite dark, and is variable in consistency and turbidity. A feature of ***vāta***, however, is that the urine has a tendency to be quite bubbly and frothy when voided, or when poured from one vessel into another. In severe ***vāttika*** conditions the urine has a greasy appearance, indicating the excretion of ***māṃsa*** and ***medas***, found in the endstage of diseases such as ***madhumeha*** (diabetes mellitus).
2. ***Odour*** and ***taste***. In all methods of examination Āyurvedic medicine requires the practitioner to utilise all his or her five senses, but in regard to the assessment of urine and faeces indirect methods (***anumāna***) were utilised for the sensation of taste. One interesting method was to place a small amount of the patient's urine in a dish and wait to see if any insects were attracted to the urine, as is

the case in ***madhumeha***, or diabetes mellitus, in which the urine contains a disproportionate amount of sugar. This technique, however, is not suited to a modern clinical setting, and thus reagent strips can be used to assess for glucose. Urine in ***kapha*** conditions will typically have a sweet smell. Urine in ***vāttika*** conditions typically displays a bitter or astringent smell, but in severe conditions can also smell quite sweet: the difference between ***kapha*** and ***vāta*** will be the volume excreted and the colour. ***Paittika*** conditions will typically have a strong, pungent and foul smelling odour.

3. ***Temperature***. In ***kaphaja*** and ***vāttika*** conditions the relative temperature of the urine will be cool, whereas in ***paittika*** conditions the urine will be quite warm.
4. ***Volume*** and ***frequency***. In both ***kaphaja*** and ***paittika*** conditions the volume tends to be copious, although the frequency is otherwise normal. In ***kapha*** conditions the voiding of urine may take an exceptionally long time and has very little force, although the frequency is otherwise normal. In ***vāttika*** conditions the volume is decreased and the frequency high, indicating a renal impairment or spasm.[21]
5. ***Symptoms***. ***Paittika*** conditions will display a burning, cutting or searing pain upon evacuation. Concomitant symptoms may include burning diarrhoea, skin eruptions and fever. ***Vāttika*** conditions display a prickling pain that migrates from place to place and varies in severity, accompanied by a sense of fullness and abdominal oedema. There may also be frequent shooting or stinging pains that arise in the perineal area, indicating spasm. Associated symptoms may be anxiety, fear, constipation and arthritis. ***Kaphaja*** conditions display symptoms such as a sense of obstruction, but not to the same extent as ***vāta***. There is usually little pain, but there may be some fluid retention and generalised oedema. Concomitant symptoms in ***kaphaja*** conditions may include a loss of appetite, nausea and sinus congestion.

In relation to disorders of the urinary tract, the designation of ***vāta***, ***pitta*** or ***kapha*** indicates the progression of the disease. ***Paittika*** diseases are acute, often involving a bacterial infection. ***Kapha*** conditions are chronic symptoms that arise from dietary and lifestyle neglect, rather than a specific pathogen, although a chronic yeast infection is a feature of ***kapha*** and ***āma***. ***Vāttika*** conditions often represent end-stage conditions, whether the result of damage caused by chronic infection or chronic abuse, and are often very challenging conditions.

A number of texts, including Dash and Junius' *A Handbook of Ayurveda*, describe an additional method in ***mūtra parīkṣā***, by the use of dropping small quantities of unrefined sesame oil in a urine sample. This technique should be performed in full sunlight, and the urine should be kept in a clear, wide-mouthed vessel. About five to ten drops of the oil are dropped into the urine sample, and after about 15 seconds the oil will begin to spread across the surface of the urine. If the oil spreads fast, the prognosis is good and there will be quick recovery from the condition. If the oil does not spread, or spreads very slowly, the prognosis is poor, and recovery may take some time. If the oil settles on the bottom of the glass, it is said that the disease is incurable.

The movement and direction in which the oil spreads may also be taken into consideration. If the oil moves in an easterly direction this is an indication of a good prognosis and a quick recovery from the condition. If the oil spreads to the south it indicates an exacerbation of the condition or an incipient fever, and that recovery may take some time. Movement in a northerly direction indicates good health, or that recovery will occur soon. Movement in a westerly direction indicates that while the condition may continue for some time, it is not serious and that health will once again be restored.

The pattern that the oil takes also tells the practitioner something about the condition. If the oil takes the appearance of a snake this indicates a ***vāttika*** disorder. If the oil develops into an umbrella-like shape, this is an indication of ***pitta***. If the oil separates into round pearl-like shapes, this is an indication of ***kapha***. Practitioners who are very skilled at ***mūtra parīkṣā*** can also see other shapes that may indicate the prognosis. Generally, shapes that suggest a plough, tortoise, buffalo, honeycomb, arrow or a sword indicate a poor prognosis. Shapes that have a circular shape or suggest a swan, lotus, or an elephant indicate a good prognosis. A pool of oil on the surface of the urine that contains tiny holes like a sieve or looks like a human body suggests spiritual possession or the fruition of negative ***karma***.

10.7 *Purīṣa parīkṣā*: EXAMINATION OF FAECES

The state of the faeces is universally regarded by many systems of traditional healing including Āyurveda as the most useful sign in determining digestive function, and as a result, the health of the patient. Ideally, the faecal material should be examined soon after expulsion, in its entirety, and for a period of several days. This represents some practical obstacles in a clinical environment, and thus patients should be instructed as to the method of collecting data regarding their bowel movements. For certain diagnostic procedures a small amount of the faecal material can be collected in a vessel. In a state of health, a bowel movement will display the following characteristics:

1. Light brown in colour
2. Solid, well-formed, voided in its entirety without breaking
3. Have a continuous size and shape, 2.5–4 cm in diameter
4. Smooth, without a twisted or nodular appearance
5. Without a large degree of undigested food.

There are several criteria when examining the stool:

1. ***Shape*** and ***consistency***: When the stool is small, voided as many pieces, irregularly shaped and has a marbled appearance, it is an indication of ***vāta***, dehydration and a lack of both exercise and fibre in the diet. When the stool is snake-like, having a small diameter, it is an indication of smooth muscle spasm, most often a combined ***vāta-pitta*** condition. When the stools are loose to liquid, this is an increase in ***pitta***, indicating gastrointestinal irritation or excessive bile excretion. When the stools are large, dense and mucoid, this is an indication of ***kapha***.
2. ***Colour***: Blackish stools indicate bleeding in the upper gastrointestinal tract, or can be from the excessive consumption of iron. Dark brown stools can either indicate blood or the presence of ***āma***. Brown stools are normal. Greenish stools indicate ***pitta***, from an increase in stomach acidity, gastric irritation and excess bile. With the use of cholagogues, however, greenish stools can also indicate the removal of ***pitta*** from the digestive tract through an increase in liver metabolism and bile. Whitish stools indicate ***kapha*** disorders such as ***agnimāndya***, hepatic torpor, or obstructive jaundice. Stools are very often coloured by naturally occurring pigments in the diet, such as the pink anthocyanins in beets and the orange carotenes in carrots and yams. As in ***mūtra parīkṣā***, anthraquinone-containing botanicals (e.g. *Rhamnus purshiana*) can also colour the faeces orange or red, and long-term usage may even temporarily stain the bowel wall, observed on colonoscopy.
3. ***Odour***: Foul-smelling faeces are related to protein putrefaction, which is a ***paittika*** disturbance, manifesting as a septic condition of the bowel. This may also be an indication of jaundice. Milky-smelling bowel movements indicate the excessive consumption of refined carbohydrates and dairy, and are often symptomatic of candidiasis, which is usually considered to be reflective of a ***kapha*** condition.
4. ***Volume*** and ***frequency***: A large volume of faecal material voided more than twice daily is indicative of ***paittika*** tendency. A small volume of faecal material voided less than once daily is an indication of ***vāta***. One or two large bowel movements a day that take much time to void is an indication of ***kapha***.
5. ***Symptoms***: Rectal bleeding is either an indication of hepatic portal congestion or from the passing of excessively dry faecal material. When concomitant with otherwise normal or liquid bowel movements it is an indication of ***pitta***, whereas rectal bleeding concomitant with dry and rough stool is an indication of ***vāta***. A sense of rectal fullness and pelvic heaviness without bleeding, but with rectal itching is an indication of ***āma*** or ***kapha***. A sense of burning or irritation is always an indication of ***pitta***, although ***vāta*** is very often involved, as in fistula-in-ano. Stool that has been passed with an explosive force and much flatulence is a combined ***vāta-pitta*** disorder. Liquid or semi-liquid bowel movements with blood and a semen-like odour is an indication of amoebic dysentery, and blood with pus and a fetid odour is an indication of bacillary dysentery, both of which are ***pittaja*** disorders.

10.8 *Nāḍī parīkṣā*: PULSE DIAGNOSIS

Nāḍī parīkṣā is described as one of the eight methods of diagnosis, but few modern college-trained Āyurvedic physicians practice it with any skill, and as a result its preservation within the framework of Āyurvedic diagnostics can almost be seen as an anomaly. Traditionally trained Āyurvedic physicians such as those of the ***aṣṭā vaidya*** families of Kerala Āyurveda, however, claim to posses this knowledge, but because these techniques are closely guarded family secrets they remain inaccessible. As a result of this situation there are a number of different and widely varying Āyurvedic pulse techniques promulgated by various teachers and practitioners, and it is difficult to determine which are valid and effective.

Many Āyurvedic physicians consider the ***Nāḍīvijñānam*** to be the most authentic text on pulse diagnosis, written by ***Maharṣi Kanada*** in about the 3rd century BCE, apparently the same person who developed the ***Vaiśeṣika Sūtra***, one of the six ***darśanas*** of the ***Vedas***.[22] The ***Nāḍīvijñānam*** is a highly detailed text that provides an in-depth knowledge of the pulses, their qualities and features. Another important text on pulse diagnosis from the medieval period is the ***Śārangadhara saṃhitā***, which contains a short treatise on the pulse. More recent is the ***Nāḍīprakaśam*** written by Sankara Sen around the turn of the last century. These three works form the primary textual link we have with what is generally supposed to be an ancient and venerable practice in India. Beyond these, there are several excellent texts on pulse diagnosis, such as the Chinese *Bin Hu Ma Xue* by Li Shi Zhen (c. 1518 CE; Huynh & Seifert 1981) and the methods of pulse assessment discussed in the fourth ***tantra*** of Tibetan *rGyud bzi* (c. 8th century CE; Finckh 1988), which is stated by some sources to be a translation of an earlier, now lost, Sanskrit text entitled the ***Amṛta Hṛdaya Aṣṭāṅga Guhyaupadeśa Tantra*** (Dash 1994). Pulse diagnosis in Chinese and Tibetan medicine appears to have a longer, continuous history of use than in India, and as a result they can be used to confirm and support the practice of pulse diagnosis in Āyurveda. Regardless of the methodology, however, it is always an important thing to realise that pulse diagnosis is ***anumāna***, an inferential method of assessment, and in and of itself cannot provide the practitioner with the exact nature of the patient's condition: it always needs to be assessed in conjunction with the case history (***āptopadeśa***) and direct observation (***pratyakṣa***). This is the skill of the master clinician – knowing what is relevant and what is extraneous.

What is the pulse?

Before we begin to delve into the specifics of ***nāḍī parīkṣā***, we need to understand the nature of the pulse. Place your index finger (not your thumb, which has its own pulse) over any artery in your body, such as the carotid or radial pulse. As you feel the pulse it may occur to you that you are feeling the movement of blood through the arteries, but in actual fact you are feeling a peristaltic muscular contraction of the artery that is initiated by the ventricular contraction of the heart. The pulse wave is like a long piece of rope stretched on the ground and flicked: the pulse wave is the 'flick' that can be seen to move down the length of the rope.

The pulse wave that is initiated in the heart functions to move the blood to the various regions of the body, and is thus reflective of the heart, the seat of consciousness. By pressing down and feeling the pulse waves you are feeling the nature of your own transient consciousness. These impulses define who and what you are at any given moment, and while they change according to factors such as emotions, activity and time of day, they also display a pattern that translates to a more generalised state of consciousness: that which is manifest as your mind and body. Thus when we examine the pulse we are examining the nature of this transient consciousness, and the patterns that are manifest within it.

Place and time

All the texts on ***nāḍī*** suggest that it is best examined first thing in the morning, sometime after awakening, and after the elimination of urine and faeces, when the lethargy of sleep has been cast off. A reading taken at this time will usually be the most accurate. Practitioners are advised to avoid reading the pulse when the patient has just exercised, eaten, been outside in the cold or warm weather, or just taken a bath or shower. Pulse diagnosis takes a great deal of concentration and as a practitioner you should not be hurried, so take your time when examining the pulse – in some traditions it would not be uncommon for a practitioner to patiently observe the pulse for several minutes. Before taking the pulse ensure that you are not too tired or hungry, and if you are having some difficulty concentrating make sure you are breathing properly. In his insightful book, *Secrets of the Pulse*, Vasant Lad recommends silently chanting the syllables SO upon inhalation, and HAM upon exhalation. The SO-HAM mantra represents the unity of consciousness and provides for enhanced concentrative powers.

Position and pressure

The pulse is generally examined by the index, middle and ring fingers of the practitioner, with the index finger positioned just below the styloid process of the radius, the projection of bone just below the root of the thumb. Care must be taken not to place the index finger on the styloid process. In Chinese pulsology the index and middle fingers are placed above and below the styloid process, respectively, and this appears to be another valid way of assessing the pulse – for the purposes of this text, however, all three fingers must be placed below the styloid process. In most people the radial artery is on the same side of the wrist as the thumb, and it is over this that the three fingers are placed.

According to the ***Nāḍīvijñānam***, the practitioner uses his or her right hand to assess the pulse of the right arm of the patient, holding the patient's hand with his or her left hand.[23] The patient's palm faces up and the arm is slightly bent at the elbow. To this end the patient may rest his or her arm comfortably on a table (Fig. 10.2A), or the practitioner may support the weight of the patient's arm by resting it across their own arm (Fig. 10.2B). In the *rGyud bzi* it is said that the pulse of the right artery is most accurate for a man, whereas the left artery is more accurate for a woman. This conforms to the ***yogic*** concept that the ***pingalā*** (masculine) ***nāḍī*** runs up the right side of the body, and the ***idā*** (feminine) ***nāḍī*** runs up the left side of the body. Generally speaking, one can use the left and right pulses to assess the relative balance between these masculine and feminine qualities in a given individual. If the right pulse is weaker than the left, then the flow of ***prāṇa*** through the ***pingalā nāḍī*** may be deficient, resulting in a decline in ***agni***. If the left pulse is weaker, then the flow of ***prāṇa*** through the ***idā nāḍī*** may be deficient, resulting in a decline in ***ojas***.

The palpating fingers should be spaced slightly apart, and a gentle and uniform pressure should be applied through the tips of the fingers until pulsation is felt. When palpating arteries that are covered by much fat and muscle tissue the third finger may need to be pressed with greater effort, the second with some force but less than the third, and the first finger pressed with the least amount of pressure. The effort should be made to ensure that the pressure of all three palpating fingers extends to the same level upon the radial artery (Fig. 10.2C).

Vega (rate)

Vega is the rate at which the pulse exerts its upward pressure on the palpating finger, and can be broadly classified according to each ***doṣa***. This process, like all movements in the body, is regulated by ***vāta***, so an abnormal pulse rate at either end of the spectrum, i.e. fast or slow, can indicate a dysfunction of ***vāta***. Generally speaking, four pulsations per breath cycle is considered normal, but this may be faster for children, a little slower for the elderly. While palpating the patient's artery the clinician should simultaneously observe the patient's breathing pattern for a few minutes. If, on average, there are more than four pulsations per breath cycle, this indicates ***pitta***, suggesting heat, fever or inflammation. An increase in the pulse rate, however, may also indicate ***vāta***, such as fear, anxiety or nervousness. The difference between ***pitta*** or ***vāta*** can be understood by noting the ***gati***, or the archetype of the pulse, described later. Less than four pulsations may indicate ***kapha***, suggesting heaviness, coldness and congestion. It may, however, represent ***vāta***, and a substantial diminishment of the life force (***jīvā***). Once again, the determination between them is made by assessing the ***gati***. Sometimes it is difficult to observe the patient's breathing pattern, and in such cases the practitioner measures the rate of pulsation against his or her own breathing cycle (and hence another requirement that pulse diagnosis be a meditative exercise).

Tāla (rhythm)

The rhythm of the pulse, or the regularity by which the pulse is felt under the palpating fingers, is an

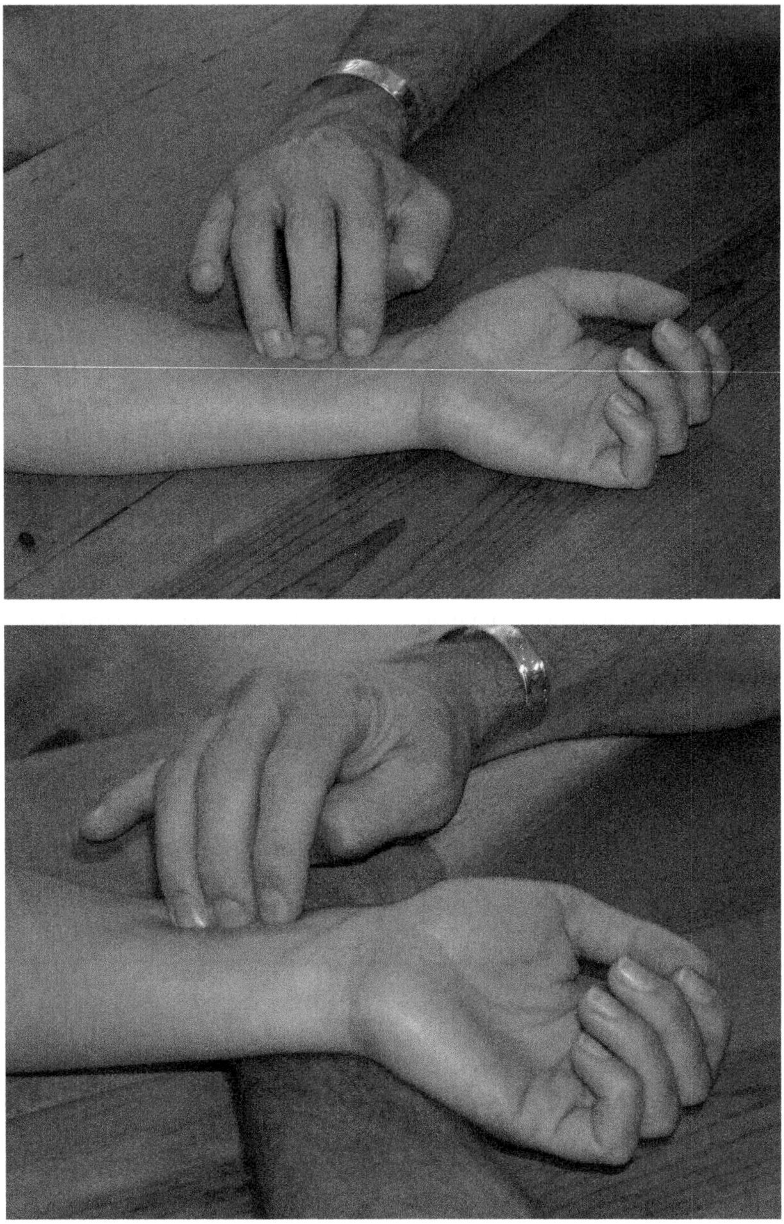

Figure 10.2A, B Radial pulse and position. Supporting the patient's arm.

Continued

assessment of ***prāṇa*** as it flows through the arteries to enliven the body. When ***vāta*** is normal the rhythm of the pulse is regular. When ***vāta*** is in an increased state the pulse becomes irregular, due to its 'dry' (***rūkṣa***) and 'light' (***laghu***) properties, making the pulse erratic and unstable. When the pulse is regularly irregular both ***vāta*** and ***kapha*** are likely involved, ***kapha*** providing an element of 'stability' (***sthira***) to the pulse. When the pulse is irregularly irregular both ***pitta*** and ***vāta*** are likely to be involved, as the 'light' (***laghu***) properties of ***pitta*** compound this same quality in ***vāta***. In many people there may be a transient increase in the heart rate with inspiration, especially with a deep breath, and a concomitant transient decrease in the heart rate with exhalation. This is called sinus arrhythmia, and is found in healthy adults and is not a sign of a dysfunction.

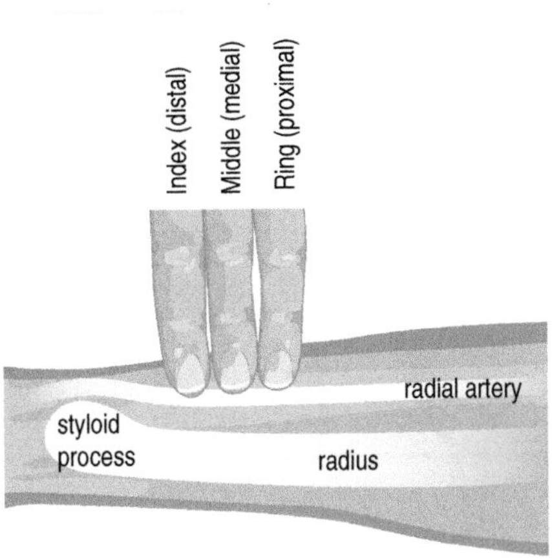

Figure 10.2C The positioning of the fingers when taking a pulse.

Balā (strength)

Balā is the'strength' of the pulse, a measure of the upward-moving force of the pulse wave under the three palpating fingers when they compress the artery. There are three basic levels to the pulse: deep, medial and superficial. The deep pulse provides indication of the status of ***soma***, or ***ojas***, the anabolic force of the body, whereas the superficial pulse corresponds to ***tejas*** or ***agni***, the catabolic force of the body. The medial pulse exists between these two levels, representing the communication and relationship between ***agni*** and ***ojas***. The actual pulse wave itself is initiated ***prāṇa***.

One way to conceptualise the difference between ***ojas*** and ***agni*** in the pulse is to understand their activities in the body. Thus, while ***agni*** functions to combust ingested food for bodily usage, its overall activity is essentially catabolic and eliminative. In contrast, ***ojas*** functions to utilise these nutrients to sustain and nourish the tissues, and therefore ***ojas*** is essentially anabolic and nutritive.

If the pulse wave is felt strongly when the artery is palpated superficially, with a light pressure of all three fingers, and a deep pressure must be exerted to stop the pulse wave, then the pulse is considered to be strong, and ***agni*** and ***ojas*** are more or less equal. In this case the medial pulse will be similar to both the superficial and deep pulses.

If the pulse is non-existent or barely palpable in the superficial position but strong in the deep position, then ***agni*** may be in a weakened state, and the patient may be suffering from cold and congestion (i.e. ***kapha***). If the pulse is weak in the superficial position, and similarly weak in the deep position, both ***agni*** and ***ojas*** may be deficient, indicating cold and congestion with deficiency (***kapha*** and ***vāta***). When the pulse is strong in the superficial position but disappears when more pressure is exerted the patient may be suffering from excess ***agni*** (***pitta***). When the pulse is both superficial and weak the patient may be suffering from heat with deficiency (***pitta*** and ***vāta***).

Gati (archetype)

The movement of the pulse in ***nāḍī parīkṣā*** is traditionally ascribed to certain animal archetypes, or ***gati***. These animal archetypes allow the practitioner to visualise factors such as rate (***vega***), rhythm (***tāla***) and strength (***balā***), along with more specific characteristics such as the width and volume of the pulse. Using these animal archetypes it becomes easier to visualise what ***doṣa*** may be influencing the pulse. The

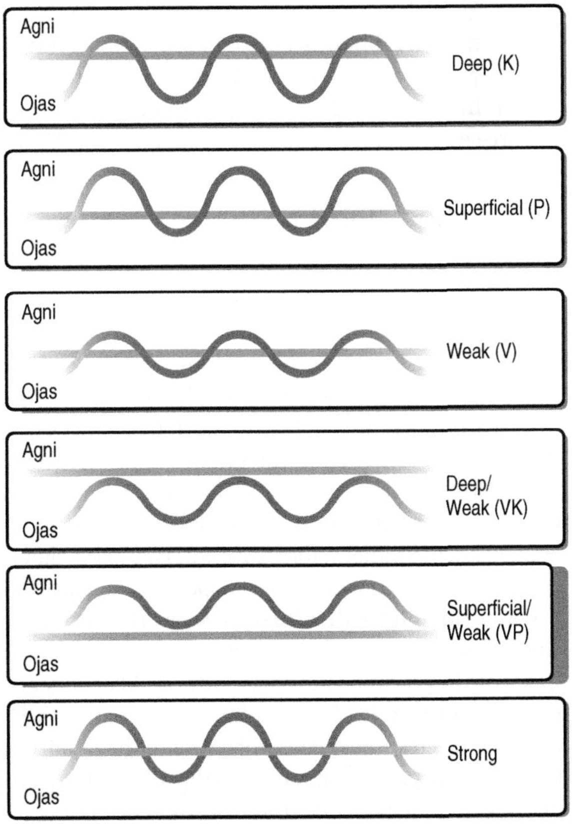

Figure 10.3 ***Balā:*** Pulse strength.

primary method to assess the ***gati*** is performed by palpating the artery with all three fingers simultaneously, pressing down with a medium pressure:

- The pulse of ***vāta*** is typically described as being that of a snake sliding along the ground: thin, subtle and empty. The pulse volume is low and difficult to detect, slipping and sliding beneath the palpating fingers.
- The pulse of ***pitta*** is described as a hopping frog: wiry, strong and abrupt. The pulse volume is high and tense, and feels hard and wiry.
- The pulse of ***kapha*** is described as a swan swimming through the water: wide, deep, and slippery. The pulse volume is full, wide and soft, gently rolling under the palpating fingers.

While there are many more animals archetypes discussed in the ***Nāḍīvijñānam***, such as a leech and elephant (some of which may even be extinct), the snake, frog and swan serve as a basic distinction between the influence of the different ***doṣas*** upon the pulse. Furthermore, it is important to note that these archetypes may occur in tandem, such that a patient might display a snake-swan pulse, indicating a combined ***vāta-kapha*** condition, a frog-snake pulse, indicating a combined ***pitta-vāta*** condition, a frog-swan pulse indicating a combined ***pitta-kapha*** condition, or even all three archetypes, indicating a ***sannipāta*** condition.

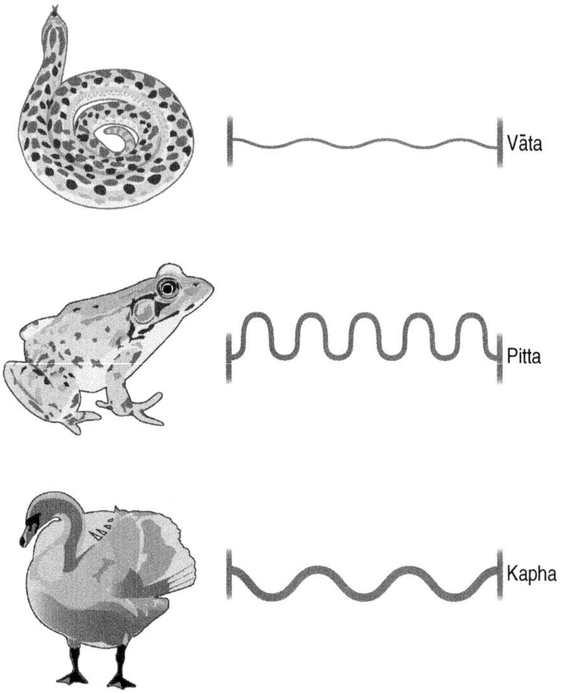

Figure 10.4 ***Gati:*** Pulse archetypes

Sthāna (location)

Each finger that is used to palpate the artery can be correlated to a specific ***doṣa***, or more specifically, a particular ***sthāna*** or region of the body that is ruled by a specific ***doṣa*** (see section 2.4 ***Sthāna***: residence of the ***doṣas***). According to the fourth stanza of the ***Nāḍīvijñānam***, when the practitioner places the index finger below the thumb (***granthi***) on the radial artery, followed by the middle and ring fingers, 'first flows ***vāta***, the middle is ***pitta***, and last is ***kapha***'. While some commentators have interpreted it differently, these explicit instructions appear to indicate that it is the ring finger that 'first' receives the peristaltic wave of the pulse. Thus, according to the ***Nāḍīvijñānam*** the ring finger indicates ***vāta***, the middle finger is ***pitta***, and the index finger is ***kapha***.[24] In my experience the specific finger does not relate to the quality of the pulse inasmuch as it relates to the different regions or ***sthānas*** ruled by each of the ***doṣas***. Thus:

- The ring finger is an assessment of ***vāta sthāna***, corresponding to the area located from the umbilicus downwards (i.e. the colon, adrenals, kidneys, bladder and reproductive organs).
- The middle finger is an assessment of ***pitta sthāna***, corresponding to the area of the body located between the umbilicus and the diaphragm (i.e. the liver, gall-bladder, spleen, pancreas and stomach).
- The index finger is an assessment of ***kapha sthāna***, corresponding to the area located from the diaphragm upwards (i.e. the lungs, heart and head).

When the right radial pulse is assessed, it may provide an indication of the health of those tissues and organs on the right side of the body. Similarly, the left radial pulse will give an indication of the health of those tissues and organs on the left side of the body. Thus the pulse on both wrists divides the body into six basic regions:

- The ***vāta*** (ring) pulse felt under the right radial artery indicates the health of tissues and organs on the lower right side of the body. Similarly, the ***vāta*** (ring) pulse under the left radial artery indicates the health of tissues and organs on the left side of the body.

- The ***pitta*** (middle) pulse under the right radial artery indicates the health of tissues and organs on the middle right side of the body. Similarly, the ***pitta*** (middle) pulse under the left radial artery indicates the health of tissues and organs on the middle left side of the body
- The ***kapha*** (index) pulse under the right radial artery indicates the health of tissues and organs on the upper right side of the body. Similarly, the ***kapha*** (index) pulse under the left radial artery indicates the health of tissues and organs on the upper left side of the body.

Using a moderate pressure, between palpating for the superficial (***agni***) and deep (***ojas***) pulses, palpate the radial artery simultaneously with all three fingers and note if the pulsation can be felt under all three. If the pulsation cannot be felt under any one of the fingers, the ***sthāna*** that corresponds with that finger may be in a weakened state. Thus, if the right artery is palpated equally with all three fingers and the pulsation is weak under the index finger, this may indicate a dysfunction in the upper part of the body, such as the right lung or pleura. If the pulse is weak in the middle, this may relate to a dysfunction of the liver or gallbladder. If the ring finger pulse is weak, the dysfunction may lie with the right adrenal, right kidney or ascending colon. These same inferences can be made with the left pulse as well. In each case, however, the practitioner will have to discern what specific tissues or organs are affected, based on an analysis of the case history (***daśavidha parīkṣā***) and other examination techniques (***aṣṭāsthāna parīkṣā***).

If a weakness is noted in any of these three areas (six locations on two wrists), or even if we want to obtain more specific information about these areas, we can use a single finger to palpate each location. Thus if we want to assess the upper right side of the body, lift off the middle and ring fingers palpating the right artery, and simply feel the right pulse with the index finger. Press down to a deep position with this finger and note the strength of the pulsation. Now release this pulse to the superficial position and note the strength of the pulse. If the pulse is strong in both the superficial and deep position, the health of the associated organs and tissues is likely good. If the pulse is weak in the superficial position then the problem may rest with the transformative and elimination aspects (i.e. ***agni***) of the tissues or organ associated with that area. Thus there may be coldness and congestion in that part of the body, but the intrinsic health (i.e. ***ojas***) of the associated organs and tissues may be fine, and simply needs to be stimulated. If the pulse is weaker in the deep position, the problem may rest with the actual health and nutrition of that organ (i.e. ***ojas***), and there may be a deficiency in that area that requires treatment. If both the superficial and deep pulses are weak in that particular location, then both ***agni*** and ***ojas*** within that tissue or organ may be in a debilitated state. If when assessing the ***sthānas*** with all three fingers you note a particularly powerful pulsation, this may indicate a higher metabolic rate (i.e.

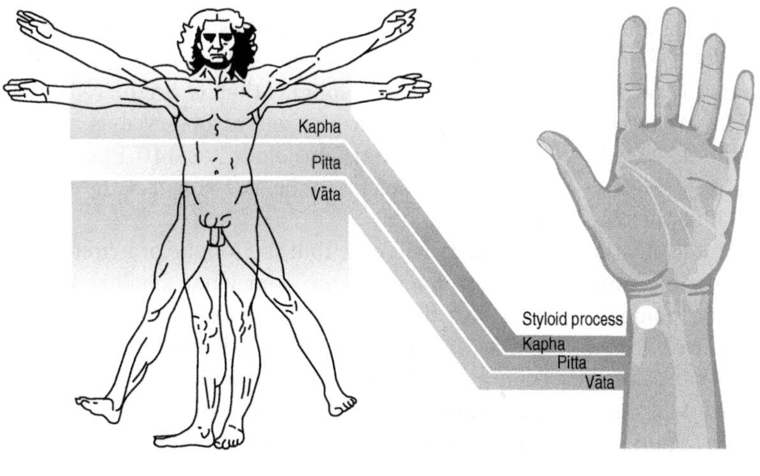

Figure 10.5 ***Sthāna: tridoṣic*** correspondence between the pulse and the body.

agni) in the associated tissues or organ, at worst, be suggestive of inflammation.

We can deepen our understanding of these individual pulse locations by applying our knowledge of ***gati***, the animal archetypes, to determine the origin or quality of this dysfunction. Thus, if the pulse in that ***sthāna*** is that of a snake (weak, thin and subtle), this may indicate a ***vāttika*** dysfunction in that area. If the pulse is a frog (wiry, tense and sharp), this may indicates a ***paittika*** dysfunction. If the pulse is a swan (slippery, wide and soft), this may indicate a ***kaphaja*** dysfunction.

Even with this relatively simplified rendering of the technique there remain many features to ***nāḍī parīkṣā***, and the practitioner must access all of these features and use them as a collective to accurately determine the nature of the pulse. To attempt to synthesise all of these aspects while learning, however, can be overwhelming. I recommend that practitioners first become proficient in determing the ***vega*** (rate), ***tāla*** (rhythm) and ***balā*** (strength) of the pulse. Later on, add the component of ***gati*** (archetype), feeling for the snake, frog and swan. Once these skills are developed, begin to incorporate them into the concept of ***sthāna*** (location), determing weaknesses and strengths in each part of the body, and the specific characteristics of the pulse wave in each pulse location that indicates the ***doṣas*** and their activities.

10.9 *Jivhā parīkṣā*: TONGUE DIAGNOSIS

The tongue (***jivhā***) is perhaps the most useful of the diagnostic techniques because it is relatively easy to read, providing detailed information of the state of not only the gastrointestinal organs, but also the assimilative, metabolic and circulatory processes of the body. Full daylight is the best condition in which to examine the tongue, but otherwise adequate lighting is acceptable. To examine the tongue properly it should be fully extended by the patient, but remain relatively relaxed, without using excessive force which will hide the true shape of the tongue and make it redder. Ideally, the tongue should be observed first thing in the morning before eating, or on an otherwise empty stomach. Certain foods, including artificially coloured foods, spices and sweets will change the colour of the coating on the tongue. Coffee and tobacco smoke will often leave a yellowish stain on the tongue, whereas pungent and salty foods like chilies and pickles, and even mouthwash, will temporarily make the tongue redder. Further, certain medications will also affect the appearance of the tongue, such as antibiotics, and may cause a peeling of the tongue coat or make it thicker.

As with the pulse and the eye, the tongue contains within itself a map of the whole organism. Just as the upper, middle and lower portions of the body contain the function of ***kapha***, ***pitta*** and ***vāta***, respectively, so too can the tongue be divided into three portions: the anterior representing ***kapha sthāna***, the middle representing ***pitta sthāna***, and the posterior (or root), representing ***vāta sthāna***. As the entire function of the tongue is controlled by ***udāna vāyu***, specific problems of the tongue, such as an inability to control tongue movement, relate to this sub-***doṣa***. In relation to specific areas on the tongue, however, certain other sub-***doṣas*** may be observed as well.

There are five aspects of tongue diagnosis: colour, shape, location, coating and movement. The following is an exposition of these five fundamental aspects of ***jivhā parīkṣā***:

Colour

This is the colour of the body of the tongue, rather than its coating, which is discussed later. If the coating on the tongue is too thick to see underneath it, then the tongue may be curled up to examine its underside. The clinical significance of the tongue colour relates to the state of ***agni***, ***ojas*** and ***vyāna vāyu***. Ideally, the tongue should have a pinkish vibrancy to it, and any deviation from this is indicative of imbalance. Once again, by referring to the ***tridoṣa lakṣaṇas*** we can understand the manifestation of ***vāta***, ***pitta*** or ***kapha***. ***Vāta*** will be noticed as a tongue that is dark red to purplish, bluish, blackish, orange or grey. ***Pitta*** will be seen as a tongue that is bright red or has a greenish hue. ***Kapha*** will be observed as a tongue that is pale or whitish in colour. Table 10.1 lists the specific signs to look for in the assessment of the colour of the tongue.

Readers will note that the tongue of extreme ***pitta*** and extreme ***vāta*** are somewhat similar, although with heat the tongue will be more reddish in colour, and with cold the tongue will appear more bluish. Failing the ability to make this distinction, rely upon techniques such as the pulse, which will be bounding and rapid with heat, and deep and slow with cold. The

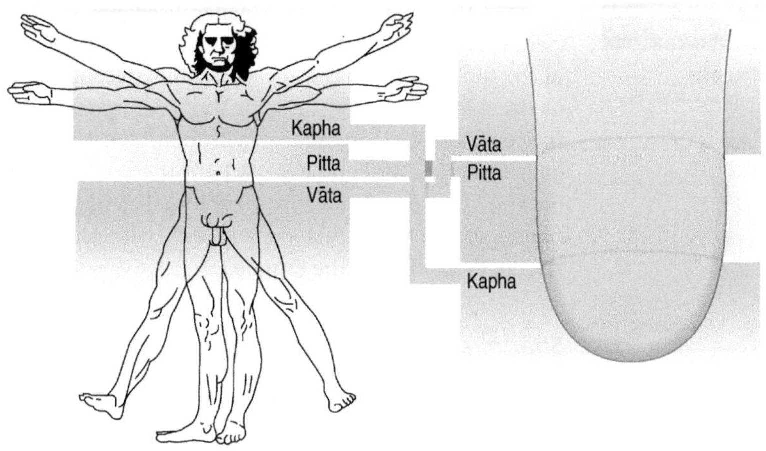

Figure 10.6 ***Sthāna:*** correspondence between the tongue and the body.

case history will also provide important indications that can help the practitioner make this distinction.

Shape

This refers to the shape of the tongue, generally, but including the sides and tip, as well as the surface. Understanding the shape of the tongue is a differentiation between thinness and thickness. Examination of the surface of the tongue means looking for cracking, furrowing, ulceration, raised papillae, deviation, swelling, bulging or depressions. Generally, ***vāttika*** tongues are thin and short, and may have cracking, furrowing, deviations, and depressions. ***Paittika*** tongues are typically long and may have raised papillae and some focal areas of ulceration. ***Kaphaja*** tongues are smooth, thick, flabby and swollen. Table 10.2 differentiates the many shapes that a tongue may take and the clinical significance of such findings.

TABLE 10.1 Clinical significance of tongue colour.

Tongue colour	Clinical significance
Pink	Normal
Pale	Cold, anaemia; coating will be dry (***vāta***) or wet (***kapha***)
Red	Heat (***pitta***) in the blood
Orange	Chronic heat (***pitta***), leading to a deficiency of blood (***vāta***); ***pitta*** aggravating ***vāta***
Dark red or reddish-purple	Extreme heat (***pitta***) and circulatory stagnation (***vāta***)
Blue or bluish-purple	Extreme cold (***vāta***) with circulatory stagnation

Shape: sides of the tongue

The sides of the tongue (Table 10.3) represent the assimilative and transformative functions of digestion. Assimilation is a measure of digestive efficiency, e.g. the digestive secretions of the lower fundus of the stomach, small intestine, liver, gall-bladder, and the exocrine pancreas, all of which are guided by ***agni***. Transformation on the other hand is a measure of how these nutrients are converted into the tissues of the body by the liver. This process is guided by both ***agni*** and ***ojas***.

Shape: tip of the tongue

The very tip of the tongue (Table 10.4) relates to the function of the heart, and the area just posterior relates to the lungs. The heart (***hṛdaya***) was traditionally thought of as the seat of the mind and emotions, and thus this region refers not only to the functional heart but also to the brain.

TABLE 10.2 Clinical significance of tongue shape.

Tongue shape	Clinical significance
Short, thin	***Vāta prakṛti***
Long, narrow	***Pitta prakṛti***
Large, thick	***Kapha prakṛti***
Furrows and fissures	Dryness (***vāta***)
Swollen	Congestion (***kapha***)
Swelling and redness	Heat (***pitta***)
Hemispheric swelling	Right side: external congestion (***pingalā nāḍī***)
	Left side: internal congestion (***ida nāḍī***)
Swollen along central axis	Nervous tension (***vāta, pitta***)
Hammer-shaped tip	***Prāṇic*** deficiency
Ulcerated, sore-covered	***Pitta sāma***

Shape: central axis of tongue

The central axis of the tongue represents the flow of ***prāṇa*** in the subtle body, along the same axis as the spinal column. ***Prāṇa*** is the animating force in the body and underlies the function of the central nervous system. Where a generalised furrow of the tongue can be seen this may indicate a generalised ***prāṇic*** deficiency. Where the furrow is deviated along the midline of the tongue, this may indicate a spinal misalignment or stress in the area of the spine that corresponds with the region on the tongue (e.g. a cranial, thoracic, lumbar or sacral misalignment). Where there is a partial furrow, this may indicate a ***prāṇic*** deficiency in the region of the body that corresponds with the same region, or ***sthāna*** of the tongue.

Shape: surface of the tongue

The tongue is a skeletal muscle covered by a mucous membrane. The projections on the tongue surface are called papillae. The majority of the papillae on the observable tongue are tightly knit filiform papillae, periodically interspersed with larger fungiform papillae that contain the taste buds. On the posterior tongue there is a v-shaped arrangement of circumvallate papillae that promote the gag-reflex when bitter, potentially poisonous substances are consumed. Generally speaking the surface of the tongue represents the bodily tissues or ***dhātus***.

Location

Location refers to specific areas on the body of the tongue that can be correlated with certain organ systems.

TABLE 10.3 Clinical significance of the sides of the tongue.

Tongue shape on sides	Clinical significance
Scalloped[25]	Malabsorption, nervous stress, anxiety (***vāta***), decreased ***ojas***
Fissured	Dryness (***vāta***), decreased ***ojas***
Swollen	Cold and congestion (***kapha***)
Swollen and Red	Heat (***pitta***)

TABLE 10.4 Clinical significance of the tip of the tongue.

Tongue shape on tip	Clinical significance
Swollen tip	Normal colour: heart congestion, dyspnoea, worry, grief (***kapha***)
	With redness: heart irritation, hypertension, anger (***pitta***)
Swollen between tip and center of tongue	Normal colour: lung congestion (***kapha***) With redness: lung inflammation (***pitta***)
Depression behind tip	Anxiety, emotional trauma, mental exhaustion

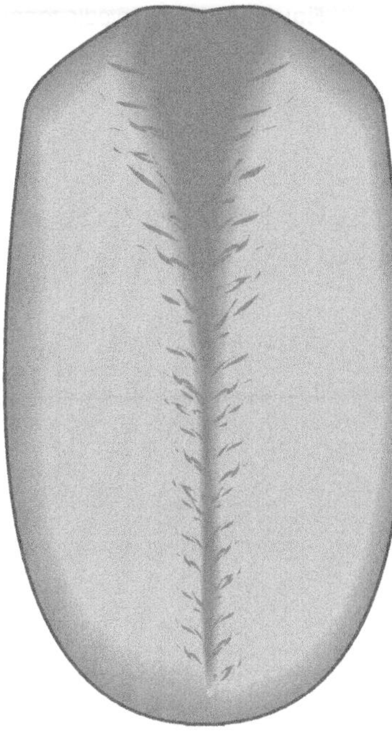

Figure 10.7 Central furrow.

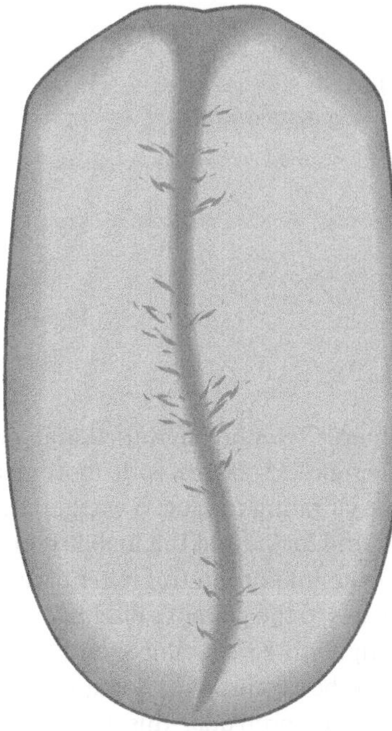

Figure 10.8 Deviated furrow.

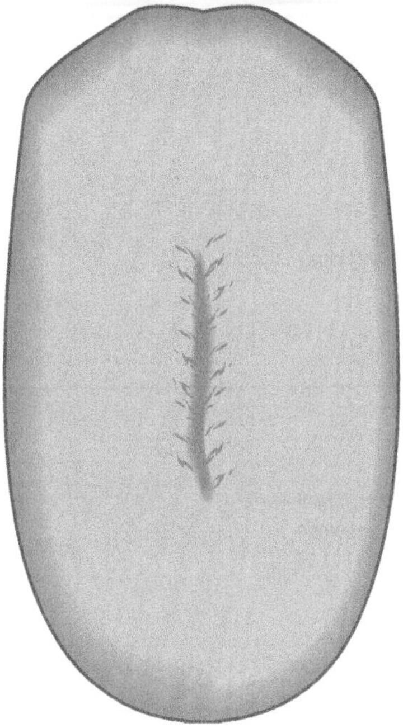

Figure 10.9 Partial furrow.

Signs such as colour, shape, moisture and coating observed within these locations provide clues as to how an organ system may be affected by ***vāta***, ***pitta*** or ***kapha***.

Coating

The coating refers to the tongue covering, also called the 'fur', and relates specifically to the function of ***agni*** (***pācaka pitta***). In association with location, however, the tongue coating will indicate the metabolic function of that organ system. Tongue coatings are identified by their color (white, whitish-yellow, yellow, dark yellow, orange, grey, brown, black), their quality (thin or thick), and their texture (dry, moist or greasy). Generally it is better to have a moist tongue than a dry tongue, and a tongue which changes from moist to dry indicates a worsening of the condition, while a coating which changes from dry to moist indicates improvement. A tongue that changes from a white to yellow coating indicates that the condition is being driven from a superficial condition deeper, from congestion (***kapha***) to inflammation (***pitta***), while the reverse indicates an improving condition, from deeper tissues to superficial areas for elimination. A coating that

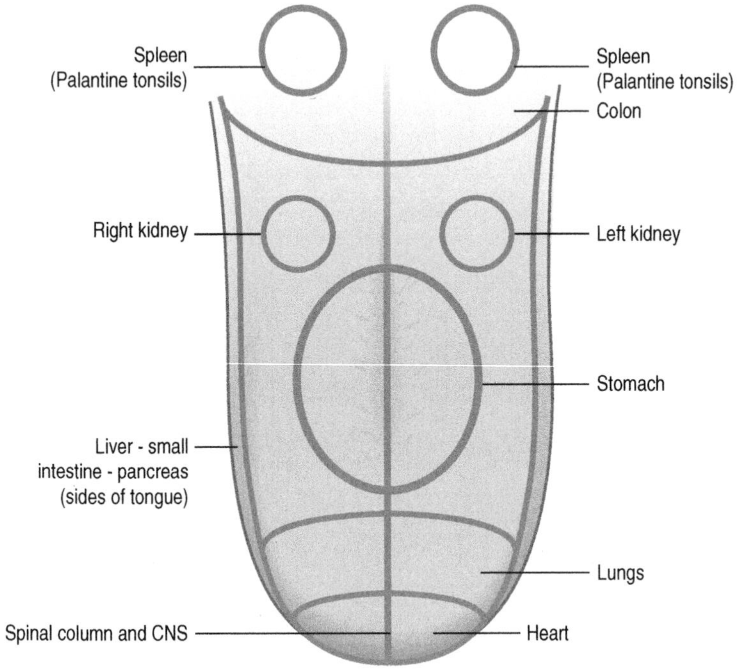

Figure 10.10 Āyurvedic tongue chart, anatomical position.

TABLE 10.5 Clinical significance of the surface of the tongue.

Surface of tongue	Clinical significance
Smooth, regular	Normal
Spots	Pale red: congestion with heat (***kapha*** aggravating ***pitta***) Red spots: heat (***pitta***) White: cold and damp (***kapha***) Purple: heat and stasis (***pitta*** aggravating ***vāta***) Black: stasis and dryness (***vāta***) Concave: cold (***vāta***) Convex: heat (***pitta***) On tip: anxiety, stress, grief On sides: anger, irritability
Fissures	Dryness (***vāta***)

becomes thicker over time indicates a worsening of the condition, while the reverse indicates improvement. Table 10.6 provides the clinical significance of each kind of tongue coating.

Movement

Movement refers to the movement of the tongue when extended for examination. As the impetus for movement is primarily ***vāta*** any dysfunctional movement is ***vāttika*** in origin. Problems with movement include a shaking or vibrating tongue, a wagging tongue that moves back and forth, and the inability to extend the tongue for examination. In this latter case, sometimes the issue relates to the patient's discomfort with allowing their tongue to be examined, and gentle encouragement may be required. In some cases where the tongue seems to protrude, this is an indication of extreme heat (***pitta kopa***).

TABLE 10.6 Tongue coating and clinical significance.

Tongue coating	Clinical significance
Clear or white, slightly moist	Normal, absence of imbalance
Absent, dry	Dryness (***vāta***)
Clear, very moist	Coldness (***kapha***)
Clear or white, thin, dry	Dryness (***vāta***)
White, thick, moist	Congestion and coldness (***kapha***)
White, thick, dry	Congestion (***kāpha***) and heat (***pitta***)
White, thick, greasy	Congestion (***kapha***) and ***āma***
White and powdery	Congestion (***kapha***) and heat (***pitta***); ***kapha*** aggravating ***pitta***
White and mouldy	Dryness (***vāta***), heat (***pitta***), congestion (***kapha***), and ***āma*** (poor prognosis)
Pale yellow	Congestion (***kapha***) with heat (***pitta***); ***kapha*** aggravating ***pitta***
Yellow	Heat (***pitta***)
Yellow and greasy	Heat (***pitta***) with ***āma***
Yellow and dry	Heat (***pitta***) with dryness (***vāta***)
	Pitta aggravating ***vāta***
Dirty yellow, brown	Heat (***pitta***) with ***āma***

ENDNOTES

21 Beverages such as tea, coffee and alcohol, however, can promote frequency, as will prescription diuretics.

22 There is some scholarly scepticism that the author of the ***Nāḍīvijñānam*** is one and the same as the author of the ***Vaiśeṣika Sūtra***. It was not uncommon for medieval writers to use the name of the great sages to add weight and significance to their own work, and as a result the ***Nāḍīvijñānam*** may be a comparatively more recent text.

23 The *rGyud bzi* states that the practitioner's left hand is used to assess the patient's right radial artery, in contradiction to what the ***Nāḍīvijñānam*** states. Further, some practitioners strongly suggest that the hand not taking the pulse should not touch the patient at all, because it will create an electrical circuit which will lead to an incorrect assessment.

24 This model places the scheme of ***nāḍī parīkṣā*** more or less in line with both Tibetan and Chinese pulsology. Using this model, it is now possible to understand the correspondences between the Chinese concept of the san jiao or 'triple burner', and the three ***sthānas*** represented by ***vāta*** (lower jiao), ***pitta*** (middle jiao) and ***kapha*** (upper jiao).

25 It is obvious that the scalloped tongue occurs because the tongue is either swollen (which indicates ***kapha***, and therefore ***mandāgni***), or because the patient unconsciously pushes his or her tongue against the teeth, causing indentation. This latter event I believe is an adaptive response to chronic stressors, and is reflective of ***vattika*** conditions. Interestingly, the palate is considered to be intimately linked to the function of the pancreas according to Āyurveda. I have come to suspect that this thrusting of the tongue upwards against the palate and the teeth occurs with hypoglycaemic patterns, associated with fight or flight mechanisms, increased ***vāta*** and decreased ***ojas***.

PART 1

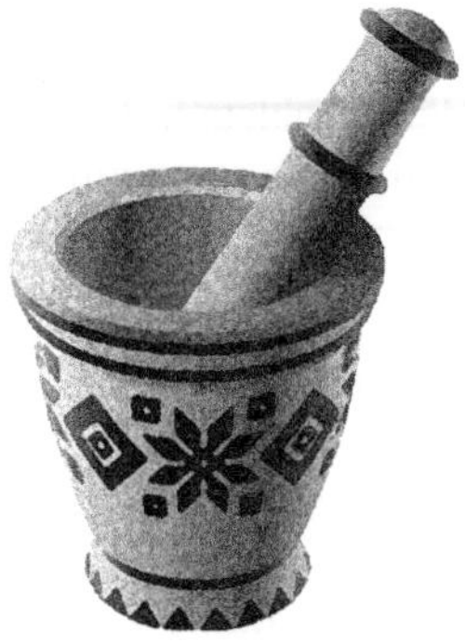

Chapter 11

TREATMENT OF DISEASE

OBJECTIVES

- To understand specialised techniques of physical and mental purification in Āyurveda.
- To understand and review therapeutic techniques to rejuvenate the body.
- To understand and review therapeutic methodologies in the treatment of disease in clinical practice.

In reviewing the text thus far you should be familiar with the dynamics of ***tridoṣa*** (Chapter 2), the structure of ***dravyguṇa*** ('pharmacology,' Chapter 6), ***vikara*** (the 'causes of disease,' Chapter 8), ***daśavidha parīkṣā*** ('case history,' Chapter 9) and the ***aṣṭāsthāna parīkṣā*** ('diagnosis techniques,' Chapter 10). Chapter 11 introduces the fundamental therapeutic approaches used in ***kāya cikitsā*** ('internal medicine'), detailing ***pañca karma***, ***rasāyana karma*** and ***śamana karma***.

As mentioned in 6.9 (***Karma***: therapeutic action), treatment strategies are described as being of two basic types:

1. ***Śodhana***: treatment strategies that seek to purify the body of the accumulated ***doṣas*** by direct means.
2. ***Śamana***: treatment strategies that seek to pacify the aggravated ***doṣas*** by indirect means.

The ***śamana*** therapies are ***bṛmhaṇa*** ('nourishing'), ***langhana*** ('depleting'), ***svedana*** ('heating'), ***stambhana*** ('cooling'), ***rūkṣana*** ('drying') and ***snehana*** ('moistening'). Unlike the ***śodhana*** or ***pañca karmas***, these therapies are suited for use on an outpatient basis, but still require an experienced hand in their administration and appropriate usage. Each of the ***śamana*** therapies is used to treat a particular ***vikṛti***, or 'disease' tendency.

11.1 THE *pañca karmas*

Śodhana karmas are commonly referred to as the ***pañca karmas***, and are ***vamana*** ('vomiting'), ***virecana*** ('purgation'), ***vasti*** ('enema'), ***nasya*** ('errhine'), and ***rakta mokṣaṇa*** ('venesection'). ***Pañca karma*** is used in different ways according to the ***prakṛti*** and the ***vikṛti***, and thus there is no standard treatment.

What follows is only an outline of the basic approaches in ***pañca karma***, not an exhaustive exposition of the many different techniques and procedures that are used. ***Pañca karma*** is a potentially debilitating therapy that must be performed under the supervision of a trained Āyurvedic physician, and is usually followed by ***rasāyana*** ('rejuvenative') treatments. ***Pañca karma*** is not a therapy that can be performed on an out-patient basis and any treatment that claims to be ***pañca karma*** and is not performed in a hospital or a similar facility cannot be ***pañca karma***.

Pañca karma is performed only after the use of the ***pūrva karmas***, specific preparatory measures that rid the body of ***āma***, including include ***dīpana*** ('enhancement of digestion') and ***pācana*** ('cooking' of ***āma***), and techniques to mobilise the vitiated ***doṣas*** for elimination, such as ***snehana*** ('oil massage') and ***svedana*** ('sudation').

After an assessment of the ***prakṛti*** and ***vikṛti*** by the physician the ***pūrva karmas*** are begun. ***Pūrva karmas*** are essential to prime the ***doṣas*** for their subsequent removal during ***pañca karma***, to promote the movement of ***āma*** and the ***doṣas*** from the 'tissues' of the body (***shakha***) to the 'digestive tract' (***koṣṭha***) for elimination. Sometimes the ***pūrva karmas*** are the only treatments employed, a technique that is especially common in the Keraliya school of Āyurveda.

11.2 *Pūrva karmas*: *āmapācana*

As mentioned previously, ***pañca karma*** is begun only once the body has been purified of ***āma***, called ***āmapācana***. To this end an Āyurvedic physician uses two distinct classes of remedies:

- ***Dīpana***: remedies that stimulate ***agni***
- ***Pācana***: remedies that have a special capacity to cook or 'digest' ***āma***.

In almost all cases an ***āmapācana*** remedy will contain aspects of both ***dīpana*** and ***pācana***. These remedies are often given along with ***ghṛta***, which has a special capacity to bring ***āma*** to the digestive tract. Normally ***ghṛta*** is contraindicated in ***āma*** conditions because it tends to weaken ***agni*** due to its ***guru*** ('heavy') and ***snigdha*** ('oily') properties, but in this case is used as a medicine to coax ***āma*** from the tissues to the digestive tract. Āyurvedic physicians employ a number of remedies in ***āmapācana***, including ***cūrṇa*** ('powders'), ***guṭikā*** ('tablets'), ***kvātha*** ('decoctions'), ***ghṛta*** ('medicated ***ghṛta*** compounds'), and ***asava/ariṣṭa*** ('natural fermentations'). These include:

- ***Cūrṇa***: ***Trikaṭu cūrṇa***, ***Avipattikāra cūrṇa***, ***Hingvaṣṭaka cūrṇa***
- ***Gulika***: ***Citrakādi vaṭī***, ***Agnituṇḍī vaṭī***, ***Gandhāka vaṭī***
- ***Kvātha***: ***Pippalyādi kvātha***, ***Jīrakādi kvātha***, ***Dhānyāpañcaka kvātha***
- ***Ghṛta***: ***Pippalyādi ghṛta***, ***Drākṣādi ghṛta***, ***Śūṇṭhī ghṛta***
- ***Asava/ariṣṭa***: ***Pippalyādyāsava***, ***Daśamūla ariṣṭa***, ***Jīrakāriṣṭa***.

While these formulas have long been used in Āyurveda, simpler formulations can also be used, composed of ***dīpanapācana*** herbs such as ***Śūṇṭhī*** dried rhizome (*Zingiber officinalis*), ***Pippalī*** fruit (*Piper longum*), ***Harītakī*** fruit (*Terminalia chebula*) and ***Yavānī*** fruit (*Trachyspermum ammi*). A number of other non-Indian herbs can also be used in ***āmapācana*** including Bayberry bark (*Myrica cerifera*), Cayenne fruit (*Capsicum annuum*), and Barberry root (*Berberis vulgaris*).

Āmapācana is given over a period of several days, up to 2 weeks, with a strict attention to diet, avoiding foods that promote ***kapha***, i.e. those that contain ***śita*** ('cold'), ***guru*** ('heavy'), ***snigdha*** ('oily'), and ***picchila*** ('sticky') properties (e.g. flour products, dairy, oily foods, excessive meat, sweets, excess fruit, etc.). When ***āmapācana*** is performed properly the appetite will be noticeably improved, eliminatory functions will normalise and there will be a feeling of lightness and renewed energy. While ***āmapācana*** is used therapeutically as a preparatory measure for ***pañca karma***, it can also be used periodically as a preventative approach to eliminate ***āma*** and enhance ***agni***.

11.3 *Pūrva karmas*: *snehana* (OLEATION)

After ***āmapācana*** has been successfully implemented the next stage in ***pūrva karma*** is ***snehana*** therapy, or oleation, used to mobilise the ***doṣas*** from their respective locations in the body so they can be eliminated during ***pañca karma***. According to Āyurveda, oil has a special capacity to move into the most minute ***srotāṃsi*** ('channels') of the body and influence the activity of the ***doṣas***. A number of different oils, both unprocessed and medicated, are used in ***snehana*** therapy, the most common of which is ***taila*** ('sesame oil') and the various medicated preparations made from it. The ***Aṣṭāñga Hṛdaya*** mentions a number of other oils, however, that can also be used in ***snehana***, including ***ghṛta***, ***vasa*** ('animal fat'), and ***majjā*** ('marrow fat'). Beyond these, Āyurvedic practitioners have added a number of other oils to take advantage of their different qualities, including coconut oil, almond oil and castor oil. In most cases, however, the oil used is ***taila*** or ***ghṛta***, often medicated with different herbs to yield a distinct therapeutic activity.

Snehana therapy has a number of indications and contraindications, depending on the signs and symptoms of the patient, the qualities of the oil to be used, and the season and climate. Generally speaking, ***snehana*** therapy is best in ***vāttika*** and ***paittika*** conditions, and is generally contraindicated in ***kaphaja*** conditions. ***Taila*** is best used in ***vāttika*** conditions, and to a lesser extent in ***kaphaja*** conditions, and is often contraindicated in ***paittika*** conditions. ***Ghṛta*** is best used in ***vāttika*** and ***paittika*** conditions, and is often contraindicated in ***kaphaja*** conditions. Both ***vasa*** and ***majjā*** are only really used in ***vāttika*** conditions, ***majjā*** being the heaviest and most nourishing of the oils. Generally speaking, ***snehana*** therapy should only be undertaken when the weather is warm and the sky is clear, and is avoided in both very hot and very cold weather.

Snehana consists of both external and internal therapies, ensuring that there is a complete penentration of the oils throughout the entire body. The following details both external and internal ***snehana***.

External *snehana*

The most common form of external ***snehana*** is ***abhyaṅga***, in which a fairly large volume of oil (250–1000 mL) is massaged over the entire body, either a plain oil such as sesame or ***ghṛta***, or a specific medicated oil. Typically the oil is applied at room temperature but may be used at higher temperatures in ***vāttika*** conditions. In such cases where warm oil is used, relatively stable oils such as sesame, olive, ***ghṛta***, ***vasa*** or ***majjā*** should be used in preference to oils rich in polyunsaturated fats such as hemp, flax, safflower and sunflower, which tend to go rancid quickly. For each patient the oil is re-used over a 3-day period before it is discarded.

While ***abhyaṅga*** can be performed on a normal massage table covered with a sheet to soak up the excess oil, specially constructed tables called ***taila droṇi*** are used in India, traditionally carved from a solid piece of wood from species such as ***Panasaḥ*** (*Artocarpus integrifolia*), ***Nimba*** (*Azadirachta indica*) or ***Ulkaṭaḥ*** (*Polyalthia longifolia*). Although there are several different kinds of ***taila droṇi***, the basic dimensions are 228 cm long by 76 cm wide.[26] The table comprises two sections: one where the head rests, and the other where the body lies. Under the head portion is a basin carved into the wood that collects the oil applied to the head, and along the sides of the body portion are channels carved into the wood that collect the excess oil, which drains into a hole at the bottom. In order to facilitate the movement of the oil downwards the table is slightly elevated at the head, and after the session the excess oil is scraped from the table into the drainage channels and collected in a vessel underneath the drainage hole. A traditionally made ***taila droṇi*** is quite expensive, even in India, and such tables are hard to come by in the West. As a result, a table can be made with other woods that are more easily obtainable – or even heat-resistant fibreglass.

The application of the oil in ***abhyaṅga*** can vary depending upon the need. In both ***vāttika*** and ***kaphaja*** conditions the oil is applied quite warm, whereas the oil in ***paittika*** conditions is applied at room temperature. When the oil is applied to the head, however, the oil is always applied at room temperature. ***Abhyaṅga*** is typically performed with two or four practitioners, one or two on each side of the patient's body working in tandem, but it can also be done with just one practitioner. The patient must be unclothed, and as a result the room must be quite warm. For the added warmth and comfort of the patient a sheet can be draped over the areas of the body not being worked on.

There are six basic positions that are used in ***abhyaṅga***, with the patient's head pointing in an easterly direction:

- Seated position: the patient sits upright and the oil is rubbed into the head, ears and neck.
- Supine position: the patient lies face up and the oil is massaged into the chest, and anterior portions of the arms, legs and feet.

- Left lateral position: the patient lies on the left side of the body, and the oil is rubbed into the right sides of the torso, arms, legs and feet.
- Prone position: the patient lies face down and the oil is massaged into the back, and posterior portions of the arms, legs and feet.
- Right lateral position: the patient lies on the right side of the body, and the oil is rubbed into the left sides of the torso, arms, legs and feet.
- Seated position: the patient again sits upright and the oil is rubbed into the head, ears and neck.

When the oil is applied to the head first, working down towards the feet, the effect is to relieve pain. ***Abhyaṅga*** can also be administered by applying the oil to the feet first, however, moving up the body and finishing with the head. This latter method is more appropriate to ground or centre the patient in mental or emotional stress.

There are a number of different massage techniques used in ***abhyaṅga*** depending upon the ***prakṛti*** and ***vikṛti*** of the patient. ***Mardana*** is the use of vigorous, deep massage strokes, used more often in ***kaphaja*** or ***pitta-kaphaja*** conditions, when the patient's body is thick and heavy. ***Sanvahana*** is the application of gentle, light massage strokes, used more often in ***vāttika*** conditions when the patient's body is thin and light. Other techniques include:

- ***pidhana***: patting and beating with the flat of the hand, used to relieve pain and spasm
- ***avapidhana***: thumb pressure, to enhance circulation
- ***uthveśtana***: circular movements, used over large joints to reduce ***vāta***
- ***paripidhana***: gently beating and rubbing the body with the bottom part of the closed fist, to invigorate the body
- ***māṃsa mardana***: rolling a smooth wooden or copper dowel with both hands over the muscles, to relieve pain and congestion.

Other massage techniques such as lymphatic drainage, myofascial release, reiki, polarity and cranial sacral therapy can all be used in ***abhyaṅga***. Care should be taken to ensure that the oil is well absorbed by the patient's skin and particular attention should be paid to the major joints of the axillary skeleton, including the shoulders, elbows, wrists, hands, hips, knees, ankles and feet.

Generally speaking, certain herbs are best used in the preparation of a medicated oil in the treatment of a specific ***doṣa*** or ***doṣas*** (see 6.11 ***Bhaiṣajya vyākhyāna:*** *principles of pharmacy*):

- To reduce ***vāta***, warming and strengthening herbs such as ***Balā*** root (*Sida cordifolia*) and ***Aśvagandhā*** root (*Withania somnifera*) can be used to medicate the oils. Formulations to reduce ***vāta*** include ***Daśamūla taila***, ***Nārāyaṇa taila*** and ***Balā taila***.
- To reduce ***pitta***, cooling and anti-inflammatory herbs such as ***Nimba*** bark (*Azadirachta indica*), ***Mañjiṣṭhā*** root (*Rubia cordifolia*) and ***Śatāvarī*** root (*Asparagus racemosa*) can be used to medicate the oil. Examples of formulations to reduce ***pitta*** include ***Candanādi taila***, ***Kṣirabalā taila*** and ***Śatāvarī ghṛta***.
- To reduce ***kapha***, pungent and clearing herbs such as ***Pippalī*** fruit (*Piper longum*), ***Guggulu*** resin (*Commiphora mukul*) and ***Śūṇṭhī*** rhizome (*Zingiber officinalis*) can be used to medicate the oil. Examples of formulations to reduce ***kapha*** include ***Sahacarādi taila*** and ***Daśamūla taila***.

Abhyaṅga is used prior to and in between each ***pañca karma*** treatment. In most circumstances, ***abhyaṅga*** is applied every 12 hours over a 4-day period before ***vamana*** ('emesis') is begun. Prior to ***virecana*** ('purgation'), ***abhyaṅga*** is again implemented every 12 hours over a 3–8 day period. Thereafter ***abhyaṅga*** preceeds the application of both ***vasti*** ('enema') and ***nasya*** ('errhine') on each separate occasion they are administered.

Other forms of external ***snehana*** include ***dhārā***, ***śiro dhārā***, ***śiro vasti***, ***picu***, ***pizhichil***, ***kati vasti***, and ***kavalagraha***. ***Dhārā*** ('dripping') is the application of a constant stream of oil over a specific area of the body, whereas ***śiro dhārā*** ('head dripping') is the application of a continuous stream of oil over the area between the hairline and the eyebrow (i.e. the ***ājñā cakra***). The kind of oil used in ***dhārā*** or ***śiro dhārā*** is dependent upon the signs and symptoms of the patient. Commonly used herbs to make medicated oils used in ***śiro dhārā*** include ***Balā*** root (*Sida cordifolia*), ***Aśvagandhā*** root (*Withania somnifera*), and ***Brāhmī*** leaf (*Bacopa monniera*), prepared in ***taila***, ***ghṛta***, milk, buttermilk or water. Important formulas include ***Candanādi taila***, ***Balā taila***, ***Jyotiṣmatī taila*** and ***Nīlībhṛṅgādi taila***. Among the more common preparations in ***śiro dhārā*** is ***Kṣirabalā taila***, which comprises:

- ***Balā*** root (*Sida cordifolia*), 4 parts (by weight)
- ***Balā*** root ***kalka*** (paste), 1 part (by weight)
- ***taila***, 4 parts (by volume)
- cow's milk, 4 parts (by volume)
- water, 64 parts (by volume).

The above ingredients are mixed together and boiled until only one-quarter of the volume remains. The preparation is then strained, cooled and bottled for later use.

Both ***dhārā*** and ***śiro dhārā*** are traditionally performed by the use of a broad-bottomed pot called a ***dhārā pātra***, made from clay, wood or metal, with a capacity of about 2–3 litres. The ***dhārā pātra*** is securely suspended over the patient's body at a distance of about 20 cm. Inside this suspended vessel is a hole through which a cotton wick is placed. The wick is tied to half a ripe coconut shell that has little grooves fashioned on its edge to allow the oil to pass underneath it, through the hole, down the wick. In this way the coconut shell regulates the flow of oil in the ***dhārā pātra*** down the wick. The distance of the cotton wick from the body should be no more than four finger-breadths (6–8 cm). To ensure that the oil moves down the wick properly it should be premoistened beforehand by soaking it in oil.

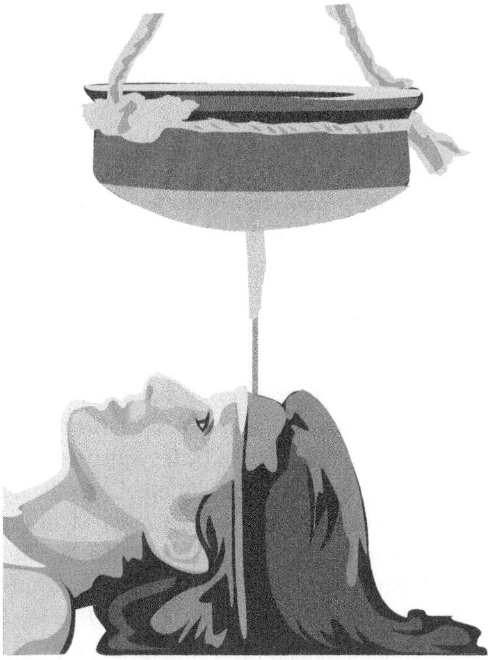

Figure 11.1 Śiro dhārā.

After ***abhyaṅga***, the ***dhārā pātra*** is positioned over the location to be treated, such as the large joints, or locations on the spine that correspond to specific ***cakras***. In ***śiro dhārā*** the ***dhārā pātra*** is positioned over the patient's forehead and a ***bandhāna*** is rolled up and loosely tied around the patient's head just at the eyebrow level or over the eyes to prevent the oil from seeping into them. The oil is then placed into the ***dhārā pātra*** and as the oil streams down onto the patient's forehead the ***dhārā pātra*** is moved back and forth so that the stream of oil slowly migrates from one side to the other. The path of the oil should not be moved back and forth across the patient's forehead in a straight line, but rather, follow a meandering zigzag path: if it is done in a straight line it is thought to disturb the mind. As the oil washes down across the body it is collected into a basin that lies below the body part being treated, or in the case of ***śiro dhārā***, a basin that is carved into or attached to the table itself. The oil is then scooped up with half of a coconut shell and poured back into the suspended ***dhārā pātra***. Thus ***dhārā*** traditionally requires two practitioners, one to regulate the stream of oil across the patient's forehead and the other to scoop the oil back into the vessel. An innovation on this traditional method is an electric pump that collects the oil from the basin and pumps it back up to the ***dhārā pātra*** with a hose, avoiding the need for two people. As the oil is collected it may need to be reheated, depending on the body part treated.

Dhārā is typically performed during the ***vāta*** dominant times of day, in the early morning or late afternoon, between 30 and 90 minutes: longer in ***vāttika*** conditions, a medium amount of time in ***paittika*** conditions, and only for a short time in ***kaphaja*** conditions. ***Śiro dhārā*** is typically administered over a period of 7–14 days, but for no more than 21 days. Although ***śiro dhārā*** is a ***pūrva karma*** it is also a stand-alone treatment, used in EENT disorders, vertigo, insomnia, headaches and to correct the flow of ***prāṇa vāyu***. It may also be used in the treatment of mental disorders such as anxiety, depression, schizophrenia and epilepsy. ***Śiro dhārā*** is contraindicated in fever and it is recommended that the patient avoid sleep for some time (3–5 hours) after treatment in order to prevent the aggravation of ***kapha***.

Śiro vasti is another ***snehana*** technique that is applied to the head. In this technique a wide leather band about 40 cm high is placed around the patient's head and stitched together to essentially make a kind of vessel. Inside this vessel is placed a paste of flour to seal the cracks that lie between the band and the patient's head. Once this is done a large volume of medicated oil is then poured over the head where it is contained by the leather band and penetrates into the scalp. In most cases patients are required to cut their hair quite short or shave their head prior to the therapy. ***Śiro vasti*** treatment usually lasts between 30 and 45 minutes and is performed in the early morning or late afternoon during the ***vāta*** time of day. ***Śiro vasti*** is used to treat diseases such as facial paralysis, insomnia, alopecia, sinus disorders, migraines and psychiatric disorders. ***Dravyas*** used to medicate the oils used in ***śiro vasti*** are similar to those used in ***śiro dhārā***. Specific medicated oils used in ***śiro vasti*** include ***Bhṛṅgarāja taila***, ***Balādhātryādi taila*** and ***Nīlībhṛṅgādi taila***.

Picu is the use of a piece of linen that has been soaked in a medicated oil and is applied over the head. A ***bandhāna*** is then tied over the top of this linen to hold it in place. The types of oil used in ***picu*** are similar to those used in ***śiro dhārā*** and ***śiro vasti***.

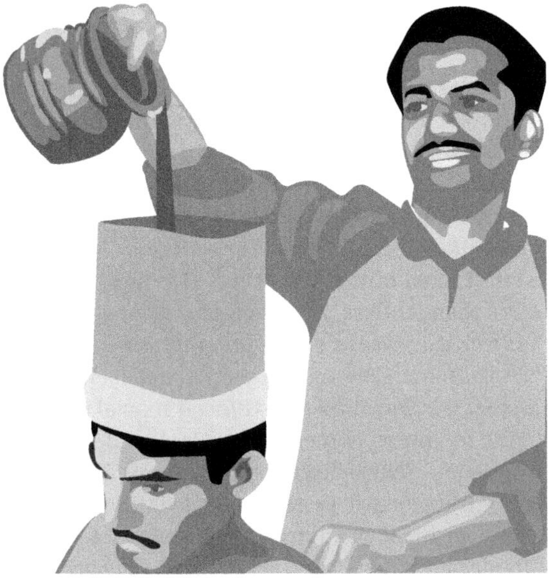

Figure 11.2 ***Śiro vasti.***

Pizhichil is somewhat similar to ***dhārā***, but is really a combination of both ***snehana*** and ***svedana*** techniques. The masseuse soaks a piece of linen in a bowl of very warm oil and wrings it out over the top of the patient. The masseuse may focus on specific areas of the body, such as the hips, or it may be a generalised application. It is best to have at least two people administering ***pizhichil***, one to administer the treatment and the other to collect the oil, warm it back up to the desired temperature, and make it available for the masseuse to use.

Kati vasti is the application of medicated oil over the ***kati***, the lumbar and sacral region of the back. A paste is made from ***urad*** bean flour and is formed into a circular wall that circumnavigates the lower back region to form a vessel. A very warm medicated oil such as ***Gandhārvahasta taila*** or ***Piṇḍa taila*** is placed inside this vessel, and is allowed to soak into the skin for 30 minutes. As the oil cools it is removed with absorbent cloths and replaced with warm oil. ***Kati vasti*** is indicated in lumbago and sciatica. This technique can also be performed on any part of the body. When it is applied in the eyes it is called ***netra vasti***, in which case simple oils such as ***ghṛta*** are used in the treatment of opthalmologic disorders, but also medicated oils such as ***Triphala ghṛta*** and herbal decoctions. Note, however, that the oils used in ***netra vasti*** are never used warm or hot. Applied over the chest this technique is called ***hṛdaya vasti***, and medicated oils such as ***Dhānvantara taila*** are applied in the treatment of heart disease.

Kavalagraha is the use of a decoction (***kaśāya kavalagraha***) or medicated oil (***sneha kavalagraha***) as a mouthwash. ***Kaśāya kavalagraha*** is used in oral diseases such as gingivitis, apthous ulcers and tooth decay. Examples of herbs used in ***kaśāya kavalagraha*** include ***Nimba*** leaf (*Azadirachta indica*), ***Guggulu*** resin (*Commiphora mukul*), ***Haridrā*** rhizome (*Curcuma longa*) and ***Triphala cūrṇa***. Used concurrently with the application of medicated oils massaged into the head and neck, ***sneha kavalagraha*** is helpful in temporomandibular joint (TMJ) syndrome.

Karṇa tarpaṇa is the instillation of a medicated oil into the ears (***karṇa***) in the treatment of disease of the ear. In the treatment of otitis media ***kapha*** and ***pitta*** reducing herbs are used to medicate the oil, such as ***Guggulu*** resin (*Commiphora mukul*), ***Haridrā*** rhizome (*Curcuma longa*) and ***Laśuna*** bulb (*Allium sativum*). In conditions such as tinnitus ***vāta*** reducing

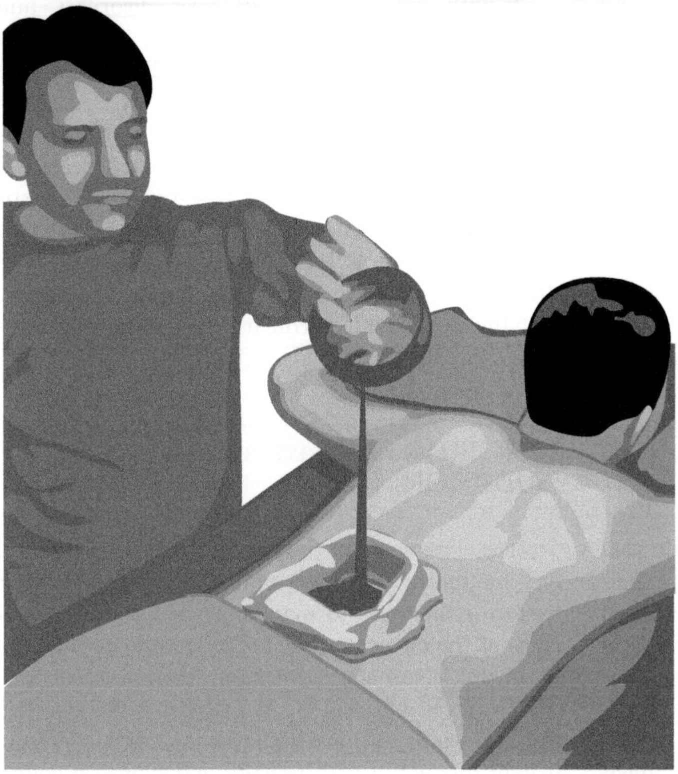

Figure 11.3 *Kati vasti.*

herbs are used to medicate the oil, such as ***Balā*** root (*Sida cordifolia*).

Because ***abhyaṅga*** and oleation therapies are primarily a treatment for ***vāta***, not all patients require oil. Two techniques, ***gharṣana*** and ***udavartana***, are best suited to relieving ***pitta*** and ***kapha***. ***Gharṣana*** makes use of special gloves of raw silk, worn by the masseuse. It is best for relieving the symptoms of excess ***kapha*** and has a stimulating and invigorating effect on the body. ***Udavartana*** is the application of certain herbal powders, such as ***Guḍūcī*** vine (*Tinospora cordifolia*), ***Guggulu*** resin (*Commiphora mukul*), ***Triphala*** or ***Trikaṭu cūrṇa*** to relieve ***kaphaja*** conditions such as lymphatic congestion, cellulite, oedema and obesity. Sometimes ***udavartana*** is used after external ***snehana***, especially in ***vāta-kapha*** or ***vāta sāma*** conditions.

Other external techniques include ***avagāha*** ('baths') and ***lepana*** ('poultice'). ***Avagāha*** includes both whole-body baths and local applications such as sitz baths. ***Lepana*** involves the use of a paste prepared from powdered medicinal plants and applied to the body. ***Śiro lepana*** ('head poultice') is the application of a herbal paste to the middle of the head in the treatment of central nervous system disorders such as multiple sclerosis, paralysis and parkinsonism. One ***śiro lepana*** recipe used in disorders of the central nervous system calls for equal parts of the recently dried finely sieved powders of ***Maṇḍūkaparṇī*** leaf (*Centella asiatica*), ***Āmalakī*** fruit (*Phyllanthus emblica*) and ***Candana*** wood (*Santalum album*), mixed together with cool milk to make a thick paste. The paste is applied over the shaved head of the patient, and is allowed to sit for 1–2 hours, once daily.

Internal *snehana*

Internal ***snehana*** therapy, or ***snehapāna*** ('oil drinking'), is the internal application of progressively larger amounts of oil, used concurrently with external oleation techniques such as ***abhyaṅga***. The purpose of ***snehapāna*** is similar to the external application of oil, to loosen and liquefy ***āma*** from the ***bāhya rogayana*** ('outer pathway') and ***madhyama rogamārga*** ('middle pathway'), and draw it to the ***añtarmārga*** ('inner pathway', gastrointestinal tract) for elimination. Additionally, ***snehapāna*** therapy lubricates the gastrointestinal tract for the elimination of ***āma*** and the ***doṣas*** during ***pañca karma***. Any kind of appropriate oil may be used for this purpose, but the safest oil is ***ghṛta***. ***Taila***, or sesame oil, is best used in the treatment of tumours, sinus ulcers, parasites and ***kaphaja*** or ***vāttika*** conditions. ***Vasa*** (muscle fats) and ***majjā*** (marrow fats) are best used in the treatment of ***vāttika*** conditions, excessive sexual activity, cachexia, exhaustion, abdominal pain, burns, earaches and headaches. In the West, olive oil is commonly used to treat gall bladder disease and also has utility in Āyurvedic medicine.

There are two forms of ***snehapāna***: ***vicaranā*** and ***acchapāna***. In ***vicaranā snehana***, only a small amount of oil is consumed, mixed with the dietary articles such as rice, broth, meat, milk, vegetables, etc. The effect is limited and takes a much longer period of time to be efficacious. It is indicated specifically in persons who have an aversion to fats and oils, when ***agni*** is weak, when ***kapha*** predominates, in a ***mṛdu koṣṭha***, or in cholelithiasis, all of which are contraindications for ***acchapāna snehana***.

Acchapāna snehana is the consumption of an oil in large volumes over a maximum period of 7 days, 50 mL the first day, with each successive day adding 50 mL until a maximum total of 350 mL of oil is consumed on the seventh day. The number of days of administration and hence the amount of oil consumed depends upon the nature of the digestive tract: when the ***koṣṭha*** ('bowel') is ***mṛdu*** ('soft'), treatment is limited to 3 days; when the ***koṣṭha*** ('bowel') is ***madhya*** ('medium'), treatment is limited to 5 days; when the ***koṣṭha*** ('bowel') is ***krūra*** ('hard'), treatment can be implemented to the maximum of 7 days (for a description of the different types of ***koṣṭhas*** see 4.1 ***Agni:*** the fire of digestion and metabolism). After the consumption of the oil, a little warm water is drunk and the patient does not eat until hunger returns and their belches are free of the taste of the oil. ***Acchapāna sneha*** is performed early in the morning or late in the afternoon, when ***vāta*** predominates. Foods to be taken the day before administration and after the digestion of the oil should be soupy, warm and bland, such as rice and ***mūng*** bean soup. The signs of properly administered ***acchapāna*** are increased appetite after therapy, fatty and semi-solid faeces, aversion to fatty foods, and lassitude. Symptoms of excessive ***snehapāna*** include lacrimation and mucus congestion, as well as a yellowish-white pallor. ***Acchapāna*** should be used with extreme care in liver disorders and cholelithiasis.

According to Hindu belief, fats and oils are generally associated with Lakṣmī, the goddess of prosperity, wealth and fortune. Thus the use of oil brings this quality of abundance to the body, and herbs medicated in oil are potentised in the way. Based on this property, fats and oils are ***bṛmhaṇa*** and are thus indicated as a ***śamana*** treatment in deficiency conditions. Where there is excess and the need for ***langhana*** therapies, both the topical and internal use of ***snehana*** therapies should be avoided or used sparingly.

11.4 *Pūrva karmas*: *svedana* (SUDATION)

The last component of the ***pūrva karmas*** is ***svedana***, or sudation therapy. ***Svedana*** therapies are used after ***snehana*** therapies to maximise the absorption and effect of the medicated oil, and to further mobilise the ***doṣas*** for elimination. ***Svedana*** therapies enhance ***agni*** and communicate its activity from the digestive tract outwards to the skin. ***Svedana*** is a particularly helpful therapy in both ***vāttika*** and ***kaphaja*** conditions, but may be contraindicated where ***pitta*** predominates, including inflammatory conditions of the nervous system such as multiple sclerosis.

Any number of ***svedana*** techniques may be used, dependent upon the condition, but they can be broadly separated into ***rūkṣa*** ('dry') and ***snigdha*** ('wet') applications. In any sudation technique, however, it is important that the head and eyes are protected from the heat. Dry sudation techniques such as a dry sauna are used in ***kaphaja*** conditions but are typically avoided when ***vāta*** is aggravated. In dry saunas a moist towel or cloth can be placed over the head to keep it cool. Wet sudation techniques are employed by the use of a ***svedana*** chamber or tent that covers the body (but not the head) of the patient lying on the massage table and into which steam is channelled. Even simple techniques such as covering the patient from the neck down with a blanket and placing a steaming pot of water underneath a chair that the patient sits on can be helpful. If a proper ***svedana*** chamber is not available a steam bath or sweat lodge is an acceptable alternative, or if these cannot be found, a hot shower. Other forms of ***svedana*** include sunbathing, which is particularly helpful in skin conditions such as leprosy and psoriasis, and vigorous exercise.

Svedana treatments can also be localised rather than the more generalised treatments described above, and can utilise steam from sources other than boiling water. One technique called ***nāḍī sveda*** involves the collection of steam from a herbal decoction, such as ***Balā*** root (***Sida cordifolia***) decocted in milk. In this case the steam is collected with a rubber surgical hose attached to a spout on a pressure cooker. The steam is then directed to the specific area that requires attention, or is generally distributed across the body. Special care must be taken not to hold the hose too close to the skin to avoid burning the patient.

Another ***svedana*** technique that is commonly used is ***piṇḍa sveda***, used after ***abhyaṅga***. ***Piṇḍa sveda*** involves the use of legumes and grains such as ***urad***, rice, oats and barley that are cooked until very soft in a previously prepared herbal decoction. Once cooked and the water evaporated away the mixture is tied in linen to make little balls or ***piṇḍa*** about the size of one's palm. Prior to treatment the ***piṇḍa*** are soaked in a very warm decoction or oil, and while they are still quite warm the ***piṇḍa*** are stroked over the body, the force of the strokes causing some of the contents and the moisture of the ***piṇḍa*** to escape onto the skin. To ensure that the application is even at least two attendants should perform the massage, standing on either side of the body, mirroring each the other's actions. As the ***piṇḍa*** loses its moisture it can be put back into oil or decoction and be used again during the session. Any number of herbs may be used to medicate the ***piṇḍa***, depending on the condition being treated and the ***doṣa*** or ***doṣas*** that predominate. ***Piṇḍa sveda*** is an invigorating and strengthening procedure that helps to both stimulate ***agni*** and promote the digestion of ***āma***. It is used therapeutically in conditions such as depression and fatigue, and in the treatment of arthritis. ***Piṇḍa sveda*** is performed on alternate days up to a maximum of 28 days.

Still another ***svedana*** method is the use of heated ***saindhava***, or rock salt, roasted until brown and applied to the body at a tolerably warm temperature. It is both stimulating as well as liquefying to ***kapha***, and promotes the elimination of ***āma***. Sometimes ***saindhava*** is added to a ***taila*** to achieve a similar effect.

11.5 *Pañca karma*: *vamana* (EMESIS)

Vamana, or emetic therapy, is usually the first of the ***pañca karmas*** to be implemented, and is a treatment given specifically to ***kapha***. If we recall from 2.4 (***Sthāna:*** residence of the ***doṣas***), ***kapha*** resides in the upper portions of the body, in the ***kapha sthāna***. ***Vamana*** therapy marshals the upward-moving activity of ***udāna vāyu***, acting from the diaphragm upwards to eliminate excess ***kapha*** via the mouth. ***Vamana*** therapy is only used during in the morning when ***kapha*** predominates, after ***snehana*** and ***svedana***.

Vamana is a technique that must be carefully supervised and is conducted only when the patient fully understands and accepts the process to be undertaken. The emetic ***dravyas*** given to induce vomiting can be harsh, and as ***vamana*** utilises the upward-moving energy of ***udāna vāyu*** it can also aggravate ***vāta***, causing ***apāna vāyu*** to move upwards and weaken ***agni*** (***udāvarta***).

Within the classical texts recommendations are given for the number of bouts of vomiting and the number of days during which ***vamana*** should be implemented. Typically, ***vamana*** is used for 3 days in ***vāttika*** conditions, with no more than four bouts of vomiting per day; 5 days in ***paittika*** conditions, with no more than six bouts of vomiting per day; and 7 days in ***kaphaja*** conditions, with no more than eight bouts of vomiting per day. In each ***vamana*** session the therapy is ceased when the patient vomits the same volume of liquid that was originally consumed immediately prior to emesis, or when the vomit itself is yellowish in colour (indicating the elimination of ***pitta***).

Vamana therapy is especially indicated by ***kaphaja*** symptoms such as sluggish digestion, a thick coating on the tongue and mucus congestion, and may be safely performed by most people if performed only occasionally, and not more than once per season. ***Vamana*** therapy is avoided in weakness, debility, malabsorption syndromes, constipation, intestinal parasites, pregnancy, fever, coryza, rhinitis, pharyngitis, tracheitis, and in the elderly. ***Vamana*** therapy is also contraindicated in those persons who have a particular aversion to or fear of vomiting. It is essential for the patient to relax during the therapy, allowing the oesophagus to be free of any kind of muscular constriction.

The evening prior to ***vamana*** therapy the patient should be directed to consume a meal of fatty and sweet foods that aggravate ***kapha***, such as gruel prepared from rice, ***urad*** bean, sesame seed, meat or fish. Upon rising the next morning, the patient is given a weak of decoction of ***Yaṣṭimadhu*** root

(*Glycyrrhiza glabra*) to drink, consuming between one and two litres. The patient is instructed to consume this preparation as quickly as possible, and after 10 minutes the patient is given a ***vamana*** formula, such as the following:

- ***Madanaphala*** fruit (*Randia dumetorium*) powder, 6–10 g
- ***Vacā*** rhizome (*Acorus calamus*) powder, 3–5 g
- honey, 20 mL
- ***saindhava***, 3–5 g
- milk or warm water, 100 mL.

The above ingredients should be mixed well and then administered immediately. In this recipe both ***Madanaphala*** and ***Vacā*** act as emetics and should be adjusted based on the age and strength of the patient, and the ***doṣa*** or ***doṣas*** that predominate. If given in full doses these herbs will promote a more profound emesis, suitable for ***kaphaja*** conditions and in those who are strong; if given in smaller quantities the emetic activity will be less, which is better in ***vātaja*** conditions, and in persons who are weak.

After the administration of the ***vamana*** formula the patient is positioned over a large bowl or bucket, and induced to vomit by having them place their index and middle fingers of the right hand down the throat, with the left hand gently massaging the stomach in a counter-clockwise direction. If this technique does not induce vomiting within a few minutes, an additional dose of the ***vamana*** formula can be administered, or another standard emetic such as Syrup of Ipecac. Upon emesis there will be voiding of much liquid, mucus (***kapha***), undigested food, and, at the end, a yellowish bilious secretion (***pitta***). After ***vamana*** therapy the patient should lie down for 10–20 minutes, and afterwards drink small amounts of a mild ***dīpanapācana*** remedy such as weak Ginger tea. After a few hours the patient can consume a small amount of rice or some vegetable soup, and make sure to rest for the remainder of the day. If vomiting is not successfully induced the result is usually ***virecana***, or purgation.

When ***vamana*** is properly administered the patient will have little difficulty in vomiting, there will be a feeling of physical lightness, enhanced sensory acuity, the appearance of hunger, and an improvement in disease symptoms. Features of inadequate or ***asamyaka vamana*** include an inability to vomit, heaviness of the body with itching, eruptions and burning sensations, and an increase in catarrh. In such cases the patient is either given the ***vamana dravyas*** again, or is required to fast for the rest of that day. Features of excess or ***atiyoga vamana*** include weakness, excessive belching, cough, hiccough, dyspnoea, dry heaves, confusion, thirst, jaw pain, throat constriction, fainting, haematemesis and diarrhoea. In such cases the patient is sprinkled with cold water after massaging them with ***ghṛta***, and given a drink prepared with sugar and honey. In cases of haematemesis the patient should be given haemostatic ***dravyas*** such as ***Nāgakeśara*** flower (*Mesua ferrea*) or ***Vāsaka*** leaf (*Adhatoda vasica*) to stop the bleeding. Additional measures include the use of ***śulapraśamana*** or antispasmodic ***dravyas*** such as ***Jīraka*** fruit (*Cuminum cyminum*) and ***Dhānyaka*** fruit (*Coriandrum sativum*), and demulcents such as ***Yaṣṭimadhu*** root (***Glycyrrhiza glabra***). In the case of diarrhoea the patient needs to be monitored for electrolyte loss, and can be given oral rehydration therapy consisting of a thin rice gruel.

11.6 *Pañca karma*: *virecana* (PURGATION)

Virecana or purgation therapy is generally instituted after ***vamana*** is complete. It is considered to be a treatment to both ***pitta*** and ***kapha***, as well as the hepatobiliary system and the small intestine, expelling the vitiated ***doṣas*** by force via the large intestine and anus. Although ***virecana*** is an important component of ***pañca karma***, it is specifically stated to be helpful in the treatment of a number of diseases, including chronic fever, skin conditions such as leprosy, certain digestive disorders such as constipation, parasites and haemorrhoids, jaundice, ophthamological disorders, inflammatory joint disease, and genitourinary tract disorders. ***Virecana*** is contraindicated in wasting diseases, fatigue, weakness, indigestion, diarrhoea, intestinal or rectal prolapse, acute fever, colds and flus, heart disease and pregnancy. Like ***vamana***, ***virecana*** is a potentially debilitating therapy and should be administered only with experienced supervision.

Specific guidelines are given in the classical texts for the types of ***virecana dravyas*** that are administered, depending upon ***balā*** ('strength'), ***vikṛti*** ('disease'), and ***prakṛti*** ('constitution') of the patient, and whether the patient has a ***krūra*** ('hard'), ***madhya*** ('medium') or ***mṛdu*** ('soft') ***koṣṭha*** ('bowel'). In the case of a ***krūra koṣṭha***, i.e. ***vāta***, ***dravyas*** used in ***virecana*** should have a ***snigdha*** ('oily') and ***uṣṇa*** ('hot') quality, such as ***Eraṇḍa*** seed oil (*Ricinus communis*) or ***Āragvadha*** fruit (***Cassia fistula***), mixed with ***dravyas*** such as ***Pippalī*** (*Piper longum*) and ***saindhava***. Initiating purgation in a ***krūra koṣṭha***, however, can be difficult, and as a result such measures are often combined with more powerful purgatives such as ***Jayapāla*** fruit (*Croton tiglium*) and ***śulapraśamana*** ('antispasmodic') ***dravyas*** such as ***Śūṇṭhī*** rhizome (*Zingiber officinalis*) to prevent griping. For a ***madhya koṣṭha***, i.e. ***kapha***, the ***dravyas*** are similarly ***uṣṇa*** but have more of a ***rūkṣa*** ('dry') quality, and are given in smaller amounts. Examples of ***dravyas*** used for a ***madhya koṣṭha*** include ***Trivṛt*** root (*Operculina turpethum*), ***Harītakī*** fruit (*Terminalia chebula*) and ***Kaṭuka*** rhizome (***Picrorrhiza kurroa***), combined with ***dīpanapācana dravyas*** such as ***Śūṇṭhī*** rhizome (*Zingiber officinalis*) and ***Pippalī*** fruit (***Piper longum***). In the case of a ***mṛdu koṣṭha***, i.e. ***pitta***, purgative ***dravyas*** such as ***Trivṛt*** are given in comparatively smaller doses, along with medications that have ***śita*** (cool) quality, such as a decoction or juice of ***Drākṣā*** fruit (*Vitis vinifera*), ***Āmalakī*** fruit (*Phyllanthus emblica*), ***Udīcya*** root (*Pavonia odorata*), and ***Candana*** bark (*Santalum album*). Among the purgative ***dravyas Trivṛt*** is considered to be the best and safest, and when used in the appropriate dosage and combined with the appropriate ***dravyas***, can be used in almost all patients. The following is an example of the appropriate use and dosage ranges of ***Trivṛt*** in formulation, for each type of patient:

- ***Krūra koṣṭha***: ***Eraṇḍa taila*** (30 mL), ***Trivṛt*** (10–15 g), ***Śūṇṭhī*** (2–3 g) and ***saindhava*** (1–2 g), taken with a little warm gruel
- ***Madhya koṣṭha***: ***Trivṛt*** (10–15 g), ***Harītakī*** (5 g) and ***Śūṇṭhī*** (2–3 g); taken with warm water
- ***Mṛdu koṣṭha***: ***Trivṛt*** (10 g) and ***Āmalakī*** (5 g); taken with sugar and tepid water.

Prior to ***virecana*** therapy the patient must have undergone a previous course of ***vamana***, followed by another course of ***snehana*** and ***svedana*** over a period of 3–8 days, depending on the nature of the bowel (i.e. fewer days for a ***mṛdu koṣṭha***, and longer for a ***krūra koṣṭha***). On the evening before treatment the patient is given food that is both ***snigdha*** ('oily) and ***uṣṇa*** ('hot') in nature. The next morning, at least 2 hours after sunrise when ***kapha*** is in its ascendancy, the patient is given the appropriate ***virecana*** recipe in the appropriate quantity, and within a few hours the patient will begin to purge. If ***virecana*** is delayed the patient can drink warm water and the abdomen is massaged in a clockwise direction: cold water is to be avoided. If the treatment causes pain and discomfort the patient can hold a hot water bottle over the abdomen. The number of bouts and volume of faecal material passed will depend upon the amount of the ***dravya*** given and the nature of the ***koṣṭha***, from 5 to 15 bouts and between a half to two litres of faecal material. During the therapy the patient should abstain from food, rest and try to stay in a positive frame of mind. If purgation is not successful, however, the patient is allowed to eat a thin rice gruel in the everning and then the ***virecana*** recipe is given again on the following day, using the same procedure. The following day after successful treatment the patient can eat again, breaking the fast by consuming a thin rice gruel, and over the next 5–7 days consuming a diet that is light and easily digestible.

When ***virecana*** is administered correctly and the treatment is successful there is an enhancement in mental and sensory acuity, lightness of the body, and improved appetite. If these symptoms are noted during treatment but the patient continues to purge, an emetic recipe is given to remove the ***virecana dravyas*** from the ***koṣṭha***. Symptoms of inadequate or ***asamyaka virecana*** are a vitiation of the ***doṣas***, lethargy and confusion, headache, weakness of appetite, vomiting, catarrh, heaviness of the abdomen and chest, body pain, constipation, skin rashes and urinary obstruction. In such cases the patient should be purged again the next day: if the cause is due to a ***krūra koṣṭha*** the patient can be treated with a herbal suppository or an enema, followed by the administration of the ***virecana*** recipe the next day. If this still does not produce a purging the patient undergoes another course of ***snehana*** and ***svedana*** over a 10-day period, and the process is repeated. Symptoms of excess or ***atiyoga virecana*** is a depletion of one, two or all three ***doṣas***, exhaustion, tremors, numbness, fainting, thirst, pallor, abdominal pain, rectal discharge or haemorrhaging, and rectal prolapse. In the treatment of ***atiyoga virecana*** the ***Cakradatta*** recommends ***dravyas*** that have a ***śita*** ('cooling') and ***grāhī*** ('astringent') property, such as ***Padmaka*** bark (*Prunus cerasoides*), ***Uśīra*** root (*Vetiveria zizanioides*), ***Nāgakeśara*** flower (*Mesua ferrea*), and ***Candana*** bark (*Santalum album*); useful formulations include ***Śaṅka bhasma***, ***Jātīphalādya cūrṇa*** and ***Kuṭaja ariṣṭa***.

While ***virecana*** is an important component of ***pañca karma*** it is also used in patients who have a small increase of the ***doṣas***, on a periodic basis, usually at the beginning of spring and autumn. In such cases mild amounts of ***virecana dravyas*** such as ***Trivṛt*** and ***Harītakī*** can be used every day for a week, along with ***dīpanapācana dravyas*** such as ***Tvak*** bark (*Cinnamomum zeylanicum*), ***Patra*** leaf (*Cinnamomum tāmala*) and ***Marica*** fruit (*Piper nigrum*).

11.7 *Pañca karma*: *vasti* (ENEMA)

Vasti or enema therapy is directed to the colon, the seat of ***vāta*** in the body. By directing treatment to the colon, ***vasti*** therapy indirectly treats the activity of all aspects of ***vāta*** in the body, including the activity of the sub-***doṣas***. The term ***vasti*** is derived from the traditional usage of an animal 'bladder' to administer the medication, although in modern practice synthetic materials are commonly used. There are two basic forms of ***vasti*** therapy: ***nirūha vasti***, or enemas prepared with herbal decoctions, and ***anuvāsana vasti***, enemas that require the use of oil. According to Caraka these two types of ***vasti*** therapy account for two components of ***pañca karma***; in contrast, Suśruta states that ***vasti*** only accounts for one aspect of ***pañca karma***, and includes ***rakta mokṣaṇa*** or 'venesection' as the fifth. There is a third type of ***vasti*** therapy not discussed in this text; it is called ***uttaravasti*** and is administered into the vagina (i.e. douche) or urethra.

Vasti therapy is implemented after ***vamana*** and ***virecana***, after ***kapha*** and ***pitta*** have been eliminated. ***Vasti*** is highly valued in Āyurvedic medicine, regarded as both an eliminative and restorative therapy, expelling excess ***vāta*** as well as normalising its function. Depending upon the type administered, ***vasti*** therapy can be used to treat a wide assortment of diseases and is also used outside of ***pañca karma*** as a stand-alone therapy. For preventative measures, the ancient texts recommend the practice of ***vasti*** approximately three times a year (i.e. once every 4 months).

Vasti therapy is traditionally administered by using an animal bladder, such as that from a deer, pig, buffalo or goat. The 'enema bag' or ***vasti putaka*** must be without holes, well cleaned, properly tanned, dry and soft before use. The medication is placed into the bladder, the sides of the bladder gathered together and tied to a nozzle (***vasti netra***), traditionally fashioned from some kind of metal such as gold, silver or copper, or from bone, bamboo, horn, or a plant stalk.

Vasti therapy is performed only after 7 days have passed since ***virecana*** treatment and the patient's digestion has returned to normal. Prior to the administration of ***vasti*** the patient undergoes ***abhyaṅga*** and ***svedana***. ***Anuvāsana vasti***, or 'oil enema', is the first type of ***vasti*** treatment to be implemented, and is used in an alternating fashion with ***nirūha vasti***, or 'decoction enema'. The length and scope of ***vasti*** therapy depends upon several factors: the benefit to be obtained, the ***vikṛti*** ('disease') and ***prakṛti*** ('constitution') of the patient, and the nature of the bowel. In a ***krūra koṣṭha***, the treatment is longer; in a ***madhya koṣṭha***, the treatments are of a medium duration; in a ***mṛdu koṣṭha***, the treatments are of a short duration. The longest ***vasti*** regimen is ***karma vasti***, consisting of alternating ***anuvāsana*** and ***nirūha vasti*** over a 24-day period, followed by 6 days of ***anuvāsana vasti*** to total 30 days. ***Kāla vasti*** consists of alternating ***anuvāsana*** and ***nirūha vasti*** for 12 days, followed by 3 days of ***anuvāsana vasti*** to total 15 days. ***Yoga vasti*** involves alternating ***anuvāsana*** and ***nirūha vasti*** for 6 days, followed by 2 days of ***anuvāsana*** to total 8 days of treatment.

The dosages used for ***anuvāsana*** and ***nirūha vasti*** can vary to a large degree, depending on factors including the patient's age and the predominant ***doṣas*** of the disease. The typical dose for ***nirūha vasti*** begins with a half a ***prasṛta*** (48 mL) for a child of 1 year, which is increased by a half a ***prasṛta*** for each year of life up to the age of 12, at which point the total volume will be equal to six ***prasṛta*** (576 mL). The volume of the medication used in ***anuvāsana*** is one-fourth, one-sixth or one-eighth the volume that is calculated for ***nirūha vasti***, for vitiations of ***vāta***, ***pitta*** and ***kapha***, respectively. Thus, the initial dose used in ***anuvāsana***

vasti for a child of 1 year is 12 mL in ***vāttika*** conditions, 8 mL in ***paittika*** conditions, and 6 mL in ***kaphaja*** conditions, and by the age of 12, the total volume of medication will be 144 mL for ***vāta***, 96 mL for ***pitta*** and 72 mL for ***kapha***. After the age of 12 the volume to be used for ***nirūha vasti*** is increased by one ***prasṛta*** (96 mL) for each year of life, up to the age of 18, at which point the total volume will be equal to 12 ***prasṛta*** (1152 mL). This dose is maintained in most people up until the age of 70, after which the total volume for ***nirūha vasti*** is decreased to 10 ***prasṛta*** (960 mL). By the age of 18 the respective doses for ***anuvāsana vasti*** are 288 mL for ***vāta***, 192 mL for ***pitta***, and 144 mL for ***kapha***, and after the age of 70 is reduced to 240 mL for ***vāta***, 160 mL for ***kapha***, and 120 mL for ***kapha***.

Anuvāsana vasti

Anuvāsana vasti is the administration of a medicated oil into the colon via the anus. It is specifically indicated when the patient suffers from ***vāttika*** conditions, such as constant hunger, dryness of the skin and mucosa, and neuromuscular disorders. It is contraindicated in acute fever, congestion and catarrh, lymphadenitis, infection, indigestion and poor appetite, poisoning, abdominal heaviness, splenomegaly, jaundice, intestinal parasites, diarrhoea, constipation, haemorrhoids, urinary diseases, obesity, diabetes and anaemia. ***Anuvāsana vasti*** is never administered on an empty stomach, and is given during the ***vāta*** time of day, i.e. early morning or late afternoon.

The prodedure for administering ***anuvāsana*** calls for the patient to undergo ***abhyaṅga*** and ***svedana*** first, followed by a small easily digestible meal and a short walk, eliminating any faeces or urine at this time. To administer the ***vasti*** the patient lies in the recovery position on his or her left side (left leg straight, right leg bent at the knee), and a sheet is draped over the patient's body for privacy and comfort, exposing only the buttocks. The medication is prepared and the ***vasti putaka*** is filled. The anus is anointed with oil, and then the nozzle or ***vasti netra*** is lubricated and then gently inserted into the anus. The practitioner then slowly squeezes the contents of the ***vasti putaka*** into the rectum with a steady and constant pressure, ensuring that only the ***dravya*** and not air is being squeezed into the rectum. As the ***vasti*** is being administered the patient is advised to not yawn, cough or sneeze. After administering the medication the patient lies in a supine position, extending the legs outwards, and then after a few minutes repeatedly brings the knees to the chest several times, and flexes the arms. During this time the feet, buttocks and abdomen are also massaged, and a hot water bottle can be applied to the abdomen. Following this the patient then assumes the recovery position by lying on the right side, directing the ***vasti dravyas*** deeper into the large intestine. The patient is then covered with a blanket and is allowed to rest for some time until the urge to eliminate is made known. Following the elimination of the oil the patient can have a normal meal. If the oil is not eliminated after 9 hours the patient can either be given a suppository or a ***virecana dravya*** to eliminate oil, or it can be retained until the ***nirūha vasti*** is given on the following day.

The ***dravyas*** used in ***anuvāsana*** are fairly simple, consisting of some kind of oil or fat such as ***taila***. The maximum amount of ***saindhava*** used is approximately one ***karṣa*** (12 g), a weight equal to 1/24 the total volume of oil administered, e.g. 12 g per 288 mL of oil for ***anuvāsana vasti***, 8 g per 192 mL of oil in ***pitta anuvāsana***, and 6 g per 144 mL of oil in ***kapha anuvāsana***.

Nirūha vasti

Nirūha vasti is used after ***anuvāsana*** on the following day, and is always administered on an empty stomach, during the ***vāta*** time of day. The procedure for administering ***nirūha vasti*** is identical to that used in ***anuvāsana***, with the exception that it be performed on an empty stomach. For practical purposes ***nirūha vasti*** is best administered during the early morning, but may also be administered in the late afternoon. ***Nirūha vasti*** is used in the treatment of conditions including chronic fever, chest pain and cardiac disorders caused by the upward movement of ***vāta***, retention of flatus and faeces, hepatomegaly and splenomegaly, intestinal parasites, lumbago, sciatica, arthritis, gout, paralysis and spasm, weakness, psychosis, genitourinary disorders and infertility. ***Nirūha vasti*** is contraindicated in the presence of ***āma***, indigestion, vomiting, anorexia, hunger, thirst, diarrhoea and dysentery, malabsorption syndromes, intestinal obstruction, haemorrhoids, asthma, cough, diabetes, ascites, skin diseases such as leprosy, and pregnancy (before the eighth month).

Unlike ***anuvāsana***, the formulations used for ***nirūha vasti*** vary to a large degree, depending on the ***vikṛti*** and ***prakṛti*** of the patient, and always contain some kind of aqueous preparation, often mixed with a herbal paste, ***saindhava***, honey and some kind of oil or fat. ***Dravyas*** used in the preparation of ***nirūha vasti*** to be used in ***vāttika*** conditions should comprise ***madhura***, ***lavaṇa*** or ***amla rasas***, such as ***Balā*** root (*Sida cordifolia*) and ***Aśvagandhā*** root (*Withania somnifera*), mixed with an oil or fat and ***saindhava*** ***Dravyas*** used in preparing ***vasti*** for ***paittika*** conditions should consist of ***madhura***, ***tikta*** and ***kaśāya rasas***, such as ***Yaṣṭimadhu*** root (*Glycyrrhiza glabra*) and ***Guḍūcī*** vine (*Tinospora cordifolia*), mixed with milk, ***ghṛta*** and sugarcane juice. ***Dravyas*** used in preparing ***vasti*** for ***kaphaja*** conditions should be composed of ***tikta***, ***kaśāya*** and ***kaṭu rasas***, such as ***Nimba*** leaf (*Azadirachta indica*) and ***Marica*** fruit (*Piper nigrum*), taken without fat or oil of any kind. ***Nirūha vasti*** can be, and is, sometimes administered more than once in a single session, the first administration targeting ***vāta***, the second ***pitta***, and lastly ***kapha***.

Although a great number of potential formulations can be used in ***nirūha vasti*** one of the more common ones used is ***Madhutailika***, consisting of:

- fresh honey, 320 mL
- ***saindhava***, 20 g
- ***taila***, 320 mL
- ***Shatapuṣpā*** herb (*Anethum graveolens*) ***cūrṇa***, 20 g
- ***Eraṇḍa*** root (*Ricinus communis*) ***kvātha***, 320 mL.

The ingredients above are mixed together in the order listed, in a pot made of gold, silver or bronze. The ***Eraṇḍa*** root decoction is added last, and should be quite warm. When the ingredients are mixed together well, and it is not too hot, the preparation is administered rectally. ***Madhutailika*** is safe for all three ***doṣas*** and can be used in both ***pañca karma*** and as a standalone treatment.

Nirūha vasti is usually retained for only a short period of time, between 5 and 15 minutes, after which it should be eliminated by having the patient sit on their heels, into a vessel that can be later examined by the attending physician. If the ***nirūha vasti*** is retained longer than 48 minutes measures are immediately taken to eliminate the retained enema by administering another ***vasti*** that has a purgative activity, composed of a solution medicated with ***dravyas*** such as ***Triphala***, ***Trikaṭu***, cow urine, honey or ***Yavakṣāra*** (*Hordeum vulgare* ash). Alternatively, a herbal suppository with laxative properties can be used, or ***virecana dravyas*** such as ***Trivṛt*** root and ***Eraṇḍa taila*** are administered. Following each ***vasti*** treatment the patient can take a bath and eat a meal: a rice gruel or ***kicari*** (see Box 11.1) for ***kaphaja*** conditions; rice cooked in milk for ***paittika*** conditions; and rice cooked in meat broth for ***vāttika*** conditions. After treatment the patient should avoid excessive exercise and emotional stimulation, sexual activity, travel and sleeping during the day.

When ***vasti*** therapy is properly administered there is an increase in the appetite, the unobstructed movement of urine, flatus and faeces, lightness of the body, enhanced mental and sensory acuity, the abatement of disease symptoms, and increased strength. Features of

Box 11.1 Preparing *kicari*

Kicari is one of the more common dietary articles used during ***pañca karma***, specifically used in ***kaphaja*** conditions. It can be consumed at other times, however, during periods of periodic fasting, or in the treatment of minor illnesses such as a cold or flu, or digestive problems. There are a great many varieties of ***kicari***, but the key ingredients consist of mung bean and rice, cooked with spices such as ginger, turmeric, coriander, cumin, black pepper and ***saindhava***. In patients with very weak digestion the rice can be a partially milled rice, or even basmati rice, and the mung beans can be the washed variety, in which the outerskins have been removed. Where the digestion is stronger, the unwashed 'whole' mung beans can be used in preference. The heaviest and most difficult to digest version of ***kicari*** is made with whole grain brown rice and whole mung bean, but is also very nutritious. To prepare ***kicari***, add one cup of mung and one cap of rice to a pot, and cover with eight cups of water. Add five or six slices of fresh ginger, one teaspoon of ***saindhava*** and bring to a boil, stirring often. Reduce to a simmer, and add two teaspoons of ground coriander seed, one teaspoon of ground cumin seed, one teaspoon of turmeric, and a half a teaspoon of fresh ground black pepper. Allow to simmer for a few hours, until it begins to thicken and the rice and mung are soft. ***Kicari*** can be eaten three times a day, over a period of 10 days to promote detoxification and restore digestion.

asamyaka or inadequate ***vasti*** therapy include a poor appetite, nausea, abdominal pain, flatulence, retention of urine, dyspnoea, coldness and stiffness. Features of ***atiyoga*** or excessive ***vasti*** therapy include numbness, exhaustion, weakness, drowsiness, psychosis and hiccough. In cases of ***atiyoga vasti*** treatments are used to enhance ***agni*** through the use of ***dīpanapācana*** and ***grāhī dravyas***.

11.8 *Nasya* (ERRHINES)

Nasya or errhine treatment is the administration of medications into the nostrils, used specifically in the treatment of disorders of the head and neck, including the brain and central nervous system, the upper respiratory system, the eyes, ears, mouth and throat, and the glandular structures of the neck. Apart from these local effects ***nasya*** also has a systemic effect through its action upon the ***idā*** and ***piṅgalā nāḍīs*** that terminate in the left and right nostrils respectively, and thus corrects and improves the flow of ***prāṇa*** in the body.

A number of different ***dravyas*** can be administered in ***nasya***, including water, oils and fats, herbal decoctions and juices, herbal powders and pastes, milk, meat broth and even animal blood, depending upon the indications. The timing of the administration of ***nasya*** is dependent upon the ***doṣa*** to be treated: thus ***kaphaja*** conditions are best treated during the ***kapha*** time of day and during spring; ***paittika*** conditions during the ***pitta*** time of day and during summer; and ***vāttika*** conditions during the ***vāta*** time of day, and during autumn. ***Nasya*** is contraindicated in patients that have just eaten food or have consumed some kind of beverage (including ***asava*** or ***ariṣṭa***), in those who have just bathed or want to bathe after administration, in acute rhinitis, dyspnoea and cough, in those that have just undergone internal ***snehapāna***, ***vamana***, ***virecana*** or ***vasti***, in children, pregnant women and the elderly, and is avoided when the weather is cloudy and cold, or excessively warm.

On the day of treatment, the patient must have an empty stomach, properly eliminated both faeces and urine, and cleansed the mouth with ***tikta*** ('bitter'), ***kaśāya*** ('astringent') and ***kaṭu*** ('pungent') ***dravyas***. The patient is then taken to a specially prepared room that is free of dust and direct breeze, and undergoes ***abhyaṅga*** with medicated oils such as ***Kshirabalā taila***, ***Dhānvantara taila*** or ***Balā taila***, paying particular attention to gently massage the face, head and neck. Upon administering ***nasya*** the patient should assume a supine position, the arms extended outwards, the feet slightly raised, and the head slightly lowered and gently tilted back. The ***nasya dravya*** is then warmed to room temperature and instilled in each nostril, closing the nostril that is not receiving the medication during administration. After instillation the patient is counselled to gently inhale the medication deep into the nose, taking long deep breaths, and remains in a supine position for approximately 2 minutes. During this time the patient is vigorously massaged over the soles of the feet, the palms of the hand, and the neck, face and ears. The patient then rolls to one side and attempts to spit out the instilled ***nasya dravyas*** until none remains. In this way, ***nasya*** can be administered two or three times in one session.

During this procedure the patient should avoid speaking, blowing the ***nasya dravyas*** out through the nose, or swallowing the medication. If the patient appears drowsy or faints cold water is sprinkled over the body. After the procedure is complete the patient sits up and gargles with warm water to remove any remaining ***kapha doṣa*** or medication. If after this procedure ***kapha doṣa*** remains, with symptoms such as headache, catarrh, or cough, ***dhūma*** ('smoke') is then administered, using herbs such as ***Yaṣṭimadhu*** root (*Glycrrhiza glabra*), ***Guggulu*** resin (*Commiphora mukul*), ***Haridrā*** rhizome (*Curcuma longa*), mixed with a little ***ghṛta*** (see 5.2 ***Dinācaryā:*** the daily regimen). After treatment the patient should avoid sleep, bathing, cold water and wind, and eat a light, easily digestible meal. ***Vāgbhaṭa*** recommends that ***nasya karma*** be performed over a 7-day period, but Suśruta indicates that the regimen can be followed for a maximum of 21 days.

When ***nasya*** is performed correctly it enhances mental and sensory acuity, promotes mental clarity and emotional happiness, clears the nasopharynx of obstruction, bestows a clear voice, promotes lightness of the body, and eliminates the symptoms of disease. Features of ***asamyaka*** or inadequate ***nasya*** therapy include mental and sensory confusion, catarrhal conditions of the head and neck, lethargy, and no abatement in disease symptoms. Features of ***atiyoga*** or excessive ***nasya*** therapy include mental confusion, headache, weakness, itching and excess salivation.

According to the ***Aṣṭāñga Hṛdaya*** there are three basic types of ***nasya***: ***virecana*** ('purgation'), ***bṛmhaṇa*** ('nourishing') and ***śamana*** ('pacifying'). In the case of ***bṛmhaṇa***, ***nasya*** is both a treatment and a preventative measure to maintain health, depending on the amount used. The dosage of the ***dravya*** used in ***nasya*** is usually quite small compared to other treatments, more if the treatment has a therapeutic objective, and less if it is being used as a preventative measure.

Virecana nasya

Virecana nasya is a powerful ***śodhana*** therapy, used more for ***kaphaja*** conditions, as well as the treatment of headache, stiffness of the neck, drowsiness, chronic rhinitis, diseases of the throat and neck, skin diseases, epilepsy, loss of consciousness, and psychosis. ***Virecana nasya*** is subdivided into two types of treatment: ***avapīḍa*** and ***pradhmāna nasya***. ***Avapīḍa nasya*** is the administration of a ***svarasa*** ('herbal juice'), ***kalka*** ('herbal paste') or ***kaśāya*** ('herbal decoction'), whereas ***pradhmāna nasya*** is the administration of a ***cūrṇa*** ('herbal powder'). Both are administered by instilling and inhaling the ***dravyas*** directly into the nose, or in the case of ***pradhmāna nasya*** specifically, blown into the nose of the patient by the practitioner with the help of a small tube, traditionally a small bone or hollow plant stalk. Both ***avapīḍa*** and ***pradhmāna nasya*** act as strong purgatives to the head, irritating the mucus membranes of the nose, sinus and pharynx and promoting a profound expectoration. This activity clears the head of blockages, and in the case of mental disorders removes obstructions and impurities of the mind and consciousness.

Depending upon the complaint a number of different ***dravyas*** are used in ***avapīḍa nasya***, including the fresh juices of **Tulasī** (*Ocimum sanctum*), **Laśuna** (*Allium sativum*) or **Śūṇṭhī** (*Zingiber officinalis*), decoctions of herbs such as ***Vacā*** rhizome (*Acorus calamus*) or ***Kuṣṭha*** root (*Saussurea lappa*), and honey and water mixed with ***saindhava***. The dose of the various ***dravyas*** used in ***avapīḍa nasya*** depends upon the nature of the condition, divided in small (***hīna***), medium (***madhya***) and large (***uttama***) doses:

- ***hīna avapīḍa nasya***: four drops
- ***madhya avapīḍa nasya***: six drops
- ***uttama avapīḍa nasya***: eight drops.

In this case, and in every case in which a drop or ***bindu*** is administered in ***nasya***, the classical texts define a drop as that which drips off the clean index finger when it is immersed in a liquid. While this technique is suitable for self-administration, for therapeutic purposes the practitioner will typically use a small dropper or absorbent cotton soaked in the ***dravya***, which is then squeezed into the nose.

In the case of ***pradhmāna nasya*** only a 'pinch' (***micyuti***) is administered in each instance, the amount of which depends upon the nature of the condition to be treated and the results to be obtained, once again, divided in small (***hīna***), medium (***madhya***) and large (***uttama***):

- ***hīna pradhmāna nasya***: two ***guñjas*** (250 mg)
- ***madhya pradhmāna nasya***: three ***guñjas*** (375 mg)
- ***uttama pradhmāna nasya***: four ***guñjas*** (500 mg).

Examples of ***dravyas*** used in ***pradhmāna nasya*** include **Pippalī** fruit (*Piper longum*), **Marica** fruit (*Piper nigrum*), **Śūṇṭhī** rhizome (*Zingiber officinalis*), **Kaṭphala** bark (*Myrica nagi*) and **Viḍaṅga** fruit (*Embelia ribes*).

Bṛmhaṇa nasya

Bṛmhaṇa nasya is a kind of 'nourishing' ***nasya*** treatment, indicated more for ***vāttika*** complaints, as well as conditions such as migraines, alopecia and premature greying, tinnitus, eye diseases, laryngitis, difficult speech, mucosal deficiency, facial paralysis, and frozen shoulder. Examples of medicaments used in ***bṛmhaṇa nasya*** include medicated oils (***sneha nasya***), meat broth, fresh animal blood, and the ***svarasa*** ('juice') of herbs that are ***madhura*** ('sweet') in taste or that otherwise reduce ***vāta***.

The most common form of ***bṛmhaṇa nasya*** is ***sneha nasya***, which can be divided into two basic forms of treatment: ***marśa*** and ***pratimarśa***. ***Marśa*** is the administration of a relatively large volume of oil by a practitioner during ***pañca karma***. ***Pratimarśa*** is the use of a much smaller volume of oil over a longer duration, self-administered by the patient and used as a method of preventative health care.

Marśa is typically used over a 7-day period, with ten, eight and six drops being the maximum (***uttama***), medium (***madhya***) and minimum (***hīna***) dosage of the indicated ***dravyas***. Like the other forms of ***nasya***, ***marśa nasya*** is stated as having a potential to cause complications and aggravate the ***doṣas***, and hence the contraindications for ***nasya*** discussed previously apply here as well; i.e. before or after food or bath, concurrent with other ***pañca karma*** therapies, in acute rhinitis, dyspnoea and cough, in children, pregnant women and the elderly, and in excessively cold, wet or warm weather.

Whereas ***marśa*** involves the application of up to eight drops of the medication in each nostril, ***pratimarśa*** is the administration of no more than two drops. It is safe for all ages, and can be used on an ongoing basis, usually first thing in the morning on an empty stomach, before bathing (see 5.2 ***Dinācaryā:*** the daily regimen). ***Pratimarśa*** may also be used at other times of the day, however, such as after strenuous exercise or sexual activity, to revitalise the mind after work or study, after the consumption of food, after vomiting, after sleeping during the day, at the end of the day or night to cleanse the ***srotāṃsi***, after the elimination of wastes, after public speaking to pacify ***vāta***, and after cleansing the oral cavity to strengthen the teeth. ***Pratimarśa*** can also be used in conjunction with ***neti*** and ***prāṇayama*** techniques such as ***nāḍī śodhana*** for added benefit.

There are a number of medications that are used in ***sneha nasya***, perhaps the most common of which is the formula ***Aṇu taila***, as well as medicated ***ghṛta*** compounds prepared with herbs such as ***Brāhmī*** leaf (*Bacopa monniera*) and ***Vacā*** rhizome (*Acorus calamus*). When ***sneha nasya*** is properly administered, the patient should be able to breath without difficulty, sleep well, and arise refreshed and experience enhanced mental and sensory acuity. With continuous usage ***bṛmhaṇa nasya*** confers the benefit of improved skin texture and complexion, stops or delays greying hair and alopecia, and strengthens the neck, shoulders and arms. Feelings of mucosal dryness and a feeling of lightness in the head are symptoms of inadequate or ***asamyaka*** administration. Itching, a feeling of heaviness in the head, excessive salivation, anorexia and rhinitis are signs of excessive or ***atiyoga sneha nasya***.

Śamana nasya

Śamana nasya is a treatment to pacify the vitiated ***doṣas***, used more for ***paittika*** conditions, as well as disease such as alopecia, eye diseases, dermatitis, boils and acne. Examples of medicaments used in ***śamana nasya*** include milk, coconut water and cool water, as well as some of the medicaments used in ***bṛmhaṇa nasya***. ***Śamana nasya*** also includes ***jala neti***: the administration of an isotonic solution of water to irrigate the nasal passages and sinuses (see 5.2 ***Dinācaryā***: the daily regimen).

11.9 *Rakta mokṣaṇa* (VENESECTION)

According to Suśruta, ***rakta mokṣaṇa*** or 'venesection' is the last of the ***pañca karmas*** to be implemented. The use of ***rakta mokṣaṇa*** is based upon the idea that the blood is a kind of ***doṣa***. In actuality, blood or ***rakta*** is a subset of ***pitta***, and when ***pitta*** is vitiated waste products remain in the blood that impair the circulation of nutrients and ***ojas***. ***Rakta mokṣaṇa*** is indicated in conditions such as skin diseases, tumours, fever and inflammatory joint disease. It is generally contraindicated in persons suffering from ***vāttika*** diseases, as well as in both pregnant and post-partum women, in anaemia, and in children and the aged.

The classical texts indicate that when ***rakta*** is healthy it is slightly ***madhura*** ('sweet') and ***lavaṇa*** ('salty') in taste, and is neither too hot nor too cold. Evidence of the five ***mahābhūtas*** ('elements') can be seen in healthy ***rakta*** by the following features: unpleasant odour (***pṛthvī***), liquid (***ap***), bright red (***tejas***), flowing (***vāyu***) and light (***ākāśa***). Symptoms of vitiated ***rakta*** are based upon the ***doṣas***. When ***rakta*** is vitiated by ***vāta*** the blood has purplish-red or bluish hue, and is thin, dry, frothy, and flows quickly. When ***rakta*** is vitiated by ***pitta*** the blood has a yellowish, green or blackish hue, a foul smell, flows quickly, and is warm to the touch. When ***rakta*** is vitiated by ***kapha*** the blood is pale in colour, oily, thick, slow moving and cool to the touch. When vitiated by two or more ***doṣas***, ***rakta*** displays the associated features in combination.

The ancient texts describe a number of methods, instruments, and locations to perform ***rakta mokṣaṇa***. Among the different implements discussed are knives of various shapes and sizes, lancets, needles, and scissors, as well as sharpened animal horns, bones, stones, or glass. Caustic alkalis and extreme heat are also used in venesection. One of the more common methods used in ***rakta mokṣaṇa*** is the use of non-poisonous leeches (*Hirudo medicinalis*), which is a comparatively safe and effective method of venesection. The location of the area to be venesected depends upon the location of the disease. In all cases only veins are venesected and never the arteries. Suśruta mentions a number of locations in the body that must not be injured or cut during any kind of surgical procedure, called ***marmas*** ('death points'). To perform ***rakta mokṣaṇa*** correctly the physician should understand these different locations.

Before ***rakta mokṣaṇa*** is begun the patient undergoes ***abhyaṅga***. Once the proper location for venesection is determined (usually local to the affected area), the physician begins the procedure. If required, a piece of gauze with a small hole cut into the middle of it, approximately 1 cm in diameter, can be applied to the area to be venesected, to direct the leech's activity. A leech is then applied to this location and is allowed to suck the blood of the patient until it becomes engorged over a 30–60 minute period of time, or until the patient begins to feel a pricking or itching sensation. A little ***saindhava*** is then applied to the leech to remove it, and the wound is cleaned with cold water and covered with anti-infective and antihaemorrhagic ***dravyas*** such as ***Haridrā*** rhizome (*Curcuma longa*) powder, ***Triphala*** and alum. The leech is then dipped in a solution of ***taila*** and ***saindhava*** and then massaged and gently squeezed so that the blood is removed from it, which is then examined for its qualities. ***Vāgbhaṭa*** states that this procedure is repeated the next day and the quality of the blood once again examined, and if determined to still contain a great volume of the vitiated ***doṣas***, the procedure is repeated again after 2 weeks have passed. If the ***rakta*** is determined to contain only a small component of the vitiated ***doṣas*** the treatment is discontinued and internal therapies to purify ***rakta*** can be given.

11.10 *Rasāyana* AND *vajīkaraṇa karma*

Once ***pañca karma*** treatment has been completed, and the patient has been allowed to rest for 7 days, ***rasāyana*** or 'rejuvenative' treatment is begun. The purpose of ***rasāyana*** is to strengthen the body and mind after the ***doṣas*** have been eliminated through ***pañca karma***. The reason why ***rasāyana*** treatment is given only after ***pañca karma*** is analogous to a piece of cloth that one wishes to dye. In order for the cloth to hold the dye and get an even distribution of the colour, the cloth must be washed beforehand, otherwise the dye will not hold and the fixative will allow the dirt to become ingrained. Likewise, unless the body has been purified prior to ***rasāyana*** treatment, ***āma*** will become strengthened and the vitiated ***doṣas*** will hold fast to the body.

There are different kinds of ***rasāyana*** therapy that can be implemented, with different goals in mind. On a mundane level, ***rasāyana*** therapy is used to tonify the body after ***pañca karma***, to improve the overall quality of health. On a supramundane level, however, ***rasāyana*** therapy is used to enhance spiritual potency, and as the tradition speaks, to achieve immortality. In this latter form of ***rasāyana*** the patient undergoes therapy to transform the ***ojas*** into ***amṛta***, the nectar of immortality.

Two kinds of ***rasāyana*** treatments are generally recognised in Āyurveda: ***kuṭīprāveśika rasāyana*** and ***vātātapika rasāyana***. In ***kuṭīprāveśika rasāyana***, the treatment is longer, requires great discipline and patience, and confers a greater benefit. It is a treatment that is generally considered to be reserved for those who wish to leave this world of ***saṃsāra***, who have disentangled themselves from the day to day responsibilities of life. In ***vātātapika*** the treatment is shorter, confers a lesser benefit, and requires little discipline other than to cultivate a healthy lifestyle and take the ***rasāyana dravya*** on a regular basis. Thus, these two forms of ***rasāyana*** therapy, ***kuṭīprāveśika*** and ***vātātapika***, are for ***brahmacaryās*** and householders respectively. A third form of rejuvenative treatment, called ***vajīkaraṇa***, is a subset of ***vātātapika***, and is implemented specifically to rejuvenate the reproductive organs, as well as treat infertility.

11.11 *Rasāyana karma*: *kuṭīprāveśika*

The term ***kuṭīprāveśika*** is derived from the word ***kuṭī***, which means 'hut', and ***prāveśika***, which means 'to enter into'. Thus ***kuṭīprāveśika*** therapy is administered to a patient residing in a specially constructed hut. The person who wishes to undergo ***kuṭīprāveśika*** therapy must reside in this hut during the course of treatment without visitors, except for visits from the physician who is administering the therapy.

The ***kuṭī*** must be constructed in an auspicious location, close to the herbs that will be used during the treatment, protected from harsh winds and the activity of other people. The structure of the hut itself actually consists of three huts, having an outer, middle and inner portion, and the main entrance faces north. The ***kuṭī*** should be constructed in such a way that there is adequate ventilation and light but the inner sanctum should be free of direct breeze and sunlight. Once constructed, the walls are painted white with slaked lime. Within the ***kuṭī***, the interior should be clean, free of pests and rodents, as well as free of any kind of distracting stimuli, such as radios, computers and televisions.

Kuṭīprāveśika rasāyana is begun during the ***uttarāyaṇa***, when the sun is in the northern hemisphere, when there are auspicious and favourable astrological indications. Before the treatment is begun the patient undergoes a short course of purification: undergoing ***abhyaṅga*** and ***svedana***, eating a gruel prepared from barley, and taking a recipe consisting of ***Harītakī*** fruit (*Terminalia chebula*), ***Āmalakī*** fruit (*Phyllanthus emblica*), ***Haridrā*** root (*Curcuma longa*), ***Vacā*** rhizome (*Acorus calamus*), ***Śūṇṭhī*** rhizome (*Zingiber officinalis*), ***Pippalī*** fruit (*Piper longum*), ***Viḍaṅga*** fruit (*Embelia ribes*), ***saindhava*** and jaggery, taken with warm water. This regimen lasts 3, 5 or 7 days, depending upon whether the patient has a ***mṛdu*** ('soft'), ***madhya*** ('medium') or ***krūra*** ('hard') ***koṣṭha*** ('bowel'). Once the ***koṣṭha*** of the patient is determined to be purifed, the patient undergoes a ritual purification and enters into the ***kuti***.

While residing in the ***kuti*** the patient is given a ***rasāyana dravya*** based upon their ***prakṛti***. This ***rasāyana*** is fed to the patient throughout the day, as much as he or she can comfortably ingest, followed by an evening meal of rice that has been boiled in milk. During the course of the therapy the patient should avoid vigorous exercise, although the practice of gentle ***hatha yoga āsanas*** may be undertaken. The patient should awaken during the ***brahmāmuhurta*** and retire with the setting sun, and maintain a positive and reverential attitude throughout the day. It is said that after eleven days of treatment the teeth and hair of the patient begin fall out, to be replaced by new hair and teeth. In total, ***kuṭīprāveśika rasāyana*** should take anywhere from 30 to 40 days.

There are many different kinds of ***rasāyana dravyas*** that are used in ***kuṭīprāveśika rasāyana***, some of which are also suitable in ***vātātapika rasāyana*** and in the treatment of various diseases: see Table 11.1.

11.12 *Rasāyana karma*: *vātātapika*

As it is not everyone that can follow through on the strict protocols of ***kuṭīprāveśika***, there is another form of ***rasāyana*** treatment called ***vātātapika***. The term ***vātātapika*** means 'sun and wind', and refers to a kind of ***rasāyana*** treatment that does not require the patient be sequestered in a specially constructed hut (and thus is exposed to sun and wind), or follow specific guidelines other than to cultivate a healthy lifestyle. ***Kuṭīprāveśika*** is treatment utilised by ***brahmacaryās*** and has a greater effect, not only to promote intelligence and longevity, but to enhance spiritual potency. Entering into the ***kuti*** and remaining there for an extended period of time is to re-enter the womb, to become 'born again'. ***Vātātapika*** on the other hand is orientated towards the maintainence of the patient's health and youthful vigour, but does not confer the same degree of benefit. Typically, ***vātātapika rasāyanas*** are relatively simple formulations, not the complex formulae like ***Cyavanaprāśa rasāyana***. If ***kuṭīprāveśika rasāyanas*** are used in ***vātātapika*** the dosage will be much less.

Perhaps the most famous of the ***vātātapika rasāyanas*** is ***Triphala cūrṇa***, the combined finely ground powders of the fruits of ***Āmalakī*** (*Phyllanthus emblica*), ***Harītakī*** (*Terminalia chebula*) and ***Bibhītaka*** (*Terminalia belerica*). ***Triphala*** is said to cleanse the ***dhātus***, improve ***agni***, nourish the ***indriyās*** ('senses') and enhance ***ojas***. The dosage used is 2–5 g, taken with ***ghṛta*** and honey once or twice daily, before meals.

Another commonly used ***vātātapika rasāyana*** is ***Nārasimha ghṛta***, a medicated ***ghṛta*** named for its ability to make a 'lion' (***simha***) out of a 'man' (***nara***). ***Nārasimha ghṛta*** is said to impart fearlessness and courage, helps to retain one's youth and vigour, increases prosperity and attractiveness, and protects one from the influence of the ***asuras*** ('demons'). The dosage is 10–12 g, taken with milk and honey.

Punarnavā root (*Boerhavia diffusa*) is another medicinal botanical used in ***vātātapika*** therapy, esteemed for its capacity to revitalise one's health, indicated by its name 'once again' (***puna***) 'new' (***navā***). The dose is 10 g of the powdered root made

TABLE 11.1 ***Kuṭīprāveśika dravyas.***

Rasāyana dravyas	**Dosage**	**Prevention and treatment**
Pippalī fruit *(Piper longum)*	Ten ***Pippalī*** are consumed with cow's milk on the first day, increased by ten on each successive day for 10 days, and thereafter reduced by ten until finished. Rice cooked with milk and ***ghṛta*** may be taken later that day after the ***Pippalī*** has been digested and can no longer be tasted	Cough, dyspnoea, consumption, diabetes, haemorrhoids, anaemia, arthritis, gout
Śilājatu	12–48 g t.i.d., taken with milk and honey for 9 to 48 days. Rice cooked with milk and ***ghṛta*** may be taken after ***Śilājatu*** has been digested	Anaemia, oedema, diabetes, tuberculosis, haemorrhoids
Cyavanaprāśa	12–48 g t.i.d. or more, with warm milk, as much as patient desires. Rice cooked with milk and ***ghṛta*** may be taken after ***Cyavanaprāśa rasāyana*** has been digested	Cough, dyspnoea, pleurisy, consumption, heart diseases, gout, dysuria, infertility, mental disorders
Agastya harītakī rasāyana	12–48 g t.i.d. or more, with warm milk, as much as patient desires. Rice cooked with milk and ***ghṛta*** may be taken after ***Agastya harītakī rasāyana*** has been digested	Cough, dyspnoea, consumption, piles, chronic fever, chronic rhinitis, sprue, premature greying, alopecia
Brahmā rasāyana	12–48 g t.i.d. or more, taken with warm milk, as much as patient desires. Rice cooked with milk and ***ghṛta*** may be taken after ***Brahmā rasāyana*** has been digested	Chronic fatigue, memory loss, senility, neurasthenia, cough

into a paste with milk, taken twice daily for 15 days, 2 months or 6 months, dependent upon the degree of rejuvenation required.

Medicinal plants that have ***rasāyana*** properties are discussed in Part II of this text.

11.13 *Vajīkaraṇa karma*: VIRILISATION THERAPY

The third type of ***rasāyana*** treatment utilised in Āyurveda is ***vajīkaraṇa rasāyana***, a term that refers to 'cultivating' (***karaṇa***) the sexual potency of a 'horse' (***vajī***). Unlike ***kuṭīprāveśika*** and ***vātātapika rasāyana***, ***vajīkaraṇa rasāyana*** targets reproductive function, and is indicated in both men and women who are infertile or wish to enjoy normal conjugal relationships without harm. Traditional Indian society has always placed a high value on progeny and an adult without children was considered to be like a tree without fruit:

> 'Stumbling walk and incomplete speech, bodies covered with dust and dirt, the mouth and face dirty and covered with saliva. In spite of all these things the child is gladdening to the heart: what other thing is equal to its sight and touch?'
>
> -***Astāñga Hṛdaya***, ***Uttarasthāna***, 40:10–11

Vajīkaraṇa or virilisation therapy has two basic goals: to enhance and strengthen the reproductive organs, and to increase the patient's desire for sexual activity. It is easy to see that the second of these goals is certainly dependent upon the first, for if the reproductive organs are deficient, the desire for sexual acitivity will be diminished. While some ***dravyas*** are certainly considered to be aphrodisiacs, ***vajīkaraṇa rasāyana*** functions to nourish the reproductive organs and increase ***ojas***. It is somewhat similar to ***vātātapika*** and many of the ***dravyas*** used in the latter therapy can be used in the former.

Unlike ***vātātapika***, however, persons suitable for ***vajīkaraṇa*** need not undergo ***pañca karma***. In this respect ***vajīkaraṇa rasāyanas*** are thought to directly target the reproductive organs, like a particular kind of seed that only one type of bird will consume (i.e. ***khalekapota***, see 4.2 **Sapta dhātus:** the seven supports). Nonetheless, ***vajīkaraṇa*** therapy should never be administered before a course of ***āmapācana***, as many of these ***dravyas*** will enhance ***āma***.

The approach taken to nurture and stimulate reproductive function is somewhat different in men and women. In addition to the nourishment of the reproductive organs, women require a greater attention to balancing ***pitta***, which plays an important role in regulating the menstrual flow (***ārtava dhātu***). Among the more important ***vajīkaraṇa rasāyanas*** for women that has this property is ***Kumārī*** juice (*Aloe vera*). The term ***Kumārī*** means 'young woman', and can be taken as the fresh juice (not the isolated gel or powdered resin) by both menstruating and post-menopausal woman to bring renewal and strength. To prepare the remedy, the Aloe leaf is split open and scraped down to the rind. This is then pounded and blended to yield a palatable texture. Typical dosages range between 25 and 50 mL of the fresh juice, once to twice daily, but can be adjusted to ensure that the bowel movements are normal. In Western herbal medicine herbs that have a similar property to decongest the uterus and liver include Yarrow leaf (*Achillea millefolium*), White Dead Nettle leaf (*Lamium album*) and Dandelion root (*Taraxacum officinalis*).

Among the most important ***dravyas*** used in Āyurveda to nourish the female reproductive organs is ***Śatāvarī*** root (*Asparagus racemosus*). Although the term ***Śatāvarī*** means 'one hundred roots,' referring to the fascicle of roots that is the habit of this plant, an alternate meaning is 'one hundred husbands', which is perhaps more descriptive of its virtue as a sexual restorative. As a ***vajīkaraṇa rasāyana*** the finely powdered root of ***Śatāvarī*** is taken in dosages of 10–15 g twice daily, mixed with milk and honey. Similarly, a medicated ***ghṛta*** can be prepared with ***Śatāvarī***, 10–15 g taken twice daily with milk. Important non-Indian herbs used as ***vajīkaraṇa rasāyanas*** for women includes Dang gui (*Angelica sinensis*), Wild Yam (*Dioscorea villosa*), Unicorn root (*Aletris farinosa*), Peony root (*Paeonia lactiflora*) and Damiana leaf (*Turnera diffusa*).

Among the most important ***vajīkaraṇa rasāyanas*** for men is ***Aśvagandhā*** root (*Withania somnifera*), whose name means to 'smell like a horse', referring to the sexual potency of a stallion. ***Aśvagandhā*** may be taken as a ***cūrṇa***, 10–15 g twice daily in milk with honey, or mixed with equal parts ***Śatāvarī***, 5–10 g each taken twice daily with milk and honey. Another useful ***vajīkaraṇa rasāyana*** is ***Tila*** seed (*Sesamum indicum*), 50 g of the ground seed taken with ***ghṛta*** and honey, once daily on an empty stomach. The ***Cakradatta*** recommends ***Vidārī*** (*Pueraria tuberosa*) as a ***vajīkaraṇa rasāyana***, 10 g of the powdered root mixed into a paste with the juice from the fresh plant and ***ghṛta***, taken once to twice daily. For suspected male infertility the Indian botanical ***Kapikacchū*** seed (*Mucana pruriens*) is highly valued, taken in doses of 10–15 g twice daily with milk and honey. In confirmed cases of male infertility and in male sexual debility, many Āyurvedic texts recommend the testicle of goat decocted with ***Tila*** seed in milk, strained, and mixed with ***ghṛta*** and ***Pippalī*** fruit (*Piper longum*) ***cūrṇa***.

11.14 *Śamana karma*: PACIFICATORY TREATMENT

When the patient is weakened by disease, and suffers from fatigue, emaciation, weakness or obesity, ***śodhana*** therapies such as ***pañca karmas*** can be too debilitating and thus a series of pacificatory, or ***śamana*** therapies are utilised. ***Śamana*** therapies are also used when the facilities to perform ***pañca karma*** are unavailable, or if ***pañca karma*** is an otherwise impractical consideration. ***Śamana karma*** comprises six components, each orientated to treat a specific ***doṣa*** or combination of the ***doṣas***, including ***langhana*** ('depleting'), ***bṛmhaṇa*** ('nourishing), ***rūkṣana*** ('drying'), ***snehana*** ('moistening'), ***stambhana*** ('cooling') and ***svedana*** ('heating').

11.15 *Śamana karma*: *langhana* THERAPY

Langhana therapies are used to normalise ***kapha*** in the body, using ***dravyas*** that are ***dīpanapācana***, exposing the body to the elements (sun and wind), engaging in strenuous exercise, fasting, and limiting the consumption of strongly nourishing foods. Some elements of ***langhana*** therapy, such as strenuous exercise, are traditionally recommended during the winter and spring, when ***kapha*** naturally accumulates. Although ***langhana*** therapy may seem contraindicated in ***vāttika*** conditions, Caraka clearly states that ***langhana*** should be used in ***vāttika*** conditions where there are indications of ***āma***. The qualities of ***langhana*** treatment are ***laghu*** ('light'), ***uṣṇa*** ('hot'), ***tikṣṇa*** ('sharp'), ***viśada*** ('clear') and ***sūkṣma*** ('subtle'). Used to excess, ***langhana*** therapies will aggravate both ***pitta*** and ***vāta***.

Herbal treatments used in ***langhana*** therapy are primarily ***tikta*** ('bitter'), ***kaśāya*** ('astringent'), and ***kaṭu*** ('pungent') in ***rasa*** ('taste'), including Indian herbs such as ***Citraka*** herb (*Plumbago zeylanica*), ***Bibhītaka*** fruit (*Terminalia belerica*), ***Guggulu*** resin (*Commiphora mukul*), ***Nimba*** leaf or bark (*Azadirachta indica*), ***Pippalī*** fruit (*Piper longum*), ***Dañtī*** root (*Baliospermum montanum*), and ***Vāsaka*** leaf (*Adhatoda vasica*). Non-Indian herbs include Bayberry bark (*Myrica cerifera*), Pipsissewa leaf (*Chimaphila umbellata*), and Cayenne fruit (*Capsicum annuum*). In terms of Chinese medicine, herbs that remove phlegm and dampness and regulate digestion may be indicated.

Snehana therapies should be avoided in ***langhana karma***, but the usage of ***gharṣana*** and ***udavartana*** therapy can be recommended, as well as ***svedana***. Some oils may be used topically and in small amounts in ***langhana karma***, such as mustard or castor oil, as well as liniments made with essential oils such as eucalyptus, wintergreen and cinnamon. Aromatherapy with clearing and pungent essential oils such as sage, cedar, pine, myrrh and camphor are best used in ***langhana*** therapy.

11.16 *Śamana karma*: *bṛmhaṇa* THERAPY

Bṛmhaṇa therapies are used to normalise ***vāttika*** and ***vātapittaja*** conditions, using foods that are nourishing and strengthening such as those implemented during ***hemañta***. When ***vāta*** symptoms predominate the ***agni*** is irregular and food should be prepared as stews and soups and, along with ***dīpanapācana dravyas***, and in some cases even digestive enzymes to ensure proper assimilation. In contrast, when ***paittika*** symptoms dominate the diet should emphasise more cooling, nourishing foods such as milk, ***ghṛta*** and coconut products. Additional therapies include ***abhyaṅga***, bathing in warm water, oatwater or medicated oils, adequate sleep, rest and relaxation, and abstinence from sexual activity. Care must be taken not to use ***bṛmhaṇa*** therapies in ***āma*** otherwise the condition being treated will be made worse and treatment more difficult. The qualities of ***bṛmhaṇa karma*** are the same as the ***guṇas*** that characterise ***kapha***, such as ***guru*** ('heavy'), ***snigdha*** ('greasy'), ***picchila*** ('slippery'), ***sthira*** ('stabilising'), ***manda*** ('slow'), and ***sāñdra*** ('solidifying'). ***Bṛmhaṇa*** therapies used to treat ***vāta*** will have a warming quality, whereas ***bṛmhaṇa karma*** in ***paittika*** conditions will have a cooling quality, and will not contain ***dravyas*** that are too ***snigdha*** ('greasy'). Used to excess, ***bṛmhaṇa*** therapies will aggravate ***kapha***.

Herbal treatments used in ***bṛmhaṇa*** therapy are primarily ***madhura*** ('sweet') and ***lavaṇa*** ('salty') in ***rasa***, including such Indian herbs as ***Śatāvarī*** root (*Asparagus racemosa*), ***Āmalakī*** fruit (*Phyllanthus emblica*), ***Balā*** leaf and root (*Sida* spp.), ***Vaṃśarocanā*** (*Bambusa arundinaceae*), ***Yaṣṭimadhu*** root (*Glycyrrhiza glabra*), ***Aṅkola*** fruit (*Alangium lamarckii*), and ***Kapikacchū*** seed (*Mucana pruriens*). Non-Indian herbs include Marshmallow root (*Althaea officinalis*), American Ginseng root (*Panax quinquefolium*), Saw Palmetto fruit (*Serenoa serrulata*), Siberian Ginseng root (*Eleuthrococcus senticosus*), Milky Oat seed (*Avena sativa*), and Damiana leaf (*Turnera diffusa*). In cases where ***pitta*** is aggravated, gentle purgatives such as Yellowdock root (*Rumex crispus*) and Dandelion root (*Taraxacum officinalis*) may be used in combination with other ***bṛmhaṇa dravyas***. In terms of Chinese medicine, herbs that sedate liver-wind, disperse liver heat, calm shen, and nurture yin and qi may be indicated.

Snehana therapies may also be indicated in ***bṛmhaṇa karma***, especially with nourishing and generally cooling oils such as coconut and ***ghṛta***, as well as medicated oils such as ***Bhṛngarāja taila*** and ***Brāhmī taila***. ***Svedana*** treatment should be mild and wet, infused with essential oils of jasmine, rose, vanilla, sandalwood, honeysuckle and ylang-ylang.

11.17 *Śamana karma*: *rūkṣana* THERAPY

Rūkṣana therapies are a treatment to ***kaphaja*** and ***paittaka*** conditions, using ***dravyas*** that have a ***tikta*** ('bitter'), ***kaśāya*** ('astringent'), and ***kaṭu*** ('pungent')

rasa, eating less food and drink, and exposure to the wind. ***Rūkṣana karma*** is in many respects similar to ***langhana*** therapies, except that it has more of a 'cooling' (***śita***) action. Used to excess, ***rūkṣana*** therapies will aggravate ***vāta***.

Although herbal treatments used in ***rūkṣana*** therapy are similar to those used in ***langhana karma***, there is a greater emphasis upon ***kaśāya*** ('astringent') ***dravyas*** such as ***Kuṭaja*** bark (*Holarrhena antidysenterica*), ***Mustaka*** root (*Cyperus rotundus*), ***Kaṭuki*** rhizome (*Picrorrhiza kurroa*), ***Vāsaka*** leaf (*Adhatoda vasica*), ***Bibhītaka*** fruit (*Terminalia belerica*), ***Mañjiṣṭhā*** root (*Rubia cordifolia*), and ***Dāruharidrā*** root (*Berberis nepalensis*). Non-Indian botanicals include Oak bark (*Quercus* spp.), Avens leaf and root (*Geum* spp.), Bayberry bark (*Myrica cerifera*), Uva ursi leaf (*Arctostaphylos uva-ursi*), Bistort root (*Bistorta* spp.), and Fir bark (*Abies* spp.) Honey may be used as an ***anupāna***. In terms of Chinese medicine, herbs that remove phlegm, dampness and dampheat may be indicated.

Snehana therapies should be avoided in ***rūkṣana karma***, but the usage of ***gharṣana*** and ***udavartana*** therapy and dry ***svedana*** may be helpful. Aromatherapy with essential oils that have a light, clear energy such as sage, cedar, pine, and camphor are all indicated in ***rūkṣana karma***.

11.18 *Śamana karma*: *snehana* THERAPY

Snehana therapies are primarily a treatment for ***vāttika*** conditions, emphasising greasy and moistening foods and treatments, while avoiding drying and light foods and therapies. The qualities of ***snehana*** therapy are ***snigdha*** ('greasy'), ***uṣṇa*** ('hot'), ***guru*** ('heavy'), and ***picchila*** ('slippery'). The primary treatment in ***snehana*** therapy is the application of medicated oils to reduce ***vāta***. Used to excess, ***snehana karma*** aggravates both ***kapha*** and ***pitta***.

Herbal treatments used in ***snehana*** therapy are primarily ***madhura*** ('sweet'), ***lavaṇa*** ('salty') and ***amla*** ('sour') in ***rasa***, including Indian herbs such as ***Āmalakī*** fruit (*Phyllanthus emblica*), ***Mātuluṅga*** fruit (*Citrus medica*), ***Aśvagandhā*** root (*Withania somnifera*), ***Śatāvarī*** root (*Asparagus racemosa*), ***Kapikacchū*** seed (*Mucana pruriens*) and ***saindhava***. Useful non-Indian herbs include sour-tasting herbs such as Rosehips (*Rosa* spp.), Orange peel (*Citrus reticulata*), and Wu Wei Zi fruit (*Schizandra chinensis*), as well sweet-tasting herbs such as American Ginseng root (*Panax quinquefolium*), Milky Oat seed (*Avena sativa*), and Shu Di Huang root (cured *Rehmannia glutinosa*). In some cases a small amount of ***kaṭu rasa*** is appropriate, used as an adjunct to primary treatment to ensure the proper digestion of the more ***guru*** ('heavy') ***dravyas***. Somewhat paradoxically, herbs that have a ***tikta*** ('bitter') ***rasa*** such as Oregon Grape root (*Mahonia aquifolium*) and Yellowdock (*Rumex crispus*) may also be used in small amounts to treat dryness, to improve the function of the liver. In terms of Chinese medicine herbs that restore qi, blood and yin may be indicated.

Additional therapies include both external and internal ***snehana*** and ***anuvāsana vasti***. Wet ***svedana*** is also used in ***snehana karma***, infused with warming and heavy essential oils as vetivert, musk, sandalwood and vanilla.

11.19 *Śamana karma*: *stambhana* THERAPY

Stambhana therapies are primarily a treatment for ***pitta***, emphasising moistening, cooling and salty foods, sufficient water, electrolytes, bathing in cool water, residing next to water, and exposure to moonlight. ***Stambhana karma*** tends to have constipating action and is thus used in ***paittika*** diseases such as diarrhoea and dysentery. The qualities of ***stambhana karma*** are ***śita*** ('cold'), ***manda*** ('slow'), ***sāñdra*** ('solidifying') and ***sthira*** ('stabilising'). Used to excess, ***stambhana*** treatments will aggravate both ***kapha*** and ***vāta***.

Herbal treatment in ***stambhana*** therapy are primarily ***madhura*** ('sweet'), ***tikta*** ('bitter'), ***kaśāya*** ('astringent') in ***rasa***, including such Indian herbs as ***Kuṭaja*** bark (*Holarrhena antidysenterica*), ***Vaṃśarocanā*** (*Bambusa arundiacea*), ***Maṇḍūkaparṇī*** leaf (*Centella asiatica*), ***Śatāvarī*** root (*Asparagus racemosa*), ***Mustaka*** root (*Cyperus rotundus*), ***Candana*** wood (*Santalum album*), ***Dāḍima*** pericarp (*Punica granatum*), and ***Yaṣṭimadhu*** (*Glycyrrhiza glabra*). Useful non-Indian herbs include astringents such as Blackberry root (*Rubus discolor*), Cranesbill Geranium root (*Geranium maculatum*), White Pond Lily root (*Nymphaea odorata*); demulcents such as Comfrey leaf (*Symphytum officinalis*) and Marshmallow root (*Althaea officinalis*); and bitter herbs such as Gentian root (*Gentiana* spp.), Dandelion root (*Taraxacum officinalis*), and Calendula flower (*Calendula officinalis*). Mineral-rich restorative herbs such as Horsetail (*Equisetum arvense*) and Nettle (*Urtica dioica*) may also be indicated in ***stambhana karma***. From a Western herbal perspective, cooling and relaxing nervines such as Skullcap (*Scutellaria* spp.), Passionflower (*Passiflora incarnata*), and Motherwort (*Leonorus cardiaca*) may also be indicated in ***stambhana karma. Saindhava*** can be particularly helpful in ***paittika*** disorders, but normal table salt is generally contraindicated. In terms of Chinese medicine, herbs used to purge toxic-heat, stabilise and bind, and tonify yin may be indicated.

Snehana and ***svedana*** therapies are generally avoided in ***stambhana karma***, or are used to a minimal extent. Useful oils include coconut and ***ghṛta***, and medicated oils such as ***Bhṛṅgarāja taila*** and ***Piṇḍa taila***. Bathing in cool water is recommended, infused with cooling and relaxing essential oils such as jasmine, rose, gardenia, vetivert and sandalwood.

11.20 *Śamana karma*: *svedana* THERAPY

Svedana therapy is primarily a treatment for combined ***vātakaphaja*** conditions, using foods and treatments with a ***kaṭu*** ('pungent') and ***amla*** ('sour') ***rasa***, drinking warm beverages, avoiding cold foods and cold environments, and the use of sweating and diaphoretic therapies. The qualities of ***svedana*** treatment are ***uṣṇa*** ('heating') and ***drava*** ('liquefying'). Used to excess, ***svedana*** treatments will aggravate ***pitta***.

Herbal treatment in ***svedana*** therapy are primarily ***kaṭu*** ('pungent') and ***lavaṇa*** ('salty') in ***rasa***, including such Indian herbs as ***Hiṅgu*** resin (*Asafoetida ferula*), ***Guggulu*** resin (*Commiphora mukul*), ***Devadāru*** wood (*Cedrus deodara*), ***Bhallātaka*** pericarp (*Semecarpus anacardium*), ***Agnimañtha*** leaf and root (*Premna integrifolia*), ***Kaṇṭakāri*** root (*Solanum xanthocarpum*), ***Tulasī*** leaf (*Ocimum sanctum*), ***Pippalī*** fruit (*Piper longum*), ***Tvak*** bark (*Cinnamomum zeylanicum*), ***Śūṇṭhī*** rhizome (*Zingiber officinalis*), and ***Elā*** fruit (*Elettaria cardamomum*). Useful non-Indian herbs include Bayberry bark (*Myrica cerifera*), Prickly Ash bark (*Zanthoxylum americanum*), Kelp frond (*Fucus* spp.), Osha root (*Ligusticum* spp.), and Cayenne fruit (*Capsicum* spp.). In terms of Chinese medicine, herbs that remove wind-damp, regulate digestion, and tonify yang and qi may be indicated.

Warm ***snehana*** treatments can be quite useful in the treatment of cold conditions such as peripheral numbness and congestive arthritis. Warming and stimulating oils such as mustard and ***Pippalyādi taila*** may be combined with ***udavartana*** and ***piṇḍa sveda. Svedana karma*** can be used in conjunction with warming and stimulating essential oils such as cinnamon, black pepper, ginger and clove.

ENDNOTE

26 In his text *Massage Therapy in Ayurveda* (1992), Vaidya Bhagwan Dash has a design to build a traditional Āyurvedic massage table.

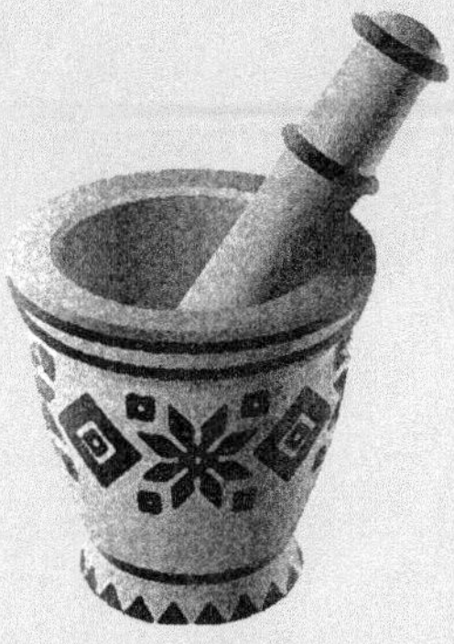

PART 2

ĀYURVEDIC MATERIA MEDICA

Agnimañtha, 'to churn the fire'
Āmalakī, 'sour'
Arjuna, 'white'
Aśvagandhā, 'smelling like a horse'
Balā, 'strength'
Bhallātaka, 'piercing like a spear'
Bhṛṅgarāja, 'ruler of the hair'
Bhūnimba, 'ground nimba'
Bibhītaka, 'intimidating'
Bilva
Brāhmī, 'consort of brahmā'
Candana, 'gladdening'
Citraka, 'the spotted one'
Devadāru, 'wood of the gods'
Elā
Gokṣura, 'cow scratcher'
Guḍūcī
Guggulu
Haridrā, 'giving yellow'
Harītakī, 'to colour yellow'
Hiṅgu
Jaṭāmāmsī, 'braided and fleshy'
Jātīphala, 'fruit of excellence'
Jyotiṣmatī, 'luminous'
Kaṇṭakāri, 'thorny'
Kapikacchū, 'monkey itcher'
Kaṭuka, 'pungent'
Kūṣmāṇḍa
Kuṣṭha, 'disease'
Kuṭaja, 'mountain born'
Maṇḍūkaparṇī, 'frog-leaved'
Mañjiṣṭhā
Mustaka
Nāgakeśara, 'serpent stamens'
Nimba, 'bestowed of health'
Nirguṇḍī
Pippalī
Punarnavā, 'once again new'
Śālaparṇī, 'leaves like śāla'
Śaṅkhapuṣpī, 'conch flower'
Śatāvarī, 'one hundred roots'
Śilājatu, 'to become like stone'
Śyonāka
Trivṛt, 'thricely twisted'
Uśīra
Vacā, 'to speak'
Vaṃśa
Vāsaka
Viḍaṅga, 'skilful'
Yavānī

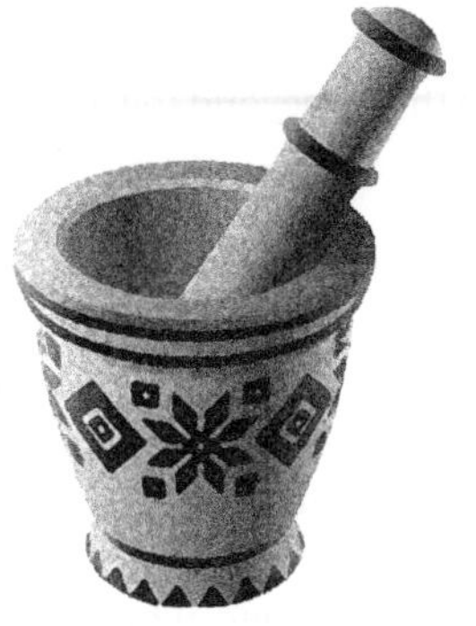

PART 2

Introduction

There are thousands of medicinal plant species found within the materia medica of Āyurveda, a tribute to the great biodiversity that the Indian subcontinent offers: from the delicate alpine meadows of the Himalayas to the broad Gangetic plain, from the semi-arid Deccan plateau to the lush tropical coastline of south India. Unfortunately the toll of misguided colonial development, population pressures and extreme poverty has led to a great decline in this biodiversity, and many Indian plants formerly gathered in the wild are now threatened or even extinct (see: www.cites.org). Although this is a matter of grave concern, Āyurveda has a long history of incorporating non-native plants into its materia medica, such as ***Madhusnuhī*** (*Smilax chinensis*) from China, brought to India by Unani physicians in the 16th century and later mentioned in the ***Bhāvaprakāśa*** as a treatment for syphilis[27]. As a Western herbalist also familiar with Chinese herbal medicine, I take a fairly liberal view that this process should be encouraged, especially in the use of cultivated and non-threatened species as substitutes or adjuncts. Thus in the following monographs I make reference to the use of non-Indian herbs in combination with more traditional Āyurvedic plants, which is reflective of my clinical approach.

In 1997 I travelled to India with samples of medicinal plants used by First Nations healers in North America. I asked several Āyurvedic physicians to taste these remedies and tell me what their impressions were. Most physicians doubted their ability to ascertain accurately the ***dravyguṇa*** alone by taste, although general characteristics can be inferred by different tastes, e.g. ***tikta rasa*** is ***śita vīrya***, ***amla rasa*** is ***uṣṇa vīrya***, etc. This inference, however, is clearly insufficient, evidenced by several exceptions in the Āyurvedic materia medica alone, such as the sour-tasting ***Āmalakī*** fruit which is classified as having a cooling (***śita***) energy (***vīrya***). Many of these physicians wanted to see the whole plant and not just the powdered herb, to see the ecology in which in grows, and wanted to know about its traditional uses. All of these are important factors in determining the profile of a medicinal plant, and thus the inclusion of non-Indian plants into the Āyurvedic materia medica must be done thoughtfully, with all the respect and due diligence required to first understand the plant within its own ethnobotanical and ecological context.

The following format has been chosen to convey precise information about each plant, and a colour plate section featuring images of the plants begins after page 302.

Sanskrit name: The most commonly used name in Sanskrit, and the etymology of the name if it is known.

Botanical name: The scientific binomial, and common botanical synonyms, and plant family.

Other names: Other Sanskrit names (in italics), as well as commonly used names in Hindi (H), Tamil (T), English (E), and Chinese (C).

Botany: Botanical description and ecology of the species concerned.

Part used: The most commonly used part(s) of the plant.

Dravyguṇa: The 'pharmacology' according to Āyurveda described in Chapter 6, divided into:

- ***Rasa***: taste.
- ***Vipāka***: post-digestive effect.

- ***Vīrya***: energy, including the ***guṇas***
- ***Karma***: action
- ***Prabhāva***: supramundane or unique attributes, if known or described.

Constituents: Recent information on major plant chemical constituents.

Medical research: Details from the scientific literature that supports or adds to the traditional uses for the particular species or its isolated constituents, divided into three components:

- ***In vitro***: medicinal properties for the particular ***dravya*** that have been elucidated through in vitro ('in glass') research (e.g. the artificial environment of a test tube or Petri dish); for example, by innoculating a fungal or bacterial culture with a herbal extract and measuring the antimicrobial effect. Researchers consider this to be among the most preliminary forms of data, and in most cases cannot be extrapolated to internal human use, although some data may be applicable to external use.
- ***In vivo***: medicinal properties for the particular ***dravya*** that have been elucidated through in vivo ('in the body') research, using experimental animals such as rats, mice, cats, pigs, dogs, monkeys, etc. Given that these animals metabolise substances differently, many of the conclusions drawn from these studies cannot be reliably extrapolated to humans.
- ***Human trials***: medicinal properties for the particular ***dravya*** that have been obtained through human clinical trials, of which there are a number of different types, including observational trials such as case–control or cohort studies, or intervention trials such as the randomised, double-blind placebo-controlled study. While medical researchers consider clinical trials to be the most reliable form of experimental evidence there are still problems with these models, particularly in context with complementary and alternative practices such as Āyurveda that tailor treatments to individual patients, usually with multiple interventions over a period of time that is beyond the length of most studies.

Toxicity: Mention of toxicity in the literature and traditional texts.

Indications: Signs, symptoms and specific disease states, from a pathophysical perspective.

Contraindications: Conditions under which the usage of the particular plant species is discouraged or inappropriate.

Medicinal uses: Additional information on clinical usage and information of general interest. Both traditonal Āyurvedic formulations and combinations with non-Indian herbs are included to illustrate the ways in which the ***dravya*** can be formulated. Indian botanicals are described by their Sanskrit names, which are defined in Appendix 3, whereas non-Indian botanicals are given with their botanical names.

Dosage: Recommended dosage levels for adults in whatever form is appropriate for administration. Please note that the doses mentioned in the extant texts of Āyurvedic medicine tend to be much larger and stronger than those mentioned in many modern sources. Please consult Chapter 6 to review the various Āyurvedic preparations, e.g. ***cūrṇa*** (powder), ***phāṇṭa*** (infusion), ***kvātha*** (decoction), etc. The ratio given for liquid extracts is the ratio of herb to solvent (w/v), and in the case of tinctures, the percentage (%) of alcohol used during preparation.

References: Works cited in the monograph.

ENDNOTE

27 Kumar and Krishnaprasad mention several medicinal plants used in Tamil (***Siddha***) medicine that are prefixed by the Tamil term 'cina,' denoting plants that originally came from China, e.g. cinailantai (*Zizyphus jujuba*) (Ancient Science of Life 1992 11(3,4):114–117). There are many other example of herbs that appear to be of Chinese origin that are now important Āyurvedic herbs, such as ***Cīnatīkṣṇa*** (*Piper cubeba*) and ***Cīnakarpūra*** (*Cinnamomum camphora*).

Agnimañtha, 'to churn the fire'

BOTANICAL NAMES: *Premna integrifolia, P. obtusifolia, P. corymbosa,* Verbenaceae

OTHER NAMES: Arni (H); Munnai (T)

Botany: ***Agnimañtha*** is a large shrub or tree attaining a height of up to 9 m, with yellowish bark, dotted with lenticels, the branches sometimes spiny. The leaves are broadly elliptic, obtuse, acuminate, and glabrous, margins entire or upper portions dentate, and give off an offensive odour when crushed. The flowers are small, greenish yellow to greenish white, borne in terminal paniculate corymbose cymes, similarly offensive in odour as the leaves, giving way to globose black drupes with a persistent saucer-shaped calyx when mature. ***Agnimañtha*** is found widespread throughout India, along the coastal regions into the plains and hills (Kirtikar & Basu 1935, Warrier et al 1995).

Part used: Leaves and root.

Dravyguṇa:

- ***Rasa***: *tikta, kaṭu, kaśāya, madhura*
- ***Vipāka***: *kaṭu*
- ***Vīrya***: *uṣṇa*
- ***Karma***: *dīpanapācana, bhedana, jvaraghna, chedana, raktaprasādana, kuṣṭaghna, mūtravirecana, mūtraviśodhana, śothahara, medohara, vedanāsthāpana, kaphavātahara* (Srikanthamurthy 2001, Warrier et al 1995).

Constituents: The limited amount of chemical research on ***Agnimañtha*** has yielded the alkaloids premnine, ganiarine, premnazole and aphelandrine, the pentacyclic terpene betulin, the flavone lutiolin, β-sitosterol, a polyisoprenoid, resin and tannin (Barik et al 1993, Kapoor 1990, Yoganarasimhan 2000).

Medical research:

- ***In vivo***: antipyretic, anti-inflammatory (Narayanan et al 2000); hypoglycaemic, hypotensive (Kapoor 1990).

Toxicity: An alcoholic extract of *Premna herbacea* was found to be safe up to a dose of 8.0 g/kg when administered orally to mice (Narayanan et al 2000).

Indications: Dyspepsia, flatulent colic, haemorrhoids, constipation, fever, catarrh, cough, bronchitis, asthma, skin diseases, urinary disease, oedema, diabetes, anaemia, neuralgia, insufficient lactation, inflammatory joint disease, tumours.

Contraindications: Pregnancy; ***pittakopa***.

Medicinal uses: ***Agnimañtha*** is an important herb for oedema, diseases of the urinary tract and diabetes. In the treatment of oedema ***Agnimañtha cūrṇa*** is combined with ***Dhānyaka*** seed (Kirtikar & Basu 1935). In the treatment of diabetes ***Agnimañtha cūrṇa*** can be combined with ***Śilājatu*** and ***Guggulu***. In the treatment of urinary tract disorders ***Agnimañtha*** may be of benefit when combined with ***Gokṣura***, or when taken alone as the fresh juice. The fresh juice can also be used along with the ***svarasa*** of ***Āmalakī*** and ***Guḍūcī*** in the treatment of diabetes, and with ***Śilājatu*** in the treatment of obesity (Sharma 2002). Nadkarni (1954) recommends an infusion of the leaves in fever, colic and flatulence. The ***Cakradatta*** recommends a formula called ***Shunthyādi*** in the treatment of urinary calculi, prepared by decocting equal parts ***Agnimañtha***, ***Śūṇṭhī***, ***Gokṣura***, ***Harītakī***, ***Pāṣāṇabheda***, ***Śigru***, ***Varuṇa*** and ***Āragvadha***, taken with ***Hiṅgu***, ***Yavakṣāra*** and salt as ***anupāna*** (Sharma 2002). ***Agnimañtha*** root is an important constituent of the famed ***Cyavanaprāśa*** fomulation.

Dosage:

- ***Svarasa***: fresh leaves, 10–25 mL b.i.d.–t.i.d.
- ***Cūrṇa***: dried root or leaves, 3–5 g b.i.d.–t.i.d.
- ***Phāṇṭa***: dried leaves, 1:4, 30–90 mL b.i.d.–t.i.d.

- ***Kvātha***: dried root, 1:4, 30–90 mL b.i.d.–t.i.d.
- ***Tincture***: dried root, 1:3, 50% alcohol, 3–5 mL b.i.d.–t.i.d.

REFERENCES

Barik BR, Bhaumik T, Patra A et al 1993 Premnazole an isoxazole alkaloid of Premna integrifolia linn. & Gmelina arborea linn. with anti-inflammatory activity. Fitoterapia. 13(4):395

Dash Bhagwan 1991 Materia medica of Ayurveda. B. Jain Publishers, New Delhi

Kapoor LD 1990 CRC Handbook of Ayurvedic medicinal plants. CRC Press, Boca Raton, p 271

Kirtikar KR, Basu BD 1935 Indian medicinal plants, 2nd edn, vols 1–4. Periodical Experts, Delhi, p 1929–1930

Nadkarni KM 1954 The Indian materia medica, with Ayurvedic, Unani and home remedies. Revised and enlarged by A. K. Nadkarni. Bombay Popular Prakasan PVP, Bombay, p 1010

Narayanan N, Thirugnanasambantham P, Viswanathan S et al 2000 Antipyretic, antinociceptive and anti-inflammatory activity of Premna herbacea roots. Fitoterapia 71(2):147–153

Sharma PV 2002 Cakradatta. Sanskrit text with English translation. Chaukhamba, Varanasi, p 318, 336

Srikanthamurthy KR 2001 Bhāvaprakāśa of Bhavamiśra, vol 1. Krishnadas Academy, Varanasi, p 231

Warrier PK, Nambiar VPK, Ramankutty C (eds) 1995 Indian medicinal plants: a compendium of 500 species, vol 4. Orient Longman, Hyderabad, p 348

Yoganarasimhan SN 2000 Medicinal plants of India, vol 2: Tamil Nadu. Self-published, Bangalore, p 440

Āmalakī, 'sour'

BOTANICAL NAMES: *Phyllanthus emblica, Emblica officinalis,* Euphorbiaceae

OTHER NAMES: ***Dhātrī***, 'nurse' (S); Amlika (H); Nelli (T); Indian Gooseberry (E)

Botany: ***Āmalakī*** is a small to medium-sized tree with a crooked trunk and spreading branches, the greyish-green bark peeling off in flakes. The branchlets are glabrous or finely pubescent, 10–20 cm long, usually deciduous; the leaves simple, subsessile and closely set along the branchlets, light green, resembling pinnate leaves. The flowers are greenish-yellow, borne in axillary fascicles, giving way to a globose fruit with a greenish-yellow flesh and six furrows, enclosing a stone with six seeds. ***Āmalakī*** is native to tropical southeastern Asia, particularly in central and southern India, Pakistan, Bangladesh, Sri Lanka, Malayasia, southern China and the Mascarene Islands. It is commonly cultivated in gardens throughout India and grown commercially as a medicinal fruit (Kirtikar & Basu 1935, Warrier et al 1995).

Part used: Fresh or dried whole fruit.

Dravyguṇa:

- ***Rasa***: primarily *amla, tikta* and *kaśāya*, but also *madhura*, noticed particularly while drinking water after one has consumed the fruit. *Kaṭu* is a minor, secondary taste, whereas *lavaṇa* is absent.
- ***Vipāka***: *madhura*
- ***Vīrya***: *śita*
- ***Karma***: *dīpanapācana, anulomana, jvaraghna, raktaprasādana, kāsahara, svāsahara, hṛdaya, cakṣuṣya, romasañjana, jīvanīya, medhya, rasāyana, tridoṣaghna*
- ***Prabhāva***: *Āmalakī* is said to be *sattvic*, bringing good fortune, love and longevity to those that consume it (Dash 1991, Dash & Junius 1983, Frawley & Lad 1986, Srikanthamurthy 2001, Warrier et al 1995).

Constituents: ***Āmalakī*** fruit contains a series of diterpenes referred to as the gibberellins, as well as the triterpene lupeol, flavonoids (e.g. kaempherol–3-*O*-β-D-glucoside, quercetin–3-*O*-β-D-glucoside), and polyphenols (e.g. emblicanin A and B, punigluconin and pedunculagin). Also present are the phyllantine and zeatin alkaloids, and a number of benzenoids, including amlaic acid, corilagin, ellagic acid, 3–6-di-*O*-galloyl-glucose, ethyl gallate, 1,6-di-*O*-galloyl-β-D-glucose, 1-di-*O*-galloyl-β-D-glucose, putranjivain A, digallic acid, phyllemblic acid, emblicol and alactaric acid. The fruits are also stated to contain significantly high amounts of ascorbic acid (vitamin C), upwards of 3.25% in the dried fruit, but this has also been disputed (Bhattacharya et al 1999, Ghosal et al 1996, Khopde et al 2001, Summanen 1999, Yoganarasimhan 2000).

Medical research:

- ***In vitro***: antiviral (El-Mekkawy et al 1995), antimicrobial (Ahmad et al 1998, Dutta et al 1998)
- ***In vivo***: anti-inflammatory (Asmawi et al 1993), immunostimulant (Suresh & Vasudevan 1994), adaptogenic (Rege et al 1999), hepatoprotective (Jeena et al 1999), pancreas-protective (Thorat et al 1995), cancer-protective (Biswas et al 1999, Nandi et al 1997, Yadav 1987), hypolipidemic (Mathur et al 1996, Mishra et al 1981, Thakur 1985)
- ***Human trials***: fresh ***Āmalakī*** demonstrated a significant hypocholesterolaemic effect in both normal and hypercholesterolaemic men aged 35–55 years (Jacob et al 1988).

Toxicity: ***Āmalakī*** is widely consumed throughout India as a medicinal food and is not considered toxic.

Indications: Dyspepsia, gastritis, biliousness, hyperacidity, hepatitis, constipation, flatulent colic, colitis, haemorrhoids, convalescence from fever, cough, asthma, skin diseases, bleeding disorders, menorrhagia, anaemia, diabetes, gout, osteoporosis, premature greying, alopecia, asthenia, mental disorders, vertigo, palpitations, cardiovascular disease, cancer.

Contraindications: Acute diarrhoea, dysentery (Frawley & Lad 1986).

Medicinal uses: ***Āmalakī*** is among the most important medicinal plants in the Āyurvedic materia medica, and along with ***Harītakī*** and ***Bibhītaka*** forms the famous ***Triphala*** formula, used to cleanse the ***dhātus*** of ***āma***, pacify all three ***doṣas***, and to promote good health and long life. A synonym for ***Āmalakī*** is ***Dhātrī*** or 'nurse', indicating that it has the power to restore health like a mother caring for her child. The fruit is the most commonly used plant part, and the fresh fruit is preferred. An excision in the unripe fruit is made and the exudate collected is used topically in conjunctivitis (Kirtikar & Basu 1935). The unripe fruits are also made into pickles and given before meals to stimulate the appetite in anorexia (Nadkarni 1954). The fresh juice of the fruit mixed with ***ghṛta*** is a ***rasāyana***; it has a beneficial activity upon the intestinal flora, and is a corrective to colon function. The fresh fruit is very hard to come by outside the subcontinent and can usually be found in Indian markets only for a few weeks during the autumn. The dried fruit is used as a decoction to treat ophthalmia when applied externally, and is used internally as a haemostatic and antidiarrhoeal (Nadkarni 1954). The boiled, reconstituted dried fruit, blended into a smooth liquid with a small quantity of ***guḍa*** added, is useful in anorexia, anaemia, biliousness, dyspepsia and jaundice. This is also an excellent restorative in chronic rhinitis and fever, with swollen and dry red lips and rashes about the mouth. The dried fruit prepared as a decoction and taken on a regular basis is useful in menorrhagia and leucorrhoea, and is an excellent post-partum restorative. Similarly, the ***Cakradatta*** recommends the fresh juice of ***Āmalakī*** with ***Āmalakī cūrṇa***, taken with ***ghṛta*** and honey as a ***vajīkaraṇa rasāyana***. In the treatment of cardiovascular disease ***Āmalakī*** is an excellent antioxidant botanical, used to treat all of the cardiovascular effects of poorly controlled diabetes and insulin resistance, including diseases of microcirculation such as macular degeneration. ***Āmalakī*** is similarly taken in polluted urban areas to keep the immune system strong. For coronary heart disease, in particular, ***Āmalakī*** can be combined with ***Arjuna***, or non-Indian botanicals such as Hawthorn, and with ***Guggulu*** for dyslipidaemia. Taken with ***Guḍūcī***, ***Kaṭuka*** and ***Bhūnimba***, ***Āmalakī*** forms an important protocol in the treatment of hepatitis and cirrhosis. ***Āmalakī*** is also an important herb to consider to protect the body against the deleterious effects of chemotherapy and radiation in conventional cancer treatments. In combination with ***Citraka***, ***Harītakī***, ***Pippalī*** and ***saindhava***, ***Āmalakī cūrṇa*** is mentioned by the ***Śāraṅgadhara saṃhitā*** in the treatment of all types of fever (Srikanthamurthy 1984). In the treatment of nausea, vomiting and poor appetite, fresh ***Āmalakī*** is crushed with ***Drākṣā*** and mixed with sugar and honey (Sharma 2002). ***Āmalakī*** fruit fried in ***ghṛta*** and reduced to a paste and mixed with fermented rice water is applied over the head to treat nosebleeds (Srikanthamurthy 1984). In the treatment of ***agnimāndya***, oedema, abdominal enlargement, haemorrhoids, intestinal parasites, diabetes and allergies, three parts ***Āmalakī cūrṇa*** is mixed with the same amount each of ***Ajamodā***, ***Harītakī*** and ***Marica*** with 1 part ***pañca lavaṇa*** macerated in buttermilk until it has fermented (Sharma 2002). Combined with equal parts ***Guḍūcī***, ***Śūṇṭhī***, ***Āragvadha*** and ***Gokṣura***, dried ***Āmalakī*** fruit is recommended by the Cakradatta as a decoction in the treatment of urinary tenesmus (Sharma 2002). ***Āmalakī*** is the primary constituent of a complex polyherbal ***lehya*** called ***Cyavanaprāśa*** that is used as a ***rasāyana***, and in the treatment of chronic lung and heart diseases, infertility and mental disorders (Sharma 2002). Another valued ***rasāyana*** that contains ***Āmalakī*** as the primary constituent is ***Brahmārasāyana***, giving the person that takes it '. . . the vigor resembling an elephant, intelligence, strength, wisdom and right attitude' (Srikanthamurthy 1995). The dried fruit made into an oil and applied to the head, and taken internally as a decoction or powder, is reputed to be useful in alopecia and adds lustre and strength to the hair. Similarly, the ***Cakradatta*** recommends a ***nasya*** of equal parts ***Āmalakī*** and ***Yaṣṭimadhu*** decocted in milk, in the treatment of alopecia (Sharma 2002). Both the fresh juice and crushed seeds are combined with ***Haridrā*** as an effective treatment for diabetes (Dash & Junius 1983, Sharma 2002). The seeds are made into a fine powder and mixed with equal parts powder of ***Aśvagandhā*** root as a ***rasāyana*** in the cold winter months (Nadkarni 1954). For scabies and skin irritations the seed is charred, powdered and mixed into sesame oil and applied externally (Nadkarni 1954).

Dosage:

- ***Cūrṇa***: 3–10 g b.i.d.–t.i.d.
- ***Kvātha***: 1:4, 60–120 mL b.i.d.–t.i.d.
- ***Tincture***: 1:3, 30% alcohol, 1–10 mL b.i.d.–t.i.d.

REFERENCES

Ahmad I et al 1998 Screening of some Indian medicinal plants for their antimicrobial properties. Journal of Ethnopharmacology 62(2):183–193

Asmawi MZ, Kankaanranta H, Moilanen E et al 1993 Anti-inflammatory activities of P. emblica Gaertn leaf extracts. Journal of Pharmacy and Pharmacology 45(6):581–584

Bhattacharya A, Chatterjee A, Ghosal S et al 1999 Anti-oxidant activity of active tannoid principles of P. emblica (amla). Indian Journal of Experimental Biology 37(7):676–680

Biswas S, Talukder G, Sharma A 1999 Protection against cytotoxic effects of arsenic by dietary supplementation with crude extract of P. emblica fruit. Phytotherapy Research: 13(6):513–516

Dash B, 1991 Materia medica of Āyurveda. B. Jain Publishers, New Delhi, p 9

Dash B, Junius M 1983 A handbook of Ayurveda. Concept Publishing, New Delhi, p 89, 90

Dutta BK, Rahman I, Das TK 1998 Antifungal activity of Indian plant extracts. Mycoses 41(11–12):535–536

El-Mekkawy S, Meselhy MR, Kusumoto IT et al 1995 Inhibitory effects of Egyptian folk medicines on human immunodeficiency virus (HIV) reverse transcriptase. Chemical and Pharmaceutical Bulletin 43(4):641–648

Frawley D, Lad V 1986 The Yoga of herbs: an Āyurveda guide to herbal medicine. Lotus Press, Santa Fe, p 157

Ghosal S, Tripathi VK, Chauhan S 1996 Active constituents of P. emblica, part 1: the chemistry and antioxidative effects of two new hydrolysable tannins, emblicanin a and b. Indian Journal of Chemistry Section B, Organic Chemistry Including Medicinal Chemistry 35:941–948

Jacob A, Pandey M, Kapoor S et al 1988 Effect of the Indian gooseberry (amla) on serum cholesterol levels in men aged 35–55 years. European Journal of Clinical Nutrition 42(11):939–944

Jeena KJ, Joy KL, Kuttan R 1999 Effect of P. emblica, Phyllanthus amarus and Picrorrhiza kurroa on *N*-nitrosodiethylamine induced hepatocarcinogenesis. Cancer Letters 136(1):11–16

Katiyar CK, Brindavanam MB, Tiwari P et al 1997 Immunomodulator products from Ayurveda: current status and future perspectives. In: Upadhyay SN (ed) Immunomodulation. Narosa Publishing House, New Delhi

Khopde SM, Pryadarshini KI, Mohan H et al 2001 Characterizing the anti-oxidant activity of amla (P. emblica) extract. Current Science 81:185–190

Kirtikar KR, Basu BD 1935 Indian medicinal plants, 2nd edn. Periodical Experts, Delhi, p 2220–2221

Mathur R, Sharma A, Dixit VP, Varma M 1996 Hypolipidaemic effect of fruit juice of P. emblica in cholesterol-fed rabbits. Journal of Ethnopharmacology 50(2):61–68

Mishra M, Pathak UN, Khan AB 1981 P. emblica Gaertn and serum cholesterol level in experimental rabbits. British Journal of Experimental Pathology 62(5):526–528

Nadkarni KM 1954 The Indian materia medica, with Ayurvedic, Unani and home remedies, revised and enlarged by AK Nadkarni. Bombay Popular Prakashan PVP, Bombay, p 481–483

Nandi P, Talukder G, Sharma A 1997 Dietary chemoprevention of clastogenic effects of 3, 4-benzo(a)pyrene by P. emblica Gaertn fruit extract. British Journal of Cancer 76(10):1279–1283

Rege NN, Thatte UM, Dahanukar SA 1999 Adaptogenic properties of six rasayana herbs used in Ayurvedic medicine. Phytotherapy Research 13(4):275–291

Sharma PV 2002 Cakradatta. Sanskrit text with English translation. Chaukhamba, Varanasi, p 71, 140, 170, 307, 327, 488

Srikanthamurthy KR 1984 Sāraṅgadhara saṃhitā. Chaukhamba Orientalia, Varanasi, p 85, 242

Srikanthamurthy KR 1995 Vāgbhaṭa's Aṣṭāñga Hṛdayam, vol 3. Krishnadas Academy, Varanasi, p 386

Srikanthamurthy KR 2001 Bhāvaprakāśa of Bhavamiśra, vol 1. Krishnadas Academy, Varanasi, p 164

Summanen JO 1999 A chemical and ethnopharmacological study on *P. emblica* (Euphorbiaceae). Dissertation, Division of Pharmacognosy, University of Helsinki Department of Pharmacy, Helsinki. Online. Available: http://ethesis.helsinki.fi/julkaisut/mat/farma/vk/summanen/achemica.pdf

Suresh K, Vasudevan DM 1994 Augmentation of murine natural killer cell and antibody dependent cellular cytotoxicity activities by *Phyllanthus emblica*, a new immunomodulator. Journal of Ethnopharmacology 44(1):55–60

Thakur CP 1985 P. emblica reduces serum, aortic and hepatic cholesterol in rabbits. Experientia 41(3):423–424

Thorat SP, Rege NN, Naik AS et al 1995 P. emblica: a novel therapy for acute pancreatitis, an experimental study. HPB Surgery 9(1):25–30

Warrier PK, Nambiar VPK, Ramankutty C eds 1995 Indian medicinal plants: a compendium of 500 species, vol 4. Orient Longman, Hyderabad, p 256

Yadav SK 1987 Protection against radiation induced chromosome damage by Emblica officinalis fruit extract. Caryologia 40(3):261–266

Yoganarasimhan SN 2000 Medicinal plants of India, vol 2: Tamil Nadu. Self-published, Bangalore, p 410

Arjuna, 'white'

BOTANICAL NAME: *Terminalia arjuna,* Combretaceae

OTHER NAMES: ***Kakubha,*** 'mountain top,' *Vīrataru,* 'hero's tree' (S); Arjun, Anjan, Kahu (H); Attumaratu, Nirmarutu, Vellaimarutu, Marutu (T); White Murdah (E)

Botany: ***Arjuna*** grows to become a very large tree with a huge buttressed trunk, widely spreading, drooping branches, and a grey bark that flakes off in large, flat pieces. The leaves are opposite, simple, oblong to elliptic, pale green above and pale brown below. The white flowers are borne in short axillary spikes or terminal panicles, giving way to an ovoid or oblong fruit with 5–7 short, hard wings. ***Arjuna*** is found throughout the subcontinent of India, from the foothills of the Himalayas southwards into Sri Lanka (Kirtikar & Basu 1935; Warrier et al 1996).

Part used: Stem bark.

Dravyguṇa:

- ***Rasa***: *kaśāya, madhura, kaṭu*
- ***Vīrya***: *śita*
- ***Karma***: *purīṣasangrahaṇiya, chedana, kāsahara, svāsahara, śoṇitasthāpana, hṛdaya, mūtravirecana, aśmaribhedana, viṣaghna, medohara, sandaniya, vajīkaraṇa, kaphapittahara* (Srikanthamurthy 2001; Warrier et al 1996).

Constituents: ***Arjuna*** contains a number of triterpenoid saponins (e.g. arjunetoside, arjunolitin, arjunoside I-IV, terminic acid, arjunic acid, arjunolic acid, arjungenin), flavonoids (arjunone, arjuno-lone, luteolin), cardenolide, gallic acid, ellagic acid, oligomeric proanthocyanidins, phytosterols, tannin, calcium, magnesium, zinc and copper (Upadhyay et al 2001, Yadav & Rathore 2001, Yoganarasimhan 2000).

Medical research:

- ***In vitro***: anti-HSV–2 (Cheng et al 2002), antitumour (Pettit et al 1996)
- ***In vivo***: cardioprotective (Sumitra et al 2001); antioxidant (Gauthaman et al 2001); hypolipidaemic, anti-atherogenic (Shaila et al 1998)
- ***Human trials***: ***Arjuna*** bark given in doses of 500 mg every 8 hours was associated with a significant decrease in the frequency of angina commensurate with significant improvements in exercise test parameters in male patients with chronic stable angina, without side-effects, compared to placebo and isosorbide mononitrate (Bharani et al 2002); ***Arjuna*** bark given in doses of 500 mg daily was found to promote significant reductions in total serum cholesterol, HDL, LDL, triglycerides and lipid peroxide levels in patients with coronary heart disease, compared to placebo and vitamin E (Gupta et al 2001); ***Arjuna*** given in doses of 500 mg every 8 hours promoted significant improvements in left ventricular ejection fraction and a reduction in the left ventricular mass in patients with postmyocardial infarction angina and ischaemic cardiomyopathy, compared to controls (Dwivedi & Jauhari 1997); ***Arjuna*** bark given in doses of 500 mg every 8 hours was associated with significant improvements in signs and symptoms of heart failure in patients with refractory chronic congestive heart failure, previous myocardial infarction and peripartum cardiomyopathy (Bharani et al 1995).

Toxicity: No data found.

Indications: Dysentery, cirrhosis, bronchitis, asthma, tuberculosis, haemorrhage, leucorrhoea, menorrhagia, coronary heart disease, cardiovascular disease, diabetes, cancer, broken bones.

Contraindications: Pregnancy, constipation, dryness, ***vātakopa***.

Medicinal uses: The tree ***Arjuna*** is perhaps best known and best studied as a remedy for the heart and cardiovascular system, first introduced into the materia medica as cardiotonic by Vāgbhaṭa (c. 6–7th century CE). For this purpose the bark is traditionally prepared as a milk decoction (***kvātha***), a process that appears to render the triterpenes more bioavailable (Tillotson 2001). The ***Aṣṭāñga Hṛdaya*** mentions ***Arjuna*** in the treatment of wounds, haemorrhages and ulcers, applied topically as a powder (Srikanthamurthy 1994). According to the ***Cakradatta***, a ***cūrṇa*** of ***Arjuna*** consumed with ***ghṛta***, milk or jaggery overcomes heart disease, chronic fever and haemorrhaging, and promotes long life (Sharma 2002). Similarly, the ***Cakradatta*** mentions a ***ghṛta*** prepared with ***Arjuna***, ***Balā***, ***Nāgabalā*** and ***Yaṣṭimadhu*** as a treatment in heart disease, chest wounds, cough, pain and arthritis (Sharma 2002). In the treatment of haemoptysis, Caraka recommends equal parts ***Arjuna*** with ***Raktacandana***, along with sugar and rice water (Nadkarni 1954). Suśruta mentions the usefulness of ***Arjuna*** as a ***vajīkaraṇa***, combined with ***Candana*** in spermatorrhoea (Nadkarni 1954). Soaked in the fresh juice of ***Vāsaka***, the ***Bhāvaprakāśa*** states that ***Arjuna*** is used in the treatment of consumption and haemoptysis (Srikanthamurthy 2000). More recently, ***Arjuna*** has gained some recognition as a major ingredient in the patented LIV–52 formula used in the treatment of liver disorders.

Dosage:

- ***Cūrṇa***: 3–5 g b.i.d.–t.i.d.
- ***Kvātha***: 1:4, 30–90 mL b.i.d.–t.i.d.
- ***Tincture***: 1:3, 50% alcohol, 3–5 mL b.i.d.–t.i.d.

REFERENCES

Bharani A, Ganguly A, Bhargava KD 1995 Salutary effect of Terminalia arjuna in patients with severe refractory heart failure. International Journal of Cardiology 49(3):191–199

Bharani A, Ganguli A, Mathur LK et al 2002 Efficacy of Terminalia arjuna in chronic stable angina: a double-blind, placebo-controlled, crossover study comparing Terminalia arjuna with isosorbide mononitrate. Indian Heart Journal 54(2): 170–175

Cheng HY, Lin CC, Lin TC 2002 Antiherpes simplex virus type 2 activity of casuarinin from the bark of Terminalia arjuna Linn. Antiviral Research 55(3):447–455

Dwivedi S, Jauhari R 1997 Beneficial effects of Terminalia arjuna in coronary artery disease. Indian Heart Journal 49(5):507–510

Gauthaman K, Maulik M, Kumari R et al 2001 Effect of chronic treatment with bark of Terminalia arjuna: a study on the isolated ischemic-reperfused rat heart. Journal of Ethnopharmacology 75(2–3):197–201

Gupta R, Singhal S, Goyle A, Sharma VN 2001 Anti-oxidant and hypocholesterolaemic effects of Terminalia arjuna tree-bark powder: a randomised placebo-controlled trial. Journal of the Association of Physicians of India 49:231–235

Kirtikar KR, Basu BD 1935 Indian medicinal plants, 2nd edn, vol 1–4. Periodical Experts, Delhi, p 1024

Nadkarni KM 1954 The Indian materia medica, with Ayurvedic, Unani and home remedies, revised and enlarged by A.K. Nadkarni. Popular Prakashan PVP, Bombay, p 1201

Pettit GR, Hoard MS, Doubek DL et al 1996 Antineoplastic agents 338. The cancer cell growth inhibitory constituents of *Terminalia arjuna* (Combretaceae). Journal of Ethnopharmacology 53(2):57–63

Shaila HP, Udupa SL, Udupa AL 1998 Hypolipidemic activity of three indigenous drugs in experimentally induced atherosclerosis. International Journal of Cardiology 67(2):119–124

Sharma PV 2002 Cakradatta. Sanskrit text with English translation. Chaukhamba, Varanasi, p 145, 303

Srikanthamurthy KR 1994 Vāgbhaṭa's Aṣṭāñga Hṛdayam, vol 1. Krishnadas Academy, Varanasi, p 206

Srikanthamurthy KR 2000 Bhāvaprakāśa of Bhāvamiśra, vol 2. Krishnadas Academy, Varanasi, p 246

Srikanthamurthy KR 2001 Bhāvaprakāśa of Bhāvamiśra, vol 1. Krishnadas Academy, Varanasi, p 297–298

Sumitra M, Manikandan P, Kumar DA et al 2001 Experimental myocardial necrosis in rats: role of arjunolic acid on platelet aggregation, coagulation and anti-oxidant status. Molecular and Cellular Biochemistry 224(1–2):135–142

Tillotson A 2001 The One Earth herbal sourcebook. Twin Streams (Kensington), New York, p 99

Upadhyay RK, Pandey MB, Jha RN et al 2001 Triterpene glycoside from Terminalia arjuna. Journal of Asian Natural Products Research 3(3):207–212

Warrier PK, Nambiar VPK, Ramankutty C eds 1996 Indian medicinal plants: a compendium of 500 species, vol 5. Orient Longman, Hyderabad, p 252–253

Yadav RN, Rathore K 2001 A new cardenolide from the roots of Terminalia arjuna. Fitoterapia 72(4):459–461

Yoganarasimhan SN 2000 Medicinal plants of India, vol 2: Tamil Nadu. Self-published, Bangalore, p 551

Aśvagandhā, 'smelling like a horse'

BOTANICAL NAME: *Withania somnifera*, Solanaceae

OTHER NAMES: Ashgandh (H); Amukkira (T); Winter Cherry (E)

Botany: ***Aśvagandhā*** is an erect branching shrub that attains a height of between 30 and 150 cm, covered in a woolly pubescence. The ovate leaves are up to 10 cm long and 2.5–5 cm wide, margins entire, arranged in an alternate fashion. The flowers are green or yellow, borne in axillary fascicles, giving rise to red globose fruits when mature. The roots are fleshy and cylindrical, the epidermis light brown and medulla white. ***Aśvagandhā*** is found throughout the drier parts of India, into West Asia and northern Africa (Kirtikar & Basu 1935, Warrier et al 1996).

Part used: Root.

Dravyguṇa:

- ***Rasa***: *tikta, kaśāya*
- ***Vipāka***: *kaṭu*
- ***Vīrya***: *uṣṇa*
- ***Karma***: *medhya, nidrājanana, stanyajanana, vedanāsthāpana, balya, vajīkaraṇa, rasāyana, vātakaphahara* (Dash 1991, Srikanthamurthy 2001, Warrier et al 1996)

Constituents: ***Aśvagandhā*** contains steroidal compounds of great interest to researchers, including ergostane type steroidal lactones, including withanolides A-Y, dehydrowithanolide-R, withasomniferin-A, withasomidienone, withasomniferols A-C, withaferin A, withanone and others. Other constituents include the phytosterols sitoindosides VII-X and β-sitosterol, as well as alkaloids (e.g. ashwagandhine, cuscohygrine, tropine, pseudotropine, isopelletierine, anaferine), a variety of amino acids, including tryptophan, and high amounts of iron (Mills & Bone 2000, Williamson 2002, Yoganarasimhan 2000).

Medical research:

- ***In vitro***: antifungal (Choudhary et al 1995), antibacterial (Arora et al 2004), anti-angiogenic (Mohan et al 2004), cholinergic (Schliebs et al 1997), GABA-nergic (Mehta et al 1991)
- ***In vivo***: adaptogenic (Bhattacharya & Muruganandam 2003), anti-oxidant (Archana & Namasivayam 1999), anti-inflammatory (al Hindawi et al 1989), neuroprotective (Parihar & Hemnani 2003), neuroregenerative (Kuboyama et al 2005), immunostimulant (Davis & Kuttan 1999, Dhuley 1998b, Ziauddin et al 1996), anti-oxidant (Bhattacharya et al 1997, Dhuley 1998a), hypoglycaemic (Hemalatha et al 2004), anti-ischaemic (Chaudhary et al 2003), cardioprotective (Gupta et al 2004, Mohanty et al 2004), anti-angiogenic (Mohan et al 2004), chemoprotective (Davis & Kuttan 1998, Diwanay et al 2004, Jena et al 2003, Kuttan 1996), myeloprotective (Davis & Kuttan 1999), radioprotective (Mathur et al 2004), antitumour (Christina et al 2004, Devi 1996, Devi et al 1995, Kaur et al 2004, Leyon & Kuttan 2004, Menon et al 1997, Sharad et al 1996), antiwithdrawal (Kulkarni & Ninan 1997)
- ***Human trials***: ***Aśvagandhā*** demonstrated hypoglycaemic and hypolipidaemic effects in non-insulin-dependent diabetic and hypercholesterolaemic patients (Andallu & Radhika 2000); a herbal formulation containing *Withania somnifera* root, *Boswellia serrata* stem, *Curcuma longa* rhizome and zinc (Articulin-F) was found to promote a significant drop in severity of pain and disability in osteoarthritic patients, with minimal side-effects (Kulkarni et al 1991); a proprietary formulation (Immu–25) containing ***Aśvagandhā*** was found to promote a significant decrease in viral loads and an increase in $CD4^+$ counts in patients with HIV (Usha et al 2003).

Toxicity: ***Aśvagandhā*** appears to be very safe, with an LD_{50} of a 50% alcohol extract determined to be 1000 mg/kg in rats (Aphale et al 1998, Williamson 2002).

Indications: Anorexia, bronchitis, asthma, consumption, leucoderma, oedema, asthenia, anaemia, exhaustion, ageing, insomnia, ADD/ADHD, infertility, impotence, repeated miscarriage, paralysis, memory loss, multiple sclerosis, immune dysfunction, immunodeficiency, cancer, rheumatism, arthritis, lumbago.

Contraindications: Caution should be used with patients on anticonvulsants, barbiturates and benzodiazepines due to its GABA-nergic and sedative properties. ***Aśvagandhā*** is traditionally avoided in lymphatic congestion, during colds and flu, or symptoms of ***āma*** (Frawley & Lad 1986).

Medicinal uses: ***Aśvagandhā*** is often considered the Indian equivalent to Ginseng (*Panax ginseng*), but unlike Ginseng, ***Aśvagandhā*** has a 'sedative' (***nidrājanana***) rather than stimulant action on the central nervous system, making it a superior medicine for exhaustion with nervous irritability. ***Aśvagandhā*** is a useful nervine, taken before bed to relax and nourish the body in deficiency diseases, but is only seen to be efficacious when taken on a sustained basis – it is not a sufficient sedative to treat acute insomnia. For poor memory, lack of concentration and in the treatment of ADD/ADHD ***Aśvagandhā*** may be used in equal proportions with ***Brāhmī*** and Ling zhi (*Ganoderma lucidum*). ***Aśvagandhā*** is widely used in any debility, emaciation or consumptive condition, in both adults and children (Kirtikar & Basu 1935, Nadkarni 1954). One rejuvenating preparation can be made by mixing ***Aśvagandhā*** with 10–15% ***Pippalī***, taken with one half part ***ghṛta*** and one part honey on an empty stomach, morning and evening. As its name 'smelling like a horse' suggests, ***Aśvagandhā*** is an important ***vajīkaraṇa dravya***, indicating the sexual potency of a stallion, used in the treatment of infertility, impotence and 'seminal depletion' (Nadkarni 1954). When mixed with equal parts ***Śatāvarī***, it is an appropriate treatment for female infertility and frigidity, useful in threatened miscarriage, and is an excellent post-partum restorative. In the treatment of uterine prolapse a paste prepared from equal parts ***Aśvagandhā***, ***Vacā***, ***Kuṣṭha***, ***Haridrā***, ***Marica*** and ***Nīlotpala*** is recommended by the ***Cakradatta*** to restore uterine tone (Sharma 2002). In the treatment of infertility in both sexes a simple decoction of ***Aśvagandhā*** in milk is indicated, taken with ***ghṛta*** as an ***anupāna*** (Sharma 2002). Similarly, a medicated ***taila*** called ***Aśvagandhādi taila*** is prepared by decocting ***Aśvagandhā***, ***Śatāvarī***, ***Kuṣṭha***, ***Jaṭāmāmsī*** and ***Bṛhatī*** in sesame oil, massaged into the breasts and genitalia to make them stronger and larger (Sharma 2002). Mixed with equal parts ***Vṛddhadāruka***, ***Aśvagandhā cūrṇa*** is allowed to sit in a pot with ***ghṛta*** for a few days, and is then administered in doses of 12 g taken with milk as a ***vajīkaraṇa rasāyana*** (Srikanthamurthy 1984). In the treatment of consumptive conditions the ***Cakradatta*** recommends a decoction of equal parts ***Aśvagandhā***, ***Guḍūcī***, ***Śatāvarī***, ***Daśamūla***, ***Balā***, ***Vāsaka***, ***Puṣkaramūla*** root and ***Ativiṣā***, taken in conjunction with a diet of milk and meat broth (Sharma 2002). A more recently developed formula by the Hospital of Integrated Medicine in Madras is ***Aśvagandhādi lehya***, used in dosages of 6–12 g in milk to strengthen the body, and promote fertility and long life (India 1978). For poor eyesight ***Aśvagandhā*** powder is mixed with equal proportions of ***Yaṣṭimadhu*** powder and the fresh juice of ***Āmalakī*** (Nadkarni 1954). Nadkarni (1954) mentions that ***Aśvagandhā*** is used in the treatment of anti-inflammatory joint disease, but it may facilitate the production of ***āma*** (Frawley & Lad 1986), and thus an eliminative regimen is best implemented prior to using this herb. Likewise, ***Aśvagandhā*** is an appropriate remedy in the treatment of asthma and bronchitis (Kirtikar & Basu 1935), but should be used concurrently with ***dravyas*** that have a ***dīpanapācana*** property to avoid the production of ***āma***. Warrier et al (1996) mention that a paste made of the roots and bruised leaves may be applied to carbuncles, ulcers and painful swellings. Based on its traditional use and the experimental data ***Aśvagandhā*** appears to be an excellent choice to support the health of patients undergoing conventional cancer treatment or suffering from immunodeficiency, to protect against injury and infection, improve immune status, and enhance recovery. Combined with ***Yaṣṭimadhu*** and used in sufficient doses ***Aśvagandhā*** may be used to wean a patient off corticosteroid therapy, or may be used in place of it.

Dosage:

- ***Cūrṇa***: 3–15 g b.i.d.–t.i.d.
- ***Kvātha***: 1:4, 60–120 mL b.i.d.–t.i.d.
- ***Tincture***: fresh root, 1:2, 95% alcohol; dried root, 1:3; 35% alcohol; 1–15 mL b.i.d. t.i.d.

REFERENCES

Al-Hindawi MK, Al-Deen IH, Nabi MH, Ismail MH 1989 Anti-inflammatory activity of some Iraqi plants using intact rats. Journal of Ethnopharmacology 26(2):163–168

Andallu B, Radhika B 2000 Hypoglycemic, diuretic and hypocholesterolemic effect of winter cherry (Withania somnifera, Dunal) root. Indian Journal of Experimental Biology 38(6):607–609

Aphale AA, Chhibba AD, Kumbhakarna NR et al 1998 Subacute toxicity study of the combination of ginseng (Panax ginseng) and ashwagandha (Withania somnifera) in rats: a safety assessment. Indian Journal of Physiology and Pharmacology 42(2):299–302

Archana R, Namasivayam A 1999 Antistressor effect of Withania somnifera. Journal of Ethnopharmacology 64(1):91–93

Arora S, Dhillon S, Rani G, Nagpal A 2004 The in vitro antibacterial/synergistic activities of Withania somnifera extracts. Fitoterapia 75(3–4):385–388

Bhattacharya SK, Muruganandam AV 2003 Adaptogenic activity of Withania somnifera: an experimental study using a rat model of chronic stress. Pharmacology, Biochemistry, and Behavior 75(3):547–555

Bhattacharya SK, Satyan KS, Ghosal S 1997 Anti-oxidant activity of glycowithanolides from Withania somnifera. Indian Journal of Experimental Biology 35(3):236–239

Chaudhary G, Sharma U, Jagannathan NR, Gupta YK 2003 Evaluation of Withania somnifera in a middle cerebral artery occlusion model of stroke in rats. Clinical and Experimental Pharmacology and Physiology 30(5–6):399–404

Choudhary MI, Dur-e-Shahwar Z, Parveen A et al 1995 Antifungal steroidal lactones from Withania coagulance. Phytochemistry 40(4):1243–1246

Christina AJ, Joseph DG, Packialakshmi M et al 2004 Anticarcinogenic activity of Withania somnifera Dunal against Dalton's ascitic lymphoma. Journal of Ethnopharmacology 93(2–3):359–361

Dash B 1991 Materia medica of Ayurveda. B. Jain Publishers, New Delhi, p 59

Dash B, Junius M 1983 A handbook of Ayurveda. Concept Publishing, New Delhi

Davis L, Kuttan G 1998 Suppressive effect of cyclophosphamide-induced toxicity by Withania somnifera extract in mice. Journal of Ethnopharmacology 62(3):209–214

Davis L, Kuttan G 1999 Effect of Withania somnifera on cytokine production in normal and cyclophosphamide treated mice. Immunopharmacology and Immunotoxicology 21(4):695–703

Devi PU 1996 Withania somnifera Dunal (Ashwagandha): potential plant source of a promising drug for cancer chemotherapy and radiosensitization. Indian Journal of Experimental Biology 34(10):927–932

Devi PU, Sharada AC, Solomon FE 1995 In vivo growth inhibitory and radiosensitizing effects of withaferin A on mouse Ehrlich ascites carcinoma. Cancer Letters 95(1–2):189–193

Dhuley JN 1998a Effect of Ashwagandha on lipid peroxidation in stress-induced animals. Journal of Ethnopharmacology 60(2):173–178

Dhuley JN 1998b Therapeutic efficacy of Ashwagandha against experimental aspergillosis in mice. Immunopharmacology and Immunotoxicology 20(1):191–198

Diwanay S, Chitre D, Patwardhan B 2004 Immunoprotection by botanical drugs in cancer chemotherapy. Journal of Ethnopharmacology 90(1):49–55

Frawley D, Lad V 1986 The yoga of herbs: an Ayurvedic guide to herbal medicine. Lotus Press, Santa Fe, p 160

Gupta SK, Mohanty I, Talwar KK et al 2004 Cardioprotection from ischemia and reperfusion injury by Withania somnifera: a hemodynamic, biochemical and histopathological assessment. Molecular and Cellular Biochemistry 260(1–2):39–47

Hemalatha S, Wahi AK, Singh PN, Chansouria J 2004 Hypoglycemic activity of Withania coagulans Dunal in streptozotocin induced diabetic rats. Journal of Ethnopharmacology 93(2–3):261–264

India, Department of Health 1978 The Ayurvedic formulary of India, Part 1. Controller of Publications, Delhi, p 27

Jena GB, Nemmani KV, Kaul CL, Ramarao P 2003 Protective effect of a polyherbal formulation (Immu–21) against cyclophosphamide-induced mutagenicity in mice. Phytotherapy Research 17(4):306–310

Kaur K, Rani G, Widodo N et al 2004 Evaluation of the antiproliferative and anti-oxidative activities of leaf extract from in vivo and in vitro raised Ashwagandha. Food and Chemical Toxicology 42(12):2015–2020

Kirtikar KR, Basu BD 1935 Indian medicinal plants, 2nd edn, vols 1–4. Periodical Experts, Delhi, p 1774, 1775, 1776

Kuboyama T, Tohda C, Komatsu K 2005 Neuritic regeneration and synaptic reconstruction induced by withanolide A. British Journal of Pharmacology 144(7):961–971

Kulkarni SK, Ninan I 1997 Inhibition of morphine tolerance and dependence by Withania somnifera in mice. Journal of Ethnopharmacology 57(3):213–217

Kuttan G 1996 Use of Withania somnifera Dunal as an adjuvant during radiation therapy. Indian Journal of Experimental Biology 34(9):854–856

Leyon PV, Kuttan G 2004 Effect of Withania somnifera on B16F–10 melanoma induced metastasis in mice. Phytotherapy Research: 18(2):118–122

Mathur S, Kaur P, Sharma M et al 2004 The treatment of skin carcinoma, induced by UV B radiation, using 1-oxo–5beta, 6beta-epoxy-witha–2-enolide, isolated from the roots of Withania somnifera, in a rat model. Phytomedicine 11(5):452–460

Mehta AK, Binkley P, Gandhi SS, Ticku MK 1991 Pharmacological effects of Withania somnifera root extract on GABA (A) receptor complex. Indian Journal of Medical Research 94:312–315

Menon LG, Kuttan R, Kuttan G 1997 Effect of rasayanas in the inhibition of lung metastasis induced by B16F–10 melanoma cells. Journal of Experimental and Clinical Cancer Research 16(4):365–368

Mills S, Bone K 2000 Principles and practice of phytotherapy. Churchill Livingstone, London, p 596

Mohan R, Hammers HJ, Bargagna-Mohan P et al 2004 Withaferin A is a potent inhibitor of angiogenesis. Angiogenesis 7(2):115–122

Mohanty I, Arya DS, Dinda A et al 2004 Mechanisms of cardioprotective effect of Withania somnifera in experimentally induced myocardial infarction. Basic and Clinical Pharmacology and Toxicology 94(4):184–190

Nadkarni KM 1954 The Indian materia medica, with Ayurvedic, Unani and home remedies, revised and enlarged by

A.K. Nadkarni. Popular Prakashan PVP, Bombay, p 1293, 1294
Parihar MS, Hemnani T 2003 Phenolic anti-oxidants attenuate hippocampal neuronal cell damage against kainic acid induced excitotoxicity. Journal of Biosciences 28(1):121–128
Schliebs R, Liebmann A, Bhattacharya SK et al 1997 Systemic administration of defined extracts from Withania somnifera (Indian Ginseng) and Shilajatu differentially affects cholinergic but not glutamatergic and GABAergic markers in rat brain. Neurochemistry International 30(2):181–190
Sharad AC, Solomon FE, Devi PU et al 1996 Antitumor and radiosensitizing effects of withaferin A on mouse Ehrlich ascites carcinoma in vivo. Acta Oncologica (Stockholm) 35(1):95–100
Sharma PV 2002 Cakradatta. Sanskrit text with English translation. Chaukhamba, Varanasi, p 134, 579, 580, 654
Srikanthamurthy KR 1984 Śāraṅgadhara saṃhitā: a treatise on Ayurveda. Chaukhamba Orientalia, Varanasi, p 100
Srikanthamurthy KR 2001 Bhāvaprakāśa of Bhāvamiśra, vol 1. Krishnadas Academy, Varanasi, p 258
Usha PR, Naidu MU, Raju YS 2003 Evaluation of the antiretroviral activity of a new polyherbal drug (Immu–25) in patients with HIV infection. Drugs in R and D 4(2):103–109
Warrier PK, Nambiar VPK, Ramankutty C (eds) 1996 Indian medicinal plants: a compendium of 500 species, vol 5. Orient Longman, Hyderabad, p 409
Williamson EM (ed) 2002 Major herbs of Ayurveda. Churchill Livingstone, London, p 322, 323
Yoganarasimhan SN 2000 Medicinal plants of India, vol 2: Tamil Nadu. Self-published, Bangalore, p 592
Ziauddin M, Phansalkar N, Patki P et al 1996 Studies on the immunomodulatory effects of Ashwagandha. Journal of Ethnopharmacology 50(2):69–76

Balā, 'strength'

BOTANICAL NAME: *Sida cordifolia,* Malvaceae

SIMILAR SPECIES: *S. acuta, S. rhombifolia, S. spinosa*

OTHER NAMES: Bariar, Barial, Jamglimedhi (H); Arivalmanaippundu, Kuruntotti (T); Country Mallow (E)

Botany: *Sida cordifolia* is a small highly branched shrub covered in a woolly pubescence. The leaves are 2.5–5 cm long, cordate, crenate, borne on long petioles up to 3.8 cm long. The yellow flowers are solitary or found in pairs in the leaf axils, the calyx 6–8 mm long, the corolla slightly extending beyond the calyx. The fruit is a schizocarp, 6–8 mm in diameter, containing 7–10 carpels. ***Balā*** is found in tropical and subtropical regions in both hemispheres, often as an invasive weed of tropical pastures (Kirtikar & Basu 1935).

Part used: Root and leaves.

Dravyguṇa: root

- ***Rasa***: *madhura*
- ***Vipāka***: *guru*
- ***Vīrya***: *śita*
- ***Karma***: *purīṣasangrahaṇiya, jvaraghna, kāsahara, raktaprasādana, hṛdaya, balya, medhya, vajīkaraṇa, jīvanīya, bṛmhaṇa, vātapittahara* (Dash 1991, Srikanthamurthy 2001, Warrier et al 1996).

Constituents: Researchers have isolated an acylsterylglycoside sitoindoside from ***Balā***, as well as small amounts of the alkaloid ephedrine, ecdysteroids (glyceryl–1-eicosanoate, 20-hydroxy,24-hydroxymethylecdysone), β-sitosterol and other phytosterols, palmatic, stearic and hexacosanoic acids, and resins. The seeds are stated to contain upwards of four times the amount of ephedrine as the rest of the plant (Darwish & Reinecke 2003, Kapoor 1990, Yoganarasimhan 2000).

Medical research:

- ***In vitro***: anti-oxidant (Auddy et al 2003), antimalarial (Banzouzi et al 2004, Karou et al 2003), antibacterial (Islam et al 2003)
- ***In vivo***: anti-inflammatory, analgesic, and hypoglycaemic (Kanth & Diwan 1999), chemoprotective (Jang et al 2003).

Toxicity: No data found.

Indications: Arrhythmia, congestive heart failure, paralysis, sciatica, neuritis, neuralgia, epilepsy, rheumatism, asthma, anorexia, fatigue, impotence, spermatorrhoea, gonorrhoea, cystitis, leucorrhoea, urinary frequency, diabetes, diarrhoea, dysentery, haemorrhoids, chronic fever.

Contraindications: ***kaphakopa***, ***āma*** (Frawley & Lad 1986). Use with caution in hypertension due to the presence of ephedrine.

Medicinal uses: Like many other species in the Malvaceae, ***Balā*** is used in Āyurveda for its soothing and mucilaginous qualities, but unlike the similar Marshmallow (*Althea officinalis*), ***Balā*** contains small amounts of ephedrine, making it a mild bronchodilator with vasoconstrictive properties (Duke 1999, Nadkarni 1954). Although remedies that promote sympathetic innervation typically aggravate ***vāta***, ***Balā*** is in fact a rejuvenative to ***vāta***, and whatever adrenergic activity the plant has is offset by its other qualities. ***Balā*** has an affinity for diseases of the nervous system and can be used in a wide variety of conditions where ***vāta*** is the main pathogenic factor (Frawley & Lad 1986). It provides a gentle stimulus while remaining a nourishing ***bṛmhaṇa dravya***. In cases of paralysis a milk decoction of ***Balā*** root is taken along with equal parts ***Aśvagandhā*** root and ***Kapikacchū***. This preparation can also be applied topically, the steam funneled off from the decoction is directed onto the affected area by a hose (***nāḍī sveda***). An excellent ***taila*** can be prepared from the root of ***Balā***, useful in ***abhyaṅga*** to treat paralysis and frozen shoulder, and is used externally for tinnitus.

A liniment made from equal parts of the ***Balā*** root and the formula ***Daśamūla*** can be used in the treatment of sciatica (Nadkarni 1954). The ***Cakradatta*** mentions ***Balā*** as a useful remedy for diseases of the heart, used with equal parts ***Nāgabalā*** and ***Arjuna***, and one quarter part ***Yaṣṭimadhu***, decocted and prepared as a ***ghṛta*** (Sharma 2002). In cases of asthma ***Balā*** can be very useful, but should be used with pungent tasting botanicals such as ***Pippalī*** or ***Elā*** to offset its strong ***kapha***-promoting qualities that may contribute to bronchial catarrh. In cases of urinary tenesmus ***Balā*** is most useful as a soothing diuretic, taken along with Kava (*Piper methysticum*) or ***Pārasikayavānī*** as an antispasmodic. The leaves of ***Balā*** are mucilaginous and cooling and may be used internally as a demulcent in chronic bronchitis, tracheitis, cystitis and bleeding haemorrhoids (Nadkarni 1954). In the treatment of Parkinsonism, ***Balā*** may be effective to manage symptoms when taken along with ***Kapikacchū*** (*Mucuna pruriens*), ***Aśvagandhā*** and ***Pārasikayavānī***. There are several similar species in the *Sida* genus, including *S. acuta, S. humilis, S. indicum, S. rhombifolia* and *S. spinosa*. Most of these are generally identified by the suffix '***balā***', such as ***Atibalā***, ***Mahābalā***, ***Nāgabalā***, etc., but unfortunately there is no general agreement as to which is which. Kirtikar & Basu (1935) describe *S. spinosa* as ***Nāgabalā*** and *S. rhombifolia* as ***Atibalā***. According to Srikanthamurthy (2001) ***Balā*** is *S. cordifolia*, ***Mahābalā*** is *S. rhombifolia*, ***Atibalā*** is a related member of the Malvaceae called *Abutilon indicum*, and ***Nāgabalā*** is *Grewia hirsuta* (Tiliaceae). The ***Bhāvaprakāśa*** mentions ***Mahābalā*** specifically in dysuria, and as a laxative, whereas ***Atibalā*** taken with milk is stated as a treatment for diabetes (Srikanthamurthy 2001). The ***Madanaphala nighaṇṭu*** mentions ***Nāgabalā*** as a treatment for ***rakta pitta***, a condition characterised by bleeding from different parts of the body (Dash 1991).

Dosage:

- ***Cūrṇa***: 1–5 g b.i.d.–t.i.d.
- ***Kvātha***: 1:4, 30–90 mL b.i.d.–t.i.d.
- ***Tincture***: 1:3, 35% alcohol, 3–5 mL b.i.d.–t.i.d.

REFERENCES

Auddy B, Ferreira M, Blasina F et al 2003 Screening of anti-oxidant activity of three Indian medicinal plants, traditionally used for the management of neurodegenerative diseases. Journal of Ethnopharmacology 84(2–3):131–138

Banzouzi JT, Prado R, Menan H et al 2004 Studies on medicinal plants of Ivory Coast: investigation of Sida acuta for in vitro antiplasmodial activities and identification of an active constituent. Phytomedicine 11(4):338–341

Darwish FM, Reinecke MG 2003 Ecdysteroids and other constituents from Sida spinosa L. Phytochemistry 62(8):1179–1184

Dash B 1991 Materia medica of Ayurveda. B. Jain Publishers, New Delhi, p 64

Duke J accessed 1999 Chemicals and their biological activities. In: *Sida rhombifolia* L. (Malvaceae) broomweed, teaplant. Agricultural Research Service (ARS), United States Department of Agriculture. Online. Available: http://www.ars-grin.gov/duke/

Frawley D, Lad V 1986 The yoga of herbs: an Ayurvedic guide to herbal medicine. Lotus Press, Santa Fe, p 162

Islam ME, Haque ME, Mosaddik MA 2003 Cytotoxicity and antibacterial activity of Sida rhombifolia (Malvaceae) grown in Bangladesh. Phytotherapy Research 17(8):973–975

Jang DS, Park EJ, Kang YH et al 2003 Compounds obtained from Sida acuta with the potential to induce quinone reductase and to inhibit 7, 12-dimethylbenz[a]anthracene-induced preneoplastic lesions in a mouse mammary organ culture model. Archives of Pharmaceutical Research 26(8):585–590

Kanth VR, Diwan PV 1999 Analgesic, anti-inflammatory and hypoglycaemic activities of Sida cordifolia. Phytotherapy Research 13(1):75–77

Kapoor LD 1990 CRC Handbook of Ayurvedic medical plants. CRC Press, Boca Raton, p 303

Karou D, Dicko MH, Sanon S et al 2003 Antimalarial activity of Sida acuta Burm. f. (Malvaceae) and Pterocarpus erinaceus Poir. (Fabaceae). Journal of Ethnopharmacology 89(2–3):291–294

Kirtikar KR, Basu BD 1935 Indian medicinal plants, 2nd edn, vols 1–4. Periodical Experts, Delhi, p 305–313

Nadkarni KM 1954 The Indian materia medica, with Ayurvedic, Unani and home remedies, revised and enlarged by A.K. Nadkarni. Popular Prakashan PVP, Bombay, p 1135, 1137

Sharma PV 2002 Cakradatta. Sanskrit text with English translation. Chaukhamba, Varanasi, p 306

Srikanthamurthy KR 2001 Bhāvaprakāśa of Bhāvamiśra, vol 1. Krishnadas Academy, Varanasi, p 250

Warrier PK, Nambiar VPK, Ramankutty C (eds) 1996 Indian medicinal plants: a compendium of 500 species, vol 5. Orient Longman, Hyderabad, p 129

Yoganarasimhan SN 2000 Medicinal plants of India, vol 2: Tamil Nadu. Self-published, Bangalore, p 497

Bhallātaka, 'piercing like a spear'

BOTANICAL NAME: *Semecarpus anacardium,* Anacardiaceae

OTHER NAMES: Bhela, Bhilawa (H); Senkottai, Erimugi (T); Marking Nut, Cashew (E)

Botany: ***Bhallātaka*** is a moderate sized semi-deciduous tree, with grey bark that exfoliates in small irregular flakes. The leaves are simple, alternate, obovate-oblong, rounded at the apex, glabrous above and pubescent below. The greenish fruits are ovoid to oblong drupes that are attached to a swollen, fleshy receptacle that sits below it and turns yellow when ripe. Although some sources indicate that ***Bhallātaka*** was brought to India from South America by the Portuguese, it is clearly mentioned and described in both the ***Suśruta*** and ***Caraka saṃhitās***, texts which antedate the Portuguese by more than a millennium. *S. anacardium* is now cultivated all over the world as a food, in moist tropical forests, and in the subcontinent ranging from the sub-Himalayas and Assam in the north, to the coast of Kerala in the south (Kirtikar & Basu 1935, Warrier et al 1996).

Part used: Pericarp of the nut, a by-product of the cashew industry.

Dravyguṇa:

- ***Rasa***: *kaśāya, madhura*
- ***Vipāka***: *madhura*
- ***Vīrya***: *uṣṇa, laghu, snigdha, tikṣṇa*
- ***Karma***: *dīpanapācana, bhedana, jvaraghna, kṛmighna, kāsahara, svāsahara, kuṣṭhaghna, medhya, vajīkaraṇa, vātakaphahara*
- ***Prabhāva***: The *Aṣṭāṅga Hṛdaya* (7th century CE) considers *Bhallātaka* fruit to be '. . . like fire in property' (Dash 1991, Nadkarni 1954, Srikanthamurthy 1994, 2001; Warrier et al 1996).

Constituents: ***Bhallātaka*** has been shown to contain the phenolic glucoside anacardoside and derivatives of anacardic acid that include a sub-class of compounds called the bhilawanols. Flavonoid constituents include semecarpuflavanone, semecarpetin, jeediflavone, galluflavanone and nallaflavanone. ***Bhallātaka*** also contains an assortment of minerals, vitamins, amino acids and a fixed oil (Gil et al 1995, Premalatha 2000, Yoganarasimhan 2000).

Medical research:

- ***In vitro***: antifungal (Sharma et al 2002), anti-inflammatory (Selvam & Jachak 2004, Tripathi & Pandey 2004), antitumour (Chakraborty et al 2004), anti-oxidant (Tripathi et al 2004b).
- ***In vivo***: anti-oxidant (Ramprasath et al 2005, Shukla et al 2000, Tripathi & Singh 2001, Tripathi et al 2004, Vijayalakshmi et al 1997b), anti-arthritic (Ramprasath et al 2005, Vijayalakshmi et al 1997a,b), anti-inflammatory (Ramprasath et al 2004, Saraf et al 1989, Selvam & Jachak 2004, Selvam et al 2004), antitumour (Arathi et al 2003, Indap et al 1983, Premalatha & Sachdanandam 1999, 2000 a–c, Sujatha & Sachdanandam 2002), anti-atherosclerotic (Sharma et al 1995), hypoglycaemic (Arul et al 2004), hypolipidaemic (Tripathi & Pandey 2004).

Toxicity: A toxicological study carried out in rats administered a Siddha milk extract of *Semecarpus anacardium* nuts showed that acute (72 hours) and sub-acute (30 days) treatment did not produce mortality at any dose level given (75–2000 mg/kg body weight), nor any marked adverse alterations in haematological and biochemical parameters (Vijayalakshmi et al 2000). The sap of the tree has been shown to be quite toxic, with one reported case in the literature of severe dermatitis, anuria and renal cortical necrosis from skin exposure (Matthai & Date 1979). Preparations of crude ***Bhallātaka*** are toxic and should be avoided.

Indications: Dyspepsia, constipation, parasites, haemorrhoids, cough, asthma, leprosy, syphilis, vitiligo, rheumatoid arthritis, sciatica, neuritis, diabetes, dysmenorrhoea, amenorrhoea, infertility, weakness, fatigue, cancer, hepatocarcinoma (aflatoxin-induced).

Contraindications: Pregnancy, lactation, ***pittakopa***.

Medicinal uses: ***Bhallātaka*** has long been considered an important remedy in the treatment of a variety of complaints including rheumatism, arthritis, neuritis, liver disorders and haemorrhoids, considered '. . . equal to mercury in action' (Nadkarni 1954). It is also considered an important remedy in the treatment of asthma, and in skin diseases such as psoriasis, and was even highly valued in syphilis. It is one of the more important remedies, along with ***Yogarājaguggulu***, in the treatment of ***āmavāta*** (rheumatoid arthritis). The pericarp contains a variety of toxic principles that can precipitate a skin rash and renal failure if the dose is too large or if the remedy is prepared incorrectly. Prepared properly, however, ***Bhallātaka*** has been shown to be remarkably non-toxic and very safe (Vijayalakshmi et al 2000). Among the many preparations that contain ***Bhallātaka*** is a ***rasāyana*** mentioned by the ***Cakradatta*** (12th century CE) called ***Amṛtabhallātaka***. To prepare this remedy 2.56 kg of ripe ***Bhallātaka*** fruit is boiled in four times the volume of water (10 litres), and reduced to 2.56 litres. The fruits are then removed, and four times the volume of milk is added (10 litres), along with one quarter part ***ghṛta*** (640 g), and is slowly reduced over a low heat until all the milk has evaporated and only the original volume of ***ghṛta*** is obtained (i.e. 640 g). An equal weight of ***guḍa*** is then added (640 g) to the preparation, mixed well, and then set aside for a week. The ***Cakradatta*** states that the dose is according to the '. . . digestive power', mentioning that this preparation is the 'king of all ***rasāyanas***', and may be used on an ongoing basis to promote strength and longevity (Sharma 2002). The English name 'marking nut' refers to its usage by ***dhobis*** (washermen) to mark laundary items, special marks that allow them to keep track of a dizzying number of items and who they belong to.

Dosage:

- ***Amṛtabhallātaka***: 2–5 g, b.i.d.–t.i.d., taken with four times the volume of milk, as an ***anupāna***.

REFERENCES

Arathi G, Sachdanandam P 2003 Therapeutic effect of Semecarpus anacardium Linn. nut milk extract on carbohydrate metabolizing and mitochondrial TCA cycle and respiratory chain enzymes in mammary carcinoma rats. Journal of Pharmacy and Pharmacology 55(9):1283–1290

Arul B, Kothai R, Christina AJ 2004 Hypoglycemic and antihyperglycemic effect of Semecarpus anacardium Linn. in normal and streptozotocin-induced diabetic rats. Methods and Findings in Experimental and Clinical Pharmacology 26(10):759–762

Chakraborty S, Roy M, Taraphdar AK, Bhattacharya RK 2004 Cytotoxic effect of root extract of Tiliacora racemosa and oil of Semecarpus anacardium nut in human tumor cells. Phytotherapy Research 8(8):595–600

Dash B 1991 Materia medica of Ayurveda. B. Jain Publishers, New Delhi, p 99

Gil RR, Lin LZ, Cordell GA 1995 Anacardoside from the seeds of Semecarpus anacardium. Phytochemistry 39(2):405–407

Indap MA, Ambaye RY, Gokhale SV 1983 Anti tumor and pharmacological effects of the oil from Semecarpus anacardium Linn. f. Indian Journal of Physiology and Pharmacology 27(2):83–91

Kirtikar KR, Basu BD 1935 Indian medicinal plants, 2nd edn, vols 1–4. Periodical Experts, Delhi, p 667

Matthai TP, Date A 1979 Renal cortical necrosis following exposure to sap of the marking-nut tree (Semecarpus anacardium). American Journal of Tropical Medicine and Hygiene 28(4):773–774

Nadkarni KM 1954 The Indian materia medica, with Ayurvedic, Unani and home remedies, revised and enlarged by A.K. Nadkarni. Popular Prakashan PVP, Bombay, p 1120

Premalatha B 2000 Semecarpus anacardium Linn. nuts–a boon in alternative medicine. Indian Journal of Experimental Biology 38(12):1177–1182

Premalatha B, Sachdanandam P 1999 Semecarpus anacardium L. nut extract administration induces the in vivo anti-oxidant defence system in aflatoxin B1 mediated hepatocellular carcinoma. Journal of Ethnopharmacology 66(2):131–139

Premalatha B, Sachdanandam P 2000a Stabilization of lysosomal membrane and cell membrane glycoprotein profile by Semecarpus anacardium linn. nut milk extract in experimental hepatocellular carcinoma. Phytotherapy Research 14(5):352–355

Premalatha B, Sachdanandam P 2000b Potency of Semecarpus anacardium Linn. nut milk extract against aflatoxin B(1)-induced hepatocarcinogenesis: reflection on microsomal biotransformation enzymes. Pharmacological Research 42(2):161–166

Premalatha B, Sachdanandam P 2000c Modulating role of Semecarpus anacardium L. nut milk extract on aflatoxin B(1) biotransformation. Pharmacological Research 41(1):19–24

Ramprasath VR, Shanthi P, Sachdanandam P 2004 Anti-inflammatory effect of Semecarpus anacardium Linn. Nut extract in acute and chronic inflammatory conditions. Biological and Pharmaceutical Bulletin 27(12):2028–2031.

Ramprasath VR, Shanthi P, Sachdanandam P 2005 Evaluation of anti-oxidant effect of Semecarpus anacardium Linn. nut extract on the components of immune system in adjuvant arthritis. Vascular Pharmacology 42(4):179–186

Saraf MN, Ghooi RB, Patwardhan BK 1989 Studies on the mechanism of action of Semecarpus anacardium in rheumatoid arthritis. Journal of Ethnopharmacology 25(2):159–164

Selvam C, Jachak SM 2004 A cyclooxygenase (COX) inhibitory biflavonoid from the seeds of Semecarpus anacardium. Journal of Ethnopharmacology 95(2–3):209–212

Selvam C, Jachak SM, Bhutani KK 2004 Cyclooxygenase inhibitory flavonoids from the stem bark of Semecarpus anacardium Linn. Phytotherapy Research 18(7):582–584

Sharma PV 2002 Cakradatta. Sanskrit text with English translation. Chaukhamba, Varanasi, p 648

Sharma A, Mathur R, Dixit VP 1995 Hypocholesterolemic activity of nut shell extract of Semecarpus anacardium (Bhilawa) in cholesterol fed rabbits. Indian Journal of Experimental Biology 33(6):444–448

Sharma K, Shukla SD, Mehta P, Bhatnagar M 2002 Fungistatic activity of Semecarpus anacardium Linn. f nut extract. Indian Journal of Experimental Biology 40(3):314–318

Shukla SD, Jain S, Sharma K, Bhatnagar M 2000 Stress induced neuron degeneration and protective effects of Semecarpus anacardium Linn. and Withania somnifera Dunn. in hippocampus of albino rats: an ultrastructural study. Indian Journal of Experimental Biology 38(10):1007–1013

Srikanthamurthy KR 1994 Vāgbhaṭa's Aṣṭāñga Hṛdayam, vol 1. Krishnadas Academy, Varanasi, p 100

Srikanthamurthy KR 2001 Bhāvaprakāśa of Bhāvamiśra, vol 1. Krishnadas Academy, Varanasi, p 196

Sujatha V, Sachdanandam P 2002 Recuperative effect of Semecarpus anacardium linn. nut milk extract on carbohydrate metabolizing enzymes in experimental mammary carcinoma-bearing rats. Phytotherapy Research 16 Suppl 1:S14–18

Tripathi YB, Singh AV 2001 Effect of Semecarpus anacardium nuts on lipid peroxidation. Indian Journal of Experimental Biology 39(8):798–801

Tripathi YB, Pandey RS 2004 Semecarpus anacardium L, nuts inhibit lipopolysaccharide induced NO production in rat macrophages along with its hypolipidemic property. Indian Journal of Experimental Biology 42(4):432–436

Tripathi YB, Reddy MM, Pandey RS et al 2004 Anti-inflammatory properties of BHUx, a polyherbal formulation to prevent atherosclerosis. Inflammopharmacology 12(2):131–152

Vijayalakshmi T, Muthulakshmi V, Sachdanandam P 1997a Effect of milk extract of Semecarpus anacardium nuts on glycohydrolases and lysosomal stability in adjuvant arthritis in rats. Journal of Ethnopharmacology 58(1):1–8

Vijayalakshmi T, Muthulakshmi V, Sachdanandam P 1997b Salubrious effect of Semecarpus anacardium against lipid peroxidative changes in adjuvant arthritis studied in rats. Molecular and Cellular Biochemistry 175(1–2):65–69

Vijayalakshmi T, Muthulakshmi V, Sachdanandam P 2000 Toxic studies on biochemical parameters carried out in rats with Serankottai nei, a siddha drug-milk extract of Semecarpus anacardium nut. Journal of Ethnopharmacology 69(1):9–15

Warrier PK, Nambiar VPK, Ramankutty C (eds) 1996 Indian medicinal plants: a compendium of 500 species, vol 5. Orient Longman, Hyderabad, p 98–102

Yoganarasimhan SN 2000 Medicinal plants of India, vol 2: Tamil Nadu. Self-published, Bangalore, p 493

Bhṛṅgarāja, 'ruler of the hair'

BOTANICAL NAME: *Eclipta alba, E. erecta, E. prostrata,* Asteraceae

OTHER NAMES: ***Keśarāja*** (S); Bungrah (H); Kaikeshi (T); Eclipta (E); Han lian cao (C)

Botany: ***Bhṛṅgarāja*** is an erect or prostrate annual branching herb, often rooting at the nodes, the stem and branches covered with short white strigose trichomes. The leaves are sessile, 2.5 to 7.5 cm long, oblong-lanceolate, acute to subacute, the base tapering, and strigose. The flower heads are 6–8 mm in diameter, solitary or with two on unequal axillary stalks. Involucral bracts, about eight to ten in number, strigose, ray florets ligulate and white, disk flowers tubular, the corollas often four-tubed. Flowers give way to compressed achenes. ***Bhṛṅgarāja*** is distributed throughout Southeast Asia, from the Punjab south to Sri Lanka, and eastwards into Burma and Malaysia (Kirtikar & Basu 1935, Warrier et al 1994).

Part used: Aerial parts, seeds, roots.

Dravyguṇa:

- ***Rasa***: *kaṭu, tikta*
- ***Vipāka***: *madhura*
- ***Vīrya***: *uṣṇa, rūkṣa*
- ***Karma***: *dīpanapācana, bhedhana, kṛmighna, jvaraghna, svāsahara, kāsahara, kuṣṭhaghna, raktaprasādana, śoṇitasthāpana, mūtravirecana, viṣaghna, medhya, rasāyana, tridoṣaghna* (Srikanthamurthy 2001, Warrier et al 1994).

Constituents: ***Bhṛṅgarāja*** contains the triterpenoid saponins eclalbasaponins I–VI, XI and XII, ecliptasaponin C and D, eclalbatin, the flavonoids apigenin and luteolin, as well as the coumestans wedelolactone, demethylwedelolactone, isodemethylwedelolactone and strychnolactone. Alkaloids include 25-β-hydroxyverazine and ecliptalbine, as well as small amounts of nicotine (0.078%) in the aerial portions. Other constituents are α-formylterthienyl, α-terthienyl, 16 related polyacetylenic thiophenes, dithienylacetyline esters I, II, and III, β-sitosterol, stigmasterol, daucosterol, stigmasterol–3-*O*-glucoside, nonacosanol, stearic acid, lacceroic acid, 3,4-dihydroxy benzoic acid, α-amyrin, ursolic acid and oleanolic acid (Abdel-Kader et al 1998, Han et al 1998, Upadhyay et al 2001, Yoganarasimhan 2000, Zhang & Chen 1996, Zhang & Guo 2001, Zhang et al 1997, 2001).

Medical research:

- ***In vitro***: antifungal (Abdel-Kader et al 1998), antimyotoxic/antivenomous (Melo et al 1994)
- ***In vivo***: hepatoprotective (Saxena et al 1993, Singh et al 2001), immunoprotective (Liu et al 2000), antimyotoxic/antivenomous (Melo et al 1994), immunomodulant (Jayathirtha & Mishra 2004), analgesic (Sawant et al 2004).

Toxicity: No data found for oral doses.

Indications: Dyspepsia, dysentery, haemorrhoids, hepatomegaly, splenomegaly, cholelithiasis, jaundice, cirrhosis, cough, bronchitis, asthma, skin diseases, ophthalmic disorders, premature greying, alopecia, odontalgia and odontopathies, oedema, anaemia, mental disorders, menorrhagia, insect, snake bites.

Contraindications: Pregnancy; severe chills (Frawley & Lad 1986).

Medicinal uses: ***Bhṛṅgarāja*** is a bitter-tasting herb that is in many respects similar to hepatic tonics such as Dandelion (*Taraxacum officinalis* root) (Nadkarni 1954), but combines this with a concomitant activity on the mind and senses, making it somewhat similar to ***Maṇḍūkaparṇī*** (Frawley & Lad 1986). Although ***Bhṛṅgarāja*** is generally listed in the older Āyurvedic ***nighaṇṭus*** as being useful to reduce vitiations of both ***kapha*** and ***vāta***, a few modern texts indicate that it can reduce all three ***doṣas***, and some even mention it as a ***rasāyana*** to ***pitta*** (Dash & Junius 1983, Frawley & Lad 1986). Traditional uses for *E. prostrata* include the treatment of cough, asthma, parasites, skin diseases, oedema, hepatosplenomegaly, dyspepsia, anorexia, wounds, ulcers, hypertension, pruritis, odontalgia (fresh root chewed or rubbed on gums), otalgia (as an ear oil in ***karṇa tarpaṇam***) and headache (Nadkarni 1954, Warrier et al 1994). The ***Mandanapala nighaṇṭu*** recommends *E. alba* in the treatment of obstinate skin diseases and in diseases of the eyes and head (Dash 1991). Both the ***Cakradatta*** and the ***Śāraṅgadhara saṃhitā*** recommend a medicated oil called ***Bhṛṅgarāja taila***, prepared with the juice of ***Bhṛṅgarāja*** mixed with a paste of ***Triphala***, ***Nīlotpala***, ***Sārivā*** and powdered iron oxide in the treatment of dandruff, premature greying, itching and alopecia (Sharma 2002, Srikanthamurthy 1984). This ***taila*** may also be used as an anti-inflammatory and vulnerary in cases of psoriasis and eczema, and finds special application when applied on the head to improve memory and mental function. A simpler preparation can be made by decocting one part ***Bhṛṅgarāja*** juice or powder in four parts ***ghṛta*** and 16 parts water until all the water has evaporated, after which the oil is cooled and filtered. This preparation finds special utility in diseases of the eye, and is used in ***netra vasti***, a method by which a mixture of wheat or bean paste is used to form a wall around the eye socket, and the oil applied over the closed eye and allowed to sit for 20–30 minutes. Internally, the ***Cakradatta*** mentions a simple formula comprising ***Bhṛṅgarāja*** juice, mixed with the powders of ***Āmalakī*** and ***Tila*** (Black sesame seed) in the treatment of alopecia and premature ageing, and to rejuvenate the senses (Sharma 2002). In cholelithiasis ***Bhrigarāja*** may be used along with appropriate antispasmodics such as Wild Yam (*Dioscorea villosa*) and carminatives such as ***Ajamodā*** (Nadkarni 1954). The expressed juice of both *E. alba* and *E. erecta* is given to infants in doses of 2–10 gtt., taken with honey for respiratory catarrh (Kirtikar & Basu 1935, Nadkarni 1954). Externally the leaves may be used as a poultice in glandular swellings, haemorrhoids and wounds to reduce inflammation and act as a drawing agent (Nadkarni 1954). Bensky & Gamble (1993) describe Eclipta prostrata as having the ability to '. . . nourish and tonify the liver and kidney yin', specific for '. . . liver and kidney yin deficiency with dizziness, blurred vision, vertigo and premature graying of the hair.' Additionally, it is used within Chinese traditional medicine to '. . . cool the blood and stop bleeding' and for '. . . yin deficiency patterns with bleeding due to heat in the blood, with such symptoms as vomiting or coughing up blood, nosebleed, blood in the stool, uterine bleeding, and blood in the urine' (Bensky & Gamble 1993).

Dosage:

- ***Cūrṇa***: dried leaves, 3–5 g b.i.d.–t.i.d.
- ***Svarasa***: 10–15 mL, b.i.d.–t.i.d.
- ***Phāṇṭa***: dried leaves, 1:4, 30–90 mL b.i.d.–t.i.d.
- ***Tincture***: dried leaves, 1:4, 50%; 3–5 mL b.i.d.–t.i.d.
- ***Taila***: 2–5 gtt. in ***nasya***; ad libitum in **abhyaṅga**, ***śirovasti***, ***kavalagraha*** etc.

REFERENCES

Bensky D, Gamble A 1993 Chinese herbal medicine materia medica revised edn. Eastland Press, Seattle, p 365

Dash B 1991 Materia medica of Ayurveda. B. Jain Publishers, New Delhi, p 82

Dash B, Junius M 1983 A handbook of Ayurveda. Concept Publishing, New Delhi, p 137

Frawley D, Lad V 1986 The yoga of herbs: an Ayurvedic guide to herbal medicine. Lotus Press, Santa, Fe p 163

Han Y, Xia C, Cheng X et al 1998 Preliminary studies on chemical constituents and pharmacological action of Eclipta prostrata L. Zhongguo Zhong Yao Za Zhi 23(11): 680–682, 703

Jayathirtha MG, Mishra SH 2004 Preliminary immunomodulatory activities of methanol extracts of Eclipta alba and Centella asiatica. Phytomedicine 11(4): 361–365

Kirtikar KR, Basu BD 1935 Indian medicinal plants, 2nd edn, vols 1–4. Periodical Experts, Delhi, p 1361, 1362

Liu X, Jiang Y, Zhao Y, Tang H 2000 Effect of ethyl acetate extract of Eclipta prostrata on mice of normal and immunosupression. Zhong Yao Cai 23(7): 407–409

Melo PA, Do Nascimento MC, Mors WB, Suarez-Kurtz G 1994 Inhibition of the myotoxic and hemorrhagic activities of crotalid venoms by Eclipta prostrata (Asteraceae) extracts and constituents. Toxicon 32(5): 595–603

Nadkarni KM 1954 The Indian materia medica, with Ayurvedic, Unani and home remedies, revised and enlarged by A.K. Nadkarni. Popular Prakashan PVP, Bombay, p 469, 472

Sawant M, Isaac JC, Narayanan S 2004 Analgesic studies on total alkaloids and alcohol extracts of Eclipta alba (Linn.) Hassk. Phytotherapy Research: PTR 18(2): 111–113

Saxena AK, Singh B, Anand KK 1993 Hepatoprotective effects of Eclipta alba on subcellular levels in rats. Journal of Ethnopharmacology 40(3): 155–161

Sharma PV 2002 Cakradatta. Sanskrit text with English translation. Chaukhamba, Varanasi, p 486, 625

Singh B, Saxena AK, Chandan BK et al 2001 In vivo hepatoprotective activity of active fraction from ethanolic extract of Eclipta alba leaves. Indian Journal of Physiology and Pharmacology 45(4): 435–441

Srikanthamurthy KR 1984 Śāraṅgadhara saṃhitā: A treatise on Ayurveda. Chaukhamba Orientalia, Varanasi, p 131

Srikanthamurthy KR 2001 Bhāvaprakāśa of Bhāvamiśra, vol 1. Krishnadas Academy, Varanasi, p 266, 267

Upadhyay RK, Pandey MB, Jha RN, Pandey VB 2001 Eclalbatin, a triterpene saponin from Eclipta alba. Journal of Asian Natural Products Research 3(3): 213–217

Warrier PK, Nambiar VPK, Ramankutty C (eds) 1994 Indian medicinal plants: a compendium of 500 species, vol 2. Orient Longman, Hyderabad, p 350–353

Yoganarasimhan SN 2000 Medicinal plants of India, vol 2: Tamil Nadu. Self-published, Bangalore, p 207

Zhao YP, Tang HF, Jiang YP et al 2001 Triterpenoid saponins *from* Eclipta prostrata L. Yao Xue Xue Bao 36(9): 660–663

Zhang M, Chen Y 1996 Chemical constituents of Eclipta alba (L.) Hassk. Zhongguo Zhong Yao Za Zhi 21(8): 480–1, 510

Zhang JS, Guo QM 2001 Studies on the chemical constituents of Eclipta prostrata (L). Yao Xue Xue Bao 36(1): 34–37

Zhang M, Chen YY, Di XH, Liu M 1997 Isolation and identification of ecliptasaponin D from Eclipta alba (L.) Hassk. Yao Xue Xue Bao 32(8): 633–634

Bhūnimba, 'ground nimba'

BOTANICAL NAME: *Andrographis paniculata,* Acanthaceae

OTHER NAMES: ***Kirātatiktā*** (S); Charayetah, Kiryat, Kalamegh, Kalpath (H); Nilavempu, Shiratkuchi (T); Green Chiretta (E); Chuan xin lian (C)

Botany: ***Bhūnimba*** is an erect, branched annual, 30–110 cm in height, with four-angled branches. The leaves are simple, glabrous and lanceolate, acute at both ends, up to 8.0 cm long and 2.5 cm broad. The small white flowers are borne in panicles or terminal racemes, giving way to linear-oblong capsules that contain numerous seeds. ***Bhūnimba*** is found wild and weedy in the plains throughout India and in the undergrowth of forests, from the Himalayan foothills southwards into Sri Lanka. It is also distributed in other locations in Southeast Asia, and has since naturalised in some areas of Central America (Kirtikar & Basu 1935, Warrier et al 1994).

Part used: Whole plant.

Dravyguṇa:

- ***Rasa***: *kaṭu, tikta*
- ***Vipāka***: *kaṭu*
- ***Vīrya***: *śita*
- ***Karma***: *dīpana, bhedana, kṛmighna, jvaraghna, chedana, raktaprasādana, dāhapraśamana, kuṣṭhaghna, sandhānīya, lekhana* (Warrier et al 1994).

Constituents: Chemical research on ***Bhūnimba*** leaves has yielded a variety of bitter tasting diterpene lactones called the andrographolides, as well as the non-bitter neoandrographolide, diterpene dimers, bis-andrographolides A–D, andrographosterol, andrographane, andrographone, a wax, and two esters containing hydroxyl groups. ***Bhūnimba*** roots have yielded apigenin–7,4′-di-*O*-methyl ether, andrographolide, 5-hydroxy–7,8,2′,3′-tetramethoxyflavone, a monohydroxy-trimethylflavone, andrographin, a dihydroxy-dimethoxyflavone, panicolin, and α-sitosterol (Matsuda et al 1994, Saxena et al 1998, Yoganarasimhan 2000).

Medical research:
- ***In vitro***: immunomodulant (Panossian et al 2002, Puri et al 1993, Shen et al 2002), antitumour (Matsuda et al 1994); hepatoprotective (Visen et al 1993), antithrombotic (Amroyan et al 1999), anti-inflammatory (Batkhuu et al 2002), antispasmodic (Burgos et al 2001), antimalarial (Najib et al 1999)
- ***In vivo***: antidiabetic, antihyperglycaemic (Zhang & Tan 2000a,b, Zhang et al 2002), hepatoprotective (Kapil et al 1993; Rana & Avadhoot 1991; Shukla et al 1992), antihypertensive (Zhang & Tan 1996, Zhang et al 1998), negatively chronotropic (Zhang et al 1998), cardioprotective (Guo et al 1996), chemopreventative (Shen et al 2000), anti-inflammatory (Shen et al 2000, Wang et al 1997), antimalarial (Najib et al 1999)
- ***Human trials***: significant improvement over placebo in the reduction of symptoms in upper respiratory tract infection (Gabrielian et al 2002, Melchior et al 2000); andrographolide isolated from *Andrographis paniculata* was demonstrated to promote an increase in $CD4^+$ lymphocyte levels in HIV–1 infected individuals (Calabrese et al 2000); compared to cotrimoxazole and norfloxacin *Andrographis paniculata* reduced the incidence of urinary tract infection post Extracorporeal Shock Wave Lithotripsy (ESWL) in the treatment of renal stones less than 3 cm (Muangman et al 1995).

Toxicity: No data found for oral doses. The powdered extract of *Andrographis paniculata* leaves was determined to have no effect on blood progesterone in pregnant rats (Panossian et al 1999).

Indications: Dyspepsia, bilious colic, hepatic sluggishness, diarrhoea, dysentery, intestinal parasites, haemorrhoids, fever, upper respiratory tract infection, cough, bronchitis, pruritis, inflammatory skin conditions, leprosy, intense thirst, burning sensations, wounds, ulcers, acute and chronic malaria.

Contraindications: ***vātakopa***, pregnancy.

Medicinal uses: ***Bhūnimba*** ('ground *nimba*') derives its name from ***Nimba***, the leaves of *Azadirachta indica*, an intensely bitter remedy that is used primarily to treat ***paittika*** disorders. Thus, ***Bhūnimba*** finds application in a similar range of conditions as ***Nimba***. It is considered synonymous with ***Kirātatiktā*** in its actions, and is used to treat ***sannipāta jvara***, a type of feverish condition in which all three ***doṣas*** are vitiated. It is also used for more straightforward ***paittika*** conditions such as ***daha*** (burning sensation), ***jvara*** (fever), ***vrana*** (ulcers), and ***tṛṣṇā*** (extreme thirst), as well as ***kaphaja*** conditions such as ***kasa*** (cough, bronchitis), ***svasa*** (asthma), and ***śotha*** (oedema). Thus ***Bhūnimba*** combines its profoundly bitter, cooling and anti-inflammatory properties with the activity of ***lekhana***, which dries up excessive moisture in the body. ***Bhūnimba*** has proved to be an important remedy in hepatic dysfunction, and given its antiviral properties, constitutes an exceptionally important remedy in viral hepatitis, as well as other forms of hepatitis induced by drugs such as acetaminophen, or accidental mushroom poisoning. Kirtikar & Basu (1935) state that the fresh juice can be extracted and taken alone or with the powders of ***Elā***, ***Tvak*** bark or ***Lavaṅga*** fruit in the treatment of poor appetite, colic, flatulence and diarrhoea, and as a treatment for intestinal parasites. Such formulations that have ***dīpanapācana*** components guard against ***vāta*** aggravation. In the treatment of malabsorption, abdominal enlargement, jaundice and diarrhoea the ***Cakradatta*** recommends ***Bhūnimbādya cūrṇa***, composed of one part each of ***Bhūnimba***, ***Kaṭuka***, ***Trikaṭu***, ***Mustaka***, and ***Indrayava***, two parts ***Citraka*** and 16 parts ***Kuṭaja*** (Sharma 2002). ***Bhūnimba*** is a popular remedy to strengthen the body during influenza epidemics or cold and flu season, to keep the immune system strong. In Chinese medicine ***Bhūnimba*** is combined with *Isatis tinctoria* and *Taraxacum officinalis* in the patent formula Chuan Xin Lian, which is used for the acute onset of colds and flus, especially with fever, sore throat, and lymphadenopathy. Nadkarni (1954) reports success with the use of ***Bhūnimba*** in treatment of malaria, in which it was considered 'superior to quinine'. The potent cooling and anti-inflammatory properties of ***Bhūnimba*** have long made it an important remedy in snake and insect bites in both Āyurvedic and Chinese medicine.

Dosage:

- ***Cūrṇa***: dried leaves, 2–3 g b.i.d.–t.i.d.
- ***Phāṇṭa***: dried leaves, 1:4, 30–60 mL b.i.d.–t.i.d.
- ***Tincture***: dried leaves, 1:4, 50%; 1–3 mL b.i.d.–t.i.d.

REFERENCES

Amroyan E, Gabrielian E, Panossian A et al 1999 Inhibitory effect of andrographolide from Andrographis paniculata on PAF-induced platelet aggregation. Phytomedicine. 6(1):27–31

Batkhuu J, Hattori K, Takano F et al 2002 Suppression of NO production in activated macrophages in vitro and ex vivo by neoandrographolide isolated from Andrographis paniculata. Biological and Pharmaceutical Bulletin 25(9):1169–1174

Burgos RA, Aguila MJ, Santiesteban ET et al 2001 Andrographis paniculata (Ness) induces relaxation of uterus by blocking voltage operated calcium channels and inhibits Ca(+2) influx. Phytotherapy Research 15(3):235–239

Calabrese C, Berman SH, Babish JG et al 2000 A phase I trial of andrographolide in HIV positive patients and normal volunteers. Phytotherapy Research 14(5):333–338

Gabrielian ES, Shukarian AK, Goukasova GI 2002 A double blind, placebo-controlled study of Andrographis paniculata fixed combination Kan Jang in the treatment of acute upper respiratory tract infections including sinusitis. Phytomedicine 9(7):589–597

Guo Z, Zhao H, Fu L 1996 Protective effects of API0134 on myocardial ischemia and reperfusion injury. Journal of Tongji Medical University 16(4):193–197

Kapil A, Koul IB, Banerjee SK, Gupta BD 1993 Antihepatotoxic effects of major diterpenoid constituents of Andrographis paniculata. Biochemical Pharmacology 46(1):182–185

Kirtikar KR, Basu BD 1935 Indian medicinal plants, 2nd edn, vols 1–4. Periodical Experts, Delhi, p 1884–1886

Matsuda T, Kuroyanagi M, Sugiyama S 1994 Cell differentiation-inducing diterpenes from Andrographis paniculata Nees. Chemical and Pharmaceutical Bulletin (Tokyo) 42(6):1216–1225

Melchior J, Spasov AA, Ostrovskij OV et al 2000 Double-blind, placebo-controlled pilot and phase III study of activity of standardized Andrographis paniculata Herba Nees extract fixed combination (Kan jang) in the treatment of uncomplicated upper-respiratory tract infection. Phytomedicine. 7(5):341–350

Muangman V, Viseshsindh V, Ratana-Olarn K, Buadilok S 1995 The usage of Andrographis paniculata following Extracorporeal Shock Wave Lithotripsy (ESWL). Journal of the Medical Association of Thailand 78(6):310–313

Nadkarni KM 1954 The Indian materia medica, with Ayurvedic, Unani and home remedies, revised and enlarged by A.K. Nadkarni. Popular Prakashan PVP, Bombay, p 102

Najib Nik A, Rahman N, Furuta T et al 1999 Antimalarial activity of extracts of Malaysian medicinal plants. Journal of Ethnopharmacology 64(3):249–254

Panossian A, Kochikian A, Gabrielian E et al 1999 Effect of Andrographis paniculata extract on progesterone in blood plasma of pregnant rats. Phytomedicine 6(3):157–161

Panossian A, Davtyan T, Gukassyan N 2002 Effect of andrographolide and Kan Jang–fixed combination of extract SHA–10 and extract SHE–3 on proliferation of human lymphocytes, production of cytokines and immune activation markers in the whole blood cells culture. Phytomedicine 9(7):598–605

Puri A, Saxena R, Saxena RP et al 1993 Immunostimulant agents from Andrographis paniculata. Journal of Natural Products 56(7):995–999

Rana AC, Avadhoot Y 1991 Hepatoprotective effects of Andrographis paniculata against carbon tetrachloride-induced liver damage. Archives of Pharmaceutical Research 14(1):93–95

Reddy MK, Reddy MV, Gunasekar D et al 2003 A flavone and an unusual 23-carbon terpenoid from Andrographis paniculata. Phytochemistry 62(8):1271–1275

Saxena S, Jain DC, Bhakuni RS, Sharma RP 1998 Chemistry and pharmacology of Andrographis species. Indian Drugs 35: 458–467

Sharma PV 2002 Cakradatta. Sanskrit text with English translation. Chaukhamba, Varanasi, p 65

Shen YC, Chen CF, Chiou WF 2000 Suppression of rat neutrophil reactive oxygen species production and adhesion by the diterpenoid lactone andrographolide. Planta Medica 66(4):314–317

Shen YC, Chen CF, Chiou WF 2002 Andrographolide prevents oxygen radical production by human neutrophils: possible mechanism(s) involved in its anti-inflammatory effect. British Journal of Pharmacology 135(2):399–406

Shukla B, Visen PK, Patnaik GK, Dhawan BN 1992 Choleretic effect of andrographolide in rats and guinea pigs. Planta Medica 58(2):146–149

Singh RP, Banerjee S, Rao AR 2001 Modulatory influence of Andrographis paniculata on mouse hepatic and extrahepatic carcinogen metabolizing enzymes and anti-oxidant status. Phytotherapy Research 15(5):382–390

Visen PK, Shukla B, Patnaik GK, Dhawan BN 1993 Andrographolide protects rat hepatocytes against paracetamol-induced damage. Journal of Ethnopharmacology 40(2):131–136

Wang HW, Zhao HY, Xiang SQ 1997 Effects of Andrographis paniculata component on nitric oxide, endothelin and lipid peroxidation in experimental atherosclerotic rabbits. Zhongguo Zhong Xi Yi Jie He Za Zhi 17(9):547–549

Warrier PK, Nambiar VPK, Ramankutty C (eds) 1994 Indian medicinal plants: a compendium of 500 species, vol 1. Orient Longman, Hyderabad, p 149

Yoganarasimhan SN 2000 Medicinal plants of India, vol 2: Tamil Nadu. Self-published, Bangalore, p 45

Zhang CY, Tan BK 1996 Hypotensive activity of aqueous extract of Andrographis paniculata in rats. Clinical and Experimental Pharmacology and Physiology 23(8):675–678

Zhang C, Kuroyangi M, Tan BK 1998 Cardiovascular activity of 14-deoxy–11,12-didehydroandrographolide in the anaesthetised rat and isolated right atria. Pharmacological Research 38(6):413–417

Zhang XF, Tan BK 2000a Anti-diabetic property of ethanolic extract of Andrographis paniculata in streptozotocin-diabetic rats. Acta Pharmacologica Sinica 21(12):1157–1164

Zhang XF, Tan BK 2000b Antihyperglycaemic and anti-oxidant properties of Andrographis paniculata in normal and diabetic rats. Clinical and Experimental Pharmacology and Physiology 27(5–6):358–363

Bibhītaka, 'intimidating'

BOTANICAL NAME: *Terminalia belerica,* Combretaceae

OTHER NAMES: ***Akṣa,*** 'eye' (S); Bahera (H); Tanni, Tanrikkai (T); Belleric Myrobalan (E)

Botany: ***Bibhītaka*** is a large deciduous tree with a buttressed trunk, thick brownish-grey bark with shallow longitudinal fissures, attaining a height of between 20 and 30 m. The leaves are crowded around the ends of the branches, alternately arranged, margins entire, elliptic to elliptic-obovate, rounded tip or subacute, midrib prominent, pubescent when young and becoming glabrous with maturity. The flowers are pale greenish-yellow with an offensive odour, borne in axillary spikes longer than the petioles but shorter than the leaves. The fruits are ovoid drupes, grey in colour, obscurely five-angled when dry, containing a kernel within. ***Bibhītaka*** is found growing wild throughout the Indian subcontinent, Sri Lanka and SE Asia, up to 1200 m in elevation, in a wide variety of ecologies. ***Bibhītaka*** is also commonly cultivated, planted along roadsides in large cities (Kirtikar & Basu 1935, Warrier et al 1996).

Part used: fruit, bark.

Dravyguṇa: Fruit

- ***Rasa***: *amla, kaśāya, madhura*
- ***Vipāka***: *madhura*
- ***Vīrya***: *uṣṇa, rūkṣa, laghu*
- ***Karma***: *chardinigrahaṇa, pācana, bhedhana* (unripe fruit), *purīṣasangrahaṇiya* (mature fruit), *kṛmighna, jvaraghna, chedana, kāsahara, svāsahara, kuṣṭhaghna, mūtravirecana, śotahara, śoṇitasthāpana, cakṣuṣya, romasañjanana, vedanāsthāpana, aśmaribhedana, madakārī* (kernel), *rasāyana, tridoṣaghna.*
- ***Prabhāva***: *Bibhītaka* is called 'intimidating' because disease shrinks in the face of its power to heal. Its synonym ***Akṣa*** (eye) indicates ***Bibhītaka's*** utility in diseases of the eye (Dash 1991, Nadkarni 1954, Srikanthamurthy 2001, Warrier et al 1996).

Constituents: ***Bibhītaka*** contains several triterpenoids, including belleric acid, β-sitosterol, and the saponin glycosides bellericoside and bellericanin. Other constituents include polyphenols (gallic acid, ellagic acid, phyllembin, ethyl galate, and chebulagic acid), lignans (termilignan, thannilignan, hydroxy-3′, 4′-[methylenedioxy] flavan, anolignan B), and a fixed yellow oil (Kapoor 1990, Nandy et al 1989, Row & Murthy 1970, Valsaraj et al 1997).

Medical research:

- ***In vitro***: anti-HIV–1 (el-Mekkawy et al 1995, Valsaraj et al 1997), antimalarial (Valsaraj et al 1997), antimutagenic (Padam et al 1996), antifungal (Valsaraj et al 1997), antibacterial (Aqil et al 2005, Rani & Khullar 2004).
- ***In vivo***: hepatoprotective (Anand et al 1997), hypocholesterolaemic, anti-atherosclerotic (Shaila et al 1995).
- ***Human trials***: anti-asthmatic, antispasmodic, expectorant, antitussive (Trivedi et al 1979).

Toxicity: No data found.

Indications: Dyspepsia, flatulence, haemorrhoids, constipation (unripe fruit), chronic diarrhoea and dysentery (dry fruit), hepatosplenomegaly, intestinal parasites, cholelithiasis, fever, sore throat, pharyngitis, laryngitis, cough, catarrh, bronchitis, asthma, skin diseases, oedema, ophthalmia, alopecia and premature greying, headache.

Contraindications: ***vātakopa*** (Frawley & Lad 1986).

Medicinal uses: ***Bibhītaka*** is a celebrated constituent of ***Triphala***, along with ***Harītakī*** and

Āmalakī, stated specifically to be a ***rasāyana*** for ***kapha***, useful for reducing excess ***medas*** (Dash & Junius 1983, Frawley & Lad 1986). It is a stimulating astringent, and has wide application in any condition marked by atony, prolapse, catarrh or haemorrhage; useful in the treatment of conditions such as uterine prolapse and menorrhagia. The mature, dried fruit of ***Bibhītaka*** is effective in the treatment of dysentery and intestinal parasites but should be taken along with purgatives such as ***Markandika*** to counteract its constipating effects; the sun-dried unripe fruit, however, is gently aperient and can be used on its own. Dash & Junius (1983) state that ***Bibhītaka*** is a good remedy for vomiting in pregnancy. Frawley & Lad (1986) mention that ***Bibhītaka*** is a useful antilithic in gall bladder and urinary diseases, liquefying and expelling the stones. The ***Cakradatta*** states that the fruit pulp mixed with ***ghṛta*** is covered with cow dung and heated in a fire, and held in the mouth to control coughing (Sharma 2002). For severe cough and asthma the ***cūrṇa*** of the dried fruit may be taken with honey (Sharma 2002). Mixed with ***saindhava***, ***Pippalī*** and buttermilk, ***Bibhītaka*** is taken in hoarseness (Sharma 2002). A decoction of the dried fruit may be taken internally and externally as an eyewash in the treatment of ophthalmological disorders (Nadkarni 1954). Vaidya Mana Bhajracharya (1997) indicates that the fresh fruit pulp is used as a collyrium in the treatment of non-traumatic corneal ulcer. Warrier et al (1996) mention that the oil from the seeds is trichogenous, and can be used topically for leucoderma and skin diseases. The kernel is typically removed before ***Bibhītaka*** is used, and specifically stated to be ***madakārī*** ('narcotic'), used topically as an analgesic in the treatment of inflammation and pain, and internally in vomiting, bronchitis and colic (Dash & Junius 1983, Kirtikar & Basu 1935). In ancient India ***Bibhītaka*** fruits were used as a form of dice (Sharma 1993).

Dosage:

- ***Cūrṇa***: 2–5 g b.i.d.–t.i.d.
- ***Kvātha***: 30–60 mL b.i.d.–t.i.d.
- ***Tincture***: crushed dried fruit, 1:4, 50%; 1–3 mL b.i.d.–t.i.d.

REFERENCES

Anand KK, Singh B, Saxena AK et al 1997 3,4,5-Trihydroxy benzoic acid (gallic acid), the hepatoprotective principle in the fruits of Terminalia belerica-bioassay guided activity. Pharmacological Research 36(4):315–321

Aqil F, Khan MS, Owais M, Ahmad I 2005 Effect of certain bioactive plant extracts on clinical isolates of beta-lactamase producing methicillin resistant Staphylococcus aureus. Journal of Basic Microbiology 45(2):106–114

Bajracharya M, Tillotson A, Abel R 1997 Ayurvedic ophthalmology: a recension of the Shalakya Tantra of Videhadhipati Janaka. Piyushabarshi Aushadhalaya Mahabouddha, Kathmandu, p 85

Dash B 1991 Materia medica of Ayurveda. B. Jain Publishers, New Delhi, p 9–10

Dash B, Junius M 1983 A handbook of Ayurveda. Concept Publishing, New Delhi, p 88

Frawley D, Lad V 1986 The yoga of herbs: an Ayurvedic guide to herbal medicine. Lotus Press, Santa Fe, p 164

Kapoor LD 1990 CRC Handbook of Ayurvedic medicinal plants. CRC Press, Boca Raton, p 321

Kirtikar KR, Basu BD 1935 Indian medicinal plants, 2nd edn, vols 1–4. Periodical Experts, Delhi, p 1018–1019

Nadkarni KM 1954 The Indian materia medica, with Ayurvedic, Unani and home remedies, revised and enlarged by A.K. Nadkarni. Popular Prakashan PVP, Bombay, p 1203–1204

Nandy AK, Podder G, Sahu NP, Mahato SB 1989 Triterpenoids and their glycosides from Terminalia belerica. Phytochemistry 28(10):2769

Padam SK, Grover IS, Singh M 1996 Antimutagenic effects of polyphenols isolated from Terminalia belerica myroblan in Salmonella typhimurium. Indian Journal of Experimental Biology 34(2):98–102

Rani P, Khullar N 2004 Antimicrobial evaluation of some medicinal plants for their anti-enteric potential against multi-drug resistant Salmonella typhi. Phytotherapy Research 18(8):670–673

Row LR and Murthy PS 1970 Chemical examination of Terminalia belerica Roxb. Indian Journal of Chemistry 8:1047–1048

Shaila HP, Udupa AL, Udupa SL 1995 Preventive actions of Terminalia belerica in experimentally induced atherosclerosis. International Journal of Cardiology 49(2):101–106

Sharma PV 1993 Essentials of Āyurveda: Ṣodaśāṅgahṛdayam. Motilal Banarsidass, Delhi, p 18

Sharma PV 2002 Cakradatta. Sanskrit text with English translation. Chaukhamba, Varanasi p 150, 158–159, 162

Srikanthamurthy KR 2001 Bhāvaprakāśa of Bhāvamiśra, vol 1. Krishnadas Academy, Varanasi, p 164

Trivedi VP, Nesamany S, Sharma VK 1979 A clinical study of the antitussive and anti-asthmatic effects of Vibhitakphal Curna (Terminalia belerica Roxb.) in the cases of Kasa-Swasa. Journal of Research in Āyurveda and Siddha 3:1–8

Valsaraj R, Pushpangadan P, Smitt UW 1997 New anti-HIV-1, antimalarial, and antifungal compounds from Terminalia bellerica. Journal of Natural Products 60(7):739–742

Warrier PK, Nambiar VPK, Ramankutty C (eds) 1996 Indian medicinal plants: a compendium of 500 species, vol 5. Orient Longman, Hyderabad, p 258

Bilva

BOTANICAL NAME: *Aegle marmelos,* Rutaceae

OTHER NAMES: ***Śrīphala*** (S); Bel (H); Kuvilam, Bilvam (T); Bael Tree (E)

Botany: ***Bilva*** is a medium-sized deciduous tree that attains a height of up to 8 m, with sharp axillary thorns up to 2.5 cm long and a yellowish-brown corky bark. The trifoliate leaves are alternately arranged, the leaflets ovate to ovate lanceolate, the lateral leaflets subsessile and the terminal leaflet on a long petiole. The flowers are greenish-white and sweet-scented, borne in axillary panicles. The oblong globose fruits that follow are 5–7.5 cm in diameter, with a grey or yellow rind enclosing a sweetish orange-coloured pulp that contains numerous seeds arranged in cells, surrounded by a slimy transparent mucilage. ***Bilva*** is native to the subcontinent of India eastwards into Cambodia, Laos, Malaysia and Indonesia, found growing wild in drier tropical forests (Kirtikar & Basu 1935, Warrier et al 1994).

Part used: Unripe fruit, leaves, bark, root.

Dravyguṇa: Unripe fruit

- ***Rasa***: *tikta, kaśāya, amla, kaṭu*
- ***Vipāka***: *laghu*
- ***Vīrya***: *uṣṇa*
- ***Karma***: *dīpanapācana, purīṣasangrahaṇiya, balya, vātakaphahara* (Dash 1991, Srikanthamurthy 2001, Warrier et al 1994).

Constituents: ***Bilva*** contains a large diversity of constituents in different parts of the plant. The fruit rind contains umbelliferone, dictamine, xanthotoxol, xanthotoxin, scoparone, isopimpinellin, sioimperatorin, *N*–2-methoxy-2-(4-methoxyphenyl) ethylcinnamamide, marmeline and its methyl ester, bergapten, marmesin, osthol and auraptin. The fruit flesh contains a mucilage, xanthotoxol, scoparone, scopoletin, umbelliferone, marmesin, skimmin, allaimperatorin, marmesolin, β-sitosterol, marmelide and psoralen. The seeds are stated to contain a fatty oil (Yoganarasimhan 2000).

Medical research:

- ***In vivo***: antidiarrhoeal (Shoba & Thomas 2001); hypoglycaemic, anti-oxidant (Upadhya et al 2004); hypolipidaemic (Rajadurai et al 2005); antitumour (Jagetia et al 2005).
- ***Human trials***: a preparation containing *Aegle marmelos* and *Bacopa monnieri* demonstrated significant improvement in irritable bowel syndrome compared to placebo (Yadav et al 1989).

Toxicity: A study which examined the treatment of male rats over an 8-week period with an extract of *Aegle marmelos* demonstrated no toxic or antifertility effects (Aritajat et al 2000).

Indications: Diarrhoea, dysentery, intestinal spasm, inflammatory bowel disease.

Contraindications: Constipation.

Medicinal uses: Although the etymology of the ancient Dravidian name ***Bilva*** is lost, the tree and in particular the trifoliate leaves are associated with the god ***Śiva***. The leaves and fruit are commonly used in Hindu religious ceremonies, and the fruit is among the objects held by the goddess ***Lakṣmī***, representing the 'fruit' (***karma***) of our actions and conditioned existence. Unripe ***Bilva*** fruit is among the most common remedies used in Āyurveda to treat both diarrhoea and dysentery, in much the same way as ***Dāḍima*** rind. It is widely believed by many practitioners that ***Bilva*** is able to cure particularly recalcitrant cases of diarrhoea when nothing else works. The unripe fruits are harvested in winter and usually dried in the sun. In the treatment of summer diarrhoea the dried fruits are decocted with carminative herbs such as

Ajamodā, strained, and then administered as a cool drink, often forming the only medication used. Similarly, the dried unripe fruit is reduced to a ***cūrṇa*** and then administered with treacle in doses of 2–3 grams. Sometimes ***Bilva*** is prepared as a conserve or jam used to treat diarrhoea or in convalescence after dysentery. In the treatment of ***grahaṇī*** or diarrhoea due to malabsorptive syndromes, the ***Cakradatta*** recommends a paste prepared from the tender fruits of ***Bilva*** with ***Śūṇṭhī*** and jaggery, prepared in buttermilk. Combined with ***Lodhra*** and ***Marica***, and mixed with honey and ***taila***, ***Bilva*** is mentioned by the ***Bhāvaprakāśa*** to be an effective treatment for dysentery (Srikanthamurthy 2000). The ***Bhāvaprakāśa*** also mentions ***Bilva*** as a key ingredient in the preparation of ***Bilva taila***, used to treat diarrhoea, malabsorption syndromes and haemorrhoids (Srikanthamurthy 2000). The mature fruits are often eaten as a medicinal food, and prepared with sugar as a cooling beverage in the heat of summer. The roots are similarly astringent as the fruit, but are also used in vitiated conditions of ***vāta*** (Warrier et al 1994), and are an ingredient in the ***Daśamūla*** ('ten roots') formula. The leaves are used in ophthalmic disorders, diabetes and asthma (Warrier et al 1994).

Dosage:

- ***Cūrṇa***: 2–12 g b.i.d.–t.i.d.
- ***Kvātha***: 1:4, 50–100 mL b.i.d.–t.i.d.

REFERENCES

Aritajat S, Kaweewat K, Manosroi J, Manosroi A 2000 Dominant lethal test in rats treated with some plant extracts. Southeast Asian Journal of Tropical Medicine and Public Health 31(suppl 1):171–173

Dash B 1991 Materia medica of Ayurveda. B. Jain Publishers, New Delhi, p 14

Haider R, Khan AK, Aziz KM et al 1991 Evaluation of indigenous plants in the treatment of acute shigellosis. Tropical and Geographical Medicine 43(3):266–270

Jagetia GC, Venkatesh P, Baliga MS 2005 Aegle marmelos (L.) Correa inhibits the proliferation of transplanted Ehrlich ascites carcinoma in mice. Biological and Pharmaceutical Bulletin 28(1):58–64

Kirtikar KR, Basu BD 1935 Indian medicinal plants, 2nd edn, vols 1–4. Periodical Experts, Delhi, p 499

Rajadurai M, Prince PS 2005 Comparative effects of Aegle marmelos extract and alpha-tocopherol on serum lipids, lipid peroxides and cardiac enzyme levels in rats with isoproterenol-induced myocardial infarction. Singapore Medical Journal 46(2):78–81

Sharma PV 2002 Cakradatta. Sanskrit text with English translation. Chaukhamba, Varanasi

Shoba FG, Thomas M 2001 Study of antidiarrhoeal activity of four medicinal plants in castor-oil induced diarrhoea. Journal of Ethnopharmacology 76(1):73–76

Srikanthamurthy KR 2000 Bhāvaprakāśa of Bhāvamiśra, vol 2. Krishnadas Academy, Varanasi, p 139

Srikanthamurthy KR 2001 Bhāvaprakāśa of Bhāvamiśra, vol 1. Krishnadas Academy, Varanasi, p 229

Upadhya S, Shanbhag KK, Suneetha G et al 2004 A study of hypoglycemic and anti-oxidant activity of Aegle marmelos in alloxan induced diabetic rats. Indian Journal of Physiology and Pharmacology 48(4):476–480

Warrier PK, Nambiar VPK, Ramankutty C (eds) 1994 Indian medicinal plants: a compendium of 500 species, vol 1. Orient-Longman, Hyderabad, p 62–63

Yadav SK, Jain AK, Tripathi SN, Gupta JP 1989 Irritable bowel syndrome: therapeutic evaluation of indigenous drugs. Indian Journal of Medical Research 90:496–503

Yoganarasimhan SN 2000 Medicinal plants of India, vol 2: Tamil Nadu. Self-published, Bangalore, p 24

Brāhmī, 'consort of Brahmā'

BOTANICAL NAME: *Bacopa monniera,* Scrophulariaceae

OTHER NAMES: ***Sarasvatī*** (S); Barami, Jalnim (H); Nirpirami, Piramiyapundu (T); Bacopa (E)

Botany: ***Brāhmī*** is a prostrate or creeping succulent annual herb, rooting at the nodes with numerous ascending branches. The leaves are oppositely arranged, margin simple, obovate-oblong, and sessile, with small black dots. The flowers are solitary, pale blue or white, borne in the leaf axils on long slender pedicles, giving rise to two-celled, two-valved ovoid capsules that contain numerous tiny seeds. ***Brāhmī*** is found throughout tropical India in damp, marshy areas (Kirtikar & Basu 1935, Warrier et al 1994). ***Brāhmī*** is sometimes found as an ornamental ground cover, and is under cultivation in India and other warm, wet locations.

Part used: Aerial portions.

Dravyguṇa:

- ***Rasa***: *tikta, kaśāya, madhura*
- ***Vipāka***: *madhura*
- ***Vīrya***: *śita*
- ***Karma***: *medhya, jīvanīya, rasāyana, kāsahara, jvaraghna, kuṣṭhaghna, anulomana, vātakaphahara, balya.*
- ***Prabhāva***: The name *Brāhmī* means 'consort of Brahmā', the active, feminine counterpart (*śakti*) to Brahmā, the lord of Creation in Hindu cosmology, suggesting that this herb has a direct ability to faciliate divine consciousness (Dash 1991, Srikanthamurthy 2001, Warrier et al 1994).

Constituents: Researchers have isolated numerous glycosidal constituents from ***Brāhmī***, including the saponins monnierin and hersaponin, dammarane-type triterpenoid, bacosaponins that include bacopasides III, IV, V, bacosides A and B (which upon acid hydrolysis yield the aglycones bacogenins A1–A5) and bacosaponins A, B and C. Other saponin glycosides include the jujubogenin bisdesmosides bacopasaponins D, E and F. Other constituents include a matsutaka alcohol derivative, a phenylethanoid glycoside, luteolin and luteolin-7-glucoside, the alkaloids brahmine, herpestine and a mixture of three bases, D-mannitol, betulic acid, β-sitosterol, stigmasterol and its esters, heptacosane, octacosane, nonacosane, triacontane, hentriacontane, dotriacontane, nicotine, and 3-formyl-4-hydroxy-2H-pyran. The presence of α-alamine, aspartic acid, glutamic acid and serine has also been reported (Cakravarty et al 2003, Garai et al 1996a, b, Hou et al 2002, Mahato et al 2000, Rastogi et al 1994, Yoganarasimhan 2000).

Medical research:

- ***In vitro***: acetylcholinesterase activity (Das et al 2002), anti-withdrawal (Sumathi et al 2002), anti-spasmodic (Dar & Channa 1999).
- ***In vivo***: nootropic (Singh & Dhawan 1982), anti-dementia (Das et al 2002), anti-epileptic (Vohora et al 2000), thyrostimulant (Kar et al 2002), anti-oxidant (Bhattacharya et al 2000, Chowdhuri et al 2002, Sumathy 2002, Tripathi et al 1996), hepato-protective (Sumathy et al 2001), anti-ulcerogenic (Sairam et al 2001).
- ***Human trials***: ***Brāhmī*** demonstrated a significant effect upon the retention of new information, decreasing the rate at which newly acquired information is forgotten, in adults aged between 40 and 65 years (Roodenrys et al 2002); ***Brāhmī*** significantly improved the speed of visual information processing, learning rate and memory consolidation, and reduced anxiety, in healthy human subjects (Stough et al 2001).

Toxicity: No data found.

Indications: Mental fatigue, poor memory, depression, psychosis, dementia, epilepsy, neuralgia, weakness, fatigue, debility, ageing, infertility, fever, skin diseases, atherosclerosis, angina, hoarseness, bronchitis, asthma, dyspepsia, flatulence, constipation, splenomegaly, ascites, urinary tenesmus, musculoskeletal inflammation, anaemia, poisoning.

Contraindications: ***pittakopa*** in high doses; use with extreme caution with antiseizure, antipsychotic and antidepressant medication.

Medicinal uses: ***Brāhmī*** is among the more important botanicals used in the treatment of ***unmāda*** ('psychosis') and ***apasmāra*** ('epilepsy'), often taken by itself in the form of the fresh juice, mixed with honey, or in complex polyherbal formulations. One remedy mentioned by the ***Cakradatta*** is ***Brāhmīghṛta***, prepared by cooking one part aged ***ghṛta*** in four parts fresh juice of ***Brāhmī***, mixed with the powders of ***Vacā***, ***Kuṣṭha*** and ***Śaṅkhapuṣpī*** (Sharma 2002). This recipe, or similar, is mentioned also in the ***Bhāvaprakāśa*** and the ***Aṣṭāñga Hṛdaya***, used in the treatment of ***unmāda***, ***apasmāra*** and spiritual possession, taken in doses of 12 g, with warm water or milk (Srikanthamurthy 1995, 2000). The ***Śāraṅgadhara saṃhitā*** recommends a similar preparation in the treatment of ***unmāda***, made up of the fresh juices of equal parts ***Brāhmī***, ***Kūṣmāṇḍa*** and ***Śaṅkhapuṣpī*** mixed with ***Kuṣṭha cūrṇa*** and honey (Srikanthamurthy 1984). A simpler preparation is made by decocting one part of the dried herb or fresh juice in four parts ***ghṛta*** and 16 water until all the water is evaporated. The resultant preparation is filtered and then applied as a ***nasya*** in doses of five drops per nostril in the treatment mental disorders. A similar preparation, but using sesame or coconut oil, results in a preparation that can be massaged into the feet, large joints and ears before sleep in the treatment of anxiety and depression. The ***Bhaiṣajyaratnāvalī*** mentions a complex formulation called ***Sārasvatariṣṭa***, a fermented beverage in which ***Brāhmī*** is the major constituent, used in the treatment of infertility, epilepsy and mental disorders, dosed between 12 and 24 mL twice daily. According to the ***Bhāvaprakāśa***, a ***lehya*** prepared from equal parts ***Brāhmī***, ***Vacā***, ***Harītakī***, ***Vāsaka*** and ***Pippalī*** mixed with honey is an effective treatment for hoarseness, enabling the patient to 'be able to sing along with the divine nymphs within seven days' (Srikanthamurthy 2000). Combined with equal parts ***Aśvagandhā*** and ***Kapikacchū***, ***Brāhmī*** may be helpful in the treatment of Parkinson's disease and epilepsy. In the treatment of Alzheimer's disease, ***Brāhmī*** may be helpful when combined with botanicals such as Ginkgo (*Ginkgo biloba*), Hawthorn (*Crataegus oxycanthoides*), Rosemary (*Rosmarinus officinalis*) and ***Haridrā***. In childhood ADD/ADHD, autism, and PDD ***Brāhmī*** may be of great help, used along with herbs such as Ling zhi (*Ganoderma lucidum*), Milky Oat seed (*Avena sativa*), Skullcap (*Scutellaria lateriflora*) and ***Aśvagandhā***. In unipolar depressive states and chronic fatigue ***Brāhmī*** may be helpful when used along with equal parts St John's Wort (*Hypericum perforatum*), Damiana (*Turnera diffusa*), Vervain (*Verbena hastata*) and American Ginseng (*Panax quinquefolium*). In the treatment of addiction and withdrawal, ***Brāhmī*** may be helpful when taken with equal parts California Poppy (*Eschscholzia californica*), Milky Oat seed (*Avena sativa*), ***Aśvagandhā*** and Skullcap (*Scutellaria lateriflora*), used in high doses as a weaning agent, or to reduce usage. In the treatment of hypothyroid conditions ***Brāhmī*** may be helpful when combined with equal parts each of ***Guggulu*** and Kelp (*Fucus vesiculosis*), with one half part each Iris root (*Iris versicolor*) and Oregon Grape root (*Mahonia aquifolium*). As a nootropic agent ***Brāhmī*** can be taken by itself or with other similar herbs such as ***Maṇḍūkaparṇī***, as the ***svarasa*** (fresh juice) or ***hima*** (infusion) to improve memory and retention by students, but only when taken regularly throughout a semester, not the evening before an exam.

Dosage:

- ***Cūrṇa***: 3–10 g b.i.d.–t.i.d.
- ***Svarasa***: 10–25 mL b.i.d.–t.i.d.
- ***Hima***: 1:4, 30–120 mL b.i.d.–t.i.d.
- ***Taila***: 1:4, ***ghṛta***, 12 g b.i.d.–t.i.d.; as ***abhyaṅga*** ad lib.; as ***nasya*** 5 gtt. in each nostril sd.
- ***Tincture***: 1:2, fresh plant; 1:4 recently dried herb, 1–10 mL b.i.d.–t.i.d.

REFERENCES

Bhattacharya SK, Bhattacharya A, Kumar A, Ghosal S 2000 Antioxidant activity of Bacopa monniera in rat frontal cortex, striatum and hippocampus. Phytotherapy Research: 14(3):174–179

Cakravarty AK, Garai S, Masuda K et al 2003 Bacopasides III-V: Three new triterpenoid glycosides from Bacopa monniera. Chemical and Pharmaceutical Bulletin (Tokyo) 51(2):215–217
Chowdhuri DK, Parmar D, Kakkar P et al 2002 Antistress effects of bacosides of Bacopa monniera: modulation of Hsp70 expression, superoxide dismutase and cytochrome P450 activity in rat brain. Phytotherapy Research 16(7):639–645
Dar A, Channa S 1999 Calcium antagonistic activity of Bacopa monniera on vascular and intestinal smooth muscles of rabbit and guinea-pig. Journal of Ethnopharmacology 66(2):167–174
Das A, Shanker G, Nath C et al 2002 A comparative study in rodents of standardized extracts of Bacopa monniera and Ginkgo biloba: anticholinesterase and cognitive enhancing activities. Pharmacology, Biochemistry, and Behavior 73(4):893–900
Dash B 1991 Materia medica of Ayurveda. B. Jain Publishers, New Delhi, p 101
Garai S, Mahato SB, Ohtani K, Yamasaki K 1996a. Dammarane-type triterpenoid saponins from Bacopa monniera. Phytochemistry 42(3):815–820
Garai S, Mahato SB, Ohtani K, Yamasaki K 1996b Bacopasaponin D – a pseudojujubogenin glycoside from Bacopa monniera. Phytochemistry 43(2):447–449
Hou CC, Lin SJ, Cheng JT, Hsu FL 2002 Bacopaside III, bacopasaponin G, and bacopasides A, B, and C from Bacopa monniera. Journal of Natural Products 65(12):1759–1763
Kar A, Panda S, Bharti S 2002 Relative efficacy of three medicinal plant extracts in the alteration of thyroid hormone concentrations in male mice. Journal of Ethnopharmacology 81(2):281–285
Kirtikar KR, Basu BD 1935 Indian medicinal plants, 2nd edn, vols 1–4. Periodical Experts, Delhi, p 1816
Mahato SB, Garai S, Cakravarty AK 2000 Bacopasaponins E and F: two jujubogenin bisdesmosides from Bacopa monniera. Phytochemistry 53(6):711–714
Rastogi S, Pal R, Kulshreshtha DK 1994 Bacoside A3: a triterpenoid saponin from Bacopa monniera. Phytochemistry 36(1):133–137
Roodenrys S, Booth D, Bulzomi S et al 2002 Chronic effects of Brahmi (Bacopa monniera) on human memory. Neuropsychopharmacology 27(2):279–281
Sairam K, Rao CV, Babu MD, Goel RK 2001 Prophylactic and curative effects of Bacopa monniera in gastric ulcer models. Phytomedicine 8(6):423–430
Sharma PV 2002 Cakradatta: Sanskrit text with English translation. Chaukhamba, Varanasi p 194
Singh HK, Dhawan BN 1982 Effect of Bacopa monniera Linn. (brahmi) extract on avoidance responses in rat. Journal of Ethnopharmacology 5(2):205–214
Srikanthamurthy KR 1984 Śāraṅgadhara saṃhitā: a treatise on Ayurveda. Chaukhamba Orientalia, Varanasi, p 53
Srikanthamurthy KR 1995 Vāgbhaṭa's Aṣṭāñga Hrydayam. vol 3. Varanasi: Krishnadas Academy, p 60
Srikanthamurthy KR 2000 Bhāvaprakāśa of Bhavamiśra. vol 2. Varanasi: Krishnadas Academy, p 263, 313
Srikanthamurthy KR 2001 Bhāvaprakāśa of Bhāvamiśra, vol 1. Krishnadas Academy, Varanasi, p 274
Stough C, Lloyd J, Clarke J et al 2001 The chronic effects of an extract of Bacopa monniera (Brahmi) on cognitive function in healthy human subjects. Psychopharmacology 156(4):481–484
Sumathi T, Nayeem M, Balakrishna K et al 2002 Alcoholic extract of 'Bacopa monniera' reduces the in vitro effects of morphine withdrawal in guinea-pig ileum. Journal of Ethnopharmacology 82(2–3):75–81
Sumathy T, Govindasamy S, Balakrishna K, Veluchamy G 2002 Protective role of Bacopa monniera on morphine-induced brain mitochondrial enzyme activity in rats. Fitoterapia 73(5):381–385
Sumathy T, Subramanian S, Govindasamy S et al 2001 Protective role of Bacopa monniera on morphine induced hepatotoxicity in rats. Phytotherapy Research 15(7):643–645
Tripathi YB, Chaurasia S, Tripathi E et al 1996 Bacopa monniera Linn. as an anti-oxidant: mechanism of action. Indian Journal of Experimental Biology 34(6):523–526
Vohora D, Pal SN, Pillai KK 2000 Protection from phenytoin-induced cognitive deficit by Bacopa monniera, a reputed Indian nootropic plant. Journal of Ethnopharmacology 71(3):383–390
Warrier PK, Nambiar VPK, Ramankutty C (eds) 1994 Indian medicinal plants: a compendium of 500 species. vol 1. Orient Longman Hyderabad, p 235
Yoganarasimhan SN 2000 Medicinal plants of India, vol 2: Tamil Nadu. Self-published, Bangalore, p 67

Candana, 'gladdening'

BOTANICAL NAME: *Santalum album*, Santalaceae

OTHER NAMES: Sandal (H); Candanam (T); Sandalwood (E); Tan xiang (C)

Botany: ***Candana*** is a medium-sized evergreen parasitic tree with slender drooping branches that, when mature, attains a height of up to 18 m. The rough bark is dark grey to brownish black with short vertical cracks, and the highly scented heartwood is yellowish brown in colour when fresh and becoming dark reddish brown with oxidation. The leaves are simple, opposite, elliptic-lanceolate and glabrous. The flowers are brownish or reddish purple borne in axillary paniculate cymes, giving rise to globose fruits. ***Candana*** is found in the dry deciduous forests of south India on stony but fertile soil, up to 1200 m in elevation. ***Candana*** and allied species are scattered widely from the Malay Archipelago to Australia and the Pacific islands, including Hawaii. In India only wild mature specimens of ***Candana*** between 30 and 50 years are considered suitable for harvesting, and this relatively slow growth complexed with a consistently high demand for this product, as well as illegal poaching, forest fires and disease, has made it a threatened species. India currently does not allow the export of any *S. album* timber. A similar species that is native to Australia and identified as *S. spicatum* is currently being used as a substitute for *S. album* (Evans 1989, Hamilton & Conrad 1990, Kirtikar & Basu 1935, Warrier et al 1996).

Part used: Dried heartwood, essential oil.

Dravyguṇa:

- ***Rasa***: *tikta*
- ***Vipāka***: *laghu*
- ***Vīrya***: *śita, rūkṣa*
- ***Karma***: *pittakaphahara, medhyam, balya, mūtraviśodhana, hṛdaya, chedana, dāhapraśamana, śoṇitasthāpana, jvaraghna, kuṣṭhaghna.*
- ***Prabhāva***: ***Candana*** is said to be ***āhlādana*** ('gives happiness') (Dash 1991, Frawley & Lad 1986, Nadkarni 1954, Srikanthamurthy 2001, Warrier et al 1996).

Constituents: The heartwood of ***Candana*** contains an essential oil called sandalwood oil, 90% of which are the sesquiterpene alcohols α and β-santalol, and 6% sesquiterpene hydrocarbons including α and β-santalenes, epi-β-santalene, and α and β-curcumenes. The α and β-santalols are responsible for the characteristic odour and colour of sandalwood oil. Other constituents in the essential oil include dihydro-β-agarofuran, santene, teresantol, borneol, teresantalic acid, santalone, santanol and tricyclo-ekasantalal. The bark contains tannins, fatty acids and a waxy material. The essential oil of *S. spicatum* is said to contain a very similar range of constituents to *S. album*, as well as the sesquiterpene furan dendrolasin that has a sweet, lemongrass fragrance (Duke 1985, Evans 1989, Walker 1968, Yoganarasimhan 2000).

Medical research:

- ***In vitro***: anti-HSV–1 and –2 (Benencia & Courreges 1999), antibacterial (Ochi et al 2005).
- ***In vivo***: chemopreventative (Banerjee et al 1993, Dwivedi et al 2003), antitumour (Dwivedi & Abu-Ghazaleh 1997), hypotensive (Bourke et al 1973).

Toxicity: Possible cytochrome P450 inducement in high doses long term (Jones et al 1994). The essential oil reported to have a 'baneful effect upon the kidneys' in larger doses, taken internally (Nadkarni 1954).

Indications: Gastric irritability, dysentery, biliousness, jaundice, cough, bronchitis, fever, inflammatory skin diseases, herpes, skin cancer, poisoning, thirst, haemorrhage, burning sensations, cystitis, menorrhagia, leukorrhoea, headache, memory loss, psychosis, depression, cardiac debility, palpitations, arrhythmia.

Contraindications: Renal disease; ***vātakopa***; concurrent usage with pharmaceuticals; beware of common adulterants to the oil, such as castor and cedar wood oil.

Medicinal uses: ***Candana*** has long been esteemed in India as not only a useful medicine, but as an important construction material that is highly resistant to decay, and as an important fragrance in Hindu ceremonies, often applied to the forehead by devout Hindus as a ***tilak*** to pacify the ***doṣas*** of the mind. To this end the ***Cakradatta*** mentions ***Candanādi lepa*** in the treatment of headache, composed of equal parts powders of ***Candana***, ***Uśīra***, ***Yaṣṭimadhu***, ***Balā***, ***Vyāghranakha*** and ***Nīlotpala***, mixed with milk, prepared as a paste and applied to the head (Sharma 2002). Several texts, including the ***Caraka saṃhitā***, ***Cakradatta*** and ***Śārańgadhara saṃhitā***, mention a complex polyherbal medicated oil that contains ***Candana*** as the chief ingredient, called ***Cañdanādya taila***, taken internally and applied topically in the treatment of spiritual possession, epilepsy, mental disorders, haemorrhage and consumptive conditions (Sharma 2002, Srikanthamurthy 1984). On a more mundane level, ***Candana*** is specific to ***paittika*** disorders, the ground powder applied topically as a paste made with cool water or milk for inflammatory skin conditions such as herpes, scabies, pruritis, prickly heat and insect bites, and internally as an emulsion in the treatment of gastric irritability, dysentery, thirst and heat stroke. In mild tachycardia (i.e. 'tobacco heart') ***Candana*** is stated to have a calming nervine effect, slowing heart rate and promoting contentment and relaxation (Nadkarni 1954). Bensky & Gamble (1986) mention that ***Candana*** is used with the Chinese herbs Dan shen (*Salvia miltorrhiza*) and Xi xin (*Asarum sieboldii*) for angina pectoris. The essential oil of ***Candana*** is a useful remedy in afflictions of the urinary tract, such as cystitis, gonorrhoea and pyelitis, and can be used in similar dosages for irritating coughs and bronchitis. The Eclectic physicians Felter and Lloyd (1893) state that the oil is specific to '. . . subacute and chronic affections of mucous tissues, particularly gonorrhoea after the active symptoms have been mitigated'. An emulsion of the wood mixed with sugar, honey and rice is used to check gastric irritability (Nadkarni 1954). When mixed with zinc oxide ointment (10%, v/v), the essential oil is a useful adjunct in the treatment of herpetic lesions, reapplied every few hours over a period of days until the inflammation ceases. Owing to its astringent and cooling qualities, ***Candana*** is a useful haemostatic and a specific to a group of diseases called ***rakta pitta***, all of which are characterised by haemorrhage, as well as ***daha***, or 'burning sensations'. To this end ***Candana*** is taken both internally and applied topically, in the latter case either as a paste mixed with cool milk or decocted and then cooled as a bath. Due to its drying (***rūkṣa***) properties a decoction of ***Candana*** is also recommended by the ***Aṣṭāñga Hṛdaya*** as ***dravya*** for ***vasanta ṛtucaryā*** (spring regimen) to relieve excess ***kapha*** (Srikanthamurthy 1994).

Dosage:

- ***Cūrṇa***: 3–5 g b.i.d.–t.i.d.
- ***Kvātha***: 1:4, 30–90 mL b.i.d.–t.i.d.
- ***Tincture***: 1:5, 50% alcohol, 1–4 mL b.i.d.–t.i.d.
- ***Essential oil***: 5–10 gtt (encapsulated, suspended in *Acacia* gum powder or similar) b.i.d.–t.i.d.

REFERENCES

Banerjee S, Ecavade A, Rao AR 1993 Modulatory influence of sandalwood oil on mouse hepatic glutathione S-transferase activity and acid soluble sulphydryl level. Cancer Letters 68(2–3):105–109

Benencia F, Courreges MC 1999 Antiviral activity of sandalwood oil against herpes simplex viruses–1 and –2. Phytomedicine 6(2):119–123

Bensky D, Gamble A 1993 Chinese herbal medicine materia medica, revised edn. Eastland Press, Seattle, p 240

Bourke EL, Matsumoto SY, Tam RF et al 1973 A hypotensive agent in Santalum ellipticum. Planta Medica 23(2):110–114

Dash B 1991 Materia medica of Ayurveda. B. Jain Publishers, New Delhi, p 32

Duke JA 1985 Handbook of medicinal herbs. CRC Press, Boca Raton, p 426

Evans WC 1989 Trease and Evan's pharmacognosy, 13th edn. Baillière-Tindall, London, p 474

Felter HW, Lloyd JU 1893 King's American dispensatory. Available: http://www.ibiblio.org/herbmed/eclectic/kings/main.html

Frawley D, Lad V 1986 The yoga of herbs: an Ayurvedic guide to herbal medicine. Lotus Press, Santa Fe, p 213

Dwivedi C, Abu-Ghazaleh A 1997 Chemopreventive effects of sandalwood oil on skin papillomas in mice. European Journal of Cancer Prevention 6(4):399–401

Dwivedi C, Guan X, Harmsen WL et al 2003 Chemopreventive effects of alpha-Santalol on skin tumor development in CD–1 and SENCAR mice. Cancer Epidemiology, Biomarkers and Prevention 12(2):151–156

Hamilton L, Conrad CE eds 1990 Proceedings of the Symposium on Sandalwood in the Pacific, April 9–11, 1990, Honolulu. USDA Forest Service, Albany

Jones GP, Birkett A, Sanigorski A et al 1994 Effect of feeding quandong (Santalum acuminatum) oil to rats on tissue lipids, hepatic cytochrome p-450 and tissue histology. Food and Chemical Toxicology 32(6):521–525

Kirtikar KR, Basu BD 1935 Indian medicinal plants, 2nd edn, vols 1–4. Periodical Experts, Delhi, p 2186

Nadkarni KM 1954 The Indian materia medica, with Ayurvedic, Unani and home remedies, revised and enlarged by AK Nadkarni. Popular Prakashan PVP, Bombay, p 1099–1102

Ochi T, Shibata H, Higuti T et al 2005 Anti-Helicobacter pylori compounds from Santalum album. Journal of Natural Products 68(6):819–824

Sharma PV 2002 Cakradatta. Sanskrit text with English translation. Chaukhamba, Varanasi, p 144, 562

Srikanthamurthy KR 1984 Śāraṅgadhara saṃhitā: a treatise on Ayurveda. Chaukhamba Orientalia, Varanasi

Srikanthamurthy KR 1994 Vāgbhaṭa's Aṣṭāñga Hrydayam, vol 1. Krishnadas Academy, Varanasi, p 37, 135

Srikanthamurthy KR 2001 Bhāvaprakāśa of Bhāvamiśra, vol 1. Krishnadas Academy, Varanasi, p 208

Walker GT 1968 Sandalwood oil: the chemistry of oil of sandalwood. Perfumery and Essential Oil Record 59:778–785

Warrier PK, Nambiar VPK, Ramankutty C (eds) 1996 Indian medicinal plants: a compendium of 500 species, vol 5. Orient Longman, Hyderabad, p 57

Yoganarasimhan SN 2000 Medicinal plants of India, vol 2: Tamil Nadu. Self-published, Bangalore, p 481

Citraka, 'the spotted one'

BOTANICAL NAMES: *Plumbago zeylanica, P. rosea,* Plumbaginaceae

OTHER NAMES: Chita, Chitri, Chiti (H); Chittiramulam, Vellai (T); White-flowered Leadwort (E)

Botany: ***Citraka*** is a perrenial and sometimes woody herb, with many stout cylindrical roots that exude a yellowish juice when cut. The leaves are thin, 3.8–7.5 cm by 2.2–3.8 cm, ovate, subacute, glabrous above and somewhat glaucous below, with a short petiole. The white (*P. zelanica*) or bright red (*P. rosea*) flowers are borne in elongated spikes, the calyx covered in sessile glands, the corolla tube slender, about four times as long as the calyx. The flower gives way to an elongated, oblong capsule. ***Citraka*** is found throughout India, Sri Lanka and the Malay Archipelago in moist, tropical locations (Kirtikar & Basu 1935, Warrier et al 1995).

Part used: Root, whole plant.

Dravyguṇa:

- ***Rasa***: *kaṭu*
- ***Vipāka***: *kaṭu*
- ***Vīrya***: *uṣṇa, rūkṣa, tikṣṇa, laghu*
- ***Karma***: *dīpanapācana, grāhī, kṛmighna, chedana, kāsahara, svāsahara, raktaprasādana, kuṣṭhaghna, mūtravirecana, śothahara, medohara, rasāyana, vātakaphahara* (Srikanthamurthy 2001, Warrier et al 1995).

Constituents: The root and root bark of ***Citraka*** contain the yellow naphthoquinone pigment plumbagin and other chemically related naphthoquinones including droserone, dihydroserone, elliptinone, nisoshinanolone, plumbazeylanone isozeylinone, napthoquinonemethylene3′ 3-diplumbagin, chitranone, maritinone, elliptinone, isoshinanolone 2-methylnaphthazarin, plumbazeylone and zeylone. Two plumbagic acid glucosides (3′-*O*-β-glucopyranosyl plumbagic acid and 3′-*O*-β-glucopyranosyl plumbagic acid methylester) have been isolated, as well as the coumarins seselin, 5-methoxyseselin, suberosin, xanthyletin and xanthoxyletin (Lin et al 2003, Yoganarasimhan 2000).

Medical research:

- ***In vitro***: antibacterial (Durga et al 1990, Wang & Huang 2005), antitumour (Prasad et al 1996), anti-oxidant (Tilak et al 2004).
- ***In vivo***: hypolipidaemic (Sharma et al 1991), anti-atherogenic (Sharma et al 1991), antibacterial (Abdul & Ramchender 1995), antitumour (Devi et al 1994, Parimala & Sachdanandam 1993), dopaminergic (Bopaiah et al 2001), anti-allergenic (Dai et al 2004)

Toxicity: The 24-hour oral LD_{50} of an ethanolic root extract of *Plumbago rosea* in mice was determined to be 1148.15 mg/kg (Solomon et al 1993). The oral LD_{50} of plumbagin in mice was stated to be 10 mg/kg (Williamson 2002).

Indications: Dyspepsia, flatulent colic, malabsorption, haemorrhoids, intestinal parasites, hepatosplenomegaly, cough, bronchitis, chronic and intermittent fever, skin diseases, amenorrhoea, anaemia, inflammatory joint disease.

Contraindications: Pregnancy, constipation, ***pittakopa***. ***Citraka*** is traditionally considered to be a potentially caustic agent with abortifacient properties and should be used with care, preferably in formulation.

Medicinal uses: The etymology of ***Citraka*** is not clear, the term 'spotted' perhaps referring to the glands on the calyx, or to the leopard, which is also called ***Citraka***, in reference to the idea that ***Citraka*** moves quickly to remove disease, like the leopard catches its prey. Krishnamurthy (1991) speculates that the term may refer to holes left on the dried primary root from fallen lateral roots. ***Citraka*** is among the most potent and active remedies to stimulate digestion and dispel accumulated ***kapha*** and ***āma***, but because of its fiery properties should be used with caution, and is most often used in formulation. It finds representation in many different formulations that are commonly used in Āyurveda, used to treat digestive disorders and oedema. It has a powerful irritant effect and no less so upon the uterus for which at one time it was used rather dangerously to procure abortion when applied topically to the cervix (Kirtikar & Basu 1935). In the treatment of malabsorptive syndromes, haemorrhoids, abdominal pain and swelling, and splenomegaly the ***Cakradatta*** recommends a simple medicated ***ghṛta*** made from ***Citraka*** (Sharma 2002). The ***Bhāvaprakāśa*** recommends ***Citrakadi guṭikā*** ('pills') in the treatment of ***grahaṇī***, or malabsorption. The ***Cakradatta*** recommends ***Citrakadya ghṛta*** as a ***vajīkaraṇa*** in both women and men, and corrector of disorders of the urinary tract. ***Citrakadya ghṛta*** is prepared by mixing 10 g each of ***Citraka***, ***Sārivā***, ***Balā***, ***Kālanusārivā***, ***Drākṣā***, ***Viśala***, ***Pippalī***, ***Indravaruni***, ***Yaṣṭimadhu*** and ***Āmalakī*** with 2.56 kg of ***ghṛta*** decocted in 10.24 litres of milk, reduced to the original volume of ***ghṛta***. When complete 640 grams each of sugar and ***Vaṃśarocanā*** are added (Sharma 2002). ***Citraka*** also makes its way into the very popular formula ***Yogarājaguggulu***, a remedy that '. . . stimulates the digestive fire, promotes energy and strength, and overcomes ***vāttika*** (***vāta***) disorders even if located in the joints and marrow' (Sharma 2002).

Dosage:

- ***Cūrṇa***: 500–1000 mg, b.i.d.–t.i.d.
- ***Ghṛta***: 3–5 g, b.i.d.–t.i.d.

REFERENCES

Abdul KM, Ramchender RP 1995 Modulatory effect of plumbagin (5-hydroxy-2-methyl-1,4-naphthoquinone) on macrophage functions in BALB/c mice. I. Potentiation of macrophage bactericidal activity. Immunopharmacology 30(3):231–236

Bopaiah CP, Pradhan N 2001 Central nervous system stimulatory action from the root extract of Plumbago zeylanica in rats. Phytotherapy Research 15(2):153–156

Dai Y, Hou LF, Chan YP et al 2004 Inhibition of immediate allergic reactions by ethanol extract from Plumbago zeylanica stems. Biological and Pharmaceutical Bulletin 27(3):429–432

Devi PU, Solomon FE, Sharada AC 1994 In vivo tumor inhibitory and radiosensitizing effects of an Indian medicinal plant, Plumbago rosea on experimental mouse tumors. Indian Journal of Experimental Biology 32(8):523–528

Durga R, Sridhar P, Polasa H 1990 Effects of plumbagin on antibiotic resistance in bacteria. Indian Journal of Medical Research 91:18–20

Kirtikar KR, Basu BD 1935 Indian medicinal plants, 2nd edn, vols 1–4. Periodical Experts, Delhi, p 1466–1467, 1469

Krishnamurthy KH 1991 Wealth of Suśruta. International Institute of Āyurveda, Coimbatore, p 407

Lin LC, Yang LL, Chou CJ 2003 Cytotoxic naphthoquinones and plumbagic acid glucosides from Plumbago zeylanica. Phytochemistry 62(4):619–622

Parimala R, Sachdanandam P 1993 Effect of Plumbagin on some glucose metabolising enzymes studied in rats in experimental hepatoma. Molecular and Cellular Biochemistry 125(1):59–63

Prasad VS, Devi PU, Rao BS, Kamath R 1996 Radiosensitizing effect of plumbagin on mouse melanoma cells grown in vitro. Indian Journal of Experimental Biology 34(9):857–858

Sharma PV 2002 Cakradatta. Sanskrit text with English translation. Chaukhamba, Varanasi, p 82, 250, 316

Sharma I, Gusain D, Dixit VP 1991 Hypolipidaemic and anti-atherosclerotic effects of plumbagin in rabbits. Indian Journal of Physiology and Pharmacology 35(1):10–14

Shoba FG, Thomas M 2001 Study of antidiarrhoeal activity of four medicinal plants in castor-oil induced diarrhoea. Journal of Ethnopharmacology 76(1):73–76

Solomon FE, Sharada AC, Devi PU 1993 Toxic effects of crude root extract of Plumbago rosea (Rakta citraka) on mice and rats. Journal of Ethnopharmacology 38(1):79–84

Srikanthamurthy KR 2001 Bhāvaprakāśa of Bhāvamiśra, vol 1. Krishnadas Academy, Varanasi, p 169

Tilak JC, Adhikari S, Devasagayam TP 2004 Anti-oxidant properties of Plumbago zeylanica, an Indian medicinal plant and its active ingredient, plumbagin. Redox Report 9(4):219–227

Wang YC, Huang TL 2005 Anti-Helicobacter pylori activity of Plumbago zeylanica L. FEMS Immunology and Medical Microbiology 43(3):407–412

Warrier PK, Nambiar VPK, Ramankutty C (eds) 1995 Indian medicinal plants: a compendium of 500 species, vol 4. Orient Longman, Hyderabad, p 321

Williamson EM (ed) 2002 Major herbs of Ayurveda. Churchill Livingstone, London, p 242

Yadav SK, Jain AK, Tripathi SN, Gupta JP 1989 Irritable bowel syndrome: therapeutic evaluation of indigenous drugs. Indian Journal of Medical Research 90:496–503

Yoganarasimhan SN 2000 Medicinal plants of India, vol 2: Tamil Nadu. Self-published, Bangalore, p 426

Devadāru, 'wood of the gods'

BOTANICAL NAME: *Cedrus deodara*, Pinaceae

OTHER NAMES: Dedwar, Deodar (H); Tevadaram, Tevadaru (T); Himalayan Cedar (E)

Botany: ***Devadāru*** is a large conifer that attains a height of between 20 and 45 m, pyramidal in shape when young but becoming irregularly shaped with age. The bark is dark, almost black in colour, the branches horizontal and spreading, the leading shoot and tips usually drooping. The needle-like leaves are stiff, about 2.5–3.8 cm long, borne in dense whorls of 20–30 per cluster. The flowers are usually monoecious, the male catkins solitary and cylindrical, producing clouds of yellow, wind-blown pollen in early spring. The egg-shaped female cones are bluish green, 10–12.5 cm long, solitary, carried on the ends of the branchlets, and release pale brown seeds with papery wings after about two years. ***Devadāru*** is found throughout the Himalayas and Hindu Kush mountain ranges, from 1000 to 3500 m in elevation, usually growing in full sunlight (Kirtikar & Basu 1935, Warrier et al 1994).

Part used: Heartwood.

Dravyguṇa:

- ***Rasa***: *tikta*
- ***Vipāka***: *kaṭu*
- ***Vīrya***: *uṣṇa*
- ***Karma***: *dīpanapācana, bhedana, kṛmighna, jvaraghna, hṛdaya, mūtravirecana, mūtraviśodhana, śotahara, vedanāsthāpana, kaphavātahara* (Srikanthamurthy 2001, Warrier et al 1994).

Constituents: The primary component of interest in ***Devadāru*** is the essential oil, which contains *p*-methylacetophenone, *p*-methyl-δ-3-tetrahydroacetophenone, alantone, the sesquiterpene alcohols himachalol, allohimachalol, α and β-himachalenes, as well as cedrol and limonene. Other constituents that have been isolated from the wood include the flavonoids deodarin, cedeodarin, cedrin, cedrinoside and quercitin, as well as the sesquiterpene himasedone, isoprimaric acid, deodadione, carboxylic acid, cedrusin, cedrusinin, matairesinol, nortrachelogenin, and a dibenzylbutyrolactollignan (Kapoor 1990, Tiwari et al 2001, Yoganarasimhan 2000).

Medical research:

- ***In vitro***: anti-oxidant (Tiwari et al 2001).
- ***In vivo***: anti-inflammatory (Shinde et al 1999a, b), analgesic (Shinde et al 1999b), antifungal (Chowdhry et al 1997), antispasmodic (Kar et al 1975), hypotensive (Kar et al 1975)

Toxicity: No data found.

Indications: Fever, dyspepsia, colic, flatulence, haemorrhoids, hiccough, bronchitis, renal and vesical calculi, stranguary, oedema, diabetes, skin diseases, ulcers, wounds, epilepsy, heart disease, pain, inflammation, headache.

Contraindications: ***pittakopa***, in large doses.

Medicinal uses: ***Devadāru*** is called the 'wood of the gods' because it grows in the Himalayan mountain range, said to be the abode of the god ***Śiva***, nurtured by the 'breastmilk' (melting snow) of his consort, ***Pārvatī*** (Sharma 1993). ***Devadāru*** is also used in Hindu religious ceremonies, mentioned in the epic ***Rāmāyaṇa*** as a fragrant wood used to build the funeral pyre. In regard to its medicinal uses, the ***Bhāvaprakāśa*** mentions that ***Devadāru*** is useful to remove ***āma*** from the ***āmāśaya*** (Srikanthamurthy 2001). To this extent ***Devadāru*** is used in the treatment of fever, particularly of the bilious variety, to rekindle ***agni*** and restore weakened hepatic secretions. ***Devadāru*** is also used as an anodyne, either singly or in combination, taken internally and applied topically. In diarrhoea ***Devadāru*** has a tonic action, restoring tone to the muscular fibres (Nadkarni 1954), and thus finds application in rectal prolapse (Kirtikar & Basu 1935). Applied topically, the powder and distilled oil is often used in the treatment of ulcers as an anti-infective and vulnerary, and has traditionally formed topical therapies targeted to leprosy (Kirtikar & Basu 1935). The ***Bhāvaprakāśa*** mentions ***Devadāru*** as one of the chief ingredients in ***Devadārvyādi kvātha***, used post-partum as a restorative and tonic (Srikanthamurthy 2000). Combined with equal parts ***Harītakī***, ***Vāsaka***, ***Śālaparṇī***, ***Śūṇṭhī*** and ***Āmalakī***, taken with honey, the ***Śāraṅgadhara saṃhitā*** recommends ***Devadāru*** in the treatment of fever, dyspnoea, cough and dyspepsia (Srikanthamurthy 1984). In the treatment of ***vāta***-type variants of headache, the ***Śāraṅgadhara saṃhitā*** recommends a ***lepa*** prepared with equal parts powders of ***Devadāru***, ***Nata***, ***Kuṣṭha***, ***Jaṭāmāmsī*** and ***Śūṇṭhī***, mixed with rice water and oil, applied over the head (Srikanthamurthy 1984).

Dosage:

- ***Cūrṇa***: 3–5 g, b.i.d.–t.i.d.
- ***Kvātha***: 1:4, 30–90 mL b.i.d.–t.i.d.
- ***Tincture***: 1:5, 50% alcohol, 1–3 mL b.i.d.–t.i.d.

REFERENCES

Chowdhry L, Khan ZK, Kulshrestha DK 1997 Comparative in vitro and in vivo evaluation of himachalol in murine invasive aspergillosis. Indian Journal of Experimental Biology 35(7): 727–734

Kapoor LD 1990 CRC Handbook of Ayurvedic medicinal plants. CRC Press, Boca Raton, p 110

Kar K, Puri VN, Patnaik GK et al 1975 Spasmolytic constituents of Cedrus deodara (Roxb.) Loud: pharmacological evaluation of himachalol. Journal of Pharmaceutical Sciences 64(2): 258–262

Kirtikar KR, Basu BD 1935 Indian medicinal plants, 2nd edn, vols 1–4. Periodical Experts, Delhi, p 2390–2391

Nadkarni KM 1954 The Indian materia medica, with Ayurvedic, Unani and home remedies, revised and enlarged by A.K. Nadkarni. Popular Prakashan PVP, Bombay, p 295

Sharma PV 1993 Essentials of Āyurveda: ṣodaśāṅgahṛdayam. Motilal Banarsidass, New Delhi, p 21

Shinde UA, Kulkarni KR, Phadke AS et al 1999a Mast cell stabilizing and lipoxygenase inhibitory activity of Cedrus deodara (Roxb.) Loud. wood oil. Indian Journal of Experimental Biology 37(3): 258–261

Shinde UA, Phadke AS, Nair AM et al 1999b Studies on the anti-inflammatory and analgesic activity of Cedrus deodara (Roxb.) Loud. wood oil. Journal of Ethnopharmacology 65(1): 21–27

Srikanthamurthy KR 1984 Śāraṅgadhara saṃhitā: a treatise on Ayurveda. Chaukhamba Orientalia, Varanasi, p 63, 242

Srikanthamurthy KR 2000 Bhāvaprakāśa of Bhāvamiśra, vol 2. Krishnadas Academy, Varanasi, p 798

Srikanthamurthy KR 2001 Bhāvaprakāśa of Bhāvamiśra, vol 1. Krishnadas Academy, Varanasi, p 210

Tiwari AK, Srinivas PV, Kumar SP, Rao JM 2001 Free radical scavenging active components from Cedrus deodara. Journal of Agricultural and Food Chemistry 49(10): 4642–4645

Warrier PK, Nambiar VPK, Ramankutty C (eds) 1994 Indian medicinal plants: a compendium of 500 species, vol 2. Orient Longman, Hyderabad, p 41–44

Yoganarasimhan SN 2000 Medicinal plants of India, vol 2: Tamil Nadu. Self-published, Bangalore, p 119

Elā

BOTANICAL NAME: *Elettaria cardamomum,* Zingiberaceae

OTHER NAMES: ***Sūkṣma Elā*** (S); Elachi (H); Elam (T); Cardamom (E)

Botany: ***Elā*** is a perennial plant with thick, fleshy rhizomes and leafy stems, attaining a height of between 1.2 and 5 m. The leaves are subsessile, 30–60 cm long and 7.5 cm wide, oblong-lanceolate, and pubescent below. The flowers are borne in panicles that arise from the base of the vegetative shoots, upright at first but eventually becoming prostrate. The flower bracts are persistent, linear-oblong, up to 5 cm in length. The calyx is 1–3 cm long, the whitish convex lip streaked with violet. The oblong seed capsule is about 2.5 cm long, and marked with fine vertical ribs. ***Elā*** exhibits considerable variation under cultivation, which has led to much confusion regarding its identification. There are two primary varieties within this species: *E. cardamomum* var. *major*, which comprises the 'wild' or indigenous Cardamom found in Sri Lanka, and *E. cardamomum* var. *minuscula*, originally derived from the former, and now comprising several cultivated races grown in Sri Lanka, South India and, more recently, Central America. Among the cultivated varietals, *Mysore* fruits have a creamy pale colour and a smooth surface; *Malabar* fruits are smaller, less smooth and have a darker colour; *Mangalore* fruits are similar in colour to *Malabar* but are rounder and have a rough pericarp; *Allepy* are narrower and the pericarp has a striated appearance, and varies in colour from buff-green to green; *Ceylon* resemble *Allepy* but are longer and usually greener. The seed capsules are dried slowly, and in some cases bleached in the sun or with burning sulphur; more often, however, an attempt is made to preserve the green colour of the capsule by soaking them in a 2% sodium carbonate solution for 10 minutes (Evans 1989, Kirtikar & Basu 1935, Warrier et al 1994).

Part used: Seeds.

Dravyguṇa:

- ***Rasa***: *kaṭu, madhura*
- ***Vipāka***: *madhura*
- ***Vīrya***: *śita, laghu, rūkṣa*
- ***Karma***: *dīpanapācana, anulomana, chardinigrahaṇa, śulapraśamana, arśoghna, chedana, kāsahara, svāsahara, hṛdaya, vajīkaraṇa, vātakaphahara* (Dash 1991, Nadkarni 1954, Srikanthamurthy 2001, Warrier et al 1994).

Constituents: ***Elā*** is noted and valued for its volatile oil, which constitutes between 2.8 and 8% of the seed's total weight (averaging about 4%). Among the many components of the oil are cineol, terpineol, terpinene, limonene, sabinene, camphene, camphor, *p*-cymene, cineol, α-ylangene, nerolidol, eugenyl-acetate and borneol. Other constituents include cardiolipin, phosphatidyl-ethanolamine, phosphatidyl-inositol, starch, gum, a yellow colouring agent, mucilage, fibre, manganese and calcium oxalate (al-Zuhair et al 1996, Duke 2003, Evans 1989, Kapoor 1990)

Medical research:

- ***In vivo***: anti-inflammatory, antispasmodic (al-Zuhair et al 1996), gastrostimulant (Vasudevan et al 2000).

Toxicity: ***Elā*** is commonly used as a culinary spice and is generally recognised as safe. Duke (2002) reports that borneol, cineol and limonene are irritants, and limonene is a photosensitiser.

Indications: Toothache, dyspepsia, colic, diarrhoea, malabsorption, haemorrhoids, colds, cough, bronchitis, asthma, hoarseness, enuresis, dysuria, spermatorrhoea, headache.

Contraindications: Duke (2002) reports that Cardamom may trigger colic in cholelithiasis; ulcers; ***pittakopa***.

Medicinal uses: ***Elā*** is lauded by Āyurvedic physicians as one of the best and safest digestive agents in the materia medica. Although it is a pungent-tasting herb it has a cool ***vīrya***, and is thus considered ***sattvic***. Unlike many stimulants it is unlikely to provoke a negative reaction in ***paittika*** conditions, and thus can be found as a mild ***dīpanapācana*** adjunct in many different Āyurvedic formulae. ***Elā*** has a long history as one of the most valuable and expensive of spices, long imported from India and Sri Lanka into the Middle East and Europe, used by both ancient Greek and Arabic physicians. ***Elā*** is an important stomachic and carminative, used in colic, flatulence and convalescence after diarrhoea, and as an adjunct to purgative formulations to reduce griping. It is added to coffee in the Middle East as a flavour and to ameliorate the negative effects of caffeine. Nadkarni (1954) mentions a compound powder containing equal parts ***Elā***, ***Śūṇṭhī***, ***Lavaṅga*** and ***Jīraka*** as a useful stomachic in atonic dyspepsia. When the powders of ***Patra*** leaf, ***Tvak*** bark and ***Elā*** are mixed together in equal proportions this is called ***Trisugandhā cūrṇa*** (the 'three aromatics'), and when these are combined with ***Nāgakeśara*** the formula is called ***Cāturjātaka cūrṇa***; both are used in the treatment of ***kaphaja*** conditions, and tend to promote dryness, lightness and heat in the body (Srikanthamurthy 1984). The ***Cakradatta*** recommends a variation of a compound called ***Elādi cūrṇa*** in the treatment of severe cases of dysuria, comprising equal parts ***Elā***, ***Pāṣāṇabheda***, ***Śilājatu*** and ***Pippalī***, mixed with water and jaggery and consumed as a ***lehya*** (Sharma 2002). The ***Bhaiṣajyaratnāvalī*** recommends another ***Elādi cūrṇa*** in the treatment of bronchitis and asthma consisting of equal parts ***Elā***, ***Lavaṅga***, ***Nāgakeśara***, ***Mustaka***, ***Candana***, ***Pippalī***, ***Kolamajja***, ***Lāja*** and ***Priyaṅgu***, taken with honey and sugar (India 1978). This latter version of ***Elādi cūrṇa*** is mentioned in the ***Cakradatta*** as a treatment for nausea and vomiting (Sharma 2002). ***Elā*** combined with equal parts ***Pippalī***, ***Gokṣura***, ***Yaṣṭimadhu***, ***Pāṣāṇabheda***, ***Reṇukā*** and ***Eraṇḍa***, and mixed with a larger proportion of ***Śilājatu***, is recommended by the ***Cakradatta*** for urinary calculi and gravel (Sharma 2002). In the treatment of fever, anorexia, vomiting, fainting, giddiness, cough, asthma, haemoptysis and chest wounds the ***Cakradatta*** recommends ***Elādi guṭikā***, comprising ***Elā*** seed, ***Tvak*** bark and ***Patra*** leaf (5 g each), ***Pippalī*** (20 g), and ***Yaṣṭimadhu***, ***Kharjūra*** and ***Drākṣā*** (40 g each), and powdered sugar, mixed with honey to make pills, 10 g daily (Sharma 2002).

Dosage:

- ***Cūrṇa***: seeds, 2–3 g, b.i.d.–t.i.d.
- ***Phāṇṭa***: crushed pods, 1:4, 30–60 mL, b.i.d.–t.i.d.
- ***Tincture***: crushed pods, 1:5, 60% alcohol, 1–2 mL, b.i.d.–t.i.d.

REFERENCES

al-Zuhair H, el-Sayeh B, Ameen HA, al-Shoora H 1996 Pharmacological studies of cardamom oil in animals. Pharmacological Research 34(1–2):79–82

Dash B 1991 Materia medica of Ayurveda. B. Jain Publishers, New Delhi, p 169

Duke J 2002 Handbook of medicinal herbs, 2nd edn. CRC Press, Boca Raton, p 154

Duke J accessed 2003 Chemicals. In: Elettaria cardamomum (L.) MATON (Zingiberaceae): Cardamom. Dr Duke's phytochemical and ethnobotanical databases. Agricultural Research Services. Available from http://www.arsgrin.gov/duke/

Evans WC 1989 Trease and Evan's Pharmacognosy, 13th edn. Baillière-Tindall, London, p 469, 470

India, Department of Health 1978 The Ayurvedic formulary of India, Part 1. Controller of Publications, Delhi, p 87

Kapoor LD 1990 CRC Handbook of Ayurvedic medicinal plants. CRC Press, Boca Raton, p 172

Kirtikar KR, Basu BD 1935 Indian medicinal plants, 2nd edn, vols 1–4. Periodical Experts, Delhi, p 2442

Nadkarni KM 1954 The Indian materia medica, with Ayurvedic, Unani and home remedies, revised and enlarged by A.K. Nadkarni. Popular Prakashan PVP, Bombay, p 475, 476

Sharma PV 2002 Cakradatta. Sanskrit text with English translation. Chaukhamba, Varanasi, p 125, 170, 310, 321

Srikanthamurthy KR 1984 Śāraṅgadhara saṃhitā: a treatise on Ayurveda. Chaukhamba Orientalia, Varanasi, p 86

Srikanthamurthy KR 2001 Bhāvaprakāśa of Bhāvamiśra, vol 1. Krishnadas Academy, Varanasi, p 216

Vasudevan K, Vembar S, Veeraraghavan K, Haranath PS 2000 Influence of intragastric perfusion of aqueous spice extracts on acid secretion in anesthetized albino rats. Indian Journal of Gastroenterology 19(2):53–56

Warrier PK, Nambiar VPK, Ramankutty C (eds) 1994 Indian medicinal plants: a compendium of 500 species, vol 2. Orient Longman, Hyderabad, p 360–364

Yoganarasimhan SN 2000 Medicinal plants of India, vol 2: Tamil Nadu. Self-published, Bangalore

Gokṣura, 'cow scratcher'

BOTANICAL NAME: *Tribulus terrestris*, Zygophyllaceae

OTHER NAMES: Gokhuru, Gokshri (H); Nerunji (T); Calthrops, Puncture-vine (E); Bai ji li (C)

Botany: **Gokṣura** is a procumbent annual or perennial herb with many spreading slender branches, the immature portions covered in a fine silky hair. The leaves are oppositely arranged, pinnate, with three to eight simple leaflets that are almost sessile to the leaf stem, with appressed hairs below, and to a lesser extent above. The solitary yellow flowers have five petals, and are borne in the leaf axils, on hairy pedicles up to 2 cm long. The fruits are globose, composed of five woody cocci that bear two pairs of sharp spines, each coccus containing several seeds. **Gokṣura** is found throughout Asia, the Middle East, Africa, and southern Europe, in sandy soils, often along roadsides and waste areas (Kirtikar & Basu 1935, Warrier et al 1996).

Part used: Fruit and root.

Dravyguṇa:

- ***Rasa***: *madhura*
- ***Vipāka***: *madhura*
- ***Vīrya***: *śita, snigdha*
- ***Karma***: *dīpanapācana, bhedana, kṛmighna, chedana, kāsahara, svāsahara, kuṣṭaghna vedanāsthāpana, mūtravirecana, aśmaribhedana, mūtraviśodhana, śothahara, dāhapraśamana, raktaprasādana, hṛdaya, vajīkaraṇa, balya, tridoṣahara.*
- ***Prabhāva***: *sattvic;* promotes clarity of mind, and corrects *apāna vāyu* (Frawley & Lad 1986, Kirtikar & Basu 1935, Nadkarni 1954, Srikanthamurthy 2001, Warrier et al 1996).

Constituents: Researchers have isolated numerous steroidal saponins from **Gokṣura**, including cistocardin, diosgenin, tribuloin, hecogenin, dioscin, and ruscogenin, as well as several unnamed steroidal constituents. Researchers have also isolated a furostanol diglycoside, the lignanamides tribulusamides A and B, *N*-trans-feruloyltyramin, terrestriamide, *N*-trans-coumaroyltyramine, and β-sitosterol (Achenbach et al 1994, Cai et al 2001, Li et al 1998, Sun et al 2002, Xu et al 2000, 2001). Kapoor (1990) reports an unidentified alkaloid in the fruit in trace amounts. Investigation of the aerial portions of **Gokṣura** has yielded the furostanol saponin methylprotodioscin and protodioscin and the sodium salt of methylprototribestin and prototribestin, L-mannitol and an inorganic salt, as well as the two β-carboline indoleamines harmane and norharmane. **Gokṣura** is a rich source of calcium (Bourke et al 1992, Duhan et al 1992, Kostava et al 2002).

Medical research:

- ***In vitro***: antispasmodic (Arcasoy et al 1998), hepatoprotective (Li et al 1998), antifungal (Bedir et al 2002), antitumour (Bedir et al 2002).
- ***In vivo***: androgenic, aphrodisiac activity (Gauthaman et al 2002); erectile stimulating (Adaikan et al 2000); antidiabetic (Li et al 2002); diuretic, antilithic (Anand et al 1994).
- ***Human trials***: a clinical trial of 406 cases of coronary heart disease treated with the saponin fraction of *Tribulus terrestris* resulted in the remission rate of 82.3%, without side-effects (Wang et al 1990).

Toxicity: The herbaceous portions of **Gokṣura** is the cause of geeldikkop in sheep and other small livestock, a condition characterized by oedema of the head, fever and jaundice (Kirtikar & Basu 1935). Two β-carboline indoleamines (harmane and norharmane) isolated from the plant material of *Tribulus terrestris* have been implicated in causing central nervous system effects in sheep that have grazed on *Tribulus* over a period of months. Researchers proposed that harmane and norharmane accumulate in tryptamine-associated neurones of the central nervous system and gradually interact irreversibly with a specific neuronal gene DNA sequence (Bourke et al 1992). Photosensitisation and cholangiohepatopathy have been noted in sheep grazing on *Tribulus terrestris* (Tapia et al 1994). A recent paper reports gynecomastia in a young male body-builder taking *Tribulus* as an anabolic agent (Jameel et al 2004).

Indications: Haemorrhoids, intestinal parasites, cough, dyspnoea, asthma, consumption, hives, dysuria, haematuria, urinary lithiasis, cystitis, nephritis, urinary tenesmus, spermatorrhoea, impotence, frigidity, infertility, venereal diseases, cardiovascular disease, gout, rheumatism, lumbago, sciatica, menorrhagia, postpartum haemorrhage, anaemia, diabetes, opthalmia, headache, insufficient lactation.

Contraindications: Dehydration (Frawley & Lad 1986); pregnancy (Bensky & Gamble 1993).

Medicinal uses: ***Gokṣura*** is an outstanding remedy in urogenital disease, promoting urine flow, soothing the mucosa, and aiding in the excretion of stones and calculi (Frawley & Lad 1986). Unlike diuretics such as Bearberry leaf (*Artostaphylos uva ursi*), ***Gokṣura*** pacifies ***vāta*** and will not promote secondary effects such as dry skin. Nadkarni (1954) mentions that both the plant and seeds are used in decoction or infusion in the treatment of spermatorrhoea, impotence, infertility, phosphaturia, dysuria, gonorrhoea, gleet, chronic cystitis, renal calculi, incontinence, gout, and postpartum haemorrhage. In most cases of cystitis a simple decoction of the fruit or the tincture will suffice, although in severe cystitis botanicals such as Marshmallow root (*Althaea officinalis*) or Corn Silk (*Zea mays*) can be used in combination for additional demulcent properties. In severe tenesmus and pain it may be used along with Kava root (*Piper methysticum*) or Henbane (*Hyocyamus niger*). For urinary lithiasis ***Gokṣura*** may be combined with Buchu herb (*Barosma betulina*) and Gravel root (*Eupatorium purpurea*). For urinary incontinence and bedwetting a combination of ***Gokṣura*** and Mullein (*Verbascum thapsus* root) may be helpful to strengthen the trigone muscle of the bladder. ***Gokṣura*** is highly esteemed as a ***vajīkaraṇa rasāyana***. In the treatment spermatorrhoea and impotence equal parts powders of ***Gokṣura***, ***Tila***, ***Kapikacchū*** and ***Aśvagandhā*** may be taken with honey, ***ghṛta*** and goat's milk, 12 g b.i.d. on an empty stomach at dawn and at dusk. For frigidity and infertility ***Gokṣura*** may be taken in equal parts ***Śatāvarī*** root and Damiana, 5–10 g b.i.d. Frawley & Lad (1986) consider ***Gokṣura*** to be a ***rasāyana*** for ***pitta***, and state that it is effective in ***vātakopa*** conditions, the harmine alkaloids most likely contribute to ***Gokṣura's*** sedative properties. It may be taken with ***Aśvagandhā*** as a tonic nervine in ***vāttika*** disorders such as nervousness and anxiety. For lumbar pain ***Gokṣura*** may be combined with ***Śūṇṭhī***, Kava (*Piper methysticum*) and Wild Yam (*Dioscorea villosa*). Warrier et al (1996) mention that the ash of the whole plant is good for external application in rheumatoid arthrtis. Topically, the oil of the seed is used in the treatment of alopecia (Frawley & Lad 1986). In Chinese medicine ***Gokṣura*** is used in the treatment of headache, vertigo and dizziness due to ascendant liver yang and wind-heat (Bensky & Gamble 1993). As a ***vajīkaraṇa***, the ***Bhāvaprakāśa*** recommends ***Gokṣurādi modaka***, composed of equal parts powders of ***Gokṣura***, ***Ikṣura bīja***, ***Aśvagandhā***, ***Śatāvarī***, ***Musalī***, ***Kapikacchū***, ***Yaṣṭimadhu***, ***Nāgabalā*** and ***Balā***. These powders are mixed togther and fried in an equal volume of ***ghṛta***, eight parts milk and two parts sugar until most of the liquid is evaporated, after which the extract is then rolled in pills, taken in dosages according the strength and needs of the individual (Srikanthamurthy 2000). In the treatment of diabetes and urinary tract disorders the ***Śārańgadhara saṃhitā*** recommends ***Gokṣurādi guggulu***, prepared by boiling four parts of ***Gokṣura*** in six times the amount of water until the original volume of water is reduced by half. The decoction is then strained from the herb, and one part ***Guggulu*** resin is added and mixed in with the decoction, to which is added one part each the powders of ***Triphala***, ***Trikaṭu*** and ***Mustaka***. The ***Śārańgadhara*** also states that ***Gokṣurādi guggulu*** is useful in menorrhagia, gout, diseases of the nervous system, and infertility (Srikanthamurthy 1984).

Dosage:

- ***Cūrṇa***: 3–6 g b.i.d.–t.i.d.
- ***Kvātha***: 30–90 mL b.i.d.–t.i.d.
- ***Tincture***: dried fruit, 1:3, 50%; 3–5 mL b.i.d.–t.i.d.

REFERENCES

Achenbach H et al 1994 Cardioactive steroid saponins and other constituents from the aerial parts of Tribulus cistoides. Phytochemistry 35(6):1527–1543

Adaikan PG, Gauthaman K, Prasad RN, Ng SC 2000 Proerectile pharmacological effects of Tribulus terrestris extract on the rabbit corpus cavernosum. Annals of the Academy of Medicine (Singapore) 29(1):22–26

Al-Ali M, Wahbi S, Twaij H, Al-Badr A 2003 Tribulus terrestris: preliminary study of its diuretic and contractile effects and comparison with Zea mays. Journal of Ethnopharmacology 85(2–3):257–260

Anand R et al 1994 Activity of certain fractions of Tribulus terrestris fruits against experimentally induced urolithiasis in rats. Indian Journal of Experimental Biology 32(8):548–552

Arcasoy HB et al 1998 Effect of Tribulus terrestris L. saponin mixture on some smooth muscle preparations: a preliminary study. Bollettino Chimico Farmaceutico 137(11):473–475

Bedir E, Khan IA 2000 New steroidal glycosides from the fruits of Tribulus terrestris. Journal of Natural Products 63(12):1699–1701

Bedir E, Khan IA, Walker LA 2002 Biologically active steroidal glycosides from Tribulus terrestris. Die Pharmazie 57(7):491–493

Bensky D, Gamble A 1993 Chinese herbal medicine materia medica, revised edn. Eastland Press, Seattle, p 425

Bourke CA et al 1992 Locomotor effects in sheep of alkaloids identified in Australian Tribulus terrestris. Australian Veterinary Journal 69(7):163–165

Cai L, Wu Y, Zhang J et al 2001 Steroidal saponins from Tribulus terrestris. Planta Medica 67(2):196–198

Duhan A et al 1992 Nutritional value of some non-conventional plant foods of India. Plant foods for human nutrition 42(3):193–200

Frawley D, Lad V 1986 The Yoga of herbs: an Ayurvedic guide to herbal medicine. Lotus Press, Santa Fe, p 169–170

Gauthaman K, Adaikan PG, Prasad RN 2002 Aphrodisiac properties of Tribulus terrestris extract (Protodioscin) in normal and castrated rats. Life Sciences 71(12):1385–1396

Jameel JK, Kneeshaw PJ, Rao VS, Drew PJ 2004 Gynaecomastia and the plant product Tribulis terrestris. Breast (Edinburgh, Scotland) 13(5):428–430

Kapoor LD 1990 CRC handbook of Ayurvedic medicinal plants. CRC Press, Boca Raton, p 325

Kirtikar KR, Basu BD 1935 Indian medicinal plants, 2nd edn, vols 1–4. Periodical Experts, Delhi, p 420–423

Kostova I, Dinchev D, Rentsch GH et al 2002 Two new sulfated furostanol saponins from Tribulus terrestris. Zeitschrift für Naturforschung 57(1–2):33–38

Li JX et al 1998 Tribulusamide A and B, new hepatoprotective lignanamides from the fruits of Tribulus terrestris: indications of cytoprotective activity in murine hepatocyte culture. Planta Medica 64(7):628–631

Li M, Qu W, Wang Y et al 2002 Hypoglycemic effect of saponin from Tribulus terrestris. Zhong Yao Cai 25(6):420–422

Nadkarni KM 1954 The Indian materia medica, with Ayurvedic, Unani and home remedies, revised and enlarged by A.K. Nadkarni. Popular Prakashan PVP, Bombay, p 1230

Srikanthamurthy KR 1984 Śāraṅgadhara saṃhitā: a treatise on Ayurveda. Chaukhamba Orientalia, Varanasi, p 109

Srikanthamurthy KR 2000 Bhāvaprakāśa of Bhavamiśra, vol 2. Krishnadas Academy, Varanasi, p 829

Srikanthamurthy KR 2001 Bhāvaprakāśa of Bhāvamiśra, vol 1. Krishnadas Academy, Varanasi, p 234

Sun W, Gao J, Tu G 2002 A new steroidal saponin from Tribulus terrestris Linn. Natural Product Letters 16(4):243–247

Tapia MO 1994 An outbreak of hepatogenous photosensitization in sheep grazing Tribulus terrestris in Argentina. Veterinary and Human Toxicology 36(4):311–313

Warrier PK, Nambiar VPK, Ramankutty C (eds) 1996 Indian medicinal plants: a compendium of 500 species, vol 5. Orient Longman, Hyderabad, p 311

Wang B, Ma L, Liu T 1990 406 cases of angina pectoris in coronary heart disease treated with saponin of Tribulus terrestris. Zhong Xi Yi Jie He Za Zhi 10(2):68, 85–87

Xu YJ, Xie SX, Zhao HF et al 2001 Studies on the chemical constituents from Tribulus terrestris. Yao Xue Xue Bao 36(10):750–753

Xu YX, Chen HS, Liang HQ et al 2000 Three new saponins from Tribulus terrestris. Planta Medica 66(6):545–550

Guḍūcī

BOTANICAL NAME: *Tinospora cordifolia,* Menispermaceae

OTHER NAMES: ***Amṛta***, 'nectar' (S); Gulancha, guḍaach (H); Amridavalli, Chintilikoti (T); Tinospora (E); Kuan jin teng (T. sinensis) (C)

Botany: ***Guḍūcī*** is a large deciduous perennial climber with large succulent stems and papery bark, sending down long, pendulous fleshy roots as it climbs. The leaves are glabrous and cordate, with seven to nine veins. ***Guḍūcī*** is monoecious with yellowish white flowers with six petals borne on racemes, the male flowers clustered in the axils of small subulate bracts, the female flowers usually solitary, with three carpels. The mature drupes are red in colour, marked with a sub-basal style-scar (Kirtikar & Basu 1935, Warrier et al 1996).

Part used: Stem.

Dravyguṇa:

- ***Rasa***: *tikta, kaśāya, madhura*
- ***Vipāka***: *madhura*
- ***Vīrya***: *langhana, uṣṇa*
- ***Karma***: *dīpanapācana, grāhī, jvaraghna, dāhapraśamana, kāsahara, kustaghna, hṛdaya, chedana, vajīkaraṇa, rasāyana, tridoṣahara* (Dash 1991, Dash & Junius 1983, Kirtikar & Basu 1935, Srikanthamurthy 2001, Warrier et al 1996).

Constituents: Researchers have isolated a variety of constituents for ***Guḍūcī***, including alkaloids, glycosides, steroids, and other compounds. Among the alkaloidal constituents are the isoquinolines berberine and jatrorrhizine, and aporphine-type alkaloids magnoflorine and tembestarine. Glycosides include the bitter tasting gilion, tinocordiside, tinocordifolioside, cordioside, syringin, syringin-apiosylglycoside, palmatosides C and F, cordifolisides A–E, and diterpenoid lactones (clerodane derivatives, tinosporon, tinosporidine, tinosporides, jateorine, columbin). Steroidal constituents consist of β-sitosterol, δ-sitosterol, tingilosterol, hydroxyl ecdysone, ecdysterone, makisterone A and giloinsterol. Other constituents include the sesquiterpenoid tinocordifolin, aliphatic compounds octacosanol, heptacosanol and nonacosan-15-one, a non-glycoside bitter principle called gilenin, and the polysaccharide arabinogalactan (Chintalwar et al 1999, Gangan et al 1994, Kapil & Sharma 1997, Singh et al 2003, Swaminathan et al 1989a, b, Yoganarasimhan 2000).

Medical research:

- ***In vitro***: immunostimulant (Kapil & Sharma 1997, Thatte et al 1992, 1994) antitumour (Jagetia et al 1998), antioxidant (Mathew & Kuttan 1997).
- ***In vivo***: immunomodulant (Bishayi et al 2002, Manjrekar et al 2000, Nagarkatti et al 1994), anti-jaundice (Rege et al 1989), antidiabetic (Grover et al 2000, Prince & Menon 1999, Stanely et al 2000, 2001), hypoglycaemic (Wadood et al 1992), antioxidant (Mathew & Kuttan 1997; Prince & Menon 1999; Stanely et al 2001), hypolipidaemic (Stanely et al 1999).
- ***Human trials***: ***Guḍūcī*** promoted a highly significant reduction in sneezing, nasal discharge, nasal obstruction and nasal pruritus in patients suffering from allergic rhinitis, compared to placebo (Badar et al 2005).

Toxicity: No data found.

Indications: Dyspepsia, vomiting, hypochondriac pain, flatulence, intestinal parasites, intermittent and chronic fever, burning sensations, cough, asthma, cardiac debility, hepatitis, jaundice, anaemia, skin diseases, thirst, debility and weakness, gout, arthritis, disorders of the genitourinary tract, diabetes.

Contraindications: Pregnancy.

Medicinal uses: According to tradition, ***Guḍūcī*** is said to have origination from the epic battle of the ***Rāmāyaṇa*** in which the God-king ***Rāma*** lays siege to the island of Lanka, home of the evil King ***Rāvaṇa***. When ***Rāvaṇa*** is finally defeated King ***Indra*** is so pleased with the result that he sprinkles ***amṛta*** (nectar) on the bodies of the slain monkeys to bring them back to life. In all the places where the nectar dribbled down from the bodies of the monkeys, the ***Guḍūcī*** plant is said to have grown. For this reason ***Guḍūcī*** is also called ***Amṛta***, but also because ***Guḍūcī*** is one of the best agents in the materia medica of India to treat ***āma*** conditions without aggravating or upsetting the ***doṣas***. To this extent ***Guḍūcī*** is ***tridoṣahara***, the ***kaśāya*** and ***tikta rasas*** pacifying ***pitta*** and ***kapha***, and the ***madhura vipāka*** and ***uṣṇa vīrya*** reducing ***vāta***. It is particularly suited in chronic debilitated conditions with autotoxicity, clearing the body of accumulated wastes (***āma***), stimulating digestion (***agni***), and restoring the energy systems of the body (***ojas***). It is widely used by Āyurvedic physicians for a variety of conditions, and finds its way into many different formulations, especially in the treatment of diabetes, in which it is often combined with ***Śilājatu***. ***Guḍūcī*** is often used along with circulatory stimulants such as ***Śūṇṭhī*** in the treatment of ***āmavāta*** (rheumatoid arthritis), to reduce the symptoms of inflammation and pain. Although classified in many ***nighaṇṭus*** as warming in energy, the balance between its bitter and sweet tastes also makes ***Guḍūcī*** specific to disorders and deficiencies of the liver, blood, and skin, and to reduce the vitiations of ***pitta***. Thus ***Guḍūcī*** is often used to treat liver disorders, including hepatitis and jaundice, as well as anaemia. The ***Bhāvaprakāśa*** mentions a series of formulations called ***Guḍūcī ghṛta***, the simplest forms prepared from a decoction of ***Guḍūcī*** dried herb or fresh juice, with ***ghṛta*** and water, in the treatment of gout, leprosy, jaundice, anaemia, splenomegaly, cough and fever (Srikanthamurthy 2000). According to the ***Cakradatta*** a similar preparation made with sesame oil is used for a similar range of conditions, including itching and ringworm (Sharma 2002). In the treatment of all types of ***jvara*** or fever, with loss of appetite, nausea, thirst and vomiting, the ***Bhāvaprakāśa*** recommends a decoction called ***Guḍūcī kvātha***, composed of equal parts ***Guḍūcī***, ***Dhānyaka***, ***Nimba***, ***Padmaka*** and ***Raktacandana*** (Srinkanthamurthy 2000). In the treatment of vomiting, the ***Cakradatta*** recommends a cold infusion (***hima***) with honey (Sharma 2002). As a rejuvenative the ***Cakradatta*** recommends ***Guḍūcyadi rasāyana***, made up of equal parts powders of ***Guḍūcī***, ***Viḍaṅga***, ***Śaṅkhapuṣpī***, ***Vacā***, ***Harītakī***, ***Kuṣṭha***, ***Śatāvarī*** and ***Apāmārga***, taken with ***ghṛta*** as an ***anupāna***. The ***Cakradatta*** states that this formula '. . . makes one capable of memorizing a thousand stanzas in only three days' (Sharma 2002).

Dosage:

- ***Cūrṇa***: 3–5 g b.i.d.–t.i.d.
- ***Kvātha***: 30–90 mL b.i.d.–t.i.d.
- ***Tincture***: fresh stem, 1:2, 95%; 2–5 mL b.i.d.–t.i.d.

REFERENCES

Badar VA, Thawani VR, Wakode PT et al 2005 Efficacy of Tinospora cordifolia in allergic rhinitis. Journal of Ethnopharmacology 96(3):445–449

Bishayi B, Roychowdhury S, Ghosh S, Sengupta M 2002 Hepatoprotective and immunomodulatory properties of Tinospora cordifolia in CC14 intoxicated mature albino rats. Journal of Toxicological Sciences 27(3):139–146

Chintalwar G, Jain A, Sipahimalani A 1999 An immunologically active arabinogalactan from Tinospora cordifolia. Phytochemistry 52(6):1089–1093

Dash B 1991 Materia medica of Ayurveda. B. Jain Publishers, New Delhi, p 14

Dash B, Junius M 1983 A handbook of Ayurveda. Concept Publishing, New Delhi, p 139

Gangan VD, Pradhan P, Sipahimalani AT, Banerji A 1994 Cordifolisides A, B, C: norditerpene furan glycosides from Tinospora cordifolia. Phytochemistry 37(3):781–786

Grover JK, Vats V, Rathi SS 2000 Anti-hyperglycemic effect of Eugenia jambolana and Tinospora cordifolia in experimental diabetes and their effects on key metabolic enzymes involved in carbohydrate metabolism. Journal of Ethnopharmacology 73(3):461–470

Jagetia GC, Nayak V, Vidyasagar MS 1998 Evaluation of the anti-neoplastic activity of guduchi (Tinospora cordifolia) in cultured HELA cells. Cancer Letters 127(1–2):71–82

Kapil A, Sharma S 1997 Immunopotentiating compounds from Tinospora cordifolia. Journal of Ethnopharmacology 58(2):89–95

Kirtikar KR, Basu BD 1935 Indian medicinal plants, 2nd edn, vols 1–4. Periodical Experts, Delhi, p 77–78

Manjrekar PN, Jolly CI, Narayanan S 2000 Comparative studies of the immunomodulatory activity of Tinospora cordifolia and Tinospora sinensis. Fitoterapia 71(3):254–257

Mathew S, Kuttan G 1997 Anti-oxidant activity of Tinospora cordifolia and its usefulness in the amelioration of cyclophosphamide induced toxicity. Journal of Experimental and Clinical Cancer Research 16(4):407–411

Nagarkatti DS, Rege NN, Desai NK, Dahanukar SA 1994 Modulation of Kupffer cell activity by Tinospora cordifolia in liver damage. Journal of Postgraduate Medicine 40(2):65–67
Prince PS, Menon VP 1999 Anti-oxidant activity of Tinospora cordifolia roots in experimental diabetes. Journal of Ethnopharmacology 65(3):277–281
Rege NN, Nazareth HM, Bapat RD, Dahanukar SA 1989 Modulation of immunosuppression in obstructive jaundice by Tinospora cordifolia. Indian Journal of Medical Research 90:478–483
Rege N, Bapat RD, Koti R 1993 Immunotherapy with Tinospora cordifolia: a new lead in the management of obstructive jaundice. Indian Journal of Gastroenterology 12(1):5–8
Sharma PV 2002 Cakradatta. Sanskrit text with English translation. Chaukhamba, Varanasi, p 169, 236, 626
Singh SS, Pandey SC, Srivastava S et al 2003 Chemistry and medicinal properties of Tinospora cordifolia (guduchi). Indian Journal of Pharmacy 35: 83–91
Srikanthamurthy KR 2000 Bhāvaprakāśa of Bhavamiśra, vol 2. Krishnadas Academy, Varanasi, p 17
Srikanthamurthy KR 2001 Bhāvaprakāśa of Bhāvamiśra, vol 1. Krishnadas Academy, Varanasi, p 402
Stanely P, Prince M, Menon VP, Gunasekaran G 1999 Hypolipidaemic action of Tinospora cordifolia roots in alloxan diabetic rats. Journal of Ethnopharmacology 64(1):53–57
Stanely P, Prince M, Menon VP 2000 Hypoglycaemic and other related actions of Tinospora cordifolia roots in alloxan-induced diabetic rats. Journal of Ethnopharmacology 70(1):9–15
Stanely P, Prince M, Menon VP 2001 Anti-oxidant action of Tinospora cordifolia root extract in alloxan diabetic rats. Phytotherapy Research 15(3):213–218
Swaminathan K, Sinha UC, Ramakumar S et al 1989a. Structure of columbin, a diterpenoid furanolactone from Tinospora cordifolia Miers. Acta Crystallographica (Section C) 45 (Pt 2): 300–303
Swaminathan K, Sinha UC, Bhatt RK et al 1989b Structure of tinosporide, a diterpenoid furanolactone from Tinospora cordifolia Miers. Acta Crystallographica (Section C) 45 (Pt 1):134–136
Thatte UM, Kulkarni MR, Dahanukar SA 1992 Immunotherapeutic modification of Escherichia coli peritonitis and bacteremia by Tinospora cordifolia. Journal of Postgraduate Medicine 38(1):13–15
Thatte UM, Rao SG, Dahanukar SA 1994 Tinospora cordifolia induces colony stimulating activity in serum. Journal of Postgraduate Medicine 40(4):202–203
Wadood N, Wadood A, Shah SA 1992 Effect of Tinospora cordifolia on blood glucose and total lipid levels of normal and alloxan-diabetic rabbits. Planta Medica 58(2):131–136
Warrier PK, Nambiar VPK, Ramankutty C (eds) 1996 Indian medicinal plants: a compendium of 500 species, vol 5. Orient Longman, Hyderabad, p 283
Yoganarasimhan SN 2000 Medicinal plants of India, vol 2: Tamil Nadu. Self-published, Bangalore, p 547–548

Guggulu

BOTANICAL NAMES: *Commiphora mukul, C. molmol, C. abyssinica,* Burseraceae

OTHER NAMES: ***Mahiṣākṣa*** (S); Gugal (H); Gukkal (T); Bdellium (E); Mo yao (C); 'Myrrh' is *C. myrrha*, called *Bola* in Sanskrit; 'Frankincense' is another similar species in the Bursuraceae called *Kuñduru* (*Boswellia serrata*)

Botany: ***Guggulu*** is a small shrubby tree, 1.2–1.8 m in height, with knotty and crooked branches that terminate in a sharp spine. The compound leaves are composed of one to three subsessile leaflets, rhomboid-ovate in shape, serrate along the upper margin and tapering at the base, the leaf surface shining and smooth, the lateral leaflets usually half the size of the terminal leaflet. The flowers are borne in fascicles of two or three, the calyx campanulate, glandular and hairy, the petals brownish red, nearly three times the length of the calyx. The flowers give way to a red drupe when ripe, 6–8 mm in diameter. ***Guggulu*** is found throughout the subcontinent of India, the Middle East and Africa, particularly in dry arid locales (Kirtikar & Basu 1935, Warrier et al 1994).

Part used: Oleogum resin, exuding from the cracks and fissures in the bark, or from incisions. Crude ***Guggulu*** may contain the oleogum resin from several different species. Warrier et al (1994) states that the best quality ***Guggulu*** is that which melts and evaporates with heat, bursts into flame when burned, and dissolves easily in hot water.

Dravyguṇa:

- ***Rasa***: *tikta, kaśāya, kaṭu*
- ***Vipāka***: *kaṭu, laghu*
- ***Vīrya***: *uṣṇa, rūkṣa*
- ***Karma***: *pācana, rasāyana, vajīkaraṇa, balya, kṛmighna, vedanāsthāpana, raktaprasādana, ārtavajanana, aśmaribhedana, sandhānīya, svarya, vātakaphahara.*
- ***Prabhāva:*** Although *Guggulu* is stated to be *uṣṇa* in *vīrya*, the *Bhāvaprakāśa* states that due to its *kaśāya rasa* it also reduces *pitta*, and is therefore *tridoṣaghna* (Srikanthamurthy 2001, Warrier et al 1994).

Constituents: The oleogum resin of ***Guggulu*** is a mixture of 30–60% water-soluble gum, 20–40% alcohol-soluble resins, and about 8% volatile oils. Among the water-soluble constituents is a mucilage, arabinose and proteins. Alcohol-soluble constituents include the commiphoric acids, commiphorinic acid and the heerabomyrrhols. Among the volatile constituents are terpenes, sesquiterpenoids, cuminic aldehyde, eugenol, myrcene, α-camphorene, the ketone steroids Z- and E-guggulsterone, and guggulsterols I, II and III. The sesquiterpenoid fraction within the essential oil contains a group of furanosesquiterpenoids that give ***Guggulu*** its primary odour. Also found in ***Guggulu*** are the lignans guggullignan I and II. (Blumenthal et al 2000, Bradley 1992, Evans 1989, Williamson 2002, Wu et al 2002, Zhu et al 2001). Gugulipid is a proprietary standardised extract of the oleogum resin that does not contain the gum or the base fraction of the resin.

Medical research:

- ***In vitro***: hypocholesterolaemic (Cui et al 2003, Urizar et al 2002, Wu et al 2002), antimicrobial (Asres et al 1998, Dolara et al 2000)
- ***In vivo***: hypocholesterolaemic (Singh et al 1990, Urizar et al 2002), antithrombotic (Olajide 1999), cardioprotective (Seth et al 1998), hypotensive (Abdul-Ghani & Amin 1997), thyrostimulant (Panda & Kar 1999), anti-inflammatory (Kimura et al 2001; Tariq et al 1986), anti-arthritic (Sharma & Sharma 1977), antitumour (al-Harbi et al 1994, Qureshi et al 1993)

- ***Human trials***: compared to placebo, Gugulipid significantly decreased total serum cholesterol, LDL, and triglycerides in patients with hypercholesterolaemia (Singh et al 1994); compared to clofibrate the use of Gugulipid in hypercholesterolaemic patients promoted a significant improvement in HDL to LDL ratios (Nityanand et al 1989); over a period of 30 days the administration of ***Guggulu*** was found to enhance weight loss in obese adults (>90 kg) eating a calorie-restricted diet, by an average of 2.25 kg (Bhatt et al 1995); over a 3-month period Gugulipid promoted slightly better results than tetracycline in the treatment of nodulocystic acne, with patients with oily faces responding best to the treatment (Thappa & Dogra 1994); ***Guggulu*** was found to be a safe and highly effective remedy in the treatment of Fasciola (liver fluke) infection over a 3-month period (Massoud et al 2001); ***Guggulu*** was found to be a safe and highly effective remedy in the treatment of schistosomiasis (Sheir et al 2001); ***Guggulu*** resin had a total curative effect in children diagnosed with fascioliasis and schistosomiasis, over a period of 4–12 weeks (Soliman et al 2004).

Toxicity: Acute (24 hour) and chronic (90 day) oral toxicity studies on *Commiphora molmol* were carried out in mice, using dosages of 0.5, 1.0 and 3 g/kg in the acute studies, and 100 mg/kg per day for the chronic study. Researchers found no significant difference in mortality in acute or chronic treatment as compared to controls, noting a significant increase in the weight of the testes, epididymides and seminal vesicles, as well as a significant increase in RBC and haemoglobin levels in the treatment group, compared to the control group (Rao et al 2001). In young male Nubian goats an oral dose of 0.25 g/kg per day was found to be non-toxic (i.e. 37.5 g in a 150 kg human) (Omer & Adam 1999). Myrrh has been reported to cause dermatitis in topical preparations used to relieve pain and swelling due to traumatic injury (Lee & Lam 1993).

Indications: Gingivitis, apthous ulcers, dyspepsia, candidiasis, chronic colitis, intestinal parasites, haemorrhoids, chronic fever, chronic upper respiratory tract infection, chronic muco-epithelial ulceration, strep throat, pharyngitis, bronchitis, cystitis, urinary calculi, spermatorrhoea, endometritis, amenorrhoea, menorrhagia, leucorrhoea, skin diseases, wounds, abrasions, chronic ulcers, arthritis, gout, lumbago, neurasthenia, diabetes, dyslipidaemia, atherosclerosis, hypothyroidism, anaemia, oedema, cancer, post-chemotherapy (to improve WBC count).

Contraindications: The ***Bhāvaprakāśa*** states that those undergoing therapy with ***Guggulu*** should avoid sour foods and drinks, uncooked foods, excessive physical and sexual activity, alcohol consumption, and excess exposure to heat and sunlight (Srikanthamurthy 2001). Generally speaking, ***Guggulu*** should be used with caution in ***pittakopa*** conditions. ***Guggulu*** is contraindicated with concurrent hypoglycaemic and lipotriptic therapies, thyrotoxicosis, thyroiditis and pregnancy. The effect of a single oral dose of Gugulipid was studied on bioavailability of single oral dose of propranolol (40 mg) and diltiazem (60 mg), and was found to significantly reduce the peak plasma concentration and area under curve of both the drugs in a small trial of healthy volunteers (Dalvi et al 1994).

Medicinal uses: ***Guggulu*** is a common ingredient in many Āyurvedic formulations, used both as a medicinal agent and excipient, such that an entire class of medicaments are called ***guggulu*** (e.g. ***Triphala guggulu***, ***Yogarāja guggulu***, ***Gokṣurādi guggulu***, etc.). In the treatment of boils and gout, the ***Bhāvaprakāśa*** recommends a preparation of ***Guggulu*** mixed with equal parts juice of ***Guḍūcī*** and ***Drākṣā*** macerated in a decoction of ***Triphala***. This preparation is evaporated in the hot sun or over heat to the correct consistency and rolled into pills of about 5 g and taken with honey (Srikanthamurthy 2001). As an antiseptic and vulnerary the ***Cakradatta*** recommends that ***Guggulu*** be mixed with a decoction of ***Triphala***, and applied topically (Sharma 2002). In the treatment of broken bones and fracture, the ***Cakradatta*** recommends an internal preparation comprising one part each ***Harītakī***, ***Trikaṭu*** and ***Triphala***, mixed with a portion of ***Guggulu*** equal to all of the above (Sharma 2002). In the treatment of sciatica the ***Cakradatta*** recommends a pill composed of 40 g ***Rāsnā*** and 50 g ***Guggulu***, mixed with ***ghṛta*** (Sharma 2002). In the treatment of ***vāttika*** disorders of muscles, bones, joints and nerves, the ***Cakradatta*** recommends a formula made up of ten parts ***Guggulu***, two parts each of ***Triphala*** and ***Pippalī***, and one part each ***Tvak*** bark and ***Elā*** seed, soaked in a decoction of ***Daśamūla***, and dried in the sun. When the appropriate consistency is obtained the mixture is then rolled into pills and dosed at 3–5 g, b.i.d.–t.i.d., taken with a diet rich in meat soups (Sharma 2002). The famous formula ***Yogarājaguggulu*** is prescribed in similar conditions. As a tincture, ***Guggulu*** is effective as a gargle in gingivitis, apthous ulcers, strep throat and pharyngitis, alone or with such herbs as Sage (*Salvia officinalis*). The tincture also has a vulnerary and antiseptic activity in gastrointestinal ulcers, both of the upper and lower tracts, although it is best avoided in active inflammation, used only after the initial inflammation has been dealt with by demulcent and vulnerary botanicals such as ***Yaṣṭimadhu***, Marshmallow (*Althaea officinalis*) and Slippery Elm (*Ulmus fulva*). Internally, the tincture improves digestion and stimulates the appetite in digestive atony, removing chronic catarrh in both the gastrointestinal and respiratory tracts. ***Guggulu*** also finds utility in urogenital infections after the active inflammation has been resolved, improving mucus membrane secretion and providing an antiseptic action against any lingering infection. In endometritis it may be combined with Purple Coneflower (*Echinacea angustifolia*), False Unicorn (*Chamaelirium luteum*), Chasteberry (*Vitex agnus castus*) and Dandelion root (*Taraxacum officinalis*) to check inflammation, remove infection and reorientate the oestrous cycle. In arthritis and gout ***Guggulu*** is particularly effective, combined with such herbs like Lignum vitae (*Guaicum officinalis*), Celery seed (*Apium graveolens*), and Devil's Claw (*Harpagophytum procumbens*), or used in formulations like ***Yogarāja guggulu***. In the treatment of dyslipidaemia, atherosclerosis and diabetes the use of the standardised extract called Gugulipid has shown promise, especially when taken with a low-carbohydrate diet and array of antioxidant minerals, vitamins and omega-3 fatty acids. For a more traditional approach, ***Guggulu*** may be combined with herbs such as ***Guḍūcī***, ***Āmalakī*** and ***Śilājatu*** in the treatment of diabetes. In chronic immunodeficiency, or in patients undergoing chemotherapy or taking corticosteroids, ***Guggulu*** may be combined with ***Aśvagandhā*** and ***Yaṣṭimadhu***.

Dosage:

- ***Cūrṇa***: 2–5 g b.i.d.–t.i.d.
- ***Tincture***: 2–5 mL (1:3 95%) b.i.d.–t.i.d.
- ***Standardized extract***: (equal to 25 mg guggulsterones), 500 mg b.i.d.–t.i.d.

REFERENCES

Abdul-Ghani AS, Amin R 1997 Effect of aqueous extract of Commiphora opobalsamum on blood pressure and heart rate in rats. Journal of Ethnopharmacology 57(3):219–222

al-Harbi MM, Qureshi S, Raza M et al 1994 Anticarcinogenic effect of Commiphora molmol on solid tumors induced by Ehrlich carcinoma cells in mice. Chemotherapy 40(5):337–347

Asres K, Tei A, Moges G et al 1998 Terpenoid composition of the wound-induced bark exudate of Commiphora tenuis from Ethiopia. Planta Medica 64(5):473–475

Bhatt AD, Dalal DG, Shah SJ et al 1995 Conceptual and methodologic challenges of assessing the short-term efficacy of Guggulu in obesity: data emergent from a naturalistic clinical trial. Journal of Postgraduate Medicine. 41(1):5–7

Blumenthal M, Goldberg A, Brinckmann J (eds) 2000 Herbal medicine: expanded Commission E monographs. American Botanical Council, Austin, p 275

Bradley PR (ed) 1992 British herbal compendium. British Herbal Medicine Association, Bournemouth, p 163

Cui J, Huang L, Zhao A et al 2003 Guggulsterone is a farnesoid X receptor antagonist in coactivator association assays but acts to enhance transcription of bile salt export pump. Journal of Biological Chemistry 278(12):10214–10220

Dalvi SS, Nayak VK, Pohujani SM et al 1994 Effect of gugulipid on bioavailability of diltiazem and propranolol. Journal of the Association of Physicians of India. 42(6):454–455

Dolara P, Corte B, Ghelardini C et al 2000 Local anaesthetic, antibacterial and antifungal properties of sesquiterpenes from myrrh. Planta Medica 66(4):356–358

Evans WC 1989 Trease and Evan's pharmacognosy, 13th edn. Baillière-Tindall, London, p 475

Kimura I, Yoshikawa M, Kobayashi S et al 2001 New triterpenes, myrrhanol A and myrrhanone A, from guggul-gum resins, and their potent anti-inflammatory effect on adjuvant-induced air-pouch granuloma of mice. Bioorganic and Medicinal Chemistry Letters 11(8):985–989

Kirtikar KR, Basu BD 1935 Indian medicinal plants, 2nd edn, vols 1–4. Periodical Experts, Delhi, p 527

Lee TY, Lam TH 1993 Allergic contact dermatitis due to a Chinese orthopaedic solution tieh ta yao gin. Contact Dermatitis 28(2):89–90

Massoud A, El Sisi S, Salama O, Massoud A 2001 Preliminary study of therapeutic efficacy of a new fasciolicidal drug derived from Commiphora molmol (myrrh). American Journal of Tropical Medicine and Hygiene 65(2):96–99

Nadkarni KM 1954 The Indian materia medica, with Ayurvedic, Unani and home remedies, revised and enlarged by A.K. Nadkarni. Popular Prakashan PVP, Bombay

Nityanand S, Srivastava JS, Asthana OP 1989 Clinical trials with gugulipid. A new hypolipidaemic agent. Journal of the Association of Physicians of India 37(5):323–328

Olajide OA 1999 Investigation of the effects of selected medicinal plants on experimental thrombosis. Phytotherapy Research 13(3):231–232

Omer SA, Adam SE 1999 Toxicity of Commiphora myrrha to goats. Veterinary and Human Toxicology 41(5):299–301

Panda S, Kar A 1999 Gugulu (Commiphora mukul) induces triiodothyronine production: possible involvement of lipid peroxidation. Life Sciences 65(12):PL137–141

Qureshi S, al-Harbi MM, Ahmed MM et al 1993 Evaluation of the genotoxic, cytotoxic, and antitumor properties of Commiphora molmol using normal and Ehrlich ascites carcinoma cell-bearing Swiss albino mice. Cancer Chemotherapy and Pharmacology 33(2):130–138

Rao RM, Khan ZA, Shah AH 2001 Toxicity studies in mice of Commiphora molmol oleo-gum-resin. Journal of Ethnopharmacology 76(2):151–154

Seth SD, Maulik M, Katiyar CK, Maulik SK 1998 Role of Lipistat in protection against isoproterenol induced myocardial necrosis in rats: a biochemical and histopathological study. Indian Journal of Physiology and Pharmacology 42(1):101–106

Sharma PV 2002 Cakradatta. Sanskrit text with English translation. Chaukhamba, Varanasi, p 94, 203, 205, 422

Sharma JN, Sharma JN 1977 Comparison of the anti-inflammatory activity of Commiphora mukul (an indigenous drug) with those of phenylbutazone and ibuprofen in experimental arthritis induced by mycobacterial adjuvant. Arzneimittelforschung nach der Zulassung 27(7):1455–1457

Sheir Z, Nasr AA, Massoud A et al 2001 A safe, effective, herbal antischistosomal therapy derived from myrrh. American Journal of Tropical Medicine and Hygiene 65(6):700–704

Singh RB, Niaz MA, Ghosh S 1994 Hypolipidemic and anti-oxidant effects of Commiphora mukul as an adjunct to dietary therapy in patients with hypercholesterolemia. Cardiovascular Drugs and Therapy 8(4):659–664

Singh V, Kaul S, Chander R, Kapoor NK 1990 Stimulation of low density lipoprotein receptor activity in liver membrane of guggulsterone treated rats. Pharmacological Research 22(1):37–44

Soliman OE, El-Arman M, Abdul-Samie ER et al 2004 Evaluation of myrrh (Mirazid) therapy in fascioliasis and intestinal schistosomiasis in children: immunological and parasitological study. Journal of the Egyptian Society of Parasitology 34(3):941–966

Srikanthamurthy KR 2000 Bhāvaprakāśa of Bhavamiśra, vol 2. Krishnadas Academy, Varanasi

Srikanthamurthy KR 2001 Bhāvaprakāśa of Bhāvamiśra, vol 1. Krishnadas Academy, Varanasi, p 211–212, 394

Tariq M, Ageel AM, Al-Yahya MA et al 1986 Anti-inflammatory activity of Commiphora molmol. Agents and Actions 17(3–4):381–382

Thappa DM, Dogra J 1994 Nodulocystic acne: oral gugulipid versus tetracycline. Journal of Dermatology 21(10):729–731

Urizar NL, Liverman AB, Dodds DT et al 2002 A natural product that lowers cholesterol as an antagonist ligand for FXR. Science 296(5573):1703–1706

Warrier PK, Nambiar VPK, Ramankutty C (eds) 1994 Indian medicinal plants: a compendium of 500 species, vol 2. Orient Longman, Hyderabad, p 164–172

Williamson EM (ed) 2002 Major herbs of Ayurveda. Churchill Livingstone, London, p 110

Wu J, Xia C, Meier J et al 2002 The hypolipidemic natural product guggulsterone acts as an antagonist of the bile acid receptor. Molecular Endocrinology 16(7):1590–1597

Zhu N, Kikuzaki H, Sheng S et al 2001 Furanosesquiterpenoids of Commiphora myrrha. Journal of Natural Products 64(11):1460–1462

Haridrā, 'giving yellow'

BOTANICAL NAME: *Curcuma longa*, Zingiberaceae

OTHER NAMES: Haldi (H); Manjal (T); Turmeric (E); Jiang huang (C)

Botany: ***Haridrā*** is a perennial herb that attains a height of up to 90 cm, with a short stem, long sheathing petiolate leaves, and a large cylindrical root with thick sessile tubers that are intensely orange-yellow when cut or broken. The leaves are simple, quite large in proportion to the stem, the petiole as long as the leaf, oblong-lanceolate, glabrous, entire and acute, 30–45 cm long to 12.5 cm wide. The yellow flowers are borne in spikes, concealed by the sheathing petioles. Thought to be native to eastern India, ***Haridrā*** is extensively cultivated throughout the tropics (Kirtikar & Basu 1935, Warrier et al 1994).

Part used: Fresh and dried root.

Dravyguṇa:

- ***Rasa***: *tikta, kaṭu,*
- ***Vipāka***: *kaṭu*
- ***Vīrya***: *uṣṇa, rūkṣa*
- ***Karma***: *dīpanapācana, grāhī, jvaraghna, kṛmighna, chedana, raktaprasādana, śothahara, cakṣuṣya, varnya, kuṣṭhaghna, sandhānīya, kaphapittahara* (Srikanthamurthy 2001, Warrier et al 1994).

Constituents: The active constituents of ***Haridrā*** are the yellow flavonoid constituents called the curcuminoids or diarylheptanoids, of which curcumin is the best studied, but also includes methoxylated curcumins. ***Haridrā*** also contains a volatile oil consisting of sesquiterpene ketones such as β-tumerone, as well as other volatile compounds including atlantone, zingiberone, α-phellandrene, sabinene, cineole and borneol. Other constituents include sugars, proteins, and resins (Evans 1989, Kapoor 1990, Mills & Bone 2000, Yoganarasimhan 2000).

Medical research:

- ***In vitro***: antioxidant (Boone et al 1992, Mortellini et al 2000, Toda et al 1985), anti-inflammatory (Brouet & Ohshima 1995; Chan 1995), antitumour (Thaloor et al 1998)
- ***In vivo***: anti-ulcerogenic (Ammon & Wahl 1991, Rafatulla et al 1990), hepatoprotective (Deshpande et al 1998, Donatus et al 1990, Kiso et al 1983, Park et al 2000, Soni et al 1992), neuroprotective (Rajakrishnan et al 1999), hypolipidaemic (Ramirez-Tortosa et al 1999, Ramprasad & Sirsi 1957), antithrombotic (Srivastava et al 1986), antioxidant (Dikshit et al 1995), anti-inflammatory (Arora et al 1971, Mukhopadhyay et al 1982, Srivastava 1989), antitumour (Kawamori et al 1999, Limtrakul et al 1997), paracidal (Allen et al 1998), antifungal, antidermatophytic (Apisariyakul et al 1995), vulnerary (Sidhu et al 1998, 1999).
- ***Human trials***: ***Haridrā*** promoted the healing and reduction of symptoms in patients diagnosed with peptic ulcer disease (Prucksunand et al 2001); ***Haridrā*** inhibited COX–2 protein induction and prostaglandin E2 production in patients with advanced colorectal cancer (Plummer et al 2001); ***Haridrā*** produced significant symptomatic relief in patients with external cancerous lesions, reducing size, odour and pruritis (Kuttan et al 1987); ***Haridrā*** promoted a reduction in signs and symptoms of chronic anterior uveitis comparable to corticosteroids, without side-effects (Lal et al 1999); a standardised extract of ***Haridrā*** was found to promote a significant reduction in the signs and symptoms of irritable bowel syndrome (IBS) in a randomised study of 207 otherwise healthy patients (Bundy et al 2004).

Toxicity: The oral LD_{50} in rats of the petroleum-ether extract of ***Haridrā*** was determined to be 12.2 g/kg (Arora et al 1971). Researchers evaluated the potential oral toxicity of curcumin taken over a 3-month period in 25 patients suffering from a variety of severe illnesses. Researchers noted that there was no treatment-related toxicity up to 8 g daily, but that beyond this, the bulky volume of the drug was unacceptable to the patients (Cheng et al 2001). ***Haridrā*** is commonly used as a culinary spice and is generally recognised as safe.

Indications: Poor appetite, dyspepsia, peptic and duodenal ulcers, gas and flatulence, constipation, candidiasis, intestinal parasites, pharyngitis, catarrh, bronchitis, asthma, anaemia, cholecystitis, cholecystalgia, jaundice, hepatitis, hepatosplenomegaly, oedema, inflammatory joint disease, sports injuries, skin diseases, parasitic skin conditions, wounds, bruises, sprains, fractures, diabetes, dyslipidaemia, cardiovascular disease, amenorrhoea, gonorrhoea, cystitis, cancer prevention and treatment.

Contraindications: ***vātakopa***, in excess.

Medicinal uses: ***Haridrā*** is one of the more familiar Indian herbs in the West, most people identifying it with the flavour of curries, although in actuality ***Haridrā*** is only a minor component in most spice mixtures, used in small proportions as a colouring agent rather than for its flavour, which is rather bitter and unpleasant. The same potency of ***Haridrā*** to color curries and other foods is also utilised in the dyeing of textiles, for which it was imported from India to the West before the advent of aniline dyes. ***Haridrā*** is still used in India as a dyeing agent, not only for textiles but also as a cosmetic, popular among Indian women as a paste to improve the texture and lustre of the skin. ***Haridrā*** also has important symbolic uses in Hindu ceremonies, especially at weddings in which it is used to draw designs on the hands and feet. The activity of ***Haridrā*** as a dyeing agent is due to the curcuminoids, which are also in large part responsible for its medicinal activities. The volatile constituents and resins, however, are also medicinal and therefore aqueous extracts are avoided in favour of the ***cūrṇa*** or a tincture. Given the quality of ***Haridrā*** as a culinary spice, however, the tincture made from the fresh rhizomes is preferred, allowing for a lower dosage, which can enhance patient compliance considerably. ***Haridrā*** is among the more common household remedies in Āyurveda. For mild colds and flus one teaspoon of the ***cūrṇa*** is mixed with one half teaspoon of ***Śūṇṭhī***, with a little honey and water, taken two to three times daily. In pharyngitis ***Haridrā cūrṇa*** can be mixed with ***Yaṣṭimadhu cūrṇa***, ***saindhava*** and water and gargled, thrice daily. For dry coughs and bronchitis, one large teaspoon of ***Haridrā cūrṇa*** can be decocted in a 150 mL of milk, taken with honey. Mixed with a pinch of ***Śūṇṭhī*** and ***Pippalī*** powders, ***Haridrā*** is mixed with a small amount of ***ghṛta***, burned and inhaled in ***dhūma*** to treat respiratory catarrh. For skin conditions including eczema, psoriasis, acne and parasitic infections (e.g. scabies) ***Haridrā*** is taken internally as well as applied externally as a paste with water or honey, or prepared as a medicated ***ghṛta***, although people with very white skin may find the transient staining somewhat unappealing. For sprains, bruises and other sports-related injuries ***Haridrā*** can be made into a paste with honey, and applied generously over the affected part and covered with plastic wrap, changing the dressing every few hours. Taken internally, ***Haridrā*** is an effective treatment to strengthen the joints and tendons, and is an exceptionally important remedy in arthritis and other joint diseases, often used with ***Guggulu*** and ***Śūṇṭhī***. In the treatment of ophthalmic disorders equal parts ***Haridrā*** and ***Triphala*** can be prepared as a medicated ***ghṛta*** and applied to the eye. The ***Cakradatta*** recommends a collyrium called ***Saugata añjana*** in ophthalmic disorders, prepared from equal parts ***Haridrā***, ***Dāruharidrā***, ***Harītakī***, ***Jaṭāmāmsī***, ***Kuṣṭha*** and ***Pippalī*** (Sharma 2002). Prepared with equal parts ***Yaṣṭimadhu*** and ***Śatāvarī***, ***Haridrā*** can be used as as a douche or medicated ***ghṛta*** in cervical dysplasia. In the treatment of haemorrhoids the ***cūrṇa*** can be mixed with mustard oil and applied topically, to accompany internal treatments. Taken as a paste prepared with ***Guḍūcī*** and ***Āmalakī***, ***Haridrā*** may be of benefit in diabetes. Combined with ***Guggulu***, ***Haridrā*** can be an effective treatment in dyslipidaemia. In the treatment of jaundice the ***Cakradatta*** recommends a milk decoction of ***Haridrā***, ***Pippalī***, ***Nimba***, ***Balā*** and ***Yaṣṭimadhu*** (Sharma 2002). In the treatment of memory loss, poor concentration, and speech disorders the ***Cakradatta*** recommends a formula called ***Kalyāṇakaleha***, consisting of ***Haridrā*** mixed with equal parts ***Vacā***, ***Kuṣṭha***, ***Śūṇṭhī***, ***Jīraka***, ***Yaṣṭimadhu*** and ***saindhava***, taken with ***ghṛta*** (Sharma 2002). In the treatment of gout with ***kaphaja*** symptoms the ***Cakradatta*** recommends a formulation of ***Haridrā***, ***Āmalakī*** and ***Mustaka*** (Sharma 2002). ***Haridrā*** is used in Chinese medicine for patterns of blood stasis and stagnant qi, with cold and deficiency, in the treatment of menstrual pain, abdominal pain and pain in the shoulders (Bensky & Gamble 1993).

Dosage:

- ***Cūrṇa***: recently dried and powdered rhizome, 3–5 g b.i.d.–t.i.d.; up to 10 g t.i.d. of the herb derived from culinary sources
- ***Svarasa***: 15–25 mL b.i.d.–t.i.d.
- ***Kvātha***: 1:4, 30–90 mL b.i.d.–t.i.d.
- ***Tincture***: fresh rhizome, 1:2, 95%, 2–5 mL b.i.d.–t.i.d.

REFERENCES

Allen PC, Danforth HD, Augustine PC 1998 Dietary modulation of avian coccidiosis. International Journal for Parasitology 28:1131–1140

Ammon HPT, Wahl MA 1991 Pharmacology of Cucuma longa. Planta Medica 57:1–7

Apisariyakul A, Vanittanakom N, Buddhasukh D 1995 Antifungal activity of turmeric oil extracted from Curcuma longa (Zingiberaceae). Journal of Ethnopharmacology 49:163–169

Arora R, Basu N, Kapoor V et al 1971 Anti-inflammatory studies on Curcuma longa (turmeric). Indian Journal of Medical Research 59:1289–1295

Bensky D, Gamble A 1993 Chinese herbal medicine materia medica, revised edn. Eastland Press, Seattle, p 272

Boone CW, Steele VE, Kelloff GJ 1992 Screening of chemopreventive (anticarcinogenic) compounds in rodents. Mutation Research 267:251–255

Brouet I, Ohshima H 1995 Curcumin, an antitumor promoter and anti-inflammatory agent, inhibits induction of nitric oxide synthetase in activated macrophages. Biochemical and Biophysical Research Communications 206:533–540

Bundy R, Walker AF, Middleton RW, Booth J 2004 Turmeric extract may improve irritable bowel syndrome symptomology in otherwise healthy adults: a pilot study. Journal of Alternative and Complementary Medicine 10(6):1015–1018

Chan MM 1995 Inhibition of tumor necrosis factor by curcumin, a phytochemical. Biochemical Pharmacology 49(11):1551–1556

Cheng AL, Hsu CH, Lin JK et al 2001 Phase I clinical trial of curcumin, a chemopreventive agent, in patients with high-risk or pre-malignant lesions. AntiCancer Research 21(4B):2895–2900

Deshpande UR, Gadre SG, Raste AS et al 1998 Protective effect of turmeric (Curcuma longa L.) extract on carbon tetrachloride-induced liver damage in rats. Indian Journal of Experimental Biology 36:573–577

Dikshit M, Rastogi L, Shukla R, Srimal RC 1995 Prevention of ischaemia-induced biochemical changes by curcumin and quinidine in the cat heart. Indian Journal of Medical Research 101:31–35

Donatus IA, Sardjoko L, Vermeulen NP 1990 Cytotoxic and cytoprotective activities of curcumin. Effects on paracetamol-induced cytotoxicity, lipid peroxidation and glutathione depletion in rat hepatocytes. Biochemical Pharmacology 39:1869–1875

Evans WC 1989 Trease and Evans' pharmacognosy, 13th edn. Baillière Tindall, London, p 468

Kapoor LD 1990 CRC Handbook of Ayurvedic medicinal plants. CRC Press, Boca Raton, p 149

Kawamori T, Lubet R, Steele VE et al 1999 Chemopreventative effect of curcumin, a naturally occurring anti-inflammatory agent, during the promotion/progression stages of colon cancer. Cancer Research 59:597–601

Kirtikar KR, Basu BD 1935 Indian medicinal plants, 2nd edn, vols 1–4. Periodical Experts, Delhi, p 2422

Kiso Y, Suzuki Y, Watanabe N et al 1983 Antihepatotoxic principles of Curcuma longa rhizomes. Planta Medica 49:185–187

Kuttan R, Sudheeran PC, Josph CD 1987 Turmeric and curcumin as topical agents in cancer therapy. Tumori 73(1):29–31

Lal B, Kapoor AK, Asthana OP et al 1999 Efficacy of curcumin in the management of chronic anterior uveitis. Phytotherapy Research 13(4):318–322

Limtrakul P, Lipigorngoson S, Namwong O et al 1997 Inhibitory effect of dietary curcumin on skin carcinogenesis in mice. Cancer Letters 116:197–203

Mills S, Bone K 2000 Principles and practice of phytotherapy. Churchill Livingstone, London, p 570

Mortellini R, Foresti R, Bassi R, Green CJ 2000 Curcumin, an antioxidant and anti-inflammatory agent, induces heme oxygenase–1 and protects endothelial cells against oxidative stress. Free Radical Biology and Medicine 28:1303–1312

Mukhopadhyay A, Basu N, Ghatak N et al 1982 Anti-inflammatory and irritant activities of curcumin analogues in rats. Agents and Actions 12:508–515

Nadkarni KM 1954 The Indian materia medica, with Ayurvedic, Unani and home remedies, revised and enlarged by A.K. Nadkarni. Popular Prakashan PVP, Bombay

Park EJ, Jeon CH, Ko G et al 2000 Protective effect of curcumin in rat liver injury induced by carbon tetrachloride. Journal of Pharmacy and Pharmacology 52:437–440

Plummer SM, Hill KA, Festing MF et al 2001 Clinical development of leukocyte cyclooxygenase 2 activity as a systemic biomarker for cancer chemopreventive agents. Cancer Epidemiology, Biomarkers and Prevention 10(12):1295–1299

Prucksunand C, Indrasukhsri B, Leethochawalit M, Hungspreugs K 2001 Phase II clinical trial on effect of the long turmeric (Curcuma longa Linn) on healing of peptic ulcer. Southeast Asian Journal of Tropical Medicine and Public Health 32(1):208–215

Rafatulla S, Tariq M, Alyahya MA et al 1990 Evaluation of turmeric (Curcuma longa) for gastric and duodenal antiulcer activity in rats. Journal of Ethnopharmacology 29:25–34

Rajakrishnan V, Viswanathan P, Rajasekharan KN, Menon VP 1999 Neuroprotective role of curcumin from curcuma longa on ethanol-induced brain damage. Phytotherapy Research 13(7):571–574

Ramirez-Tortosa MC, Mesa MD, Aguilera MC et al 1999 Oral administration of a turmeric extract inhibits LDL oxidation and has hypocholesterolemic effects in rabbits with experimental atherosclerosis. Atherosclerosis 147:371–378

Ramprasad C, Sirsi M 1957 Curcuma longa and bile secretion. Quantitative changes in the bile constituents induced by sodium curcuminate. Journal of Scientific and Industrial Research 16C:108–110

Sharma PV 2002 Cakradatta. Sanskrit text with English translation. Chaukhamba, Varanasi, p 199, 235, 543

Sidhu GS, Singh AK, Thaloor D et al 1998 Enhancement of wound healing by curcumin in animals. Wound Repair and Regeneration 6(2):167–177

Sidhu GS, Mani H, Gaddipati JP et al 1999 Curcumin enhances wound healing in streptozotocin induced diabetic rats and genetically diabetic mice. Wound Repair and Regeneration 7(5):362–374

Soni KB, Rajan A, Kuttan R 1992 Reversal of aflatoxin induced liver damage by turmeric and curcumin. Cancer Letters 66:115–121

Srikanthamurthy KR 2001 Bhāvaprakāśa of Bhāvamiśra, vol 1. Krishnadas Academy, Varanasi, p 191

Srivastava R 1989 Inhibition of neutrophil response by curcumin. Agents and Actions 28:298–303

Srivastava R, Puri V, Srimal RC, Dhawan BN 1986 Effect of curcumin on platelet aggregation and vascular prostacyclin synthesis. Arzneimittel Forschung 36:715–717

Thaloor D, Singh AK, Sidhu GS et al 1998 Inhibition of angiogenic differentiation of human umbilical vein endothelial cells by curcumin. Cell Growth and Differentiation 9:305–312

Toda S, Miyase T, Arich H et al 1985 Natural anti-oxidants. Antioxidative compounds isolated from rhizome of Curcuma longa L. Chemical and Pharmaceutical Bulletin 33:1725–1728

Warrier PK, Nambiar VPK, Ramankutty C (eds) 1994 Indian medicinal plants: a compendium of 500 species, vol 2. Orient Longman, Hyderabad, p 259

Yoganarasimhan SN 2000 Medicinal plants of India, vol 2: Tamil Nadu. Self-published, Bangalore, p 171

Harītakī, 'to colour yellow'

BOTANICAL NAME: *Terminalia chebula*, Combretaceae

OTHER NAMES: ***Abhayā*** 'fearless' (S); Hara, Harad (H); Katukkay (T); Chebulic myrobalan (E); He zi (C)

Botany: ***Harītakī*** is a medium to large deciduous tree attaining a height of up to 30 m, with widely spreading branches and a broad roundish crown. The leaves are elliptic-oblong, with an acute tip, cordate at the base, margins entire, glabrous above with a yellowish pubescence below. The flowers are monoecious, dull white to yellow, with a strong unpleasant odour, borne in terminal spikes or short panicles. The fruits are glabrous, ellipsoid to ovoid drupes, yellow to orange brown in colour, containing a single angled stone. ***Harītakī*** is found throughout deciduous forests of the Indian subcontinent, on dry slopes up to 900 m in elevation (Kirtikar & Basu 1935, Warrier et al 1996).

Part used: Fruit; seven types are recognised (i.e. ***vijayā***, ***rohiṇī***, ***pūtanā***, ***amṛta***, ***abhayā***, ***jīvantī*** and ***cetakī***), based on the region the fruit is harvested as well as on the colour and shape of the fruit. Generally speaking the ***vijayā*** variety is preferred, which is traditionally grown in the Vindhya mountain range of central India and has a roundish as opposed to a more angular shape (Srikanthamurthy 2001).

Dravyguṇa: Fresh fruit

- ***Rasa***: *kaśāya, tikta, amla, kaṭu, madhura*
- ***Vipāka***: *madhura*
- ***Vīrya***: *uṣṇa*
- ***Karma***: *dīpanapācana, bedhana (cūrṇa), grāhī (kvātha, tincture), kṛmighna, mūtravirecana, jvaraghna, svāsahara, kāsahara, kuṣṭhaghna, śothahara, medhya, vedanāsthāpana, sandhānīya, cakṣuṣya, hṛdaya, rasāyanam, tridoṣaghna.*
- ***Prabhāva***: named for the god *Śiva* (*Harī*), who brings 'fearlessness' (*abhayā*) in the face of death and disease, and because it purifies the mind of attachments (Dash 1991, Dash & Junius 1983, Frawley & Lad 1986, Warrier et al 1996).

Constituents: Researchers have isolated a number of glycosides from ***Harītakī***, including the triterpenes arjunglucoside I, arjungenin, and the chebulosides I and II. Other constituents include a coumarin conjugated with gallic acids called chebulin, as well as other phenolic compounds including ellagic acid, 2, 4-chebulyl-β-D-glucopyranose, chebulinic acid, gallic acid, ethyl gallate, punicalagin, terflavin A, terchebin, luteolin, and tannic acid (Creencia et al 1996, Kapoor 1990, Saleem et al 2002, Williamson 2002, Yoganarasimhan 2000).

Medical research:

- ***In vitro***: antibacterial (Ahmad et al 1998, Jagtap & Karkera 1999, Malekzadeh et al 2001, Phadke & Kulkarni 1989, Sato et al 1998), antifungal (Dutta et al 1998), antiviral (Badmaev & Nowakowski 2000, El-Mekkawy et al 1995, Yukawa et al 1996), antitumour (Creencia et al 1996, Kaur et al 1998, Saleem et al 2002)
- ***In vivo***: hepatoprotective (Sohni & Bhatt 1996), antibacterial (Suguna et al 2002), antiamoeba (Sohni et al 1995), antiviral, immunomodulant (Yukawa et al 1996), vulnerary (Suguna et al 2002), hypolipidaemic (Thakur et al 1988), anti-ulcerogenic (Nadar & Pillai 1989)
- ***Human trials***: a mouth rinse prepared with a 10% solution of ***Harītakī*** siginificantly inhibited salivary bacterial counts (Jagtap & Karkera 1999).

Toxicity: Feeding trials in rats with *Terminalia chebula* produced hepatic lesions that included central vein abnormalities and marked renal lesions (Arseculeratne et al 1985). This same study also suggested that *Withania somnifera* produces similar renal lesions, an effect that has not been observed in any other studies.

Given the long history of usage and popularity of ***Harītakī***, this single study cannot be reliably extrapolated to human usage.

Indications: Gingivitis, stomatitis, asthma, cough, dyspnoea, dyspepsia, gastroenteritis, ulcers, diarrhoea, constipation, IBS, haemorrhoids, candidiasis, parasites, malabsorption syndromes, biliousness, hepatomegaly, splenomegaly, ascites, vesicular and renal calculi, urinary discharges, tumours, skin diseases, leprosy, intermittent fever, rheumatism, arthritis, gout, neuropathy, paralysis, memory loss, epilepsy, depression, leucorrhoea, diabetes, cardiovascular disease, anorexia, wounds.

Contraindications: Pregnancy, dehydration, emaciation, ***pittakopa*** (Frawley & Lad 1985). ***Caraka*** indicates that ***Harītakī*** is contraindicated in weak digestion, fatigue due to excessive sexual activity, with alcoholic drinks, and in hunger, thirst and heat stroke (Sharma & Dash 1988).

Medicinal uses: The Sanskrit name ***Harītakī*** is rich with meaning, referring to the yellowish dye (***harita***) that it contains, as well as indicating that it grows in the abode of the god ***Śiva*** (*Hari*, i.e. the Himalayas), and that it cures (***hārayet***) all disease (Dash 1991). Its other commonly used Sanskrit name, ***Abhayā***, refers to the 'fearlessness' it provides in the face of disease. According to the ***Bhāvaprakāśa***, ***Harītakī*** is derived from a drop of nectar from Indra's cup, similar to ***Guḍūcī*** (Srikanthamurthy 2001). Although the fresh fruit is difficult to obtain in the West, the fruit can be reconstituted by simmering in water and used in a similar fashion. Above all, ***Harītakī*** is considered to mitigate ***vāta*** and eliminate ***āma***, the latter indicated by constipation, a thick greyish tongue coating, abdominal pain and distension, foul faeces and breath, flatulence, weakness, and a slow pulse. The fresh fruit is ***dīpana*** and the powdered dried fruit made into a paste and taken with jaggery is ***malaśodhana***, removing impurities and wastes from the body. ***Harītakī*** is an efficacious purgative when taken as a powder, but when the whole dried fruit is boiled the resulting decoction is ***grāhī***, useful in the treatment of diarrhoea and dysentery. The fresh or reconstituted fruit fried in ***ghṛta*** and taken before meals is ***dīpanapācana***. If this latter preparation is taken with meals it increases ***buddhi*** ('intellect'), nourishes the ***indriyās*** ('senses') and is ***mutrāmalaśodhana*** (purifies the digestive and genitourinary tract). Taken after meals, ***Harītakī*** 'quickly cures diseases caused by the aggravation of ***vāyu***, ***pitta*** and ***kapha*** as a result of unwholesome food and drinks' (Dash 1991). ***Harītakī*** is a ***rasāyana*** to ***vāta***, increasing awareness, and has a nourishing, restorative effect on the central nervous system. ***Harītakī*** improves digestion, promotes the absorption of nutrients, and regulates colon function. ***Harītakī*** is very useful in prolapsed organs, improving the strength and tone of the supporting musculature. It may be taken with other hepatic restoratives such as ***Haridrā*** or ***Dāruharidrā***, and with carminatives such as ***Elā*** or ***Ajamodā*** in dyspepsia and biliousness. In gastrointestinal candidiasis it may be taken along with ***Haridrā***, Barberry root (*Berberis vulgaris*), Pau D'Arco (*Tabebuia avellanedae*), or used by itself for this purpose. In cases of gastroenteritis and dysentery four parts ***Harītakī*** may be decocted with two parts ***Dhānyaka*** seed, two parts ***Śātapuṣpā*** seed, one part ***Ajamodā*** seed, one part ***Śūṇṭhī*** rhizome, and one part ***Yaṣṭimadhu*** for prompt relief. In the treatment of piles and vaginal discharge, a decoction of ***Harītakī*** may be used as an antiseptic and astringent wash (Nadkarni 1954). A fine paste of the powder may be applied on burns and scalds (Nadkarni 1954). A cold infusion of ***Harītakī*** is an effective mouth rinse and the powder a good dentifrice in the treatment of apthous stomatitis, periodentitis, and dental caries (Kirtikar & Basu 1935, Nadkarni 1954). In the treatment of sciatica, lumbago and general lower back pain ***Harītakī*** may be combined with ***Guggulu***, Black Cohosh (*Cimicifuga racemosa* rhizome), ***Pippalī***, ***Elā*** and ***Tvak*** bark. In combination with ***Guggulu***, ***Harītakī*** is useful in the treatment of gout. ***Harītakī*** is the primary constituent of ***Agastya Rasāyana leha*** (confection), formulated by the sage Agastya, father of the ***Siddha*** school of medicine. It is an excellent formula to improve digestion, remove waste and impurities from the body, and stimulate the regeneration of tissues, although the taste may prove to be a challenge for many Westerners. ***Harītakī*** is perhaps best known as a constituent of the formula ***Triphala***, usually containing equal proportions of ***Harītakī***, ***Bibhītaka*** and ***Āmalakī***.

Dosage:

- ***Cūrṇa***: 1–10 g b.i.d.–t.i.d.
- ***Kvātha***: 30–120 mL b.i.d.–t.i.d.
- ***Tincture***: 1:5, 30% alcohol, 1–5 mL b.i.d.–t.i.d.

REFERENCES

Arseculeratne SN, Gunatilaka AA, Panabokke RG 1985 Studies of medicinal plants of Sri Lanka. Part 14: Toxicity of some traditional medicinal herbs. Journal of Ethnopharmacology 13(3):323–335

Ahmad I, Mehmood Z, Mohammad F 1998 Screening of some Indian medicinal plants for their antimicrobial properties. Journal of Ethnopharmacology 62(2):183–193

Badmaev V, Nowakowski M 2000 Protection of epithelial cells against influenza A virus by a plant derived biological response modifier Ledretan-96. Phytotherapy Research 14(4):245–259

Creencia E, Eguchi T, Nishimura T, Kakinuma K 1996 Isolation and structure elucidation of the biologically active components of Terminalia chebula Retzius (Combretaceae). KIMIKA 12:1–10

Dash B 1991 Materia medica of Ayurveda. B. Jain Publishers, New Delhi, p 8

Dash B, Junius M 1983 A handbook of Ayurveda. Concept Publishing, New Delhi, p 84–87

Dutta BK, Rahman I, Das TK 1998 Antifungal activity of Indian plant extracts. Mycoses 41(11–12):535–536

El-Mekkawy S et al 1995 Inhibitory effects of Egyptian folk medicines on human immunodeficiency virus (HIV) reverse transcriptase. Chemical and Pharmaceutical Bulletin 43(4):641–648

Frawley D, Lad V 1986 The Yoga of herbs: an Ayurvedic guide to herbal medicine. Lotus Press, Santa Fe, p 174

Jagtap AG, Karkera SG 1999 Potential of the aqueous extract of Terminalia chebula as an anticaries agent. Journal of Ethnopharmacology 68(1–3):299–306

Kapoor LD 1990 CRC handbook of Ayurvedic medicinal plants. CRC Press, Boca Raton, p 332

Kaur S Grover IS, Singh M, Kaur S 1998 Antimutagenicity of hydrolyzable tannins from Terminalia chebula in Salmonella typhimurium. Mutagen Research 419(1–3):169–179

Kirtikar KR, Basu BD 1935 Indian medicinal plants, 2nd edn, vols 1–4. Periodical Experts, Delhi, p 1020–1021

Kurokawa M, Nagasaka K, Hirabayashi T et al 1995 Efficacy of traditional herbal medicines in combination with acyclovir against herpes simplex virus type 1 infection in vitro and in vivo. Antiviral Research 27(1–2):19–37

Malekzadeh F, Ehsanifar H, Shahamat M 2001 Antibacterial activity of black myrobalan (Terminalia chebula Retz) against Helicobacter pylori. International Journal of Antimicrobial Agents 18(1):85–88

Nadar TS, Pillai MM 1989 Effect of Āyurvedic medicines on beta-glucuronidase activity of Brunner's glands during recovery from cysteamine induced duodenal ulcers in rats. Indian Journal of Experimental Biology 27(11):959–962

Nadkarni KM 1954 The Indian materia medica, with Ayurvedic, Unani and home remedies, revised and enlarged by A.K. Nadkarni. Popular Prakashan PVP, Bombay, p 1207–1210

Phadke SA, Kulkarni SD 1989 Screening of in vitro antibacterial activity of Terminalia chebula, Eclipta alba and Ocimum sanctum. Indian Journal of Medical Sciences 43(5):113–117

Saleem A, Husheem M, Harkonen P, Pihlaja K 2002 Inhibition of cancer cell growth by crude extract and the phenolics of Terminalia chebula retz. fruit. Journal of Ethnopharmacology 81(3):327–336

Sato Y, Oketani H, Singyouchi K et al 1997 Extraction and purification of effective antimicrobial constituents of Terminalia chebula RETS. against methicillin-resistant Staphylococcus aureus. Biological and Pharmaceutical Bulletin 20(4):401–404

Sharma RK, Dash B 1988 Agnivesa's Caraka Saṃhitā: text with English translation and critical exposition based on Cakrapani Datta's Āyurvedic Dipika, vol 3. Chaukhambha Orientalia, Varanasi, p 14

Sohni YR, Bhatt RM 1996 Activity of a crude extract formulation in experimental hepatic amoebiasis and in immunomodulation studies. Journal of Ethnopharmacology 54(2–3):119–124

Sohni YR, Kaimal P, Bhatt RM 1995 The antiamoebic effect of a crude drug formulation of herbal extracts against Entamoeba histolytica in vitro and in vivo. Journal of Ethnopharmacology 45(1):43–52

Srikanthamurthy KR 2001 Bhāvaprakāśa of Bhāvamiśra, vol 1. Krishnadas Academy, Varanasi, p 159, 160

Suguna L, Singh S, Sivakumar P et al 2002 Influence of Terminalia chebula on dermal wound healing in rats. Phytotherapy Research 16(3):227–231

Thakur CP, Thakur B, Singh S et al 1988 The Āyurvedic medicines Haritaki, Amala and Bahira reduce cholesterol-induced atherosclerosis in rabbits. International Journal of Cardiology 21(2):167–175

Warrier PK, Nambiar VPK, Ramankutty C (eds) 1996 Indian medicinal plants: a compendium of 500 species, vol 5. Orient Longman, Hyderabad, p 263

Williamson EM (ed) 2002 Major herbs of Ayurveda. Churchill Livingstone, London, p 299

Yoganarasimhan SN 2000 Medicinal plants of India, vol 2: Tamil Nadu. Self-published, Bangalore, p 541

Yukawa TA, Kurokawa M, Sato H et al 1996 Prophylactic treatment of cytomegalovirus infection with traditional herbs. Antiviral Research 32(2):63–70

Hiṅgu

Botanical name: *Ferula foetida, F. narthex, F. rubricaulis,* etc., Apiaceae

Other names: Hing (H); Perungayam, Gayam (T); Asafoetida, Devil's Dung (E)

Botany: ***Hiṅgu*** is a herbaceous perennial attaining a height of up to 3 m, with a fleshy forked taproot much like a carrot or parsnip, the cortex black and the whitish medulla exuding a thick, milky foetid juice when cut. The leaves are alternate, pinnately decompound, on wide, sheathing petioles. The pale greenish-yellow flowers are borne at the top of the stem in simple or compound umbels. ***Hiṅgu*** is found growing wild in the northwest of India, Nepal and Tibet, extending westwards into Afghanistan, Iran, the Middle East and southern Europe. ***Hiṅgu*** has since naturalised in the Americas (Kirtikar & Basu 1935, Warrier et al 1995).

Part used: Dried resinous exudate of the root.

Dravyguṇa:

- ***Rasa***: *kaṭu, tikta*
- ***Vipāka***: *kaṭu*
- ***Vīrya***: *uṣṇa*
- ***Karma***: *pācana, anulomana, kṛmighna, chedana, svāsahara, ārtavajanana, kaphavātahara* (Srikanthamurthy 2001, Warrier et al 1995).

Constituents: A number of constituents have been isolated from ***Hiṅgu***, including a volatile oil, a gum, a resin, and other constituents generally considered to be impurities. The volatile oil contains the sulfur compounds foetisulfides A–D, and foetithiophene A and B, responsible for the characteristically pungent, sulfurous odour of ***Hiṅgu***. The resin contains asaresinol ferulate and free ferulic acid. The gum contains glucoronic acid, galactose, arabinose, rhamnose and protein. Other constituents in ***Hiṅgu*** include the sesquiterpene coumarins assafoetidnol A and B, gummosin, polyanthin, badrakemin, neveskone, samarcandin and galbanic acid (Abd El-Razek et al 2001, Duan et al 2002, Evans 1989, Kapoor 1990).

Medical research:

- ***In vitro***: antispasmodic (Sadraei et al 2001), antibacterial (Tamemoto et al 2001).
- ***In vivo***: anticonvulsant (Sayyah et al 2002), erectile stimulating (El-Thaher et al 2001), antioxidant, chemopreventative (Saleem et al 2001).

Toxicity: The TD_{50} value for a seed acetone extract of *F. gummosa* was determined to be 375.8 mg/kg in mice (Sayyah et al 2002). ***Hiṅgu*** is widely used as a culinary spice and is generally regarded as safe. Most Āyurvedic authorities, however, recommend that ***Hiṅgu*** undergo a purification process whereby it is fried in oil (e.g. ***ghṛta***) to reduce any potential toxicity.

Indications: Poor appetite, gas and flatulence, constipation, candidiasis, parasites, malabsorption syndromes, bronchitis, whooping cough, asthma, pneumonia, otitis media, epilepsy, chorea, dysmenorrhoea, amenorrhoea, nervous irritability and anxiety, inflammatory joint disease.

Contraindications: ***pittakopa***.

Medicinal uses: ***Hiṅgu*** is an excellent representative of the many herbs of India that serve both as a culinary spice and as an active medicinal agent. To this end, ***Hiṅgu*** is often used as an ingredient in food, a small amount of the crushed resin dissolved and fried in ***ghṛta***, often with medicaments such as ***Ajamodā***, ***Trikaṭu***, ***Triphala*** and ***saindhava***, and then consumed with rice. The most commonly used classical remedy is ***Hingvastak cūrṇa***. Such formulas are commonly used to treat poor appetite, colic, abdominal bloating, gas, flatulence, and malabsorption, and when consumed on a regular basis, ***Hiṅgu*** is effective in intestinal candidiasis and parasites. Given that digestive weakness is the aetiology of several different pathologies in Āyurveda, including conditions such as ***āmavāta*** (rheumatoid arthritis), ***Hiṅgu*** has a potentially wide application in the treatment of many diseases. Apart from its specific activity to enhance digestion, however, ***Hiṅgu*** is also an effective antispasmodic in the respiratory, genitourinary and nervous systems. For lung complaints such as asthma, chronic bronchitis, whooping cough, and pneumonia, ***Hiṅgu*** can be taken internally, burned with ***ghṛta*** and the smoke inhaled (***dhūma***), or the resin dissolved in oil and then applied to the chest as a rubifacient plaster. Similarly, the resin can be dissolved in oil and applied warm in otitis media. In the treatment of skin parasites such as ring worm the same oil can be applied topically, and Nadkarni (1954) states that it is an effective vulnerary. In the treatment of dysmenorrhoea ***Hiṅgu*** is commonly used by herbalists to relieve uterine spasm, as well as treat the nervous irritability that often accompanies the condition. As a nervine antispasmodic ***Hiṅgu*** is also used internally in the treatment of epilepsy and seizure, often mixed with other pungent herbs such as ***Vacā*** and ***Pippalī***. Its use in epilepsy, however, extends beyond its antispasmodic activity, as it is also used as a protective charm, the resin contained in a sachet and hung around the neck to ward off negative spiritual influences. Orthodox Hindus will often use ***Hiṅgu*** in place of garlic as a culinary spice, based on the idea that garlic (***Laśuna***) is thought to disturb the mind, whereas ***Hiṅgu*** does not. Generally speaking, ***Hiṅgu*** is a remedy specific to ***vāta***, or phrased in Western terms, " . . . cases exhibiting nervous depression, with more or less feebleness, and particularly if associated with gastric derangements with constipation, flatulence, and tardy or imperfect menstruation" (Felter & Lloyd 1893). Due to its pungent and warming characteristics, however, ***Hiṅgu*** is also used in ***kaphaja*** conditions, but should be avoided in cases of intense heat or acute ulceration (i.e. ***pittakopa***). Like garlic, the sulfurous compounds in ***Hiṅgu*** are excreted through the urine, breast milk, breath and sweat.

Dosage:

- ***Cūrṇa***: fried in oil, 1–2 g b.i.d.–t.i.d.
- ***Tincture***: 1:5, 80%, 1–2 mL b.i.d.–t.i.d.

REFERENCES

Abd El-Razek MH, Ohta S, Ahmed AA, Hirata T 2001 Sesquiterpene coumarins from the roots of Ferula assa-foetida. Phytochemistry 58(8):1289–1295

Dash B, Junius M 1983 A handbook of Ayurveda. Concept Publishing, New Delhi

Duan H, Takaishi Y, Tori M et al 2002 Polysulfide derivatives from Ferula foetida. Journal of Natural Products 65(11):1667–1669

El-Thaher TS, Matalka KZ, Taha HA, Badwan AA 2001 Ferula harmonis 'zallouh' and enhancing erectile function in rats: efficacy and toxicity study. International Journal of Impotence Research 13(4):247–251

Evans WC 1989 Trease and Evans' pharmacognosy, 13th edn. Baillière Tindall, London, p 476

Felter HW, Lloyd JU 1893 King's American dispensatory. Available: http://www.ibiblio.org/herbmed/eclectic/kings/main.html.

Kapoor LD 1990 CRC Handbook of Ayurvedic medicinal plants. CRC Press, Boca Raton, p 185

Kirtikar KR, Basu BD 1935 Indian medicinal plants, 2nd edn, vols 1–4. Periodical Experts, Delhi, p 1216–1217

Nadkarni KM 1954 The Indian materia medica, with Ayurvedic, Unani and home remedies, revised and enlarged by A.K. Nadkarni. Popular Prakashan PVP, Bombay, p 540

Sadraei H, Asghari GR, Hajhashemi V et al 2001 Spasmolytic activity of essential oil and various extracts of Ferula gummosa Boiss. on ileum contractions. Phytomedicine 8(5):370–376

Saleem M, Alam A, Sultana S 2001 Asafoetida inhibits early events of carcinogenesis: a chemopreventive study. Life Sciences 68(16):1913–1921

Sayyah M, Mandgary A, Kamalinejad M 2002 Evaluation of the anticonvulsant activity of the seed acetone extract of Ferula gummosa Boiss. against seizures induced by pentylenetetrazole and electroconvulsive shock in mice. Journal of Ethnopharmacology 82(2–3):105–109

Srikanthamurthy KR 2001 Bhāvaprakāśa of Bhāvamiśra, vol 1. Krishnadas Academy, Varanasi, p 174

Tamemoto K, Takaishi Y, Chen B et al 2001 Sesquiterpenoids from the fruits of Ferula kuhistanica and antibacterial activity of the constituents of F. kuhistanica. Phytochemistry 58(5):763–767

Warrier PK, Nambiar VPK, Ramankutty C (eds) 1995 Indian medicinal plants: a compendium of 500 species, vol 3. Orient Longman, Hyderabad, p 263

Jaṭāmāmsī, 'braided and fleshy'

BOTANICAL NAMES: *Nardostachys grandiflora, N. jatamansi,* Valerianaceae

OTHER NAMES: ***Māmsī*** (S); Jatamamsi (H); Jatamashi (T); Indian Spikenard (E)

Botany: ***Jaṭāmāmsī*** is an erect perennial herb attaining a height of 10–60 cm, with a long woody rootstalk covered in reddish brown fibres that are derived from the petioles of the withered leaves. The leaves are mostly basal and elongated, up to 20 cm in length by 2.5 cm wide, with longitudinal veins, glabrous to slightly pubescent. The flowers are pale pink or blue, borne in dense crowded cymes. ***Jaṭāmāmsī*** is found in the fragile ecosystems of the subalpine and alpine meadows of the Himalayan mountain range, between 3500 and 4500 m in elevation. When dried, the fleshy aromatic rhizome is fringed with reddish brown fibres that appear like a braid, a feature which appears to be the origin of the name ***Jaṭāmāmsī***. Due to unregulated harvesting in Nepal ***Jaṭāmāmsī*** is now a threatened species and is listed in CITES Appendix II (Kirtikar & Basu 1935, Mulliken 2000, Nepal 2002, Warrier et al 1995).

Part used: Rhizome.

Dravyguṇa:

- ***Rasa***: *tikta, kaśāya, madhura*
- ***Vipāka***: *kaṭu*
- ***Vīrya***: *śita*
- ***Karma***: *dīpana, kāsahara, svāsahara, dāhapraśamana, raktaprasādana, kuṣṭhaghna, romasañjana, vedanāsthāpana, nidrājanana, medhya, balya, vajīkaraṇa, pittavātahara* (Srikanthamurthy 2001, Warrier et al 1995).

Constituents: ***Jaṭāmāmsī*** contains the commercially important Spikenard oil used in perfumery, described as a sweet, woody and spicy-animal odour. Spikenard oil consists a variety of constituents including hydrocarbons (α-pinene, β-pinene, limonene, aristolene, dihydroazulenes, α-gurjunene, β-gurjunene, α-patchoulene, β-patchoulene, seychellene, seychelane, β-maaliene), alcohols (calarenol, nardol, valerianol, patchouli alcohol, maliol), aldehydes (valerianal), ketones (valeranone [jatamansone], a β-ionone, 1-hydroxyaristolenone, aristolenone), and oxides (1,8-cineole). The rhizome also contains the terpenoid ester nardostachysin, the coumarins angelicin and jatamansin, β-sitosterol, a resin, gum, starch and sugar (Chatterjee et al 2000, Kapoor 1990, Lawless 1995, Rucker et al 1978)

Medical research:

- ***In vivo***: serotinergic, dopaminergic (Prabhu et al 1994); anticonvulsant, hypnotic (Rucker et al 1978); neuroprotective (Salim et al 2003); hepatoprotective (Ali et al 2000); antioxidant (Salim et al 2003, Tripathi et al 1996).

Toxicity: The oral LD_{50} of the isolated sesquiterpene valeranone is reported to be greater than 3160 mg/kg in rats and mice (Rucker et al 1978). ***Jaṭāmāmsī*** is generally regarded as safe.

Indications: Dyspepsia, colic, flatulence, pharyngitis, cough, bronchitis, asthma, insomnia, neurosis, depression, anxiety, confusion, memory loss, convulsions, epilepsy, tenesmus and spasm, nephropathies, muscle pain, lumbago, dysmenorrhoea, burning sensations, skin diseases, ulcers, angina, palpitations, hypertension.

Contraindications: Use with extreme care or otherwise avoid with the use of barbiturates, benzodiazepines, antiepileptics, antipsychotics, antidepressants and antihypertensives.

Medicinal uses: ***Jaṭāmāmsī*** is often used interchangeably with ***Tagara*** or ***Nata***, and in many respects is similar to the European Valerian (*Valeriana officinalis*) in activity. The taste and odour of ***Jaṭāmāmsī***, however, is far more agreeable and its essential oil (called 'Nard oil') has long been an important ingredient in perfumery all over the world. Unlike Valerian ***Jaṭāmāmsī*** has a cooling property, making it appropriate for vitiations of ***pitta***, but combines this activity with an antispasmodic and sedative activity, making it suitable to treat afflictions of ***vāta***. ***Jaṭāmāmsī*** acts primarily upon the nervous system, inducing a natural sleep, without any adverse effect upon awakening, and appears to lack the stimulating effects that a certain number of people experience with Valerian. The most common usage of ***Jaṭāmāmsī*** is as a nervine sedative in the treatment of insomnia, or to treat chronic irritability and nervousness, with exhaustion and debility. To this end ***Jaṭāmāmsī*** can be prepared as a medicated ***taila*** and applied topically in ***abhyaṅga***, and taken internally combined with herbs such as ***Aśvagandhā*** and ***Brāhmī*** to nourish and relax the nervous system. This relaxant property extends into its usage as a mildly acting anodyne, indicated in muscle pain, headaches and dysmenorrhoea, in combination with ***Guggulu*** and ***Śūṇṭhī***. As a treatment for epilepsy seizure disorders ***Jaṭāmāmsī*** may be useful in petit mal, but taken alone is probably insufficient for more severe conditions. It can be combined with ***Aśvagandhā***, ***Vacā***, ***Brāhmī***, and the potentially toxic ***Pārasikayavānī***, as well as with Western herbs such as Black Cohosh (*Actaea racemosa*) and Lobelia (*Lobelia inflata*) for added effect. For Parkinsonism (***kampavāta***), ***Jaṭāmāmsī*** can be used with herbs such as ***Kapikacchū***, ***Aśvagandhā***, ***Pārasikayavānī*** and ***Balā***. In the treatment of benzodiazepine addiction ***Jaṭāmāmsī*** can be an effective weaning agent, but with other addictions such as heroin or tobacco it is probably insufficient without combining it with botanicals such as ***Aśvagandhā***, Milky Oats (*Avena sativa*), California Poppy (*Eschscholzia californica*), Skullcap (*Scutellaria lateriflora*), and Lobelia (*Lobelia inflata*). In the treatment of flatulent colic and abdominal cramping and pain, ***Jaṭāmāmsī*** can be combined with ***Ajamodā*** and ***Śūṇṭhī***. Similarly, ***Jaṭāmāmsī*** can be used in bronchial afflictions, to ease spasmodic coughing, used in combination with ***Vāsaka*** and ***Puṣkaramūla***. ***Jaṭāmāmsī*** is also utilised in hypertension, with ***Arjuna*** in the treatment of arrhythmia and palpitation, and with ***Arjuna*** and ***Jātīphala*** in angina pectoris.

Dosage:

- ***Cūrṇa***: recently dried rhizome, 1–5 g b.i.d.–t.i.d.
- ***Hima***: 60–120 mL b.i.d.–t.i.d.
- ***Tincture***: fresh plant, 1:2, 95%; recently dried rhizome, 1:4, 50%; 1–5 mL b.i.d.–t.i.d.
- ***Taila***: in ***abhyaṅga***, ad lib.
- ***Essential oil***: 2–3 gtt b.i.d.–t.i.d.

REFERENCES

Ali S, Ansari KA, Jafry MA et al 2000 Nardostachys jatamansi protects against liver damage induced by thioacetamide in rats. Journal of Ethnopharmacology 71(3):359–363

Chatterjee A, Basak B, Saha M et al 2000 Structure and stereochemistry of nardostachysin, a new terpenoid ester constituent of the rhizomes of Nardostachys jatamansi. Journal of Natural Products 63(11):1531–1533

Evans WC 1989 Trease and Evans' pharmacognosy, 13th edn. Baillière Tindall, London

Kapoor LD 1990 CRC Handbook of Ayurvedic medicinal plants. CRC Press, Boca Raton, p 239

Kirtikar KR, Basu BD 1935 Indian medicinal plants, 2nd edn, vols 1–4. Periodical Experts, Delhi, p 1307–1308

Lawless J 1995 The illustrated encyclopedia of essential oils. Element, Rockport, MA, p 184

Mulliken TA 2000 Implementing CITES for Himalayan medicinal plants Nardostachys grandiflora and Picrorhiza kurrooa. In: TRAFFIC Bulletin 18:63–72

Nadkarni KM 1954 The Indian materia medica, with Ayurvedic, Unani and home remedies, revised and enlarged by A.K. Nadkarni. Popular Prakashan PVP, Bombay

Nepal, Ministry of Forests and Soil Conservation 2002 Nepal Biodiversity Strategy. Ministry of Forests and Soil Conservation, Nepal p 29

Prabhu V, Karanth KS, Rao A 1994 Effects of Nardostachys jatamansi on biogenic amines and inhibitory amino acids in the rat brain. Planta Medica 60(2):114–117

Rucker G, Tautges J, Sieck A et al 1978 Isolation and pharmacodynamic activity of the sesquiterpene valeranone from Nardostachys jatamansi DC. Arzneimittelforschung nach der Zulassung 28(1):7–13

Salim S, Ahmad M, Zafar KS et al 2003 Protective effect of Nardostachys jatamansi in rat cerebral ischemia. Pharmacology, Biochemistry, and Behavior 74(2):481–486

Srikanthamurthy KR 2001 Bhāvaprakāśa of Bhāvamiśra, vol 1. Krishnadas Academy, Varanasi, p 220

Tripathi YB, Tripathi E, Upadhyay A 1996 Antilipid peroxidative property of Nardostachys jatamansi. Indian Journal of Experimental Biology 34(11):1150–1151

Warrier PK, Nambiar VPK, Ramankutty C (eds) 1995 Indian medicinal plants: a compendium of 500 species, vol 4. Orient Longman, Hyderabad, p 104

Jātīphala, 'fruit of excellence'

BOTANICAL NAME: *Myristica fragrans*, Myristicaceae

OTHER NAMES: ***Madaśaunda***, 'intoxicating fruit' (S); Jaiphal (H); Jatamaram, Jatikkai (T); Nutmeg (E); Rou dou kou (C)

Botany: ***Jātīphala*** is a moderate-sized evergreen aromatic tree, usually dioecious, with greyish black bark that contains a reddish juice in the cambium layer. The leaves are elliptic to oblong lanceolate, thin and leathery, shiny above and dull below, the margin entire and tip acute. The flowers are creamy-yellow in colour, fragrant, borne in racemes, the male flowers with a stalked staminal column and 10–14 anthers, the ovary of the female flowers sessile. The globose fruits are 3.5–5 cm long, covered in a fleshy pericarp that splits into two when mature, the fragrant seed oblong and hard, covered in a reddish aril. ***Jātīphala*** is native to the Maluku Spice Islands of Indonesia, but has long since been cultivated in the warmer, tropical regions of the subcontinent of India (Kirtikar & Basu 1935, Warrier et al 1995).

Part used: Seed (***Jātīphala***) and arils (***Jatipatra***, Mace).

Dravyguṇa:

- ***Rasa***: *tikta, kaṭu, kaśāya*
- ***Vipāka***: *kaṭu*
- ***Vīrya***: *uṣṇa*
- ***Karma***: *dīpanapācana, grāhī, kṛmighna, kāsahara, hṛdaya, vedanāsthāpana, nidrājanana, madakārī, vajīkaraṇa, vātakaphahara* (Srikanthamurthy 2001, Warrier et al 1995).

Constituents: ***Jātīphala*** is noted for its essential oil, comprising between 5 and 15% of fruit, containing various constituents including pinene and camphene (80%), dipentene (8%), myristicin (4%), safrole (0.6%), eugenol and isoeugenol (0.2%), as well as methylleugenol, methylisoeugenol, elemicin, isomelecin, methoxyeugenol, cymene, geraniol, linalool, and terpineol. Researchers have also identified four neolignans in ***Jātīphala***, the fragnasols A, B, C and dehydrodiisoeugenol. ***Jātīphala*** also contains a mixture of fats (lauric, myristic, stearic, hexadecenoic, oleic and linoleic acids), epicatechin and cyanidin, proteins, carbohydrates, calcium, phosphorus, iron, magnesium, sodium, potassium, zinc, vitamin A, riboflavin and niacin. The arils (i.e. 'Mace') are stated to contain a variety of neolignins similar to the seed including fragransol C and D, as well as myristicanol A and B, nectandrin B, verrucosin, dihydroguaiaretic acid, and the resorcinols malabaricone B and malabaricone C (Duke 1986, Evans 1989, Juhasz 2000, Kapoor 1990, Orabi et al 1991, Park 1998, Yoganarasimhan 2000).

Medical research:

- ***In vitro***: antispasmodic (Grover et al 2002); antifungal, antibacterial (Orabi et al 1991).
- ***In vivo***: antidiarrhoeal (Grover et al 2002), hepatoprotective (Morita et al 2003), hypotensive (Grover et al 2002), hypolipidaemic (Ram et al 1996, Sharma et al 1995), antithrombotic (Ram et al 1996), analgesic (Grover et al 2002), anti-inflammatory (Olajide et al 1999, Ozaki et al 1989), antitumour (Hussain & Rao 1991, Jannu et al 1991).
- ***Human trials***: a dosage of four to six tablespoons of Nutmeg powder successfully controlled diarrhoea associated with medullary carcinoma of the thyroid, and also helped to correct drug-resistant hypercalcemia to one third of its original level (Duke 1989).

Toxicity: Several cases of intoxication have been reported after an ingestion of approximately 5 g of ***Jātīphala***, corresponding to 1–2 mg myristicin/kg body weight, which is a major constituent in the essential oil. Such doses and larger are reported to be more or less intoxicating, with symptoms such as visual hallucinations, headache, dizziness and tachycardia. Researchers have hypothesised that myristicin and elemicin can be readily modified into amphetamines by the body. In toxicological studies with rats no toxic effects were observed with the administration of myristicin perorally at a dose of 10 mg/kg. The oral LD_{50} for the potentially carcinogenic safrole is 1950 mg/kg in rats. The oral LD_{50} for Nutmeg oil is 2600 mg/kg in rats, 4620 mg/kg in mice, and 6000 mg/kg in hamsters (Duke 1989, Hallstrom & Thuvander 1997).

Indications: Dyspepsia, colic, flatulence, diarrhoea, dysentery, insomnia, muscle pain, fibromylagia, rheumatism, lumbago, dysmenorrhoea, cough, bronchitis, asthma, angina, hypertension, dyslipidaemia, impotence.

Contraindications: Use with extreme care or otherwise avoid with the use of barbiturates, benzodiazepines, antiepileptics, antipsychotics, antidepressants and antihypertensives. Avoid oral usage in mucoepithelial ulceration.

Medicinal uses: The origin of the name ***Jātīphala***, the 'fruit of excellence' or 'high caste fruit', is unknown, but is likely a reference to its rich essential oil content and its pleasant and distinct aroma. ***Jātīphala*** is now widely used throughout the world as both a culinary spice and medicinal agent. In Āyurvedic medicine it is most commonly used as an adjunct to other formulas to improve their taste or odour, and as a ***dīpanapācana*** agent to enhance the uptake of the other constituents in the formula. It is often used along with, or instead of, similarly aromatic herbs such as ***Tvak*** bark, ***Lavaṅga*** fruit, and ***Śūṇṭhī*** rhizome to treat a variety of digestive disorders, including nausea and dyspepsia. One of the most important uses for ***Jātīphala*** is in both infectious and chronic diarrhoea, for which it acts to slow the number of motions, ease intestinal griping, and kill parasites. To this end a compound called ***Jātīphaladi cūrṇa*** is often prescribed, taken in doses of 10–12 g with honey as an ***anupāna***; also used to treat malabsorption, bronchitis, asthma, consumption and rhinitis caused by ***vāta*** and ***kapha*** (Srikanthamurthy 1984). Prepared as a medicated oil or the taken as the essential oil diluted in a base oil, ***Jātīphala*** can be used in ***abhyaṅga*** as an analgesic and antispasmodic in the treatment of myalgia and rheumatism. Prepared in a saturated fat such as ***ghṛta*** or lard ***Jātīphala*** is used topically in the treatment of haemorrhoids (Felter & Lloyd 1893, Nadkarni 1954). Taken internally, ***Jātīphala*** is a very good antispasmodic in the treatment of chronic inflammatory conditions of the muscles such as fibromyalgia. In sufficient doses ***Jātīphala*** acts as a delayed onset sedative that begins to act 3–5 hours later, and is particularly useful for night-time wakening, particularly that associated with muscle pain and rheumatism. To this end, ***Jātīphala*** mixed with more immediate-acting hypnotics such as the Himalayan Poppy (*Meconopsis grandis*) and ***Jaṭāmāmsī*** instead of the sleeping pills, antidepressants and anti-inflammatories commonly used to treat fibromyalgia. Taken with antispasmodics such as Black Cohosh (*Cimicifuga racemosa*), Kava (*Piper methysticum*), and Lobelia (*Lobelia inflata*), ***Jātīphala*** can be similarly taken during the day to relieve fibromyalgia pain. ***Jātīphala*** is also considered to be an important agent in the treatment of heart disease and angina, and in the treatment of hypertension and dyslipidaemia may be of benefit when taken with ***Guggulu***, ***Arjuna*** and ***Laśuna***. As an expectorant, ***Jātīphala*** finds its way into several different formulations in the treatment of bronchitis, asthma and consumptive conditions, and its virtues extolled in both hemispheres in the treatment of intermittent fever (Felter & Lloyd 1893). As a ***vajīkaraṇa***, ***Jātīphala*** is believed to awaken the sexual passions in both men and women in the treatment of impotence and frigidity, in combination with other ***vajīkaraṇa dravyas*** such as ***Aśvagandhā***, ***Gokṣura*** and ***Śatāvarī***.

Dosage:

- ***Cūrṇa***: freshly powdered seed, 1–5 g b.i.d.–t.i.d.
- ***Tincture***: freshly crushed seed, 1:3, 50% alcohol, 1–5 mL b.i.d.–t.i.d.
- ***Taila***: in ***abhyaṅga***, ad lib.

REFERENCES

Duke JA 1985 Handbook of medicinal herbs. CRC Press, Boca Raton, p 319–321

Evans WC 1989 Trease and Evans' pharmacognosy, 13th edn. Baillière Tindall, London p 452

Felter HW, Lloyd JU 1893 King's American Dispensatory. Available: http://www.ibiblio.org/herbmed/eclectic/kings/main.html

Hallstrom H, Thuvander A 1997 Toxicological evaluation of myristicin. Natural Toxins 5(5):186–192

Hussain SP, Rao AR 1991 Chemopreventive action of mace (Myristica fragrans, Houtt) on methylcholanthrene-induced carcinogenesis in the uterine cervix in mice. Cancer Letters 56(3):231–234

Grover JK, Khandkar S, Vats V et al 2002 Pharmacological studies on Myristica fragrans – antidiarrheal, hypnotic, analgesic and hemodynamic (blood pressure) parameters. Methods and Findings in Experimental and Clinical Pharmacology 24(10):675–680

Jannu LN, Hussain SP, Rao AR 1991 Chemopreventive action of mace (Myristica fragrans, Houtt) on DMBA-induced papillomagenesis in the skin of mice. Cancer Letters 56(1):59–63

Juhasz L, Kurti L, Antus S 2000 Simple synthesis of benzofuranoid neolignans from Myristica fragrans. Journal of Natural Products 63(6):866–870

Kapoor LD 1990 CRC Handbook of Ayurvedic medicinal plants. CRC Press, Boca Raton, p 238

Kirtikar KR, Basu BD 1935 Indian medicinal plants, 2nd edn, vols 1–4. Periodical Experts, Delhi, p 2141

Morita T, Jinno K, Kawagishi H et al 2003 Hepatoprotective effect of myristicin from nutmeg (Myristica fragrans) on lipopolysaccharide/d-galactosamine-induced liver injury. Journal of Agricultural and Food Chemistry 51(6):1560–1565

Nadkarni KM 1954 The Indian materia medica, with Ayurvedic, Unani and home remedies, revised and enlarged by A.K. Nadkarni. Popular Prakashan PVP, Bombay, p 833

Olajide OA, Ajayi FF, Ekhelar AI et al 1999 Biological effects of Myristica fragrans (nutmeg) extract. Phytotherapy Research 13(4):344–345

Orabi KY, Mossa JS, el-Feraly FS 1991 Isolation and characterization of two antimicrobial agents from mace (Myristica fragrans). Journal of Natural Products 54(3):856–869

Ozaki Y, Soedigdo S, Wattimena YR, Suganda AG 1989 Anti-inflammatory effect of mace, aril of Myristica fragrans Houtt., and its active principles. Japanese Journal of Pharmacology 49(2):155–163

Park S, Lee DK, Yang CH 1998 Inhibition of fos-jun-DNA complex formation by dihydroguaiaretic acid and in vitro cytotoxic effects on cancer cells. Cancer Letters 127(1–2):23–28

Ram A, Lauria P, Gupta R, Sharma VN 1996 Hypolipidaemic effect of Myristica fragrans fruit extract in rabbits. Journal of Ethnopharmacology 55(1):49–53

Sharma A, Mathur R, Dixit VP 1995 Prevention of hypercholesterolemia and atherosclerosis in rabbits after supplementation of Myristica fragrans seed extract. Indian Journal of Physiology and Pharmacology 39(4):407–410

Srikanthamurthy KR 1984 Śārṅgadhara saṃhitā: A treatise on Ayurveda. Chaukhamba Orientalia, Varanasi, p 92

Srikanthamurthy KR 2001 Bhāvaprakāśa of Bhāvamiśra, vol 1. Krishnadas Academy, Varanasi, p 220

Warrier PK, Nambiar VPK, Ramankutty C (eds) 1995 Indian medicinal plants: a compendium of 500 species, vol 4. Orient Longman, Hyderabad, p 90

Yoganarasimhan SN 2000 Medicinal plants of India, vol 2: Tamil Nadu. Self-published, Bangalore, p 370

Jyotiṣmatī, 'luminous'

BOTANICAL NAME: *Celastrus paniculatus*, Celastraceae

OTHER NAMES: Malkanguni, Malkuki, Malkungi (H); Valulavai (T); Staff tree (E)

Botany: ***Jyotiṣmatī*** is a large deciduous climbing shrub with long slender branches attaining a height of up to 18 m, the bark reddish brown and covered in elongated white lenticels. The leaves are simple, ovate to obovate, leathery and smooth, alternately arranged on short petioles. The greenish white flowers are borne in terminal drooping panicles giving rise to depressed-globose capsules, bright yellow and three-lobed, each containing three to six seeds enclosed in an orange-red aril. ***Jyotiṣmatī*** is found throughout India, from the sub-Himalayan tract in India eastwards into southern China, Malaysia, Indonesia and Australia. It is now cultivated in these areas, and more recently in Africa, but wild populations in India are reported to be at risk (Kirtikar & Basu 1935, Nayar & Sastry 1987, Warrier et al 1994).

Part used: Seeds, bark, leaves.

Dravyguṇa:

- ***Rasa***: *kaṭu, tikta*
- ***Vipāka***: *kaṭu*
- ***Vīrya***: *uṣṇa, snigdha, tikṣṇa*
- ***Karma***: *dīpanapācana, anulomana, jvaraghna, chedana, kāsahara, hṛdaya, mūtravirecana, ārtavajanana, medhya, vajīkaraṇa, vātakaphahara* (Srikanthamurthy 2001, Warrier et al 1994).

Constituents: ***Jyotiṣmatī*** contains the sesquiterpene esters malkanguniol, malkangunin, celapanine, and celapanigine, dihydroagarofuran sesquiterpenoids, the alkaloids celastrine and paniculatine, and a sesquiterpene polyol ester. Quinone-methide and phenolic triterpenoids isolated from the root bark have been identified as celastrol, pristimerin, zeylasterone and zeylasteral. The seeds contain a brownish yellow oil, with a higher proportion of acetic and benzoic acids in addition to other fatty acids, as well as a crystalline substance thought to be a tetracasanol and sterol (Gamlath et al 1990, Kapoor 1990, Yoganarasimhan 2000).

Medical research:
- ***In vitro***: antioxidant (Russo et al 2001).
- ***In vivo***: nootropic (Gattu et al 1997, Kumar & Gupta 2002; Nalini et al 1995), sedative (Kapoor 1990), analgesic, anti-inflammatory (Ahmad et al 1994).

Toxicity: The oil of ***Jyotiṣmatī*** administered to rats at the highest dose of 5 g/kg did not produce any toxic effect or impair motor coordination (Nalini et al 1995).

Indications: Dyspepsia, arthritis, rheumatism, paralysis, sprains, sores, ulcers, asthma, mental impairment, mental exhaustion, poor memory and concentration, senile dementia, epilepsy, psychosis.

Contraindications: The ***Bhāvaprakāśa*** states that ***Jyotiṣmatī*** is an emetic, and is contraindicated in nausea and vomiting, and in conditions where emesis is contraindicated (Srikanthamurthy 2001). Given its ***uṣṇa*** and ***tikṣṇa vīrya***, ***Jyotiṣmatī*** is contraindicated in ***pittakopa*** conditions. Applied topically in large amounts the expressed oil may cause skin irritation.

Medicinal uses: ***Jyotiṣmatī*** means 'luminous', perhaps in reference to the brightly coloured fruit, or more likely to its effect of enhancing cognitive function and the natural luminosity of the 'intellect' (***buddhi***). ***Jyotiṣmatī*** is a warming herb, used internally as a decoction with botanicals such as ***Jātīphala*** and ***Tvak*** bark in the treatment of ***vāttika*** and ***kaphaja*** afflictions of the muscles and joints, including rheumatism, gout and paralysis (Nadkarni 1954). As the expressed or medicated oil ***Jyotiṣmatī*** is used for topical application as a rubifacient and stimulant. As a poultice the seeds are also used to heal indolent ulcers and sores, as well as infectious skin conditions such as scabies (Kirtikar & Basu 1935). The medicated oil is also used when applied to the head to enhance the mind and memory (Nadkarni 1954). Internally, the decoction can be used in the treatment of intellectual impairment and cognitive dysfunction, in combination with botanicals such as ***Vacā***, ***Brāhmī***, ***Jaṭāmāmsī*** and ***Maṇḍūkaparṇī***. Several texts report the benefit of the expressed oil in beriberi, a disease of the peripheral nervous system associated with a thiamine deficiency, in doses of 10–15 drops (Kirtikar & Basu 1935). Similarly, a smaller dose of 4–10 drops of the expressed oil can be used in mental exhaustion, taken earlier in the day to accommodate any possible stimulant activity. In combination with botanicals such as ***Kapikacchū*** and ***Aśvagandhā***, ***Jyotiṣmatī*** may be helpful as a ***vajīkaraṇa rasāyana*** in the treatment of sexual debility. The ***Aṣṭāñga Hṛdaya*** recommends ***Jyotiṣmatī*** to be smoked (***dhūma***) as a ***tikṣṇa dravya*** in the treatment of ***kaphaja*** conditions of the head and neck, and can also be used as an adjunct therapy in 'psychosis' (***unmāda***) (Srikanthamurthy 1994). In the treatment of amenorrhea and delayed menses the ***Cakradatta*** recommends a combination of ***Jyotiṣmatī*** leaves and ***Japā*** flower (Sharma 2002).

Dosage:

- ***Cūrṇa***: freshly powdered seed, 1–3 g b.i.d.–t.i.d.
- ***Tincture***: freshly crushed seed, 1:5, 50%, 1–3 mL b.i.d.–t.i.d.
- ***Taila***: in ***abhyañga***, ***śirodhara***, ***śirovasti***, ad lib.

REFERENCES

Ahmad F, Khan RA, Rasheed S 1994 Preliminary screening of methanolic extracts of Celastrus paniculatus and Tecomella undulata for analgesic and anti-inflammatory activities. Journal of Ethnopharmacology 42(3):193–198

Gamlath CB, Gunatilaka AAL, Tezuka Y et al 1990 Quinone-methide, phenolic and related triterpenoids of plants of Celastraceae: further evidence for the structure of celastranhydride. Phytochemistry-Oxford 29:3189–3192

Gattu M, Boss KL, Terry AV, Buccafusco JJ 1997 Reversal of scopolamine-induced deficits in navigational memory performance by the seed oil of Celastrus paniculatus. Pharmacology, Biochemistry, and Behavior 57(4):793–799

Kapoor LD 1990 CRC handbook of Ayurvedic medicinal plants. CRC Press, Boca Raton, p 111

Kirtikar KR, Basu BD 1935 Indian medicinal plants, 2nd edn, vols 1–4. Periodical Experts, Delhi, p 574–576

Kumar MH, Gupta YK 2002 Anti-oxidant property of Celastrus paniculatus willd.: a possible mechanism in enhancing cognition. Phytomedicine 9(4):302–311

Nadkarni KM 1954 The Indian materia medica, with Ayurvedic, Unani and home remedies, revised and enlarged by A.K. Nadkarni. Popular Prakashan PVP, Bombay, p 296

Nalini K, Karanth KS, Rao A, Aroor AR 1995 Effects of Celastrus paniculatus on passive avoidance performance and biogenic amine turnover in albino rats. Journal of Ethnopharmacology 47(2):101–108

Nayar MP, Sastry ARK (eds) 1987 Red data book of Indian plants, vol 1. Botanical Survey of India, Calcutta

Russo A, Izzo AA, Cardile V et al 2001 Indian medicinal plants as antiradicals and DNA cleavage protectors. Phytomedicine 8(2):125–132

Sharma PV 2002 Cakradatta. Sanskrit text with English translation. Chaukhamba, Varanasi, p 579

Srikanthamurthy KR 1994 Vāgbhaṭa's Aṣṭāñga Hṛdayam, vol 1. Krishnadas Academy, Varanasi, p 267

Srikanthamurthy KR 2001 Bhāvaprakāśa of Bhāvamiśra, vol 1. Krishnadas Academy, Varanasi, p 186

Warrier PK, Nambiar VPK, Ramankutty C (eds) 1994 Indian medicinal plants: a compendium of 500 species, vol 2. Orient Longman, Hyderabad, p 47

Yoganarasimhan SN 2000 Medicinal plants of India, vol 2: Tamil Nadu. Self-published, Bangalore, p 120

Kaṇṭakāri, 'thorny'

BOTANICAL NAME: *Solanum xanthocarpum, S. surattense,* Solanaceae

OTHER NAMES: ***Vyāghrī***, 'tigress' (S); Birhatta (H); Kandangattiri, Papparapalli (T); Yellowberried Nightshade

Botany: ***Kaṇṭakāri*** is a highly branched perennial herb, with an irregularly shaped stem that is somewhat woody at the base, covered in whitish hairs, with shining yellowish prickles that are up to 1.3 cm long. The leaves are up 5–10 cm in length and between 2.5 and 6 cm wide, ovate to elliptic, deeply lobed, covered in whitish hairs and prickles along the midrib and veins. The purple or blue flowers are borne in axillary cymes, giving rise to small globose berries that are yellowish white, with green veins, containing small yellowish brown seeds. ***Kaṇṭakāri*** is found throughout tropical India and Southeast Asia (Kirtikar & Basu 1935).

Part used: Whole plant, root.

Dravyguṇa:

- ***Rasa***: *kaṭu, tikta*
- ***Vipāka***: *kaṭu*
- ***Vīrya***: *uṣṇa, rūkṣa*
- ***Karma***: *dīpanapācana, anulomana, kṛmighna, jvaraghna, chedana, kāsahara, svāsahara, mūtravirecana, aśmaribhedana, hṛdaya, ārtavajanana, vātakaphahara* (Srikanthamurthy 2001, Warrier et al 1996)

Constituents: The limited amount of chemical research on ***Kaṇṭakāri*** has yielded the steroidal glycosides carpesterol, indioside, β-sitosterol, dioscin, methyl protoprosapogenin A, methyl protodioscin and protodioscin. In addition researchers have isolated the sesquiterpene solavetivone, a novel solafuranone, scopoletin, esculin, esculetin, *N*-(*p*-transcoumaroyl) tyramine, and *N*-trans-feruloyltyramine, as well as the alkaloids solanine, solanidine, solasonine, solamargine, and solaurine (Chiang et al 1991, Gan et al 1993, Kapoor 1990, Syu et al 2001, Yoganarasimhan 2000).

Medical research:

- ***Human trials***: *Solanum xanthocarpum* and *Solanum trilobatum* were demonstrated to promote a significant improvement in the ventilatory function of asthmatic individuals, without side effects (Govindan et al 1999, 2004).

Toxicity: No data found.

Indications: Dyspepsia, colic, flatulence, constipation, haemorrhoids, intestinal parasites, fever, catarrh, cough, bronchitis, pharyngitis, asthma, urolithiasis, oedema, skin diseases, inflammatory joint disease, sciatica, cardiovascular disease, amenorrhoea, dysmenorrhoea, epilepsy.

Contraindications: ***pittakopa***.

Medicinal uses: ***Kaṇṭakāri*** is a warming, stimulating herb, with a ***dīpanapācana*** activity that is useful to correct digestion and remove catarrh, commonly used in the treatment of fever (***jvara***), digestive weakness and respiratory conditions. For fever with pain in the chest ***Kaṇṭakāri*** is decocted with ***Gokṣura***, and taken with red rice (Sharma 2002). In the treatment of cough the ***Cakradatta*** recommends a decoction of ***Kaṇṭakāri*** and ***Harītakī***, taken with honey and a paste of ***Trikaṭu*** (Sharma 2002). Similarly, a medicated ***ghṛta*** prepared with the fresh juice of ***Kaṇṭakāri*** and powders of ***Rāsnā***, ***Balā***, ***Gokṣura*** and ***Trikaṭu*** is used to treat the different types of cough as well as hoarseness (Sharma 2002). In the treatment of colic ***Kaṇṭakāri*** is decocted with ***Balā***, ***Punarnavā***, ***Gokṣura***, and ***Bṛhatī***, taken with ***Hiṅgu*** and rock salt (Sharma 2002). In the treatment of haemorrhoids ***Kaṇṭakāri*** is prepared as a medicated

ghṛta called ***Simhyamṛta ghṛta***, prepared by decocting it along with ***Guḍūcī***, and a smaller proportion of ***Citraka***, ***Triphala***, ***Pūtikā*** bark, ***Indrayava***, ***Gambhāri*** and ***Viḍaṅga*** (Sharma 2002). As a 'simple' (remedy), a decoction of ***Kaṇṭakāri*** taken with honey is stated to be effective in all forms of dysuria and urolithiasis (Sharma 2002). In the treatment of parasites ***Kaṇṭakāri*** is used with antihelminthic herbs such as ***Viḍaṅga***, and purgatives such as ***Trivṛt***.

Dosage:

- ***Cūrṇa***: 3–5 g b.i.d.–t.i.d.
- ***Kvātha***: 30–90 mL b.i.d.–t.i.d.

REFERENCES

Chiang HC, Tseng TH, Wang CJ et al 1991 Experimental antitumor agents from Solanum indicum L. AntiCancer Research 11(5):1911–1917

Gan KH, Lin CN, Won SJ 1993 Cytotoxic principles and their derivatives of Formosan Solanum plants. Journal of Natural Products 56(1):15–21

Govindan S, Viswanathan S, Vijayasekaran V, Alagappan R 1999 A pilot study on the clinical efficacy of Solanum xanthocarpum and Solanum trilobatum in bronchial asthma. Journal of Ethnopharmacology 66(2):205–210

Govindan S, Viswanathan S, Vijayasekaran V, Alagappan R 2004 Further studies on the clinical efficacy of Solanum xanthocarpum and Solanum trilobatum in bronchial asthma. Phytotherapy Research 18(10):805–809

Kapoor LD 1990 CRC Handbook of Ayurvedic medicinal plants. CRC Press, Boca Raton, p 305

Kirtikar KR, Basu BD 1935 Indian medicinal plants, 2nd edn, vols 1–4. Periodical Experts, Delhi, p 1759–1760

Nadkarni KM 1954 The Indian materia medica, with Ayurvedic, Unani and home remedies, revised and enlarged by A.K. Nadkarni. Popular Prakashan PVP, Bombay

Sharma PV 2002 Cakradatta. Sanskrit text with English translation. Chaukhamba, Varanasi, p 4, 88, 155, 163, 257, 311

Srikanthamurthy KR 1994 Vāgbhaṭa's Aṣṭāṅga Hṛdayam, vol 1. Krishnadas Academy, Varanasi

Srikanthamurthy KR 2001 Bhāvaprakāśa of Bhāvamiśra, vol 1. Krishnadas Academy, Varanasi, p 233

Syu WJ, Don MJ, Lee GH, Sun CM 2001 Cytotoxic and novel compounds from Solanum indicum. Journal of Natural Products 64(9):1232–1233

Warrier PK, Nambiar VPK, Ramankutty C (eds) 1996 Indian medicinal plants: a compendium of 500 species, vol 5. Orient Longman, Hyderabad, p 164

Yoganarasimhan SN 2000 Medicinal plants of India, vol 2: Tamil Nadu. Self-published, Bangalore, p 505

Kapikacchū, 'monkey itcher'

BOTANICAL NAME: *Mucuna pruriens*, Papilionaceae (Fabaceae)

OTHER NAMES: ***Ātmaguptā***, 'concealed self' (S); Goncha, Kevancha, Khujani (H); Punaikkali (T); Cowitch, Cowhage (E)

Botany: ***Kapikacchū*** is a climbing annual with slender, pubescent branches. The leaves are trifoliate, attached by a long petiole up to 12 cm long, the leaflets ovate, elliptic to rhomboid ovate, 7–15 cm long, the terminal leaflet slightly larger, the leaf surface pubescent above and densely covered in silvery-grey hairs below, margin entire. The purple flowers are borne in elongated racemes of up to 30 flowers, giving rise to curved pods with longitudinal ribs, covered in brown or grey bristles, 5–7.5 cm long, each containing four to six black ovoid seeds. ***Kapikacchū*** is found throughout India, Africa and Southeast Asia (Kirtikar & Basu 1935, Warrier et al 1995).

Part used: Seeds.

Dravyguṇa:

- ***Rasa***: *amla, tikta, kaśāya, madhura*
- ***Vipāka***: *guru*
- ***Vīrya***: *uṣṇa*
- ***Karma***: *medhya, balya, vajīkaraṇa, vātapittahara* (Srikanthamurthy 2001, Warrier et al 1995).

Constituents: The most prominent constituent in ***Kapikacchū*** is L-dopa (3,4-dihydroxy-L-phenylalanine or 3-hydroxy-L-tyrosine), present in concentrations that range from a low of 1.81% for an accession named *M. pruriens* var. *utilis* grown in the USA, to a high of 7.64% for an accession named *M. pruriens* var. *cochinchinensis* grown in Bénin. It appears that L-dopa synthesis in the various cultivars is higher in plants grown at low latitudes, near the equator. Researchers have also identified a number of hallucinogenic indoles such as bufotenine, *N,N*-dimethyltryptamine and other tryptamines including serotonin, the latter of which is found in high concentrations in the bristles on the seed pods, which can cause profound skin irritation similar to a Nettle rash (hence the name 'itcher of monkeys'). Other constituents include physostigmine, cyanogenic glycosides, trypsin and amylase inhibitors, tannins, lectins, and phytic acid. Several alkaloids have also been identified, including nicotine, mucunine, mucunadine, prurienine, prurienidine, prurieninine, as well as an oil composed of stearic, palmatic, myristic, arachidic, oleic, and linoleic acids, phytosterols and lecithin (Burgos et al 2002, Kapoor 1990, St-Laurent et al 2002, Szabo & Tabbet 2002, Yoganarasimhan 2000).

Medical research:

- ***In vitro***: antioxidant (Tripathi & Upadhyay 2002)
- ***In vivo***: antidiabetic (Rathi et al 2002), antivenom (Aguiyi et al 2001)
- ***Human trials***: Used after 28 days of ***pañca karma*** therapy, a formula comprising *Mucuna pruriens, Hyoscyamus reticulatus, Withania somnifera* and *Sida cordifolia*, decocted in cow's milk, promoted a significant improvement in symptoms of Parkinson's disease (Nagashayana et al 2000). An extract of *Mucuna pruriens* was found to promote statistically significant reductions in Hoehn and Yahr Stage scores and the Unified Parkinson's Disease Rating Scale (UPDRS) scores in patients with Parkinson's disease (Manyam et al 1995). Compared with standard L-dopa/carbidopa, 30 g of *Mucuna pruriens* extract given to patients suffering from Parkinson's disease led to a more rapid onset of action and longer effect without a concomitant increase in dyskinesia (Katzenschlager et al 2004).

Toxicity: A study examining the oral toxicity of *Mucuna pruriens* on albino rats for 30 days showed no toxic effect up to a dose of 600 mg/kg (Tripathi & Upadhyay 2002). ***Kapikacchū*** contains phytic acid, which binds to minerals in the gut thereby inhibiting their absorption, as well as lectins, which can promote gastrointestinal upset and inflammation. Some studies have shown GI upset to be a minor side-effect of higher doses.

Indications: Weakness, debility, consumption, wasting, asthenia, infertility, frigidity, spasm, tremor, chorea, Parkisonson's disease, dementia.

Contraindications: Pre-existing sensitivities to legumes, inflammatory bowel disease and irritable bowel syndrome.

Medicinal uses: ***Kapikacchū*** has long been valued in Āyurveda as one of the most effective ***vajīkaraṇa dravyas***, used in both men and women, but specifically male sexual dysfunction, such as erectile dysfunction, premature ejaculation and sperm pathologies. To this end ***Kapikacchū*** is often combined with botanicals such as ***Gokṣura*** and ***Aśvagandhā*** for men, and with ***Gokṣura*** and ***Śatāvarī*** in the treatment of frigidity and leucorrhea in women. As an all-purpose ***vajīkaraṇa rasāyana*** the ***Bhāvaprakāśa*** recommends a formulation for a ***vaṭī*** ('pill') called ***Vānārī vaṭī***, made by decocting one ***kuḍava*** (approx. 192 g) of the seed-pods in one ***prastha*** (approx. 768 mL) of cow's milk until the milk becomes thick. The seeds are then removed from the pods and pounded, fried in ***ghṛta***, and mixed with twice their weight in jaggery. The resultant preparation is then rolled into small pills and dosed at about 3–4 g, twice daily (Srikanthamurthy 2000). ***Kapikacchū*** is also widely used in the treatment of almost any ***vāta*** disorder used to strengthen the mind and body in debilitated states, used in combination with botanicals such as ***Aśvagandhā***, ***Āmalakī***, ***Brāhmī*** and ***Jaṭāmāmsī***. It is an important remedy in many spasmodic afflictions, both topically and internally, including paralysis, hemiplegia and ***kampavāta*** (paralysis agitans). In the treatment of Parkinson's disease ***Kapikacchū*** has shown benefit in clinical trials, used singly or in combination with botanicals such as ***Aśvagandhā***, ***Balā***, and ***Pārasikayavānī***. Mixed with equal parts powders of ***Arjuna*** and ***Nāgabalā***, ***Kapikacchū*** seed powder is fried in ***ghṛta*** and cooked with milk and sugar to make ***Kakubhādi modaka***, used in the treatment of cough, bronchitis and consumption (Sharma 2002). As a member of the Fabaceae ***Kapikacchū*** contains many of the same constituents found in beans that can promote gastrointestinal distress, and thus measures should be taken to include herbs with a ***pācana*** activity in formulation, such as ***Śūṇṭhī***. The seeds are traditionally referred to as an antivenomous remedy against scorpion sting and snakebite, which has been validated by modern research. The hairs scraped from the pods are traditionally used topically as an irritant in fainting, and internally as a decoction in the treatment of intestinal parasites.

Dosage:

- ***Cūrṇa***: freshly powdered dried seed, 3–10 g b.i.d.–t.i.d.
- ***Tincture***: crushed seeds, 1:4, 25% alcohol, 3–15 mL

REFERENCES

Aguiyi JC, Guerranti R, Pagani R, Marinello E 2001 Blood chemistry of rats pretreated with Mucuna pruriens seed aqueous extract MP101UJ after Echis carinatus venom challenge. Phytotherapy Research 15(8):712–714

Burgos A, Matamoros I, Toro E 2002 Evaluation of velvet bean (Mucuna pruriens) meal and Enterolobium ciclocarpum fruit meal as replacements for soybean meal in diets for dual-purpose cows. In: Flores M, Eilittä M, Myhrman R et al (eds) Food and feed from Mucuna: current uses and the way forward. Cover Crops Internal Clearinghouse (CIDICCO), Tegucigalpa, Honduras, p 228–237

Kapoor LD 1990 CRC handbook of Ayurvedic medicinal plants. CRC Press, Boca Raton, p 236

Katzenschlager R, Evans A, Manson A et al 2004 Mucuna pruriens in Parkinson's disease: a double blind clinical and pharmacological study. Journal of Neurology, Neurosurgery and Psychiatry 75(12):1672–1677

Kirtikar KR, Basu BD 1935 Indian medicinal plants, 2nd edn, vols 1–4. Periodical Experts, Delhi, p 778–780

Manyam BV 1995 An alternative medicine treatment for Parkinson's disease: results of a multicenter clinical trial. HP-200 in Parkinson's Disease Study Group. Journal of Alternative and Complementary Medicine 1(3):249–255

Nadkarni KM 1954 The Indian materia medica, with Ayurvedic, Unani and home remedies, revised and enlarged by A.K. Nadkarni. Popular Prakashan PVP, Bombay

Nagashayana N, Sankarankutty P, Nampoothiri MR et al 2000 Association of L-DOPA with recovery following Ayurveda medication in Parkinson's disease. Journal of the Neurological Sciences 176(2):124–127

Rathi SS, Grover JK, Vats V 2002 The effect of Momordica charantia and Mucuna pruriens in experimental diabetes and their effect on key metabolic enzymes involved in carbohydrate metabolism. Phytotherapy Research 16(3):236–243

Sharma PV 2002 Cakradatta: Sanskrit text with English translation. Chaukhamba, Varanasi, p 134

Srikanthamurthy KR 2000 Bhāvaprakāśa of Bhāvamiśra, vol 2. Krishnadas Academy, Varanasi, p 834

Srikanthamurthy KR 2001 Bhāvaprakāśa of Bhāvamiśra, vol 1. Krishnadas Academy, Varanasi, p 248

St-Laurent L, Livesey J, Arnason JT, Bruneau A 2002 Variation in L-dopa concentration in accessions of Mucuna pruriens (L.) DC. and in Mucuna brachycarpa Rech. In: Flores M, Eilittä M, Myhrman R et al (eds) Food and feed from Mucuna: current uses and the way forward. Cover Crops Internal Clearinghouse (CIDICCO), Tegucigalpa, Honduras, p 352–374

Szabo NJ, Tebbett IR 2002 The chemistry and toxicity of Mucuna species. In: Flores M, Eilittä M, Myhrman R et al (eds) Food and feed from Mucuna: current uses and the way forward. Cover Crops Internal Clearinghouse (CIDICCO), Tegucigalpa, Honduras, p 120–141

Tripathi YB, Upadhyay AK 2002 Effect of the alcohol extract of the seeds of Mucuna pruriens on free radicals and oxidative stress in albino rats. Phytotherapy Research 16(6):534–538

Warrier PK, Nambiar VPK, Ramankutty C (eds) 1995 Indian medicinal plants: a compendium of 500 species, vol 4. Orient Longman, Hyderabad, p 68

Yoganarasimhan SN 2000 Medicinal plants of India, vol 2: Tamil Nadu. Self-published, Bangalore, p 366

Kaṭuka, 'pungent'

BOTANICAL NAME: *Picrorrhiza kurroa*, Scrophulariaceae

OTHER NAMES: Kutki (H); Katukurogani (T); Picrorrhiza (E); Hu huang lian (C)

Botany: ***Kaṭuka*** is a small pubescent perennial herb that spreads by elongated creeping rhizomes, about the thickness of the little finger. The leaves are basal, leathery, spatulate in shape with serrated margins, the tip rounded, about 5–10 cm in length. The white or bluish flowers are borne on stems as a terminal spicate raceme, longer than the leaves and for the most part naked. The fruits are ovoid capsules. ***Kaṭuka*** is native to alpine regions in the Himalayas, from Kashmir to Sikkim, 2700 to 4500 m in elevation. Unregulated overharvesting has made ***Kaṭuka*** a threatened species in Nepal and is listed in CITES Appendix II (Kirtikar & Basu 1935, MOPE 2001, Warrier et al 1995).

Part used: Rhizome. Two varieties are described: a white variety, which is intensely bitter, and a black variety, which is less so (Kirtikar & Basu 1935).

Dravyguṇa:

- ***Rasa***: *tikta, kaṭu*
- ***Vipāka***: *kaṭu*
- ***Vīrya***: *śita, rūkṣa*
- ***Karma***: *dīpanapācana, bhedana, kṛmighna, jvaraghna, kāsahara, svāsahara, raktaprasādana, kuṣṭhaghna, pittakaphahara* (Srikanthamurthy 2001, Warrier et al 1995).

Constituents: The best studied constituents of ***Kaṭuka*** are its glycosides, such as picrorhizin, which is stated to be its bitter-tasting principle, and specifically, a glycosidal fraction referred to as picroliv, standardised to contain a mixture of at least 60% kutkoside and the iridoid glycoside picroside I. Since the isolation of picroliv, however, a number of related iridoid glycosides have been described, including picrosides II, III and IV, pikuroside and 6-feruloyl catalpol. Other constituents isolated from ***Kaṭuka*** root include a group of phenylethanoid glycosides called scrosides A–C, the phenol glycoside androsin, the catechol apocynin, nine cucurbitacin glycosides, D-mannitol, kutkiol, kutkisterol, and glucosidovanilloyl glucose (Duke 2002, Jia et al 1999, Li et al 1998, Kapoor 1990, Smit et al 2000, Stuppner & Wagner 1989).

Medical research:

- ***In vitro***: anti-HBsAg (Mehrotra et al 1990), antioxidant (Chander et al 1992), anti-inflammatory (Engels et al 1992).
- ***In vivo***: hepatoprotective (Chander et al 1998, Dwivedi et al 1992, Jeena et al 1999, Mittal 1998, Rajeshkumar & Kuttan 2000, Santra et al 1998, Saraswat et al 1997, 1999, Singh et al 1992), immunostimulant (Puri et al 1992, Sharma et al 1994), anti-anaphylaxis (Baruah et al 1998, Dorsch et al 1991), antimicrobial (Mittal 1998; Chander et al 1998), antioxidant (Gaddipati et al 1999, Rastogi et al 2001, Singh et al 2000), cardioprotective (Senthil Kumar et al 2001), antidiabetic (Joy & Kuttan 1999), antitumour (Joy et al 2000, Rajeshkumar & Kuttan 2001).
- ***Human trials***: ***Kaṭuka*** root powder promoted significant improvements in serum bilirubin, SGOT and SGPT compared to placebo in patients diagnosed with acute viral hepatitis (HBsAg negative) (Vaidya et al 1996).

Toxicity: The potential toxicity of ***Kaṭuka*** has not been well studied, but from a survey of the literature, both ancient and modern, ***Kaṭuka*** appears to be relatively non-toxic. Duke (2002) reports that the curcubitans may be responsible for '. . . diarrhea, gas and griping', and have an oral LD_{50} of 10.9 mg/kg in mice.

Indications: Bilious dyspepsia, hepatic torpor, constipation, fever, cough, bronchitis, asthma, allergies, burning sensation, inflammatory skin conditions, infection, jaundice, hepatitis, cirrhosis, oedema, inflammatory joint disease, cancer.

Contraindications: In large doses ***Kaṭuka*** may act as a purgative, and should be avoided during pregnancy. In addition, the exceptionally cooling and drying nature of ***Kaṭuka*** make it contraindicated in ***vātakopa***, without utilising proper adjuncts in formulation. Mills & Bone (2000) state that ***Kaṭuka*** acts as a potent immunostimulant, and thus may be contraindicated in autoimmune disease and immune dysregulation.

Medicinal uses: ***Kaṭuka*** is an archetypal bitter herb in Āyurvedic medicine, with a linear relationship between its intensely bitter taste (***tikta rasa***) and its cold and dry energies (***śita rūkṣa vīrya***). Thus ***Kaṭuka*** is indicated primarily in ***pitta*** (hot) and ***kapha*** (wet) conditions, and should be used only in small doses or for short periods of time in ***vāttika*** states. Why exactly ***Kaṭuka*** is called 'pungent' is not entirely clear, as ***kaṭu*** is at best an ***anu rasa***, or secondary taste – in some texts ***Kaṭuka*** is classified as having an ***uṣṇa vīrya***, and this may explain the discrepancy. As a bitter herb, ***Kaṭuka*** is obviously important in liver and spleen dysfunction, used in simple states of hepatic torpor and bilious dyspepsia, as well as in hepatosplenomegaly, drug-induced liver injury, viral hepatitis, jaundice, cirrhosis and liver flukes, usually in combination with aromatic ***dīpanapācana*** herbs to reduce any possible griping. In the treatment of viral hepatitis ***Kaṭuka*** may be of benefit when combined with other antiviral botanicals such as ***Bhūnimba***, Wu wei zi (*Schizandra chinensis*), St John's Wort (*Hypericum perforatum*) and Osha (*Ligusticum porteri*). In the treatment of jaundice and other liver disorders, the ***Cakradatta*** recommends a decoction of ***Kaṭuka*** with equal parts ***Triphala***, ***Guḍūcī***, ***Vacā***, ***Kirātatiktā*** and ***Nimba***, taken with honey (Sharma 2002). ***Kaṭuka*** is also used more generally in a variety of digestive disorders, such as constipation, in which it is used in small amounts combined with ***dīpanapācana*** remedies such as ***Triphala***, ***Hingvatsak*** and ***saindhava***. In the treatment of malabsorption (***grahaṇī***), with bloody diarrhoea and haemorrhoids, the ***Cakradatta*** recommends a ***cūrṇa*** called ***Nāgarādya cūrṇa*** composed of equal parts ***Kuṣṭha***, ***Śūṇṭhī***, purified ***Ativiṣā***, ***Mustaka***, ***Dhātaki***, ***Rasāñjana***, ***Kuṭaja***, ***Bilva*** and ***Pāṭhā***, mixed with honey and taken with ***peya*** (rice water) (Sharma 2002). In the treatment of ***udara*** (intestinal parasites) and secondary anaemia the ***Cakradatta*** recommends ***Kaṭuka*** decocted with equal parts ***Punarnavā***, ***Nimba***, ***Paṭola***, ***Śūṇṭhī***, ***Guḍūcī***, ***Devadāru*** and ***Harītakī***. This remedy is also stated to be useful in cough and dyspnoea (Sharma 2002). As a cooling, anti-inflammatory remedy, ***Kaṭuka*** is important in ***pittakopa*** conditions, with symptoms of heat and burning, as well as in inflammatory and infectious skin conditions. In the treatment of ***paittika jvara*** (fever) for example, the ***Cakradatta*** recommends that ***Kaṭuka*** be decocted with equal parts ***Indrayava***, ***Kaṭphala***, ***Mustaka***, and ***Pāṭhā*** (Sharma 2002). In the treatment of inflammatory joint diseases such as gout, particularly with symptoms of burning and heat, ***Kaṭuka*** is combined with equal parts ***Paṭola***, ***Śatāvarī***, ***Triphala*** and ***Guḍūcī*** (Sharma 2002). ***Kaṭuka*** is also important in typically ***kaphaja*** conditions such as cough and bronchitis, in combination with herbs such as ***Bibhītaka***, ***Vāsaka***, and ***Yaṣṭimadhu***, and usually with ***dīpanapācana*** remedies such as ***Trikaṭu*** to offset its cooling energy. In the treatment of oedema ***Kaṭuka*** is mentioned in formulation with botanicals such as ***Harītakī***, ***Devadāru***, and ***Pippalī***. More recently, ***Kaṭuka*** has been used by Western herbalists as an potent immunostimulant, in combination with herbs such as Purple Coneflower (*Echinacea angustifolia*) and ***Bhūnimba***, in the treatment of chronic viral infection and immunodeficiency.

Dosage:

- ***Cūrṇa***: dried rhizome, 2–3 g b.i.d.–t.i.d.
- ***Tincture***: dried rhizome, 1:4, 60% alcohol, 1–3 mL

REFERENCES

Baruah CC, Gupta PP, Nath A et al 1998 Anti-allergic and anti-anaphylactic activity of picroliv–a standardised iridoid glycoside fraction of Picrorhiza kurroa. Pharmacological Research 38(6):487–492

Chander R, Kapoor NK, Dhawan BN 1992 Picroliv, picroside-I and kutkoside from Picrorhiza kurrooa are scavengers of superoxide anions. Biochemical Pharmacology 44(1):180–183

Chander R, Singh K, Visen PK et al 1998 Picroliv prevents oxidation in serum lipoprotein lipids of Mastomys coucha infected with Plasmodium berghei. Indian Journal of Experimental Biology 36(4):371–374

Dorsch W, Stuppner H, Wagner H et al 1991 Anti-asthmatic effects of Picrorhiza kurroa: androsin prevents allergen- and PAF-induced bronchial obstruction in guinea pigs. International Archives Of Allergy And Applied Immunology 95(2–3):128–133

Dwivedi Y, Rastogi R, Garg NK, Dhawan BN 1992 Effects of picroliv, the active principle of Picrorhiza kurroa, on biochemical changes in rat liver poisoned by Amanita phalloides. Zhongguo Yao Li Xue Bao 13(3):197–200

Duke JA 2002 Handbook of medicinal herbs, 2nd edn. CRC Press, Boca Raton, p 568

Engels F, Renirie BF, Hart BA et al 1992 Effects of apocynin, a drug isolated from the roots of Picrorhiza kurroa, on arachidonic acid metabolism. FEBS Letters 305(3):254–256

Gaddipati JP, Mani H, Banaudha KK et al 1999 Picroliv modulates the expression of insulin-like growth factor (IGF)-I, IGF-II and IGF-I receptor during hypoxia in rats. Cellular and Molecular Life Sciences 56(3–4):348–355

Jeena KJ, Joy KL, Kuttan R 1999 Effect of Emblica officinalis, Phyllanthus amarus and Picrorrhiza kurroa on N-nitroso-diethylamine induced hepatocarcinogenesis. Cancer Letters 136(1):11–16

Jia Q, Hong MF, Minter D 1999 Pikuroside: a novel iridoid from Picrorhiza kurroa. Journal of Natural Products 62(6):901–903

Joy KL, Kuttan R 1999 Anti-diabetic activity of Picrorrhiza kurroa extract. Journal of Ethnopharmacology 67(2):143–8

Joy KL, Rajeshkumar NV, Kuttan G, Kuttan R 2000 Effect of Picrorrhiza kurroa extract on transplanted tumors and chemical carcinogenesis in mice. Journal of Ethnopharmacology 71(1–2):261–266

Kapoor LD 1990 CRC handbook of Ayurvedic medicinal plants. CRC Press, Boca Raton, p 263

Kirtikar KR, Basu BD 1935 Indian medicinal plants, 2nd edn, vols 1–4. Periodical Experts, Delhi, p 1825–1826

Li JX, Li P, Tezuka Y, Namba T, Kadota S 1998 Three phenylethanoid glycosides and an iridoid glycoside from Picrorhiza scrophulariiflora. Phytochemistry 48(3):537–542

Mehrotra R, Rawat S, Kulshreshtha DK 1990 In vitro studies on the effect of certain natural products against hepatitis B virus. Indian Journal of Medical Research 92:133–8

Mills S, Bone K 2000 Principles and practice of phytotherapy. Churchill Livingstone, London, p 154

Mittal N, Gupta N, Saksena S 1998 Protective effect of Picroliv from Picrorhiza kurroa against Leishmania donovani infections in Mesocricetus auratus. Life Sciences 63(20):1823–1834

MOPE 2001 Nepal's State of the Environment. Ministry of Population and Environment, Kathmandu p annex 1–2. Available: http://www.mope.gov.np/environment/state2001.php

Nadkarni KM 1954 The Indian materia medica, with Ayurvedic, Unani and home remedies, revised and enlarged by A.K. Nadkarni. Popular Prakashan PVP, Bombay

Puri A, Saxena RP, Sumati et al 1992 Immunostimulant activity of Picroliv, the iridoid glycoside fraction of Picrorhiza kurroa, and its protective action against Leishmania donovani infection in hamsters. Planta Medica 58(6):528–532

Rajeshkumar NV, Kuttan R 2000 Inhibition of N-nitrosodiethyl-amine-induced hepatocarcinogenesis by Picroliv. Journal of Experimental and Clinical Cancer Research 19(4):459–465

Rajeshkumar NV, Kuttan R 2001 Protective effect of Picroliv, the active constituent of Picrorhiza kurroa, against chemical carcinogenesis in mice. Teratogenesis, Carcinogenesis, and Mutagenesis 21(4):303–313

Rastogi R, Srivastava AK, Rastogi AK 2001 Long term effect of aflatoxin B(1) on lipid peroxidation in rat liver and kidney: effect of picroliv and silymarin. Phytotherapy Research 15(4):307–310

Santra A, Das S, Maity A et al 1998 Prevention of carbon tetrachloride-induced hepatic injury in mice by Picrorhiza kurrooa. Indian Journal of Gastroenterology 17(1):6–9

Saraswat B, Visen PK, Patnaik GK, Dhawan BN 1997 Protective effect of picroliv, active constituent of Picrorhiza kurrooa, against oxytetracycline induced hepatic damage. Indian Journal of Experimental Biology 35(12):1302–1305

Saraswat B, Visen PK, Patnaik GK, Dhawan BN 1999 Ex vivo and in vivo investigations of picroliv from Picrorhiza kurroa in an alcohol intoxication model in rats. Journal of Ethnopharmacology 66(3):263–269

Senthil Kumar SH, Anandan R, Devaki T, Santhosh Kumar M 2001 Cardioprotective effects of Picrorrhiza kurroa against isoproterenol-induced myocardial stress in rats. Fitoterapia 72(4):402–405

Sharma ML, Rao CS, Duda PL 1994 Immunostimulatory activity of Picrorhiza kurroa leaf extract. Journal of Ethnopharmacology 41(3):185–192

Sharma PV 2002 Cakradatta. Sanskrit text with English translation. Chaukhamba, Varanasi, p 12, 65, 114, 234, 347

Singh AK, Mani H, Seth P et al 2000 Picroliv preconditioning protects the rat liver against ischemia-reperfusion injury. European Journal of Pharmacology 395(3):229–239

Singh V, Visen PK, Patnaik GK 1992 Effect of picroliv on low density lipoprotein receptor binding of rat hepatocytes in hepatic damage induced by paracetamol. Indian Journal of Biochemistry and Biophysics. 29(5):428–432

Smit HF, van den Berg AJ, Kroes BH 2000 Inhibition of T-lymphocyte proliferation by cucurbitacins from Picrorhiza scrophulariaeflora. Journal of Natural Products 63(9):1300–1302

Srikanthamurthy KR 2001 Bhāvaprakāśa of Bhāvamiśra, vol 1. Krishnadas Academy, Varanasi, p 182

Stuppner H, Wagner H 1989 New cucurbitacin glycosides from Picrorhiza kurrooa. Planta Medica 55(6):559–563

Vaidya AB, Antarkar DS, Doshi JC et al 1996 Picrorhiza kurroa (Kutaki) Royle ex Benth as a hepatoprotective agent: experimental and clinical studies. Journal of Postgraduate Medicine 42(4):105–108

Warrier PK, Nambiar VPK, Ramankutty C (eds) 1995 Indian medicinal plants: a compendium of 500 species, vol 4. Orient Longman, Hyderabad, p 269–272

Kūṣmāṇḍa

BOTANICAL NAMES: *Benincasa hispida, B. cerifera,* Cucurbitaceae

OTHER NAMES: Petha, Kondha, Kudimah (H); Sambal pushani, Pushanikkai (T); Wax Gourd, Winter Melon (E); Dong gua (C)

Botany: ***Kūṣmāṇḍa*** is a large trailing plant with stout angular stems and stiff hairs. The cordate leaves are large, up to 12 cm in diameter, with five to seven lobes, mostly glabrous above with stiff hairs below. The flowers are yellow, monoecious, the male peduncle longer than the female. The fruit is a cylindrical gourd that grows up to 45 cm in length and can weigh up to 35 kg. It is hairy and is covered in a waxy, chalky coating that protects it against pests and gives it an exceptionally long shelf-life. ***Kūṣmāṇḍa*** is found throughout Asia in tropical regions, cultivated as both a food and medicine (Kirtikar & Basu 1935, Warrier et al 1994).

Part used: Unripe, maturing and ripened fruit, seeds.

Dravyguṇa:

- ***Rasa***: *madhura*
- ***Vipāka***: *guru* (unripe fruit), *laghu* (ripe fruit)
- ***Vīrya***: *śita, rūkṣa* (unripe fruit); ripe fruit has an almost neutral *vīrya*
- ***Karma***: unripe fruit is *bhedana, jvaraghna, raktaprasādana, śoṇitasthāpana, dāhapraśamana, vajīkaraṇa, balya, vātapittahara;* maturing fruit is *kaphakopa;* mature fruit and seed is *dīpana, mūtravirecana, medhya, tridoṣaghna* (Dash 1991, Srikanthamurthy 2001, Warrier et al 1994).

Constituents: Researchers have isolated a number of triterpene glycosides from ***Kūṣmāṇḍa***, including alnusenol and multiflorenol, as well as a flavonoid C-glycoside, a benzyl glycoside, and β-sitosterol. Other constituents include proteins, sugars and fats, as well as a cucumisin-like serine protease (Uchikoba et al 1998, Yoganarasimhan 2000, Yoshizumi et al 1998).

Medical research:

- ***In vivo***: anti-ulcerogenic (Grover et al 2001); anti-allergenic (Grover et al 2001, Kumar & Ramu 2002, Yoshizumi et al 1998); nootropic (Kumar & Nirmala 2003); anti-withdrawal (Grover et al 2000).

Toxicity: Chronic toxicity studies carried out for 3 months in experimental animals revealed no deleterious effect of fresh juice of *B. hispida* on various haematological and biochemical parameters (Grover et al 2001).

Indications: Dyspepsia, colic, intestinal parasites, fever, dry cough, purulent bronchitis, asthma, consumption, wasting, oedema, thirst, burning sensations, haemorrhage, urinary calculi, cystitis, leucorrhoea, epilepsy, psychosis.

Contraindications: Diarrhoea (Bensky & Gamble 1993).

Medicinal uses: *Kūṣmāṇḍa* is both a medicinal plant and a vegetable, consumed widely throughout Asia. In India ***Kūṣmāṇḍa*** is highly valued as a nutritive food, used during convalescence in wasting diseases, and prepared as a confection in the treatment in ulceration of the lungs and intestines. The fresh fruit of the juice is used in haemoptysis and internal bleeding (Nadkarni 1954). The ***Cakradatta*** recommends a ***lehya*** called ***Vāsākhaṇḍakūṣmāṇḍaka***, prepared from ***Kūṣmāṇḍa*** pulp, ***Vāsaka*** and ***dīpanapācana dravyas*** in the treatment of internal haemorrhaging, chest wounds, cough, dyspnoea, consumption, angina and back pain (Sharma 2002). In Chinese medicine the seeds are similarly used in lung conditions with a yellowish sputum, as well as in yellowish mucosal discharges of the bowels and uterus (Bensky & Gamble 1993). ***Kūṣmāṇḍa*** is also an important remedy in the treatment of ***unmāda*** ('psychosis') and ***apasmāra***

('epilepsy'). The ***Cakradatta*** recommends the fresh juices of ***Kūṣmāṇḍa***, ***Brāhmī***, ***Vacā***, ***Śaṅkhapuṣpī*** and ***Kuṣṭha***, taken with honey, in the treatment of ***unmāda*** (Sharma 2002). Similarly, the ***Bhāvaprakāśa*** recommends that 18 parts the fresh juice of ***Kūṣmāṇḍa*** be decocted in one part ***ghṛta***, with a paste of ***Yaṣṭimadhu***, down to one part ***ghṛta***, in the treatment of ***apasmāra*** (Srikanthamurthy 2000). In the treatment of difficult cases of intestinal colic the ***Bhāvaprakāśa*** recommends that the freshly dried ***Kūṣmāṇḍa*** fruit be heated until red hot over a mild fire, reduced to a powder, and taken with a little ***Śūṇṭhī*** (Srikanthamurthy 2000). In the treatment of cystitis the ***Cakradatta*** recommends the fresh juice of ***Kūṣmāṇḍa*** with ***Yavakṣāra*** and sugar (Sharma 2002). Much like pumpkin seeds, the seeds of ***Kūṣmāṇḍa*** are consumed in the treatment of intestinal parasites.

Dosage:

- ***Cūrṇa***: dried pulp and/or seed, 2–10 g b.i.d.–t.i.d.
- ***Svarasa***: 30–120 mL b.i.d.–t.i.d.

REFERENCES

Bensky D, Gamble A 1993 Chinese herbal medicine materia medica, revised edn. Eastland Press, Seattle, p 135

Dash B 1991 Materia medica of Ayurveda. B Jain Publishers, New Delhi, p 317–318

Grover JK, Rathi SS, Vats V 2000 Preliminary study of fresh juice of Benincasa hispida on morphine addiction in mice. Fitoterapia 71(6):707–709

Grover JK, Adiga G, Vats V, Rathi SS 2001 Extracts of Benincasa hispida prevent development of experimental ulcers. Journal of Ethnopharmacology 78(2–3):159–164

Kapoor LD 1990 CRC Handbook of Ayurvedic medicinal plants. CRC Press, Boca Raton

Kirtikar KR, Basu BD 1935 Indian medicinal plants, 2nd edn, vols 1–4. Periodical Experts, Delhi, p 1127

Kumar A, Nirmala V 2003 Nootropic activity of methanol extract of Benincasa hispida fruit. Indian Journal of Pharmacy 35:194–201

Kumar A, Ramu P 2002 Effect of methanolic extract of Benincasa hispida against histamine and acetylcholine induced bronchospasm in guinea pigs. Indian Journal of Pharmacology 34:365–366

Nadkarni KM 1954 The Indian materia medica, with Ayurvedic, Unani and home remedies, revised and enlarged by A.K. Nadkarni. Popular Prakashan PVP, Bombay, p 186

Sharma PV 2002 Cakradatta: Sanskrit text with English translation. Chaukhamba, Varanasi, p 130, 184

Srikanthamurthy KR 2000 Bhāvaprakāśa of Bhāvamiśra, vol 2. Krishnadas Academy, Varanasi, p 313, 426

Srikanthamurthy KR 2001 Bhāvaprakāśa of Bhāvamiśra, vol 1. Krishnadas Academy, Varanasi, p 388

Uchikoba T, Yonezawa H, Kaneda M 1998 Cucumisin like protease from the sarcocarp of Benincasa hispida var. Ryukyu. Phytochemistry 49(8):2215–2219

Warrier PK, Nambiar VPK, Ramankutty C (eds) 1994 Indian medicinal plants: a compendium of 500 species, vol 1. Orient Longman, Hyderabad, p 261

Yoganarasimhan SN 2000 Medicinal plants of India, vol 2: Tamil Nadu. Self-published, Bangalore, p 75

Yoshizumi S, Murakami T, Kadoya M et al 1998 Medicinal foodstuffs. XI. Histamine release inhibitors from wax gourd, the fruits of Benincasa hispida Cogn. Yakugaku Zasshi 118(5):188–192

Kuṣṭha, 'disease'

BOTANICAL NAMES: *Saussurea lappa, Aucklandia lappa,* Asteraceae

OTHER NAMES: Kuth, Kur (H); Kostam, Goshtam (T); Costus (E); Mu xiang (C)

Botany: ***Kuṣṭha*** is a robust erect perennial herb with a stout stem attaining a height of up to 2 m, and roots up to 60 cm long that have a distinctive, characteristic odour. The leaves are membranous and irregularly toothed, the basal leaves quite large, up to 1.2 m in length, triangularly shaped with a winged stalk, the terminal lobe up to 30 cm across. The upper leaves arise from the stem and are smaller, with two clasping lobes at the base. The bluish-purple flowers are borne in axillary and terminal clusters, giving rise to compressed achenes. ***Kuṣṭha*** is native to the Himalayas, from Kashmir to Sikkim, northwards into Tibet and eastwards into Yunnan province in China, between elevations of 2500 and 4000 m. ***Kuṣṭha*** is currently threatened with extinction due to unregulated harvesting and is listed in CITES Appendix I (Kirtikar & Basu 1935, MOPE 2001, Warrier et al 1996).

Part used: Root.

Dravyguṇa:

- ***Rasa***: *tikta, kaṭu, madhura*
- ***Vipāka***: *madhura*
- ***Vīrya***: *uṣṇa*
- ***Karma***: *dīpanapācana, jvaraghna, chedana, kāsahara, svāsahara, mūtravirecana, raktaprasādana, kuṣṭhaghna, vedanāsthāpana, stanyajanana, vajīkaraṇa, rasāyana, vātakaphahara* (Nadkarni 1954, Srikanthamurthy 2001, Warrier et al 1996).

Constituents: ***Kuṣṭha*** contains an essential oil used in perfumery called costus oil, comprising upwards of 1.5% of the dried plant, that has a woody, musty, lingering smell. Costus oil is composed mostly of sesquiterpene lactones, including dihydrocostus lactone (15%) and costos lactone (10%), other constituents including aplotaxene (20%), δ-costen (6%), β-costen (6%), and costic acid (14%), and also smaller amounts of camphene, phellandrene, caryophyllene and selinene. Non-volatile constituents include amino acid-sesquiterpene adducts saussureamines A–E, a lignan glycoside, the alkaloid saussurine, a bitter principle, a resin, tannin, fixed oil, inulin and sugar (De Kraker et al 2001, Kapoor 1990, Lawless 1995, Yoshikawa et al 1993).

Medical research:

- ***In vitro***: anti-inflammatory (Cho et al 2000, Gokhale et al 2002, Matsuda et al 2003), anti-HBsAg (Chen et al 1995), antitumour (Jeong et al 2002, Ko et al 2004, 2005).
- ***In vivo***: anti-ulcer (Yoshikawa et al 1993)
- ***Human trials***: in healthy volunteers a decoction of *Saussurea lappa* was found to accelerate gastric emptying and increase endogenous motilin release, an amino acid peptide that regulates upper GI motility (Chen et al 1994).

Toxicity: Costus oil isolated from *Saussurea lappa* is associated with several cases of allergic contact dermatitis (Cheminat et al 1981).

Indications: Dyspepsia, biliousness, gastrointestinal spasm, diarrhoea, dysentery, fever, bronchitis, asthma, skin diseases, dysmenorrhoea, muscle spasm, gout, autotoxicity.

Contraindications: ***pittakopa***. Bensky & Gamble (1993) stated that ***Kuṣṭha*** is contraindicated in yin deficiency and dryness.

Medicinal uses: The name ***Kuṣṭha*** refers to an ancient Vedic plant god mentioned in the ***Atharva veda*** as a remedy for ***takman***, the archetypal disease of excess or ***jvara*** (fever). In ancient India ***Kuṣṭha*** was considered to be a divine plant derived from heavenly sources, growing high in the Himalayas, considered to be the brother of the divine ***Soma*** (Zysk 1998). From its Sanskrit name it could be inferred that ***Kuṣṭha*** is a specific for skin disease (i.e. ***kuṣṭha***), and indeed it is used as such, primarily as ***raktaprasādana***, or alterative. Although it is not considered among the most important plants in the treatment of skin disease it is used in a variety of skin conditions, from leprosy, ulcers and ringworm to leucoderma and simple pruritis. More importantly, ***Kuṣṭha*** is a ***rasāyana*** for ***vāta***, helping to normalise and strengthen digestion, cleanse the body of toxic accumulations, enhance fertility and reduce pain. As a bitter tasting herb ***Kuṣṭha*** acts on the liver and gall bladder, stimulating bile synthesis and excretion, and as an aromatic, acts as a carminative to ease cramping and intestinal colic. Generally speaking, ***Kuṣṭha*** is an important remedy in any kind of spasm or pain, be it smooth or skeletal muscle, primarily due to its ability to normalise ***vāta***. In the treatment of cramping and spasm of the abdomen or musculature the ***Cakradatta*** recommends a topical preparation called ***Kuṣṭhadi taila***, comprising ***taila*** and vinegar, mixed with powders of ***Kuṣṭha*** and ***saindhava***, and massaged into the affected tissues (Sharma 2002). Mixed with equal parts powders of ***Hiṅgu***, ***Trikaṭu***, ***Yavakṣāra*** and ***saindhava***, ***Kuṣṭha*** is mixed with ***Mātuluṅga*** juice and taken internally to alleviate abdominal pain (Sharma 2002). Similarly, ***Kuṣṭha*** is used in Chinese medicine mixed with Bai zhu (*Atractylodes macrocephala*) for epigastric pain and bloating (Bensky & Gamble 1993). In the treatment of diarrhoea and dysentery ***Kuṣṭha*** can be taken along with ***Kuṭaja***, ***Harītakī***, ***Śūṇṭhī***, ***Mustaka***, and ***Dāruharidrā***. In the treatment of ***ūrusthambha*** (paraplegia), the ***Cakradatta*** recommends ***Kuṣṭhādya taila***, composed of ***Kuṣṭha***, ***Śriveṣṭaka*** resin, ***Udīcya***, ***Sarala*** wood, ***Devadāru***, ***Nāgakeśara***, ***Ajagandhā*** and ***Aśvagandhā*** decocted in mustard oil, taken internally with honey (Sharma 2002). In the treatment of ***vāttika*** headache the ***Śāraṅgadhara saṃhitā*** recommends a paste of ***Kuṣṭha cūrṇa*** prepared with rice water and castor oil, applied topically (Srikanthamurthy 1984). In the treatment of toothache, gum swelling and bleeding, ***Kuṣṭha*** is mixed with equal parts ***Dārvī***, ***Mañjiṣṭhā***, ***Pāṭhā***, ***Kaṭuka***, ***Haridrā***, ***Tejanī***, ***Mustaka*** and ***Lodhra***, and applied to the gums (Srikanthamurthy 1984). In the treatment of ***vāttika udara roga*** in which ***apāna vāyu*** moves upwards, characterised by abdominal bloating and pain, and accompanied by joint pain, bodyache and lethargy, the ***Bhāvaprakāśa*** recommends ***Kuṣṭhadi cūrṇa***, composed of equal parts ***Kuṣṭha*** along with ***dīpanapācana*** remedies such as ***Hiṅgu***, ***Cavya***, ***Citraka*** and ***Śūṇṭhī*** (Srikanthamurthy 2000). In the treatment of ***vāttika*** anorexia, ***Kuṣṭha cūrṇa*** is taken with equal parts ***Sauvarcala*** (Sanchal salt), ***Jīraka***, ***Marica***, ***Viḍa*** (black salt) and sugar, with ***taila*** and honey as an ***anupāna*** (Sharma 2002). In the treatment of ***unmāda*** ('psychosis'), the ***Cakradatta*** recommends a combination of equal parts ***Kuṣṭha*** with ***Brāhmī***, ***Kūṣmāṇḍa***, ***Vacā*** and ***Śaṅkhapuṣpī***, taken with honey (Sharma 2002). To keep children healthy and strong, the ***Cakradatta*** recommends a ***lehya*** prepared from equal parts ***Kuṣṭha***, ***Vacā***, ***Brāhmī***, and ***Svarṇa*** (purified gold), prepared with honey and ***ghṛta***, (Sharma 2002). As a refreshing mouth rinse, the ***Cakradatta*** recommends ***Kuṣṭhadi kavala***, comprised of equal parts infusion of ***Kuṣṭha***, ***Elāvaluka***, ***Elā***, ***Mustaka***, ***Dhānyaka*** and honey (Sharma 2002). In the treatment of asthma, a tincture of ***Kuṣṭha*** is stated to be particularly effective to relieve bronchial spasm (Kirtikar & Basu 1935, Nadkarni 1954).

Dosage:

- ***Cūrṇa***: freshly dried root, 3–5 g b.i.d.–t.i.d.
- ***Phāṇṭa***: freshly crushed root, 1:4, 30–60 mL b.i.d.–t.i.d.
- ***Tincture***: freshly dried root, 1:4, 50% alcohol, 1–5 mL

REFERENCES

Bensky D, Gamble A 1993 Chinese herbal medicine materia medica, revised edn. Eastland Press, Seattle, p 237–238

Cheminat A, Stampf JL, Benezra C et al 1981 Allergic contact dermatitis to costus: removal of haptens with polymers. Acta Dermato-Venereologica 61(6):525–529

Chen HC, Chou CK, Lee SD et al 1995 Active compounds from Saussurea lappa Clarks that suppress hepatitis B virus surface antigen gene expression in human hepatoma cells. Antiviral Research 27(1–2):99–109

Chen SF, Li YQ, He FY 1994 Effect of Saussurea lappa on gastric functions. Zhongguo Zhong Xi Yi Jie He Za Zhi 14(7):406–408

Cho JY, Baik KU, Jung JH, Park MH 2000 In vitro anti-inflammatory effects of cynaropicrin, a sesquiterpene lactone, from Saussurea lappa. European Journal of Pharmacology 398(3):399–407

De Kraker JW, Franssen MC, De Groot A et al 2001 Germacrenes from fresh costus roots. Phytochemistry 58(3):481–487

Gokhale AB, Damre AS, Kulkami KR, Saraf MN 2002 Preliminary evaluation of anti-inflammatory and anti-arthritic activity of S. lappa, A. speciosa and A. aspera. Phytomedicine 9(5):433–437

Jeong SJ, Itokawa T, Shibuya M et al 2002 Costunolide, a sesquiterpene lactone from Saussurea lappa, inhibits the VEGFR KDR/Flk–1 signaling pathway. Cancer Letters 187(1–2):129–133

Kapoor LD 1990 CRC handbook of Ayurvedic medicinal plants. CRC Press, Boca Raton, p 300

Kirtikar KR, Basu BD 1935 Indian medicinal plants, 2nd edn, vols 1–4. Periodical Experts, Delhi, p 1420–1422

Ko SG, Koh SH, Jun CY et al 2004 Induction of apoptosis by Saussurea lappa and Pharbitis nil on AGS gastric cancer cells. Biological and Pharmaceutical Bulletin 27(10):1604–1610

Ko SG, Kim HP, Jin DH et al 2005 Saussurea lappa induces G2-growth arrest and apoptosis in AGS gastric cancer cells. Cancer Letters 220(1):11–19

Lawless J 1995 The illustrated encyclopedia of essential oils. Element, Rockport MA, p 219

Matsuda H, Toguchida I, Ninomiya K et al 2003 Effects of sesquiterpenes and amino acid-sesquiterpene conjugates from the roots of Saussurea lappa on inducible nitric oxide synthase and heat shock protein in lipopolysaccharide-activated macrophages. Bioorganic and Medicinal Chemistry 11(5):709–715

MOPE 2001 Nepal's State of the Environment. Ministry of Population and Environment, Kathmandu p annex 1–2. Available: http://www.mope.gov.np/environment/state2001.php

Nadkarni KM 1954 The Indian materia medica, with Ayurvedic, Unani and home remedies, revised and enlarged by A.K. Nadkarni. Popular Prakashan PVP, Bombay, p 1112

Sharma PV 2002 Cakradatta. Sanskrit text with English translation. Chaukhamba, Varanasi, p 107, 165, 184, 245, 267, 595, 656

Srikanthamurthy KR 1984 Śāraṅgadhara saṃhitā: a treatise on Ayurveda. Chaukhamba Orientalia, Varanasi, p 235, 242

Srikanthamurthy KR 2000 Bhāvaprakāśa of Bhavamiśra, vol. 2. Krishnadas Academy, Varanasi, p 519

Srikanthamurthy KR 2001 Bhāvaprakāśa of Bhāvamiśra, vol 1. Krishnadas Academy, Varanasi, p 186,

Warrier PK, Nambiar VPK, Ramankutty C (eds) 1996 Indian medicinal plants: a compendium of 500 species, vol 5. Orient Longman, Hyderabad, p 80–83

Yoshikawa M, Hatakeyama S, Inoue Y, Yamahara J 1993 Saussureamines A, B, C, D, and E, new anti-ulcer principles from Chinese Saussureae Radix. Chemical and Pharmaceutical Bulletin (Tokyo) 41(1):214–216

Zysk KG 1998 Asceticism and healing in ancient India: medicine in the Buddhist monastery. Motilal Banarsidass, Delhi, p 19

Kuṭaja, 'mountain born'

BOTANICAL NAMES: *Holarrhena antidysenterica, H. pubescens,* Apocynaceae

OTHER NAMES: ***Indrayava***, 'Indra's seeds' (S); Kurchi, Kuda (H); Kutashappalai, Veppalai (T); Kurchi tree, Conessi tree (E)

Botany: ***Kuṭaja*** is a shrub or small tree with pale coloured bark that exudes a whitish latex when cut. The leaves are simple, broadly ovate to elliptic, glabrous or pubescent, with 10–14 pairs of conspicuous nerves, oppositely arranged on short petioles. The flowers are white, without odour, borne in terminal flat-topped cymes, giving rise to long narrow fruits that are tipped with a crown of brown hairs. ***Kuṭaja*** is found throughout India and Southeast Asia, in deciduous forests up to 900 m (Kirtikar & Basu 1935, Warrier et al 1995).

Part used: Bark (***Kuṭaja***), seeds (***Indrayava***).

Dravyguṇa:

- ***Rasa***: *kaśāya, tikta*
- ***Vipāka***: *laghu*
- ***Vīrya***: *śita*
- ***Karma***: *dīpana, chardinigrahaṇa, purīṣasangrahaṇīya, kṛmighna, jvaraghna, kāsahara, svāsahara, śoṇitasthāpana, kuṣṭhaghna, kaphahara* (Dash 1991, Srikanthamurthy 2001, Warrier et al 1995).

Constituents: Researchers have isolated only a few classes of constituents from ***Kuṭaja***, mostly alkaloids, as well as steroidal alkaloids and steroids. Among the alkaloidal constituents are conessine, conessimine, kurchine, conamine, conimine, conessidine, conarrhimine, holarrhimine, holarrhine and kurchicine. Steroidal alkaloids include antidysentericine and regholarrhenines A–F. Recently isolated steroidal compounds include pubadysone, puboestrene and pubamide. Other constituents include β-sitosterol, a triterpene alcohol, lupeol, gum, lettoresinols A and B, and tannins (Kapoor 1990, Kumar and Ali 2000, Siddiqui et al 2001, Williamson 2002, Yoganarasimhan 2000).

Medical research:

- ***In vitro***: antibacterial (Aqil et al 2005, Chakraborty & Brantner 1999, Kavitha et al 2004, Rani & Khullar 2004, Voravuthikunchai et al 2004).
- ***In vivo***: anti-amoebic, antidysentery (Duke 2002, Williamson 2002); antidiarrhoeal (Kavitha et al 2004); immunomodulant (Atal et al 1986).

Toxicity: No data found.

Indications: Dyspepsia, diarrhoea, dysentery, amoebic dysentery, intestinal parasites, haemorrhoids, fever, malaria, asthma, pneumonia, jaundice, hepatosplenomegaly, internal haemorrhaging, menorrhagia, rheumatism, skin diseases.

Contraindications: Constipation, ***vātakopa***.

Medicinal uses: ***Kuṭaja*** is an exceptionally important and useful remedy in diarrhoea and dysentery, and for this purpose the bark is preferred, which in addition to containing antimicrobial alkaloids also contains tannins that help to astringe the gut mucosa. Among the best remedies to treat infectious diarrhoea is ***Kuṭaja ariṣṭa***, a fermented preparation mentioned in the ***Bhaiṣajyaratnāvalī***, taken in dosages of 12–24 mL in the treatment of dysentery, bloody diarrhoea, malabsorptive syndromes, and fever (India 1978). In the treatment of diarrhoea the ***Cakradatta*** recommends a ***cūrṇa*** composed of equal parts ***Trikaṭu***, ***Indrayava***, ***Nimba***, ***Bhūnimba***, ***Bhṛṅgarāja***, ***Citraka***, ***Kaṭuka***, ***Pāṭhā***, ***Dāruharidrā*** and purified ***Ativiṣā***, the total of which is mixed with an equal quantity of ***Kuṭaja***, taken in doses of 3–5 g with rice water or honey (Sharma 2002). Simpler formulations mentioned by the ***Cakradatta*** include a decoction of ***Indrayava***, ***Kuṭaja*** and ***Mustaka***, 30–120 mL, taken with sugar and honey, or ***Kuṭaja*** and ***Dāḍima*** pericarp (*Punica granatum*) prepared as a thick extract by decoction, taken in teaspoonful doses with buttermilk (Sharma 2002). In the treatment of haemorrhoids the ***Cakradatta*** recommends ***Kuṭajaleha***, ***Kuṭajārasakriyā***, and ***Kuṭajādya ghṛta***, the latter of which is prepared by medicating ***ghṛta*** with equal parts ***Kuṭaja***, ***Nāgakeśara***, ***Nīlotpala***, ***Lodhra***, and ***Dhātaki***, taken in doses of 3–12 g (Sharma 2002). Beyond its ability to check the secretions of the digestive tract, ***Kuṭaja*** is also widely used as an antihaemorrhagic. In the treatment of menorrhagia ***Kuṭaja*** can be combined with herbs such as ***Arjuna***, ***Bilva*** and ***Nīlotpala***, or non-Indian herbs such as Shepherd's Purse (*Capsella bursa-pastoris*) and Cranesbill (*Geranium maculatum*). For pthisis and tuberculosis ***Kuṭaja*** can be used to check bleeding, in combination with herbs such as ***Vāsaka***, ***Āmalakī***, ***Puṣkaramūla*** and ***Arjuna***. Combined with equal parts ***Āmalakī***, ***Arjuna*** and ***Nimba***, ***Kuṭaja*** is taken as a powder with honey for the ***paittika*** variants of polyuria, indicated by polyuria with symptoms of burning sensations, the urine coloured deep yellow to red, with a pungent odour (Sharma 2002).

Dosage:

- ***Cūrṇa***: bark and/or seed, 3–8 g b.i.d.–t.i.d.
- ***Tincture***: bark, 1:3, 70% alcohol, 2–5 mL b.i.d.–t.i.d.

REFERENCES

Aqil F, Khan MS, Owais M, Ahmad I 2005 Effect of certain bioactive plant extracts on clinical isolates of beta-lactamase producing methicillin resistant Staphylococcus aureus. Journal of Basic Microbiology 45(2):106–114

Atal CK, Sharma ML, Kaul A, Khajuria A 1986 Immunomodulating agents of plant origin. I: Preliminary screening. Journal of Ethnopharmacology 18(2):133–141

Chakraborty A, Brantner AH 1999 Antibacterial steroid alkaloids from the stem bark of Holarrhena pubescens. Journal of Ethnopharmacology 68(1–3):339–344

Dash B 1991 Materia medica of Ayurveda. B. Jain Publishers, New Delhi, p 49

Duke JA 2002 Handbook of medicinal herbs, 2nd edn. CRC Press, Boca Raton, p 219

India, Department of Health 1978 The Ayurvedic formulary of India, Part 1. Controller of Publications, Delhi, p 7

Kapoor LD 1990 CRC handbook of Ayurvedic medicinal plants. CRC Press, Boca Raton, p 205–206

Kavitha D, Shilpa PN, Devaraj SN 2004 Antibacterial and antidiarrhoeal effects of alkaloids of Holarrhena antidysenterica WALL. Indian Journal of Experimental Biology 42(6):589–594

Kirtikar KR, Basu BD 1935 Indian medicinal plants, 2nd edn, vols 1–4. Periodical Experts, Delhi, p 1570

Kumar A, Ali M 2000 A new steroidal alkaloid from the seeds of Holarrhena antidysenterica. Fitoterapia 71(2):101–104

Nadkarni KM 1954 The Indian materia medica, with Ayurvedic, Unani and home remedies, revised and enlarged by A.K. Nadkarni. Popular Prakashan PVP, Bombay

Rani P, Khullar N 2004 Antimicrobial evaluation of some medicinal plants for their anti-enteric potential against multi-drug resistant Salmonella typhi. Phytotherapy Research 18(8):670–673

Sharma PV 2002 Cakradatta: Sanskrit text with English translation. Chaukhamba, Varanasi, p 47, 53, 90, 326

Siddiqui BS, Usmani SB, Ali ST et al 2001 Further constituents from the bark of Holarrhena pubescens. Phytochemistry 58(8):1199–1204

Srikanthamurthy KR 2001 Bhāvaprakāśa of Bhāvamiśra, vol 1. Krishnadas Academy, Varanasi, p 183, 245

Voravuthikunchai S, Lortheeranuwat A, Jeeju W et al 2004 Effective medicinal plants against enterohaemorrhagic Escherichia coli O157:H7. Journal of Ethnopharmacology 94(1):49–54

Warrier PK, Nambiar VPK, Ramankutty C (eds) 1995 Indian medicinal plants: a compendium of 500 species, vol 3. Orient Longman, Hyderabad, p 156

Williamson EM (ed) 2002 Major herbs of Ayurveda. Churchill Livingstone, London, p 173

Yoganarasimhan SN 2000 Medicinal plants of India, vol 2: Tamil Nadu. Self-published, Bangalore, p 272

Maṇḍūkaparṇī, 'frog-leaved'

BOTANICAL NAME: *Centella asiatica,* Apiaceae

OTHER NAMES: ***Brāhmī***, 'consort of Brahmā', ***Brahmāmaṇḍuki***, 'frog-leaved Brahmā' (S); Bemgsag (H); Vallarai (T); Indian Penny-wort (E); Luei Gong Gen (C); 'Gotu Kola' is derived from the Sinhala name

Botany: ***Maṇḍūkaparṇī*** is a slender herbaceous creeping perennial, with long stems, rooting at the nodes. The leaves are obicularly reniform, crenate, on long petioles. The small flowers are white, pink or purple, borne in fascicled umbels, giving rise to a fleshy compressed fruit with two mericarps (Kirtikar & Basu 1935, Warrier et al 1994).

Part used: Leaves.

Dravyguṇa:

- ***Rasa***: *tikta, kaṭu*
- ***Vipāka***: *kaṭu*
- ***Vīrya***: *śita*
- ***Karma***: *dīpana, jvaraghna, raktaprasādana, mūtravirecana, kuṣṭaghna, hṛdaya, medhya, rasāyana.*
- ***Prabhāva***: also called *Brāhmī* (consort of Brahmā) because it aids in the development of *Brahman*, the Supreme Reality, strengthening nervous function, and promoting longevity, intelligence and memory (Dash 1991, Dash & Junius 1983, Frawley & Lad 1986, Srikanthamurthy 1994, 2001, Warrier et al 1994).

Constituents: ***Maṇḍūkaparṇī*** contains a variety of constituents of which the triterpenoids have attracted the most attention from researchers. These include asiaticoside A and B, madecassoside, braminoside, brahmiside, brahminoside, thankuniside, isothankuniside, as well as triterpene acids such as asiatic acid, 6-hydroxy asiatic acid, madecassic acid, madasiatic acid, brahmic acid, isobrahmic acid, betulinic acid and isothankunic acid. ***Maṇḍūkaparṇī*** also contains flavones, including quercitin, kaempferol and astragalin, the alkaloid hydrocotylin, and phytosterols stigmasterol and sitosterol. The fresh and recently dried plant contains an essential oil comprising, primarily, sesquiterpenoids such as β-caryophyllene, α-humulene and germacrene. Additional constituents include tannins, amino acids, B-complex vitamins and a resin (Heinerman 1984, Williamson 2002, Yoganarasimhan 2000).

Medical research:

- ***In vitro***: neuroprotective (Mook-Jung et al 1999), antitumuor (Babu et al 1995, Lin et al 1972).
- ***In vivo***: nootropic, anxiolytic (Leung & Foster 1996); GABA-nergic (Chatterjee et al 1992); antimicrobial (Oliver-Bever 1986), CNS-depressant (Ramaswamy et al 1970); antiulcer (Chatterjee et al 1992); antioxidant (Shukla et al 1999b); anti-inflammatory (Chen et al 1999); vulnerary (Maquart et al 1999, Shukla et al 1999a, Suguna et al 1996).
- ***Human trials***: ***Maṇḍūkaparṇī*** promoted significant improvements in cooperation, memory, concentration, attention, vocabulary and social adjustment in mentally challenged children, compared to placebo (Appa Rao 1973); ***Maṇḍūkaparṇī*** significantly reduced the number of circulating endothelial cells asiatica in patients with post-phlebitic syndrome (Montecchio et al 1991) and significantly and safely promoted improvement in patients with chronic venous hypertensive microangiopathy (Cesarone et al 1994). ***Maṇḍūkaparṇī*** was found to significantly reduce ankle oedema and foot swelling, and improve capillary filtration rate and microcirculatory parameters in patients with venous insufficiency (Cesarone et al 1992). A titrated extract of ***Maṇḍūkaparṇī*** promoted clinical improvement in 5 of 12 patients with chronic hepatic disorders (Darnis et al 1979). ***Maṇḍūkaparṇī*** was efficacious in the treatment of chronic or subchronic systemic scleroderma with limited skin involvement, and in progressive and/or advanced focal

scleroderma (Guseva et al 1998). In the treatment of keloids madecassol (asiaticoside) extracted from **Maṇḍūkaparṇī** compared favourably with compression bandaging, and provided more lasting results than either intralesional cortisone or radiation therapy (Bosse et al 1979); a topical extract of *Centella asiatica* was found to be useful in *Pseudofolliculitis barbae* (razor bumps) when used as a shaving lubricant (Spencer 1985).

Toxicity: No relevant data found.

Indications: Gastric ulceration and inflammation, dysentery, jaundice, hepatitis, fever, bronchitis, alopecia, eczema, psoriasis, leprous ulcers, venereal diseases, burns, anxiety, poor memory, ADD/ADHD, senility, Alzheimer's disease, epilepsy, chronic fatigue, premature aging, hypertension, anaemia, diabetes, oedema, varicosities, phlebitis, venous insufficiency, immunodeficiency, autoimmune disorders, cancer.

Contraindications: A water-soluble fraction of *Centella asiatica* was reported to inhibit hepatic enzymes responsible for barbiturate metabolism (Leung & Foster 1996), and has been found to have a GABAnergic activity (Chatterjee et al 1992). **Maṇḍūkaparṇī** is thus contraindicated with the concurrent use of drugs such as benzodiazepines, barbituates or antiepileptics. Contact dermatitis has been reported in some patients using preparations of fresh or dried parts of the plant (Eun & Lee 1985). Although the triterpene constituents have shown to lack any kind of teratogenic effect (Bosse et al 1979), relaxation of the rat uterus has been documented for brahmoside and brahminoside, and therefore **Maṇḍūkaparṇī** is thus avoided in pregnancy (Ramaswamy et al 1970). Hyperglycaemic and hypercholesterolaemic effects have been reported for asiaticoside in humans (Newall et al 1996), and caution should be exercised with the concomitant use of hypolipidaemic and hypoglycaemic therapies. Frawley & Lad (1986) report that high doses of **Maṇḍūkaparṇī** may cause a loss of consciousness and headaches and that they may aggravate pruritis. The majority of Āyurvedic texts tend to indicate that **Maṇḍūkaparṇī** is contraindicated in **vāttika** conditions (Warrier et al 1995).

Medicinal uses: **Maṇḍūkaparṇī** is a common green vegetable throughout Southeast Asia, from India to the Phillipines, sometimes eaten raw as a side dish, or prepared as a juice. It is said to be a favourite food of elephants in Sri Lanka. Modern clinical research has supported many of the time-honoured properties attributed to **Maṇḍūkaparṇī**. Plant geneticists have recently termed **Maṇḍūkaparṇī** as an 'araliaceous hydrocotyloid' (Downie et al 2000), for although it is a member of the Apiaceae, it bears many similarities both botanically and in therapeutic action with other genera of the Araliaceae, such as Ginseng (*Panax ginseng*). For internal administration the fresh plant is considered best, either as a juice, or more recently, as a fresh plant tincture. Dried plant preparations are used in Āyurveda and should not be considered as useless; however care should be taken to carefully source the herb as **Maṇḍūkaparṇī** grows quite well along the edges of rivers and sewer outfalls and could be contaminated with heavy metals, faecal coliforms or parasites. **Maṇḍūkaparṇī** is a useful treatment in a range of mental and cerebrovascular conditions including epilepsy, stroke, dementia, memory loss, poor concentration, and attention deficit disorder. Some texts state that **Maṇḍūkaparṇī** is the same as **Brāhmī** (*Bacopa monniera*) in action, some even suggesting that they are one and the same. They are, however, different plants with a different range of activities, but both are active as agents to enhance mental function. Generally speaking, **Maṇḍūkaparṇī** is used in cognitive dysfunction where **pitta** is the predominant **doṣa**, best used as the fresh juice, 25 mL twice daily. In skin conditions such as psoriasis and eczema, benefit can be obtained by using **Maṇḍūkaparṇī** with hepatics such as **Bhṛṅgarāja**, **Mañjiṣṭhā**, **Dāruharidrā** and Yellowdock (*Rumex crispus*). **Maṇḍūkaparṇī** may also be used topically in salves and balms to treat chapped lips, herpetic lesions, leprosy, scrofula, seborrheic dermatitis, 'dish pan' hands, eczema, psoriasis and insect bites and stings. As an alternative to antibiotics, **Maṇḍūkaparṇī** could be taken internally with **Kaṭuka** and **Bhūnimba**, or Western herbs such as Goldenseal (*Hydrastis canadensis* root) and Purple Coneflower (*Echinacea* spp.) in the treatment of infectious conditions. For wounds **Maṇḍūkaparṇī** can be combined with Comfrey (*Symphytum officinalis* root), applied topically and taken internally to speed healing and recovery. ***Maṇḍūkaparṇī***, along with other immunomodulants such as Huang qi (*Astragalus membranaceus*) and ***Aśvagandhā***, should be considered an adjunct in the treatment of immunodeficiency diseases. The ***Aṣṭāṅga Hṛdaya*** mentions the usefulness of ***Maṇḍūkaparṇī*** in the treatment of ***sannipātaja udara*** (abdominal enlargement in which all three ***doṣas*** are active), after purgative therapies have been initiated, taken as the fresh juice for a period of a month (Srikanthamurthy 1995).

Dosage:

- ***Cūrṇa***: 3–10 g b.i.d.–t.i.d.
- ***Svarasa***: 25 mL b.i.d.–t.i.d.
- ***Phāṇṭa***: 30–120 mL b.i.d.–t.i.d.
- ***Tincture***: fresh plant 1:2, 95% alcohol; dry plant 1:3, 50% alcohol, 1–5 mL b.i.d.–t.i.d.
- ***Ghṛta***: 2 gtt. s.d. taken as nasya for nervous disorders.
- ***Taila***: ad lib. in ***abhyaṅga*** etc. for nervous system disorders.

REFERENCES

Appa Rao MVR, Srinivasan K, Rao KT 1973 The effect of Mandookaparni (Centella asiatica) on the general mental ability (medhya) of mentally retarded children. Journal of Indian Medicine 8:9–16

Babu TD, Kuttan G, Padikkala J 1995 Cytotoxic and antitumor properties of certain taxa of Umbelliferae with special reference to Centella asiatica (L.) Urban. Journal of Ethnopharmacology 48(1):53–57

Bosse JP, Papillon J, Frenette G et al 1979 Clinical study of a new antikeloid agent. Annals of Plastic Surgery 3(1): 13–21

Cesarone MR, Laurora G, De Sanctis MT, Belcaro G 1992 Activity of Centella asiatica in venous insufficiency. Minerva Cardioangiologica 40(4):137–143

Cesarone MR, Laurora G, De Sanctis MT et al 1994 The microcirculatory activity of Centella asiatica in venous insufficiency. A double-blind study. Minerva Cardioangiologica 42(6):299–304

Chatterjee TK, Cakraborty A, Pathak M, Sengupta GC 1992 Effects of plant extract Centella asiatica (Linn.) on cold restraint stress ulcer in rats. Indian Journal of Experimental Biology 30(10):889–891

Chen YJ, Dai YS, Chen BF et al 1999 The effect of tetrandrine and extracts of Centella asiatica on acute radiation dermatitis in rats. Biological and Pharmaceutical Bulletin 22(7):703–706

D'Amelio F 1987 Gotu Kola. Cosmetics and Toiletries 102(6):49–50

Darnis F, Orcel L, De Saint-Maur PP, Mamou P 1979 Use of a titrated extract of Centella asiatica in chronic hepatic disorders. La Semaine Des Hopitaux 55(37–38):1749–1750

Dash B 1991 Materia medica of Ayurveda. B. Jain Publishers, New Delhi, p 102

Dash B, Junius M 1983 A handbook of Ayurveda. Concept Publishing, New Delhi, p 103

Downie S, Watson MF, Spalik K, Katz-Downie DS 2000 Molecular systematics of Old World Apioideae (Apiaceae): relationships among some members of tribe Peucedaneae sensu lato, the placement of several island-endemic species, and resolution within the apioid superclade. Canadian Journal of Botany 78:506–528

Eun HC, Lee AY 1985 Contact dermatitis due to madecassol. Contact Dermatitis 13(5):310–313

Frawley D, Lad V 1986 The yoga of herbs: an Ayurvedic guide to herbal medicine. Lotus Press, Santa Fe, p 170–171

Guseva NG, Starovoitova MN, Mach ES 1998 Madecassol treatment of systemic and localized scleroderma. Terapevticheskii Arkhiv 70(5):58–61

Heinerman J 1984 An herb for our time: the scientific rediscovery of Gotu Kola. Unpublished manuscript p 85

Kirtikar KR, Basu BD 1935 Indian medicinal plants, 2nd edn, vols 1–4. Periodical Experts, Delhi, p 1192

Leung AY, Foster S 1996 Encyclopedia of common natural ingredients used in food, drugs and cosmetics, 2nd edn. John Wiley, New York, p 284–285

Lin YC, Yang TI, Chen JY, Yang CS 1972 Search for biologically active substances in Taiwan medicinal plants. 1. Screening for antitumor and antimicrobial substances. Zhonghua Minguo Wei Sheng Wu Xue Za Zhi 5(1):76–81

Maquart FX, Chastang F, Simeon A et al 1999 Triterpenes from Centella asiatica stimulate extracellular matrix accumulation in rat experimental wounds. European Journal of Dermatology 9(4):289–296

Montecchio GP, Samaden A, Carbone S 1991 Centella asiatica Triterpenic Fraction (CATTF) reduces the number of circulating endothelial cells in subjects with post phlebitic syndrome. Haematologica 76(3):256–259

Mook-Jung I, Shin JE, Yun SH 1999 Protective effects of asiaticoside derivatives against beta-amyloid neurotoxicity. Journal of Neuroscience Research 58(3):417–425

Newall C, Anderson L, Phillipson JD 1996 Herbal medicines: a guide for professionals. The Pharmaceutical Press, London, p 170–172

Oliver-Bever B 1986 Medicinal plants in tropical West Africa. Cambridge University Press, Cambridge, p 67

Ramaswamy AS, Pariyaswamy SM, Basu N 1970. Pharmacological studies on Centella asiatica Linn. Journal of Research in Indian Medicine 4:160–175

Shukla A, Rasik AM, Jain GK et al 1999a In vitro and in vivo wound healing activity of asiaticoside isolated from Centella asiatica. Journal of Ethnopharmacology 65(1):1–11.

Shukla A, Rasik AM, Dhawan BN 1999b Asiaticoside-induced elevation of anti-oxidant levels in healing wounds. Phytotherapy Research 13(1):50–54

Spencer TS 1985 Pseudofolliculitis barbae or razor bumps and shaving. Cosmetics and Toiletries 100:47–49

Srikanthamurthy KR 1994 Vāgbhaṭa's Aṣṭāṅga Hṛdayam, vol 1. Krishnadas Academy, Varanasi, p 90

Srikanthamurthy KR 1995 Vāgbhaṭa's Aṣṭāṅga Hṛdayam, vol 3. Krishnadas Academy, Varanasi, p 438

Srikanthamurthy KR 2001 Bhāvaprakāśa of Bhāvamiśra, vol 1. Krishnadas Academy, Varanasi, p 274

Suguna L, Sivakumar P, Chandrakasan G 1996 Effects of Centella asiatica extract on dermal wound healing in rats. Indian Journal of Experimental Biology 34(12):1208–1211

Warrier PK, Nambiar VPK, Ramankutty C (eds) 1994 Indian medicinal plants: a compendium of 500 species, vol 2. Orient Longman, Hyderabad, p 52, 54–55
Williamson EM (ed) 2002 Major herbs of Ayurveda. Churchill Livingstone, London, p 103
Yoganarasimhan SN 2000 Medicinal plants of India, vol 2: Tamil Nadu. Self-published, Bangalore, p 122

Mañjiṣṭhā

BOTANICAL NAME: *Rubia cordifolia,* Rubiaceae

OTHER NAMES: Manjit (H); Manjitti, Shevvelli (T); Indian Madder (E); Qian cao gen (C)

Botany: ***Mañjiṣṭhā*** is a perennial herbaceous climber, branches and stems quadangular, the mature portions covered in a whitish bark that is rather rough and grooved, the roots long and cylindrical, covered in a reddish bark, medulla deep red in colour. The leaves are variable, margins entire, 3–9 cm long by 1–4 cm wide, arranged in whorls of three to eight (usually four), the petioles of one pair often longer than the other, cordate-ovate to ovate-lanceolate, with five to seven veins that arise from the base. The small white or greenish flowers are borne in terminal panicles or cymes, giving rise to a purplish-black globose fruit containing two small seeds. ***Mañjiṣṭhā*** is found in hilly areas, up to 3750 m in elevation, in tropical Africa and Southeast Asia, north and eastwards into Tibet and China (Kirtikar & Basu 1935, Warrier et al 1996).

Part used: Root, stem.

Dravyguṇa:

- ***Rasa***: *madhura, tikta, kaśāya*
- ***Vipāka***: *kaṭu*
- ***Vīrya***: *uṣṇa*
- ***Karma***: *dīpanapācana, purīṣasangrahaṇīya, jvaraghna, kṛmighna, mūtravirecana, aśmaribhedana, raktaprasādana, śoṇitasthāpana, śothahara, kuṣṭaghna, viṣaghna, sandhānīya, vedanāsthāpana, cakṣuṣya, balya, rasāyana, kaphapittahara* (Dash 1991, Frawley & Lad 1986, Srikanthamurthy 2001, Warrier et al 1996).

Constituents: ***Mañjiṣṭhā*** contains a variety of quinones including the anthraquinones cordifoliol and cordifodiol, the quinoidal dimers naphthohydroquinone anhydride, furomollugin, mollugin, and rubilactone, as well as naphthoic acid esters. ***Mañjiṣṭhā*** has also been shown to contain the iridoid glycosides 6-methoxygeniposidic acid, manjishtin, garancin and alazarin. Triterpenoids include oleananes rubiprasin A–C and arboranes rubiarbonol A–F. Researchers have also isolated bicyclic hexapeptides RA-VII and RA-X to RA-XVI, as well as β-sitosterol and daucosterol (Abdullah et al 2003, Hassanean et al 2000, Ho et al 1996, Hua et al 1992, Itokawa et al 1993, Kapoor 1990, Morita et al 1992, Qiao et al 1990, Takeya et al 1993, Wang et al 1992, Williamson 2002).

Medical research:

- ***In vitro***: antioxidant (Pandey et al 1994, Tripathi et al 1997, 1998), anti-HBsAg (Ho et al 1996), antispasmodic (Gilani et al 1994), antithrombotic (Tripathi et al 1993).
- ***In vivo***: GABA-nergic, serotinergic, antiseizure (Kasture et al 2000).

Toxicity: The oral LD_{50} is stated to be greater than 175 g/kg in mice (Bensky & Gamble 1993).

Indications: Dyspepsia, colic, diarrhoea, dysentery, intestinal parasites, haemorrhoids, jaundice, hepatitis, splenitis, intermittent fever, pharyngitis, cough, oedema, skin diseases, wounds, ulcers, broken bones, amenorrhea, dysmenorrhoea, metrorrhagia, haemorrhage, urinary tenesmus, inflammatory joint disease, neuralgia, pain, diabetes, cancer.

Contraindications: ***vātakopa***.

Medicinal uses: ***Mañjiṣṭhā*** is revered as a potent alterative or ***raktaprasādana*** in Āyurvedic medicine, acting on the liver and kidneys to mobilise toxins from the tissues and blood for elimination. It is particularly useful to break up congestion and stagnation in tissues by enhancing circulation (hence it has an ***uṣṇa vīrya***), and thus finds utility in a range of conditions, from tumours to chronic infection. The traditional indication to use ***Mañjiṣṭhā*** in blood disorders can be inferred from its intensely red pigment, which resembles the colour of blood. Thus ***Mañjiṣṭhā*** can be used whenever there is inflammation or bleeding, from inflammatory skin conditions, such as acne, to dysfunctional uterine bleeding. ***Manijishta*** is still used in countries like India to dye cloth, and when applied topically or taken internally, this dye can temporarily colour the skin and urine red. ***Mañjiṣṭhā*** is valued in both urinary lithiasis and cholelithiasis, and stated to be effective in both calcium phosphate and oxalate stones of the bladder (Nadkarni 1954). ***Mañjiṣṭhā*** is similarly indicated in haematuria, with herbs such as ***Gokṣura*** and ***Agnimañtha***. Taken internally with herbs such as ***Yastimadhu***, ***Guḍūcī***, ***Kaṭuki*** and ***Candana***, ***Mañjiṣṭhā*** may be effective in peptic ulcer (***amlapitta***). In the treatment of consumptive conditions with epistaxis ***Mañjiṣṭhā*** may be effective when used in combination with herbs such as ***Arjuna***, ***Āmalakī***, ***Vāsaka*** and ***Puṣkaramūla***. In the treatment of rheumatoid arthritis, lupus and gout ***Mañjiṣṭhā*** is often applied topically as a medicated oil, often in the form of preparation called ***Piṇḍa taila***, composed of ***Mañjiṣṭhā***, ***Sarjasa*** resin, ***Sārivā*** and beeswax, decocted in water and sesame oil. The ***Cakradatta*** recommends a formula similarly useful in the internal treatment of inflammatory joint disease, comprising equal parts ***Mañjiṣṭhā***, ***Āmalakī***, ***Harītakī***, ***Bibhītaka***, ***Nimba***, ***Vacā***, ***Kaṭuka***, ***Guḍūcī*** and ***Dāruharidrā*** in decoction or as a ***cūrṇa*** (Sharma 2002). In the treatment of vomiting of blood or bleeding from the nose the ***Cakradatta*** recommends a medicated ***ghṛta*** prepared with ***Mañjiṣṭhā***. As its name might suggest, this herb is also indicated in ***mañjiṣṭhā prameha***, a polyuria in which the urine is bright red – for this purpose the ***Cakradatta*** recommends a combination of ***Mañjiṣṭhā*** and ***Raktacandana*** (Sharma 2002). In the treatment of wounds ***Mañjiṣṭhā*** can be applied singly as a powder or with equal parts herbs, such as ***Triphala***, ***Haridrā***, ***Nimba*** and ***Yaṣṭimadhu***. In the same fashion, ***Mañjiṣṭhā*** is also applied to ulcers and tumours in combination with a variety of medicaments. To prevent miscarriage the ***Cakradatta*** recommends a milk decoction of ***Mañjiṣṭhā***, ***Śatāvarī***, ***Tila*** and ***Aṣmantaka***, taken for the first 7 months of pregnancy in susceptible women (Sharma 2002). Prepared as a medicated ***ghṛta*** with ***Triphala***, ***Mañjiṣṭhā*** can be used in conjunctivitis and glaucoma. In the patients having undergone chemotherapy for lung and oesophageal cancer presenting with haemoptysis, ***Mañjiṣṭhā*** can be combined with ***Aśvagandhā*** and ***Yaṣṭimadhu*** to promote healing. Chinese herbal medicine corroborates many of the traditional Āyurvedic uses for ***Mañjiṣṭhā***, using it in the treatment of bleeding disorders and in blood stasis, and in pain from trauma or joint pain (Bensky & Gamble 1993).

Dosage:

- ***Cūrṇa***: 3–5 g b.i.d.–t.i.d.
- ***Kvātha***: 1:4, 30–120 mL b.i.d.–t.i.d.
- ***Tincture***: dried root, 1:3, 50% alcohol, 1–5 mL b.i.d.–t.i.d.
- ***Taila***: ad lib. in ***abhyaṅga*** etc. for inflammatory joint disorders.

REFERENCES

Abdullah ST, Ali A, Hamid H et al 2003 Two new anthraquinones from the roots of Rubia cordifolia Linn. Die Pharmazie 58(3):216–217

Bensky D, Gamble A 1993 Chinese herbal medicine materia medica, revised edn. Eastland Press, Seattle, p 258

Dash B 1991 Materia medica of Ayurveda. B. Jain Publishers, New Delhi, p 78

Frawley D, Lad V 1986 The yoga of herbs: an Ayurvedic guide to herbal medicine. Lotus Press, Santa Fe, p 178

Gilani AH, Janbaz KH, Zaman M et al 1994 Possible presence of calcium channel blocker(s) in Rubia cordifolia: an indigenous medicinal plant. Journal of the Pakistan Medical Association 44(4):82–85

Hassanean HA, Ibraheim ZZ, Takeya K, Itorawa H 2000 Further quinoidal derivatives from Rubia cordifolia L. Die Pharmazie 55(4):317–319

Ho LK, Don MJ, Chen HC et al 1996 Inhibition of hepatitis B surface antigen secretion on human hepatoma cells. Components from Rubia cordifolia. Journal of Natural Products 59(3):330–333

Hua HM, Wang SX, Wu LJ et al 1992 Studies on naphthoic acid esters from the roots of Rubia cordifolia L. Yao Xue Xue Bao 27(4):279–282

Itokawa H, Ibraheim ZZ, Qiao YF, Takeya K 1993 Anthraquinones, naphthohydroquinones and naphthohydroquinone dimers from Rubia cordifolia and their cytotoxic activity. Chemical and Pharmaceutical Bulletin (Tokyo) 41(10):1869–1872

Kapoor LD 1990 CRC handbook of Ayurvedic medicinal plants. CRC Press, Boca Raton, p 292

Kasture VS, Deshmukh VK, Chopde CT 2000 Anticonvulsant and behavioral actions of triterpene isolated from Rubia cordifolia Linn. Indian Journal of Experimental Biology 38(7):675–680

Kirtikar KR, Basu BD 1935 Indian medicinal plants, 2nd edn, vols 1–4. Periodical Experts, Delhi, p 1303–1304

Morita H, Yamamiya T, Takeya K, Itokawa H 1992 New antitumor bicyclic hexapeptides, RA-XI, -XII, -XIII and -XIV from Rubia cordifolia. Chemical and Pharmaceutical Bulletin (Tokyo) 40(5):1352–1354

Nadkarni KM 1954 The Indian materia medica, with Ayurvedic, Unani and home remedies, revised and enlarged by A.K. Nadkarni. Popular Prakashan PVP, Bombay, p 1076

Pandey S, Sharma M, Chaturvedi P, Tripathi YB 1994 Protective effect of Rubia cordifolia on lipid peroxide formation in isolated rat liver homogenate. Indian Journal of Experimental Biology 32(3):180–183

Qiao YF, Wang SX, Wu LJ 1990 Studies on antibacterial constituents from the roots of Rubia cordifolia L. Yao Xue Xue Bao 25(11):834–839

Sharma PV 2002 Cakradatta: Sanskrit text with English translation. Chaukhamba, Varanasi, p 236, 326, 585

Srikanthamurthy KR 2001 Bhāvaprakāśa of Bhāvamiśra, vol 1. Krishnadas Academy, Varanasi, p 190

Takeya K, Yamamiya T, Morita H, Itokawa H 1993 Two antitumor bicyclic hexapeptides from Rubia cordifolia. Phytochemistry 33(3):613–615

Tripathi YB, Sharma M 1998 Comparison of the anti-oxidant action of the alcoholic extract of Rubia cordifolia with rubiadin. Indian Journal of Biochemistry and Biophysics 35(5):313–316

Tripathi YB, Pandey S, Shukla SD 1993 Antiplatelet activating factor property of Rubia cordifolia Linn. Indian Journal of Experimental Biology 31(6):533–535

Tripathi YB, Sharma M, Manickam M 1997 Rubiadin, a new antioxidant from Rubia cordifolia. Indian Journal of Biochemistry and Biophysics 34(3):302–306

Wang SX, Hua HM, Wu LJ 1992 Studies on anthraquinones from the roots of rubia cordifolia. Yao Xue Xue Bao 27(10):743–747

Warrier PK, Nambiar VPK, Ramankutty C (eds) 1996 Indian medicinal plants: a compendium of 500 species, vol 5. Orient Longman, Hyderabad, p 17

Williamson EM (ed) 2002 Major herbs of Ayurveda. Churchill Livingstone, London, p 258

Yoganarasimhan SN 2000 Medicinal plants of India, vol 2: Tamil Nadu. Self-published, Bangalore

Mustaka

BOTANICAL NAME: *Cyperus rotundus,* Cyperaceae

OTHER NAMES: Motha (H); Korai (T); Nut Grass (E); Xiang fu (C)

Botany: *Mustaka* is a perennial, herbaceous sedge attaining a height of up to 75 cm, with elongated, slender stolons interspersed by aromatic tubers, 1–3 cm in length, the cortex black, the medulla reddish-white. The leaves are shorter than the stem, glabrous, linear, dark green, finely acuminate, flat, with a single vein. The flowers are borne in spikes arranged as simple or compound umbels, each spike in turn composed of several spikelets containing small flowers with a reddish-brown husk. The fruit is an obovoid, greyish-brown, three-angled nut that is black when mature. ***Mustaka*** is stated to be native to India, but is now found all over the world and is considered by many to be an invasive weed of wet, marshy places (Kirtikar & Basu 1935, Warrier et al 1994).

Part used: Tuber.

Dravyguṇa:

- ***Rasa***: *tikta, kaśāya*
- ***Vipāka***: *kaṭu*
- ***Vīrya***: *śita*
- ***Karma***: *dīpanapācana, purīṣasangrahaṇīya, jvaraghna, chedana, kṛmighna, mūtravirecana, aśmaribhedana, kuṣṭaghna, śoṇitasthāpana, sandhānīya, ārtavajanana, stanyajanana, vedanāsthāpana, medhya, kaphapittahara* (Srikanthamurthy 2001, Warrier et al 1994).

Constituents: ***Mustaka*** contains an essential oil that provides for the characteristic odour and taste of the herb, mostly consisting of sesquiterpene hydrocarbons, epoxides, ketones, monoterpenes and aliphatic alcohols. Sesquiterpenes include β-selinene, isocurcumenol, nootkatone, aristolone, isorotundene, cypera-2,4(15)-diene, and norrotundene, as well as the sesquiterpene alkaloid rotundines A–C. Other constituents include the ketone cyperadione, and the monoterpenes cineole, camphene and limonene. ***Mustaka*** has also been shown to contain miscellaneous triterpenes including oleanolic acid and β-sitosterol, as well as flavonoids, sugars and minerals (Ha et al 2002, Jeong et al 2000, Kapoor 1990, Sonwa & Konig 2001, Williamson 2002).

Medical research:

- ***In vitro***: antitoxic (Daswani et al 2001), antimalarial (Weenen et al 1990), GABA nergic (Ha et al 2002), antioxidant (Seo et al 2001).
- ***In vivo***: antitoxic (Daswani et al 2001).
- ***Human trials***: obese patients given an extract of ***Mustaka*** over a 90-day period were found to have experienced a reduction in weight, as well as a similar reduction in serum triglycerides and cholesterol (Williamson 2002).

Toxicity: The LD_{50} of an ethanolic extract was determined to be 1500 mg/kg (Williamson 2002).

Indications: Nausea and vomiting, dyspepsia, colic, flatulence, diarrhoea, dysentery, intestinal parasites, fever, malaria, cough, bronchitis, renal and vesical calculi, urinary tenesmus, skin diseases, wounds, amenorrhoea, dysmenorrhoea, deficient lactation.

Contraindications: ***vātakopa***, constipation.

Medicinal uses: ***Mustaka*** is an important medicinal plant in Āyurvedic medicine, a bitter tasting aromatic herb that acts to enkindle ***agni***, dispel ***āma***, and relieve intestinal spasm. Overall, ***Mustaka*** helps to normalise excessive secretion, and in this way tends to have a constipating activity that makes it particularly effective in diarrhoea. While it is used in formulation to treat dysentery, it is particularly useful after initial treatment, used over the medium term to restore digestive health and combat any lingering infection. It is also used in non-infective digestive disorders, however, marked by intestinal spasm, bloating, and a tendency to loose motions. The ***Cakradatta*** recommends a variety of formulations containing ***Mustaka*** in the treatment of diarrhoea, depending on the severity and associated symptoms. For severe diarrhoea ***Mustaka*** is combined with herbs such as ***Kuṭaja***, ***Bilva***, ***Dāḍima***, and ***Dhātaki***, along with antimicrobial botanicals such as ***Kaṭuka***, ***Guḍūcī*** and ***Dāruharidrā***, and antispasmodic herbs such as ***Vacā*** and ***Elā***. For diarrhoea with symptoms of burning sensation and thirst, ***Mustaka*** is combined with cooling botanicals such as ***Candana***, ***Dhānyaka*** and ***Balāka***. In diarrhoea with symptoms of ***āma***, in which the bowel movements have a foul odour and are accompanied by severe colic, ***Mustaka*** is combined with botanicals such as ***Harītakī***, ***Śūṇṭhī***, ***Hiṅgu*** and ***Pippalī***. In the treatment of intestinal parasites the ***Cakradatta*** recommends ***Mustādi kvātha***, which consists of a decoction of ***Mustaka***, ***Mūṣākarṇi***, ***Triphala***, ***Śigru*** and ***Devadāru***, with the pastes of ***Pippalī*** and ***Viḍaṅga*** (Sharma 2002). In the treatment of cough, bronchitis and asthma ***Mustaka*** can be combined with botanicals such as ***Vāsaka***, ***Haridrā***, ***Bibhītaka***, ***Pippalī***, ***Kaṇṭakāri***, and ***Puṣkaramūla***. In the treatment of inflammatory joint disease (***āmavāta***) ***Mustaka*** is used as an adjunct to herbs such as ***Guggulu***, ***Guḍūcī***, ***Citraka***, ***Śūṇṭhī*** and ***Triphala***, to relieve pain and enkindle ***agni***. In the treatment of diabetes ***Mustaka*** is used in conjunction with herbs such as ***Triphala***, ***Devadāru***, ***Guḍūcī***, ***Guggulu***, ***Haridrā*** and ***Śilājatu***. The antispasmodic properties of the root also make it helpful in gynaecological disorders such as premenstrual tension, dysmenorrhoea, endometritis, all more or less attended by loose motions or diarrhoea. ***Mustaka*** is also taken internally and applied topically as a fresh plant poultice as a galactagogue.

Dosage:

- ***Cūrṇa***: 3–5 g b.i.d.–t.i.d.
- ***Kvātha***: 1:4, 30–90 mL b.i.d.–t.i.d.
- ***Tincture***: dried root, 1:3, 50% alcohol, 1–5 mL b.i.d.–t.i.d.

REFERENCES

Daswani PG, Birdi TJ, Antia NH 2001 Study of the action of Cyperus rotundus root decoction on the adherence and enterotoxin production of diarrhoeagenic Escherichia coli. Indian Journal of Pharmacology 33:116–117

Ha JH, Lee KY, Choi HC et al 2002 Modulation of radioligand binding to the GABA(A)-benzodiazepine receptor complex by a new component from Cyperus rotundus. Biological and Pharmaceutical Bulletin 25(1):128–130

Jeong SJ, Miyamoto T, Inagaki M et al 2000 Rotundines A–C, three novel sesquiterpene alkaloids from Cyperus rotundus. Journal of Natural Products 63(5):673–675

Kapoor LD 1990 CRC Handbook of Ayurvedic medicinal plants. CRC Press, Boca Raton, p 292

Kirtikar KR, Basu BD 1935 Indian medicinal plants, 2nd edn, vols 1–4. Periodical Experts, Delhi, p 2638–2639

Seo WG, Pae HO, Oh GS et al 2001 Inhibitory effects of methanol extract of Cyperus rotundus rhizomes on nitric oxide and superoxide productions by murine macrophage cell line, RAW 264.7 cells. Journal of Ethnopharmacology 76(1):59–64

Sharma PV 2002 Cakradatta: Sanskrit text with English translation. Chaukhamba, Varanasi, p 110

Sonwa MM, Konig WA 2001 Chemical study of the essential oil of Cyperus rotundus. Phytochemistry 58(5):799–810

Srikanthamurthy KR 2001 Bhāvaprakāśa of Bhāvamiśra, vol 1. Krishnadas Academy, Varanasi, p 220

Warrier PK, Nambiar VPK, Ramankutty C (eds) 1994 Indian medicinal plants: a compendium of 500 species, vol 2. Orient Longman, Hyderabad, p 296–299

Weenen H, Nkunya MH, Bray DH et al 1990 Antimalarial activity of Tanzanian medicinal plants. Planta Medica 56(4):368–370

Williamson EM (ed) 2002 Major herbs of Ayurveda. Churchill Livingstone, London, p 122–124

Nāgakeśara, 'serpent stamens'

BOTANICAL NAMES: *Mesua ferrea, M. nagassarium,* Clusiaceae

OTHER NAMES: ***Nagapuṣpa***, 'serpent flowers' (S); Nagkesar (H); Nagappu, Nanku (T); Ironwood (E)

Botany: ***Nāgakeśara*** is a medium to large sized tree that can attain a height of between 18 and 30 m, with reddish-brown to greyish coloured bark that peels off in thin flakes, the wood extremely hard. The leaves are simple, lanceolate, acute, leathery, covered in a waxy bloom below, red when young, oppositely arranged, 7–13 cm long by 2–4 cm wide. The flowers are white with a floral fragrance, up to 7.5 cm in diameter, with numerous golden-colored stamens shorter than the length of the petals, the style twice as long as the stamens, borne singly or in pairs, axillary or terminal. The fruits are ovoid with a conical point, 2.5–5 cm long, with a woody pericarp that contains one to four seeds. ***Nāgakeśara*** is found throughout Southeast Asia in tropical evergreen forests up to 1500 m in elevation (Kirtikar & Basu 1935, Warrier et al 1995).

Part used: Flowers.

Dravyguṇa:

- ***Rasa***: *kaśāya, tikta*
- ***Vipāka***: *kaṭu*
- ***Vīrya***: *uṣṇa, rūkṣa*
- ***Karma***: *dīpanapācana, purīṣasangrahaṇīya, jvaraghna, chedana, mūtravirecana, mūtraviśodhana, śoṇitasthāpana, hṛdaya, viṣaghna, vedanāsthāpana, vajīkaraṇa, tridoṣaghna* (Srikanthamurthy 2001, Warrier et al 1995).

Constituents: The flowers of *Mesua ferrea* contain a yellow-coloured highly fragrant essential oil, the stamens specifically containing mesuanic acid, α-amyrin, β-amyrin, β-sitosterol, and the biflavonoids mesuaferrone A and B. Researchers have also isolated a group of xanthones from *M. ferrea*, including euxanthone, dehydrocycloguanadin, jacareubin, and mesuaxanthones A and B. The seed contains the coumarin mesaugin, the lactones mesuol, mesuone, and mammeisin, as well as a fixed oil comprising oleic, stearic, palmatic and linoleic acids (Gopalkrishnan et al 1980, Kapoor 1990, Yoganarasimhan 2000).

Medical research:

- ***In vitro***: antibacterial (Kapoor 1990).
- ***In vivo***: CNS depressant (Gopalkrishnan et al 1980), anti-inflammatory (Gopalkrishnan et al 1980), anti-asthmatic (Kapoor 1990).

Toxicity: There have been some reports of aflatoxins in the seed oil, probably from poor storage conditions (Roy & Chourasia 1989).

Indications: Vomiting, halitosis, ulcer, dysentery, bleeding haemorrhoids, fever, cough, pharyngitis, asthma, haemoptysis, skin diseases, buring sensations, cystitis, cardiac debility, headache, leucorrhoea, impotency.

Contraindications: No data found.

Medicinal uses: ***Nāgakeśara*** is valued as a pleasantly fragrant herb that can help to improve the odour of formulations, with an astringent, ***pācana*** property that acts to clear away congestion and ***āma***. Although classified as mildly warming ***Nāgakeśara*** is an important herb to use for ***pittakopa*** conditions such as dysentery and burning sensations. ***Vāttika*** conditions are also stated to be pacified by it (Warrier et al 1995), probably by virtue of its ***dīpanapācana*** property as well as due to the pleasing, uplifting fragrance of the essential oil. The ***Aṣṭāñga Hṛdaya*** includes ***Nāgakeśara*** in a list of medicinal plants that are used to counter the effects of poison, treat skin rashes and itching, and reduce all three ***doṣas*** (Srikanthamurthy 1994). In the treatment of haemorrhoids ***Nāgakeśara*** is used in a variety of formulations depending on the causative factor. For haemorrhoids associated with ***kapha***, four parts ***Nāgakeśara*** can be mixed with seven parts ***Śūṇṭhī***, six parts ***Pippalī***, five parts ***Marica***, three parts ***Patra*** leaf, two parts ***Tvak*** bark and one part ***Elā*** (Sharma 2002). For bleeding haemorrhoids ***Nāgakeśara*** can be prepared as a medicated ***ghṛta*** mixed with equal parts ***Kuṭaja***, ***Nīlotpala***, ***Lodhra***, and ***Dhātaki***, taken in doses of 3–12 g (Sharma 2002). For a more simplified approach, the ***cūrṇa*** of ***Nāgakeśara*** is mixed with butter and sugar and taken internally in the treatment of haemorrhoids and dysentery (Sharma 2002). Nadkarni states that this preparation is similarly useful in thirst, gastric irritation, excessive perspiration, and cough (1954). Prepared as a medicated ***ghṛta Nāgakeśara*** can also be applied topically in haemorrhoids, and can be similarly applied in the treatment of burning and tingling sensations of the feet (Nadkarni 1954, Sharma 2002). In the treatment of skin diseases and obesity a ***cūrṇa*** of ***Nāgakeśara*** can be mixed with equal parts ***Śiriṣa***, ***Lāmajjaka***, and ***Lodhra***, applied in ***udavartana abhyaṅga*** (Sharma 2002). ***Nāgakeśara*** is stated to be useful in symptoms of gonorrhoea and renal diseases, and can be used as a substitute for ***Cavya*** in the treatment of diseases of the urinary tract (Kapoor 1990, Nadkarni 1954).

Dosage:

- ***Cūrṇa***: 3–5 g b.i.d.–t.i.d.
- ***Hima***: 30–90 mL bi.d.–t.i.d.

REFERENCES

Gopalkrishnan C, Shankaranarayanan D, Nazimudeen SK et al 1980 Anti-inflammatory and CNS depressant activities of xanthones from Calophyllum inophyllum and Mesua ferrea. Indian Journal of Pharmacology 12(3):181–191

Kapoor LD 1990 CRC Handbook of Ayurvedic medicinal plants. CRC Press, Boca Raton, p 228–229

Kirtikar KR, Basu BD 1935 Indian medicinal plants, 2nd edn, vols 1–4. Periodical Experts, Delhi, p 274–5

Nadkarni KM 1954 The Indian materia medica, with Ayurvedic, Unani and home remedies, revised and enlarged by A.K. Nadkarni. Popular Prakashan PVP, Bombay, p 794–795

Roy AK, Chourasia HK 1989 Aflatoxin problems in some medicinal plants under storage. International Journal of Crude Drug Research 27(3):156–160

Sharma PV 2002 Cakradatta: Sanskrit text with English translation. Chaukhamba, Varanasi, p 83, 89, 90, 204, 338

Srikanthamurthy KR 1994 Vāgbhaṭa's Aṣṭāñga Hṛdayam, vol 1. Krishnadas Academy, Varanasi, p 202, 207

Srikanthamurthy KR 2001 Bhāvaprakāśa of Bhāvamiśra, vol 1. Krishnadas Academy, Varanasi, p 217

Warrier PK, Nambiar VPK, Ramankutty C (eds) 1995 Indian medicinal plants: a compendium of 500 species, vol 4. Orient Longman, Hyderabad, p 27–30

Yoganarasimhan SN 2000 Medicinal plants of India, vol 2: Tamil Nadu. Self-published, Bangalore, p 353

Nimba, 'bestower of health'

BOTANICAL NAMES: *Azadirachta indica, Melia azadirachta,* Meliaceae

OTHER NAMES: Nim, Nimb (H); Vempu, Veppu (T); Neem, Margosa (E)

Botany: ***Nimba*** is a medium to large evergreen tree, attaining a height of between 15 and 20 m, with a straight trunk, widely spreading branches, and greyish tubercled bark. The leaves are alternate and imparipinately compound, with 7–17 leaflets arranged in pairs, often with a terminal leaflet, ovate to lanceolate, sickle-shaped with an uneven base and serrate margins, 6–8 cm long, 1–3 cm wide. The flowers are cream to yellow in colour, borne in axillary panicles, giving rise to a single seeded ellipsoid drupe that is greenish-yellow when ripe. ***Nimba*** is widely cultivated in tropical and subtropical regions all over the world, and is thought to be native to the subcontinent (Kirtikar & Basu 1935).

Part used: Bark, leaves (***Nimbapatra***), seeds (***Nimbaphala***).

Dravyguṇa:

- ***Rasa***: *kaśāya, tikta*
- ***Vipāka***: *kaṭu*
- ***Vīrya***: *śita*
- ***Karma***: *dīpanapācana, vamana, purīṣasangrahaṇīya, kṛmighna, jvaraghna, chedana, dāhapraśamana, raktaprasādana, kuṣṭhaghna, mūtravirecana, mūtraviśodhana, sandhānīya, viṣaghna, pittakaphahara* (Srikanthamurthy 2001, Warrier et al 1994).

Constituents: ***Nimba*** is a fairly well researched medicinal plant, and as a result a number of constituents have been isolated from it. Among these are bitter-tasting terpenes called limonoids, including azadirachtin, nimbanal, nimbidiol, margocin, margocinin and related compounds, as well as a variety of other terpenoids including isoazadirolide, nimbocinolide, gedunin, margosinone and nimbonone. More recently, researchers have isolated a series of tetranortriterpenoids including azadirachtol, 1α, 2α-epoxy-17β–hydroxyazadiradione, 1α, 2α-epoxynimolicinol, and 7-deacetylnimolicinol. Other constituents include the flavonoids kaempferol, quercetin, quercitrin, rutin, and myricetin, as well as β-sitosterol, a tannin, a gum, and a series of polysaccharides named CSP-II and -III, CSSP-I, -II, and -III, etc. (Duke 2003, Hallur et al 2002, Kapoor 1990, Luo et al 2000, Malathi et al 2002, Williamson 2002).

Medical research:

- ***In vitro***: negatively ionotropic/chronotropic (Kholsa et al 2002), hypotensive (Chattopadhyay 1997), antiviral (Badam et al 1999; Parida et al 2002), antifungal (Fabry et al 1996), antibacterial (Almas 1999, Alzoreky & Nakahara 2003).
- ***In vivo***: hepatoprotective (Arivazhagan et al 2000; Bhanwra et al 2000), anti-ulcerogenic (Bandyopadhyay et al 2002), hypoglycaemic (Kholsa et al 2000), hypotensive (Koley & Lal 1994), immunostimulant (Mukherjee et al 1999, Njiro & Kofi-Tsekpo 1999, Upadhyay et al 1992), anti-inflammatory (Chattopadhyay et al 1998), antitumour (Kumar et al 2002; Tepsuwan et al 2002), anxiolytic (Jaiswal et al 1994), antifertility (Kasturi et al 2002, Mukherjee et al 1999, Parshad et al 1994), antiviral (Parida et al 2002).
- ***Human trials***: a lyophilised powder of ***Nimba*** extract administered over 10 days, 30–60 mg twice daily, caused a significant decrease in gastric acid secretion and pepsin activity, and when taken for between 6 and 10 weeks almost completely healed lesions in patients suffering from duodenal, gastric and oesophageal ulcers (Bandyopadhyay et al 2004). An extract of ***Nimba*** was found to lower total serum cholesterol and LDL-cholesterol levels in non-malarial patients, while increasing triacylglycerol and HDL-cholesterol in malarial patients (Njoku et al 2001). A ***Nimba*** mouth rinse was found to be active against *Streptococcus mutans*

and reversed incipient carious lesions (Vanka et al 2001); a dental gel containing ***Nimba*** leaf extract (25 mg/g) was found to significantly reduce the plaque index and bacterial count compared to chlorhexidine gluconate (0.2% w/v) mouthwash (Pai et al 2004). A paste prepared from ***Nimba*** and ***Haridrā*** was found to promote a 97% cure rate in scabies within 3 to 15 days of treatment, with no toxic or adverse reactions (Charles & Charles 1992); a 2% ***Nimba*** oil mixed in coconut oil applied to the exposed body parts of human volunteers provided complete protection from mosquito bites over a 12-hour period (Sharma et al 1993).

Toxicity: A cumulative oral dose of the crude bark extract of ***Nimba***, of 1–9 g/kg in mice over a 15-day period, was well tolerated and below the LD_{50} (Bandyopadhyay et al 2002). The seed oil of ***Nimba*** was determined to have a 24-hour oral LD_{50} of 14 ml/kg in rats and 24 ml/kg in rabbits. The lungs and central nervous system appeared to be the target organs of toxicity. In comparison, a mustard seed oil was determined to have an oral LD_{50} of 80 ml/kg (Gandhi et al 1988). Chewing sticks made from ***Azadirachta indica*** were observed to be susceptible to post-harvest spoilage and are not advisable for oral hygiene measures if not fresh (Etebu et al 2003).

Indications: Dyspepsia, ulcers, intestinal parasites, haemorrhoids, liver diseases, fever, malarial fever, cough, bronchitis, asthma, tuberculosis, skin diseases, inflammatory joint disease, cystitis, amenorrhoea, diabetes, tumours, conjunctivitis and ophthalmic disorders generally.

Contraindications: ***vātakopa***.

Medicinal uses: The name ***Nimba*** is an ancient name, derived from the Sanskrit phrase ***'nimbati svāsthyamdadati'***, meaning 'bestower of good health'. ***Nimba*** is a sacred tree in India, associated with Lakṣmī, the goddess of abundance and good fortune, and *Surya*, the sun. It has a bitter taste and a cooling energy, acting to remove congestion and reduce inflammation, and is thus reserved for afflictions of ***pitta*** and ***kapha***. Although one study indicates an anxiolytic effect, the ***Bhāvaprakāśa*** states specifically that it is 'bad for the heart', and 'unpleasant for the mind' (Srikanthamurthy 2001). ***Nimba*** is an important herb in fever, used in simple formulations such as a soup prepared with ***Paṭola*** (Sharma 2002). It is also used in more complex formulations such as ***Nimbādi kvātha***, used in the treatment of ***masūrikā***, or chicken pox, composed of equal parts ***Nimba***, ***Harītakī***, ***Kaṭuka***, ***Vāsaka***, ***Uśīra***, ***Āmalakī***, ***Candana***, ***Parpaṭa***, ***Durālabhā***, ***Paṭola***, and ***Raktacandana*** (Sharma 2002). In the treatment of jaundice the ***Cakradatta*** recommends a buffalo milk decoction of ***Nimba***, ***Haridrā***, ***Pippalī***, ***Balā*** and ***Yaṣṭimadhu*** (Sharma 2002). In the treatment of acid reflux and vomiting associated with gastritis, as well as colic and fever, the ***Cakradatta*** recommends a decoction of ***Nimba***, ***Guḍūcī***, ***Triphala*** and ***Paṭola***, taken cool with honey (Sharma 2002). In the treatment of ***unmāda*** ('psychosis') ***Nimba*** leaves are reduced to a powder with ***Vacā***, ***Hiṅgu***, ***Sarṣapa*** seed and the discarded skin of a snake, and burned as an incense (Sharma 2002). In the treatment of gout and eczema ***Nimba*** is mixed with equal parts ***Triphala***, ***Mañjiṣṭhā***, ***Vacā***, ***Kaṭuka***, ***Guḍūcī*** and ***Dāruharidrā***, taken as a ***cūrṇa*** or ***kvātha*** (Sharma 2002). In combination with ***Punarnavā***, ***Kaṭuka***, ***Guḍūcī***, ***Devadāru***, ***Harītakī***, ***Paṭola***, and ***Śūṇṭhī***, ***Nimba*** is stated to be an effective treatment for intestinal parasites associated with anaemia and dyspnoea (Sharma 2002). Mixed with ***Haridrā***, ***Nimba*** has been shown to be an effective remedy in the treatment of scabies, and similar formulations can be used in ***udavartana abhyaṅga*** in the treatment of obesity and oedema. ***Nimba*** is also used in premature ageing and greyness associated with anger and physical strain, used as a simple medicated ***taila*** in ***nasya*** therapy for a period of 1 month (Sharma 2002). ***Nimba*** flowers are traditionally used in Tamil cookery, stir-fried with pepper, mustard seed, and ***Hiṅgu*** in ghee, after which water, tamarind paste, curry leaves and salt are added as the base of a spicy, flavourable ***dīpanapācana*** soup. ***Nimba*** has recently undergone much investigation for its insecticidal properties against disease-carrying insects such as mosquitoes and common agricultural pests such as flies, beetles, worms, cockroaches and moths, but appears to cause little harm to beneficial insects such as wasps, butterflies, bees, spiders and earthworms (Vietmeyer 1992). Organic farmers can thus take advantage of ***Nimba's*** insecticidal properties to good advantage, and people can apply the diluted oil (2%) to ward off mosquitos, without fear of harm. Some studies suggest that ***Nimba*** may act as a contraceptive, but this application is still in the experimental stage.

Dosage:

- ***Cūrṇa***: bark, leaf, 1–2 g b.i.d.–t.i.d.
- ***Svarasa***: leaf, 6–12 mL b.i.d.–t.i.d.
- ***Hima***: leaf, 30–90 mL b.i.d.–t.i.d.
- ***Kvātha***: bark, 30–60 mL b.i.d.–t.i.d.
- ***Seed oil***: topically only, 2–50% v/v in a carrier oil.

REFERENCES

Almas K 1999 The antimicrobial effects of extracts of Azadirachta indica (Neem) and Salvadora persica (Arak) chewing sticks. Indian Journal of Dental Research 10(1):23–26

Alzoreky NS, Nakahara K 2003 Antibacterial activity of extracts from some edible plants commonly consumed in Asia. International Journal of Food Microbiology 80(3):223–230

Arivazhagan S, Balasenthil S, Nagini S 2000 Garlic and Neem leaf extracts enhance hepatic glutathione and glutathione dependent enzymes during N-methyl-N'-nitro-N-nitrosoguanidine (MNNG)-induced gastric carcinogenesis in rats. Phytotherapy Research 14(4):291–293

Badam L, Joshi SP, Bedekar SS 1999 In vitro antiviral activity of Neem (Azadirachta indica. A. Juss) leaf extract against group B coxsackieviruses. Journal of Communicable Diseases 31(2):79–90

Bandyopadhyay U, Biswas K, Chatterjee R et al 2002 Gastroprotective effect of Neem (Azadirachta indica) bark extract: possible involvement of H(+)-K(+)-ATPase inhibition and scavenging of hydroxyl radical. Life Sciences 71(24):2845–2865

Bandyopadhyay U, Biswas K, Sengupta A et al 2004 Clinical studies on the effect of Neem (Azadirachta indica) bark extract on gastric secretion and gastroduodenal ulcer. Life Sciences 75(24):2867–2878.

Bhanwra S, Singh J, Khosla P 2000 Effect of Azadirachta indica (Neem) leaf aqueous extract on paracetamol-induced liver damage in rats. Indian Journal of Physiology and Pharmacology 44(1):64–68

Charles V, Charles SX 1992 The use and efficacy of Azadirachta indica ADR (Neem) and Curcuma longa ('Turmeric') in scabies. A pilot study. Tropical and Geographical Medicine 44(1–2):178–181

Chattopadhyay RR 1997 Effect of Azadirachta indica hydroalcoholic leaf extract on the cardiovascular system. General Pharmacology 28(3):449–451

Chattopadhyay RR 1998 Possible biochemical mode of anti-inflammatory action of Azadirachta indica A. Juss. in rats. Indian Journal of Experimental Biology 36(4):418–420

Duke JA (accessed 2003) Chemicals and their biological activities. In: Azadirachta indica A. JUSS. (Meliaceae): Neem. Agricultural Research Service (ARS), United States Department of Agriculture. Available: http://www.ars-grin.gov/duke/

Etebu E, Tasie AA, Daniel-Kalio LA 2003 Post-harvest fungal quality of selected chewing sticks. Oral Diseases 9(2):95–98

Fabry W, Okemo P, Ansorg R 1996 Fungistatic and fungicidal activity of east African medicinal plants. Mycoses 39(1–2):67–70

Gandhi M, Lal R, Sankaranarayanan A et al 1988 Acute toxicity study of the oil from Azadirachta indica seed (Neem oil). Journal of Ethnopharmacology 23(1):39–51

Hallur G, Sivramakrishnan A, Bhat SV 2002 Three new tetranortriterpenoids from Neem seed oil. Journal of Natural Products 65(8):1177–1179

Jaiswal AK, Bhattacharya SK, Acarya SB 1994 Anxiolytic activity of Azadirachta indica leaf extract in rats. Indian Journal of Experimental Biology 32(7):489–491

Kapoor LD 1990 CRC Handbook of Ayurvedic medicinal plants. CRC Press, Boca Raton, p 60

Kasturi M, Ahamed RN, Pathan KM 2002 Ultrastructural changes induced by leaves of Azadirachta indica (Neem) in the testis of albino rats. Journal of Basic and Clinical Physiology and Pharmacology 13(4):311–328

Khosla P, Bhanwra S, Singh J et al 2000 A study of hypoglycaemic effects of Azadirachta indica (Neem) in normal and alloxan diabetic rabbits. Indian Journal of Physiology and Pharmacology 44(1):69–74

Khosla P, Gupta A, Singh J 2002 A study of cardiovascular effects of Azadirachta indica (Neem) on isolated perfused heart preparations. Indian Journal of Physiology and Pharmacology 46(2):241–244

Kirtikar KR, Basu BD 1935 Indian medicinal plants, 2nd edn, vols 1–4. Periodical Experts, Delhi, p 536–537

Koley KM, Lal J 1994 Pharmacological effects of Azadirachta indica (Neem) leaf extract on the ECG and blood pressure of rat. Indian Journal of Physiology and Pharmacology 38(3):223–225

Kumar A, Rao AR, Kimura H 2002 Radiosensitizing effects of Neem (Azadirachta indica) oil. Phytotherapy Research 16(1):74–77

Luo XD, Wu SH, Ma YB, Wu DG 2000 A new triterpenoid from Azadirachta indica. Fitoterapia 71(6):668–672

Malathi R, Rajan SS, Gopalakrishnan G, Suresh G 2002 Azadirachtol, a tetranortriterpenoid from Neem kernels. Acta Crystallographica (Section C) 58(Pt 12):708–710

Mukherjee S, Garg S, Talwar GP 1999 Early post implantation contraceptive effects of a purified fraction of Neem (Azadirachta indica) seeds, given orally in rats: possible mechanisms involved. Journal of Ethnopharmacology 67(3):287–296

Nadkarni KM 1954 The Indian materia medica, with Ayurvedic, Unani and home remedies, revised and enlarged by A.K. Nadkarni. Popular Prakashan PVP, Bombay

Njiro SM, Kofi-Tsekpo MW 1999 Effect of an aqueous extract of Azadirachta indica on the immune response in mice. Onderstepoort Journal of Veterinary Research 66(1):59–62

Njoku OU, Alumanah EO, Meremikwu CU 2001 Effect of Azadirachta indica extract on plasma lipid levels in human malaria. Bollettino Chimico Farmaceutico 140(5):367–370

Pai MR, Acharya LD, Udupa N 2004 Evaluation of antiplaque activity of Azadirachta indica leaf extract gel: a 6-week clinical study. Journal of Ethnopharmacology 90(1):99–103

Parida MM, Upadhyay C, Pandya G, Jana AM 2002 Inhibitory potential of Neem (Azadirachta indica Juss) leaves on dengue virus type–2 replication. Journal of Ethnopharmacology 79(2): 273–278

Parshad O, Singh P, Gardner M et al 1994 Effect of aqueous Neem (Azadirachta indica) extract on testosterone and other blood constituents in male rats: a pilot study. West Indian Medical Journal 43(3):71–74

Sharma PV 2002 Cakradatta: Sanskrit text with English translation. Chaukhamba, Varanasi p 6, 120, 168, 190, 236, 265, 347, 469, 490

Sharma VP, Ansari MA, Razdan RK 1993 Mosquito repellent action of Neem (Azadirachta indica) oil. Journal of the American Mosquito Control Association 9(3):359–360

Srikanthamurthy KR 2001 Bhāvaprakāśa of Bhāvamiśra, vol 1. Krishnadas Academy, Varanasi, p 242

Tepsuwan A, Kupradinun P, Kusamran WR 2002 Chemopreventive potential of Neem flowers on carcinogen-induced rat mammary and liver carcinogenesis. Asian Pacific Journal of Cancer Prevention 3(3):231–238

Upadhyay SN, Dhawan S, Garg S, Talwar GP 1992 Immunomodulatory effects of Neem (Azadirachta indica) oil. International Journal of Immunopharmacology 14(7):1187–1193

Vanka A, Tandon S, Rao SR et al 2001 The effect of indigenous Neem (Azadirachta indica) mouth wash on Streptococcus mutans and lactobacilli growth. Indian Journal of Dental Research 12(3):133–144

Vietmeyer ND (ed) 1992 Neem: a tree for solving global problems. National Academy Press, Washington, p 39–59

Warrier PK, Nambiar VPK, Ramankutty C (eds) 1994 Indian medicinal plants: a compendium of 500 species, vol 1. Orient Longman, Hyderabad, p 227

Williamson EM (ed) 2002 Major herbs of Ayurveda. Churchill Livingstone, London, p 57

Nirguṇḍī

Botanical name: *Vitex negundo*, Verbenaceae

Other names: Sambhalu, Sanduvar (H); Nallavavili (T); Indian Privet, Five-leaved Chastetree (E)

Botany: ***Nirguṇḍī*** is a large shrub or small tree with thin grey bark, quadangular branchlets covered with a fine white hair, which attains a height of about 3 m. The leaves are oppositely arranged, with three to five leaflets, the leaflets lanceolate, acute, glabrous above with a white, fine hair below, the terminal leaflet longer than the others on a long petiole, 5–10 cm in length by 1.6–3.2 cm wide, the lateral leaflets on very short petioles. The bluish purple flowers are borne in axillary or terminal panicles up to 30 cm long, giving rise to black globose drupes with four seeds when ripe. ***Nirguṇḍī*** is the name given to specimens with a bluish purple flower; ***Sinduvara*** is the name for the identical plant with a white flower. ***Nirguṇḍī*** is found throughout India, in waste areas and along water courses, extending westwards into Iran and Eastern Africa, and eastwards into Malaysia and China (Kirtikar & Basu 1935, Srikanthamurthy 2001, Warrier et al 1996).

Part used: Whole plant.

Dravyguṇa:

- ***Rasa***: *kaśāya, tikta, kaṭu*
- ***Vipāka***: *laghu*
- ***Vīrya***: *uṣṇa*
- ***Karma***: *dīpanapācana, kṛmighna, jvaraghna, chedana, mūtravirecana, raktaprasādana, ārtavajanana, sandhānīya, vedanāsthāpana, cakṣuṣya, romasañjanana, viṣaghna, medhya, rasāyana, vātakaphahara (leaf), pittahara (flower)* (Srikanthamurthy 2001, Warrier et al 1996).

Constituents: A variety of constituents have been isolated from the different plants of ***Nirguṇḍī***, including an essential oil, flavonoids and triterpenes. The leaf is reported to contain an essential oil comprising monoterpenes terpinen-4-ol, *p*-cymene, α-terpineol and sabinene, and sesquiterpenes β-caryophyllene, globulol, spathulenol, β-farnesene and bis[1, 1-dimethyl]methylphenol. Other constituents include the alkaloids nishidine and hydrocotylene, the flavonoids casticin, chrysophenol-D, luteolin and isoorientin, the triterpenoids betulinic acid, ursolic acid, 3β-acetoxyolean-12-en-27-oic acid, 2α,3α-dihydroxyoleana-5,12-dien-28-oic acid, 2β,α-diacetoxyoleana-5,12-dien-28-oic acid, and 2α, 3β-diacetoxy-18-hydroxyoleana-5,12-dien-28-oic acid, β-sitosterol, the aliphatic alcohol *n*-hentriacontanol, and *p*-hydroxybenzoic acid (Chandramu et al 2003, Chawla et al 1992, Shafi et al 1998, Yoganarasimhan 2000).

Medical research:

- ***In vitro***: antibacterial (Perumal et al 1998), antivenom (Alam & Gomes 2003).
- ***In vivo***: CNS-depressant, analgesic, anticonvulsant (Gupta et al 1999); hepatoprotective (Avadhoot & Rana 1991); anti-inflammatory (Jana et al 1999); anti-allergenic (Nair & Saraf 1995); insect repellent (Hebbalkar et al 1992); antivenom (Alam & Gomes 2003); antifertility (Bhargava et al 1989).

Toxicity: An alcoholic extract of the leaves is stated to have an LD_{50} of 1500 mg/kg (Avadhoot & Rana 1991).

Indications: Dyspepsia, colic, flatulence, dysentery, haemorrhoids, hepatosplenomegaly, intestinal parasites, fever, cough, bronchitis, skin diseases, ear infection, alopecia, ophthalmic disorders, dysmenorrhoea, PMS, injuries and wounds, inflammatory joint disease, pain, epilepsy, poor memory, psychosis, drug withdrawal.

Contraindications: ***Nirguṇḍī*** should be used with caution with the concurrent use of psychotropic drugs, including analgesics, sedatives, antidepressants, anticonvulsants and antipsychotics. *Vitex negundo* is quite similar botanically to the better studied *V. agnus castus*, and thus may have a similar range of contraindications, including the concurrent use of progesterogenic drugs and hormone replacement therapies (Mills & Bone 2000).

Medicinal uses: ***Nirguṇḍī*** is used in a variety of ways, both internally and externally, depending upon the plant part used. Taken internally, the juice (***svarasa***) of the fresh leaf is used in a variety of digestive disorders, from dyspepsia to parasites, and helps to resolve ***kaphaja*** and ***vāttika*** fevers, catarrh, cough and bronchitis. The leaf juice also displays an alterative property that makes it useful in skin conditions such as eczema and psoriasis, and in inflammatory joint disorders such as arthritis and gout. Applied externally, the ***svarasa*** is used in the treatment of otitis media, joint inflammation, wounds, snake and insect bites, ulcers, bruises, sprains, and orchitis, to relieve both pain and inflammation. The juice is also used in bacterial and parasitic skin conditions. The freshly dried leaves can be made into a strong infusion and used in much the same way as the fresh juice, and specifically, are smoked in the treatment of ***kaphaja*** conditions such as headache and catarrh (Nadkarni 1954). The fresh juice prepared as a medicated ***ghṛta*** is mentioned in the treatment of cough, consumptive conditions and chest wounds (Sharma 2002, Srikanthamurthy 1995). Prepared as medicated ***ghṛta*** with the fresh juices of ***Maṇḍūkaparṇī***, ***Brāhmī***, ***Bhṛṅgarāja*** and ***Āmalakī***, ***Nirguṇḍī*** leaf juice can be used in the treatment of alopecia and poor eyesight, as well as to enhance intelligence and treat mental disorders. Combined with the powders of ***Uśīra***, ***Trikaṭu***, barley, and mung bean, and crushed with goat's urine, ***Nirguṇḍī cūrṇa*** is fashioned into suppositories (***vartti***), mixed with water and used as a collyrium in the treatment of epilepsy, psychosis and unconsciousness (Sharma 2002, Sharma & Dash 1988). The ***Madanapahala nighaṇṭu*** states specifically that ***Nirguṇḍī*** is a promoter of memory (Dash 1991), and this traditional usage as a ***medhya rasāyana*** parallels the modern usage of Chasteberry (***Vitex agnus castus***) as a dominergic agent, helpful in weaning patients off addictive drugs such as heroin. Prepared as a medicated oil with ***Mustaka***, ***Uśīra***, ***Devadāru***, ***Mañjiṣṭhā***, ***Viḍaṅga***, ***Khadira*** and ***Yaṣṭimadhu***, ***Nirguṇḍī*** is used as a mouthwash in the treatment of periodontal disease and to relieve tooth pain (Sharma 2002). The fresh juice of ***Nirguṇḍī*** mixed with sesame oil, ***saindhava***, soot, jaggery and honey is recommended by the ***Cakradatta*** in the treatment of purulent discharges of the ear (Sharma 2002). The root bark is mentioned in the treatment of rheumatism, haemorrhoids, and irritable bladder, used in much the same way as the leaf (Nadkarni 1954). The flowers are somewhat different from the rest of the plant, however, and have a cooling energy, used in ***paittika***-specific disorders such as bleeding diarrhoea and haemorrhage (Warrier et al 1996).

Dosage: Leaves

- ***Cūrṇa***: 3–5 g b.i.d.–t.i.d.
- ***Svarasa***: 12–25 mL b.i.d.–t.i.d.
- ***Hima***: 30–90 mL b.i.d.–t.i.d.
- ***Tincture***: recently dried leaf, 1:3, 2–5 mL b.i.d.–t.i.d.

REFERENCES

Alam MI, Gomes A 2003 Snake venom neutralization by Indian medicinal plants (Vitex negundo and Emblica officinalis) root extracts. Journal of Ethnopharmacology 86(1):75–80

Avadhoot Y, Rana AC 1991 Hepatoprotective effect of Vitex negundo against carbon tetrachloride-induced liver damage. Archives of Pharmacal Research 14(1):96–98

Bhargava SK 1989 Antiandrogenic effects of a flavonoid-rich fraction of Vitex negundo seeds: a histological and biochemical study in dogs. Journal of Ethnopharmacology 27(3):327–339

Chandramu C, Manohar RD, Krupadanam DG, Dashavantha RV 2003 Isolation, characterization and biological activity of betulinic acid and ursolic acid from Vitex negundo L. Phytotherapy Research 17(2):129–134

Chawla AS, Sharma AK, Handa SS, Dhar KL 1992 Chemical investigation and anti-inflammatory activity of Vitex negundo seeds. Journal of Natural Products 55(2):163–167

Dash B 1991 Materia medica of Ayurveda. B. Jain Publishers, New Delhi, p 55

Gupta M, Mazumder UK, Bhawal SR 1999 CNS activity of Vitex negundo Linn. in mice. Indian Journal of Experimental Biology 37(2):143–146

Hebbalkar DS, Hebbalkar GD, Sharma RN et al 1992 Mosquito repellent activity of oils from Vitex negundo Linn. leaves. Indian Journal of Medical Research 95:200–203

Jana U, Chattopadhyay RN, Shaw P 1999 Anti-inflammatory activity of Zingiber officinale Rosc., Vitex negundo Linn. and Tinospora cordifolia (Willid) Miers in albino rats. Indian Journal of Pharmacology 31:232–233

Kirtikar KR, Basu BD 1935 Indian medicinal Plants, 2nd edn, vols 1–4. Periodical Experts, Delhi, p 1937–1938

Mills S, Bone K 2000 Principles and practice of phytotherapy. Churchill Livingstone, London, p 332

Nadkarni KM 1954 The Indian materia medica, with Ayurvedic, Unani and home remedies, revised and enlarged by A.K. Nadkarni. Popular Prakashan PVP, Bombay, p 1280

Nair AM, Saraf MN 1995 Inhibition of antigen and compound 48/80 induced contractions of guinea pig trachea by the ethanolic extract of the leaves of Vitex negundo Linn. Indian Journal of Pharmacology 27:230–233

Perumal SR, Ignacimuthu S, Sen A 1998 Screening of 34 Indian medicinal plants for antibacterial properties. Journal of Ethnopharmacology 62(2):173–182

Shafi MP, Geetha Nambiar MK, Jirovetz L et al 1998 Analysis of the essential oils of the leaves of the medicinal plants Vitex negundo var. negundo and Vitex negundo var. purpurescens from India. Acta Pharmaceutica 48: 179–186

Sharma PV 2002 Cakradatta: Sanskrit text with English translation. Chaukhamba, Varanasi, p 143, 192, 500, 517

Sharma RK, Dash B 1988 Agnivesa's Caraka Saṃhitā: text with English translation and critical exposition based on Cakrapani Datta's Āyurveda Dipika, vol 3. Chaukhambha Orientalia, Varanasi, p 452

Srikanthamurthy KR 1995 Vāgbhaṭa's Aṣṭāñga Hṛdayam, vol 3. Krishnadas Academy, Varanasi, p 225

Srikanthamurthy KR 2001 Bhāvaprakāśa of of Bhāvamiśra, vol 1. Krishnadas Academy, Varanasi, p 217, 245

Warrier PK, Nambiar VPK, Ramankutty C (eds) 1996 Indian medicinal plants: a compendium of 500 species, vol 5. Orient Longman, Hyderabad, p 387

Yoganarasimhan SN 2000 Medicinal plants of India, vol 2: Tamil Nadu. Self-published, Bangalore, p 585

Pippalī

BOTANICAL NAME: *Piper longum,* Piperaceae

OTHER NAMES: Pipli, Pipal (H); Pippili, Tippili (T); Long Pepper (E)

Botany: ***Pippalī*** is a slender aromatic climber with a perennial woody root, an erect rootstalk, with many jointed branches, the nodes swollen and sometimes rooting. The leaves are entire, glabrous, with reticulate venation, the lower leaves ovate, cordate, on long petioles, the upper leaves smaller, similarly cordate but oblong-oval, petioles short or absent. The creamy coloured flowers are are borne in solitary penduncu-late cylindrical spikes, the male flowers longer and more slender than the female spikes, the latter giving way to a cylindrical cluster of small ovoid fruits about 4 cm in length, that passes from green to orange-red in colour when ripe, becoming black upon drying. ***Pippalī*** is found growing wild throughout the hotter regions of Southeast Asia in evergreen forests, but is also cultivated extensively (Kirtikar & Basu 1935, Warrier et al 1995).

Part used: Fruit (***Pippalī***), root (***Pippalīmūla***).

Dravyguṇa: Fruit

- ***Rasa***: *kaṭu*
- ***Vipāka***: *madhura*
- ***Vīrya***: *uṣṇa, snigdha, tikṣṇa*
- ***Karma***: *dīpanapācana, bhedana, kṛmighna, jvaraghna, chedana, kāsahara, svāsahara, kuṣṭhaghna, mūtravirecana, medohara, hṛdaya, medhya, vajīkaraṇa, rasāyana, vātakaphahara* (Srikanthamurthy 2001, Warrier et al 1995).

Constituents: ***Pippalī*** fruit contains a number of constituents, including a volatile oil, alkaloids, isobutylamides, lignans and esters. The volatile oil is responsible for the characteristic odour of ***Pippalī***, consisting of caryophyllene, pentadecane, bisaboline, thujine, terpinoline, zingiberine, *p*-cymene, *p*-methoxyacetophenone, dihydrocarveol and others. The pungency, however, is due primarily to the alkaloidal constituents, including piperine, methylpiperine, pipernonaline, piperettine, asarinine, pellitorine, piperundecalidine, piperlongumine, piperlonguminine and others, as well as isobutylamides such as retrofractamide, brachystamide and longamide that provide for the characteristic tingling sensation and sialogogue properties of ***Pippalī***. Other constituents include the lignans sesamin, pulviatilol and fargesin, the esters tridecyl-dihydro-*p*-coumarate, eicosanyl-(E)-*p*-coumarate, and Z–12-octadecenoic-glycerol-monoester, fatty acids including palmatic, linoleic and linolenic acids, amino acids including L-tyrosine, L-cysteine and DL-serine, as well as minerals such as calcium, phosphorous and iron (Williamson 2002, Yoganarasimhan 2000).

Medical research:

- ***In vitro***: anti-amoebic (Ghoshal & Lakshmi 2002, Ghoshal et al 1996), giardicidal (Tripathi et al 1999), insecticidal (Yang et al 2002).
- ***In vivo***: anti-amoebic (Ghoshal & Lakshmi 2002, Ghoshal et al 1996), giardicidal (Tripathi et al 1999), immunostimulant (Agarwal et al 1994), absorption/bioavailability enhancement (Atal et al 1981, Khajuria et al 2002), anti-ulcerogenic (Agrawal et al 2000), hepatoprotective (Koul and Kapil 1993), antitumour (Pradeep & Kuttan 2002).
- ***Human trials***: a formula consisting of *Piper longum* and *Butea monosperma* given to patients suffering from giardiasis completely eliminated the parasite from the stool in 92% of the treatment group, and simultaneously decreased the presence of mucus, pus cells and RBCs (Agarwal et al 1997).

Toxicity: A series of acute (24 hour) and chronic (90 day) oral toxicity studies were carried out on an ethanolic extract of *Piper longum* fruit in mice. Acute dosages were 0.5, 1.0 and 3 g/kg, while the chronic dosage was 100 mg/kg daily. The extract caused no significant acute or chronic mortality compared to controls, although researchers noted that the extract caused a significant increase in the weight of the lungs and spleen, as well as reproductive organs, without any negative effects upon sperm count or motility (Shah et al 1998). Duke (1985) states that piperine and other ***Piper*** alkaloids are chemically similar to a mutagenic urinary safrole metabolite, and thus there is theoretical concern for carcinogenicity, although feeding trials with *Piper nigrum* in experimental animals have failed to produce any negative effects at doses of 50 g/3 kg in the diet (Shwaireb et al 1990). A few studies have associated the incidence of oesophageal cancer with *Piper nigrum*, thought to be due to an irritative effect upon the oesophageal mucosa (Ghadirian et al 1992).

Indications: Poor appetite, dyspepsia, flatulent colic, constipation, dysentery, haemorrhoids, cholelithiasis, jaundice, splenomegaly, intestinal parasites, fever, hiccough, pharyngitis, coryza, cough, bronchitis, asthma, skin diseases, cystitis, coma, paralysis, epilepsy, amenorrhoea, post-parturient, arthritis, gout, lumbago, circulatory problems.

Contraindications: Due to its warming nature ***Pippalī*** is contraindicated in severe ***pittakopa*** conditions.

Medicinal uses: ***Pippalī*** is without a doubt the most celebrated and widely used pungent remedy in Āyurvedic medicine, used as a simple home remedy in the treatment of disorders such as dyspepsia, coryza and bronchitis, and also as an important ***rasāyana dravya***. In ***kuṭīprāveśika rasāyana***, the most potent ***rasāyana*** technique, the ***Cakradatta*** recommends that ten fruits be consumed with cow's milk on the first day, increased by ten fruits on each successive day for 10 days, and thereafter reduced by ten until finished (Sharma 2002). The ***Cakradatta*** also states that the daily consumption of ***Pippalī*** in the amount of five, seven, eight or ten fruits daily, taken with honey, also acts as a ***rasāyana***, although the effect is less than in the former technique. Both these methods, however, are stated to be effective for a wide range of conditions, including anorexia, dyspepsia, malabsorption, haemorrhoids, bronchitis, asthma, consumption, throat disorders, chronic fever, anaemia, oedema and paralysis. The ***Bhāvaprakāśa*** ascribes different therapeutic properties to ***Pippalī*** depending upon the ***anupāna***. Taken with honey ***Pippalī*** specifically reduces ***medas*** (fat) and accumulations of ***kapha***, and is stated to be a good treatment for fever, cough and bronchitis, with ***vajīkaraṇa*** and ***medhya rasāyana*** properties (Srikanthamurthy 2001). Taken with twice the amount of jaggery the ***Bhāvaprakāśa*** states that ***Pippalī*** is suited to the treatment chronic fever, dyspepsia, asthma, heart diseases and intestinal parasites (Srikanthamurthy 2001). Although generally considered to be a pungent, warming herb, the effect is stated to be so mild that ***Pippalī*** can be used in the treatment of fever, although it is best reserved in ***vāta*** or ***kapha*** variants, with predominant symptoms such as body pain and catarrh, as opposed to a very high temperature. Although difficult to obtain in the West, the fresh green fruit is stated to have a ***śita*** and ***snigdha vīrya***, and is used specifically to reduce ***pitta*** (Srikanthamurthy 2001). ***Pippalī*** is most often found as part of the famous ***Trikaṭu*** formulation, composed of equal parts ***Pippalī***, ***Śūṇṭhī*** and ***Marica***, used in the treatment of anorexia, dyspepsia, pharyngitis, catarrhal conditions, ***āma***, coldness and poor circulation. ***Trikaṭu*** and ***Pippalī*** are found in literally hundreds of formulas as an adjunct to enhance the bioavailability or modify the effect of the other constituents in the formula. Prepared as a medicated ***ghṛta***, the ***Cakradatta*** states that ***Pippalī*** is useful in the treatment of flatulent colic, splenomegaly and hepatic torpor (Sharma 2002). Prepared as a medicated oil, ***Pippalī*** is decocted with equal parts ***Bilva***, ***Śatapuṣpā***, ***Vacā***, ***Kuṣṭha***, ***Citraka***, ***Devadāru***, ***Śaṭī***, ***Yaṣṭimadhu***, ***Puṣkaramūla*** and ***Madana***, used as an enema in severe haemorrhoids, rectal prolapse, dysentery, dysuria, and weakness of the lower back and legs (Sharma 2002). As a post-parturient emmenagogue to expel the placenta and to relieve pain the ***Cakradatta*** recommends ***Pippalī cūrṇa*** be taken with wine (Sharma 2002).

Dosage:

- ***Cūrṇa***: 2–3 g b.i.d.–t.i.d.
- ***Ghṛta***: 3–6 g b.i.d.
- ***Tincture***: dried fruit, 1:3, 1–2 mL b.i.d.–t.i.d.

REFERENCES

Agarwal AK, Singh M, Gupta N et al 1994 Management of giardiasis by an immuno-modulatory herbal drug Pippali rasayana. Journal of Ethnopharmacology 44(3):143–146

Agarwal AK, Tripathi DM, Sahai R et al 1997 Management of giardiasis by a herbal drug Pippali rasayana: a clinical study. Journal of Ethnopharmacology 56(3):233–236
Agrawal AK, Rao CV, Sairam K et al 2000 Effect of Piper longum Linn, Zingiber officinalis Linn and Ferula species on gastric ulceration and secretion in rats. Indian Journal of Experimental Biology 38(10):994–998
Atal CK, Zutshi U, Rao PG 1981 Scientific evidence on the role of Ayurvedic herbals on bioavailability of drugs. Journal of Ethnopharmacology 4(2):229–232
Chatterjee A, Dutta CP 1967 Alkaloids of Piper longum Linn. I. Structure and synthesis of piperlongumine and piperlonguminine. Tetrahedron 23(4):1769–1781
Duke JA 1985 Handbook of medicinal herbs. CRC Press, Boca Raton, p 383
Ghadirian P, Ekoe JM, Thouez JP 1992 Food habits and esophageal cancer: an overview. Cancer Detection and Prevention 16(3):163–168
Ghoshal S, Lakshmi V 2002 Potential antiamoebic property of the roots of Piper longum Linn. Phytotherapy Research 16(7):689–691
Ghoshal S, Prasad BN, Lakshmi V 1996 Antiamoebic activity of Piper longum fruits against Entamoeba histolytica in vitro and in vivo. Journal of Ethnopharmacology 50(3):167–170
Khajuria A, Thusu N, Zutshi U 2002 Piperine modulates permeability characteristics of intestine by inducing alterations in membrane dynamics: influence on brush border membrane fluidity, ultrastructure and enzyme kinetics. Phytomedicine 9(3):224–231
Kirtikar KR, Basu BD 1935 Indian medicinal plants, 2nd edn, vols 1–4. Periodical Experts, Delhi, p 2128
Koul IB, Kapil A 1993 Evaluation of the liver protective potential of piperine, an active principle of black and long peppers. Planta Medica 59(5):413–417
Nadkarni KM 1954 The Indian materia medica, with Ayurvedic, Unani and home remedies, revised and enlarged by A.K. Nadkarni. Popular Prakashan PVP, Bombay
Pradeep CR, Kuttan G 2002 Effect of piperine on the inhibition of lung metastasis induced B16F–10 melanoma cells in mice. Clinical and Experimental Metastasis 19(8):703–708
Shah AH, Al-Shareef AH, Ageel AM, Qureshi S 1998 Toxicity studies in mice of common spices, Cinnamomum zeylanicum bark and Piper longum fruits. Plant Foods for Human Nutrition 52(3):231–239
Sharma PV 2002 Cakradatta: Sanskrit text with English translation. Chaukhamba, Varanasi p 88, 273, 353, 589
Shwaireb MH, Wrba H, El-Mofty MM, Dutter A 1990 Carcinogenesis induced by black pepper (Piper nigrum) and modulated by vitamin A. Experimental Pathology 40(4):233–238
Srikanthamurthy KR 2001 Bhāvaprakāśa of Bhāvamiśra, vol 1. Krishnadas Academy, Varanasi, p 166, 167
Tripathi DM, Gupta N, Lakshmi V et al 1999 Antigiardial and immunostimulatory effect of Piper longum on giardiasis due to Giardia lamblia. Phytotherapy Research 13(7):561–565
Warrier PK, Nambiar VPK, Ramankutty C (eds) 1995 Indian medicinal plants: a compendium of 500 species, vol 4. Hyderabad, Orient Longman, p 290
Williamson EM (ed) 2002 Major herbs of Ayurveda. Churchill Livingstone, London, p 226
Yang YC, Lee SG, Lee HK et al 2002 A piperidine amide extracted from Piper longum L. fruit shows activity against Aedes aegypti mosquito larvae. Journal of Agricultural and Food Chemistry 50(13):3765–3767
Yoganarasimhan SN 2000 Medicinal plants of India, vol 2: Tamil Nadu. Self-published, Bangalore, p 416

Punarnavā, 'once again new'

BOTANICAL NAMES: *Boerhavia repens, B. diffusa,* Nyctaginaceae

OTHER NAMES: ***Śvetapunarnavā, Raktapunarnavā*** (S); Sant, Gadahpurna (H); Mukkurattai (T); Red Spiderling, Spreading Hogweed (E)

Botany: ***Punarnavā*** is a herbaceous perennial with a large root and highly branched stems that are prostrate or ascending to a height of up to a metre. The leaves are simple, ovate-oblong, acute or obtuse at the tip and rounded or subcordate at the base, glabrous above, white with minute scales below. The small rose or white coloured flowers are borne in small umbels arranged in corymbone, axillary and terminal panicles, giving way to a detachable indehiscent seed with a thin pericarp. ***Punarnavā*** is found throughout the subcontinent of India as a weed of wastelands and roadsides, and is also found in similar tropical and subtropical environs in Africa and the Americas. The Sanskrit name ***Śvetapunarnavā*** refers to *B. repens* (with white flowers), whereas ***Raktapunarnavā*** refers to *B. diffusa* (with red flowers) (Kirtikar & Basu 1935, Warrier et al 1994).

Part used: Roots, aerial parts.

Dravyguṇa:

The various ***nighaṇṭus*** typically differentiate between ***Śvetapunarnavā*** and ***Raktapunarnavā***, and based on this, provide differing and sometimes contradictory accounts of the ***dravyguṇa***.

- ***Rasa***: *tikta, madhura, kaṭu, kaśāya (Śvetapunarnavā); tikta (Raktapunarnavā)*
- ***Vipāka***: *madhura (Śvetapunarnavā); kaṭu (Raktapunarnavā)*
- ***Vīrya***: *uṣṇa, rūkṣa (Śvetapunarnavā); śita, laghu (Raktapunarnavā)*
- ***Karma***: *dīpana, bhedana (Svetapunarnavā), stambhana (Raktapunarnavā), sulapraśamana, kṛmighna, chedana, svāsahara, mūtravirecana, mūtraviśodhana, śotahara, hṛdaya, viṣaghna, ārtavajanana, rasāyana, tridoṣahara;* the *Bhāvaprakāśa* states that *Raktapunarnavā* increases *vāta*, and thus *Śvetapunarnavā* is preferred in *vātaja* conditions (Dash 1991, Kirtikar & Basu 1935, Srikanthamurthy 2001, Warrier et al 1994).

Constituents: Among the first constituents isolated from ***Punarnavā*** was the sulfate of an alkaloid named punarnavine, and since then a variety of constituents have been described, including rotenoid analogues (boeravinone A–F, punarnavoside), lignans (liriodendrin, syringaresinol mon-β-D-glucoside), xanthones (boerhavine, dihydroisofuranoxanthone), C-methylflavone, hentriacontane, β-sitosterol, ursolic acid, potassium nitrate, and amino acids (Kapoor 1990, Williamson 2002, Yoganarasimhan 2000).

Medical research:
- ***In vitro***: immunomodulant (Mehrotra et al 2002).
- ***In vivo***: hepatoprotective (Chandan et al 1991); antibacterial (Singh et al 1986); adaptogenic (Sharma et al 1990); hypoglycaemic (Chude et al 2001); anti-amoebic, immunomodulant (Sohni & Bhatt 1996).

Toxicity: The LD_{50} for an ethanolic extract of the root and whole plant is 1000 mg/kg in adult albino rats (Williamson 2002).

Indications: Dyspepsia, gastritis, ulcer, constipation (***Śvetapunarnavā***), diarrhoea and dysentery (***Raktapunarnavā***), intestinal parasites, fistula, jaundice, cirrhosis, splenomegaly, fever, cough, bronchitis, asthma, pleurisy, urinary tenesmus, renal diseases, gonorrhoea, oedema, ascites, scrotal enlargement, haemorrhage, scabies, lumbago, myalgia, leucorrhoea, dysmenorrhoea, heart disorders, heart valve stenosis, anaemia, epilepsy, debility and fatigue, ophthalmia.

Contraindications: Pregnancy; the ***Bhāvaprakāśa*** states the ***Raktapunarnavā*** is contraindicated in ***vātakopa*** conditions. Due to its potential GABA-nergic activity ***Punarnavā*** may be contraindicated with concurrent use of tranquilisers, antidepressants and antiseizure drugs. Nadkarni (1954) states that in high doses ***Punarnavā*** may act as an emetic.

Medicinal uses: ***Punarnavā*** is an important ***rasāyana dravya*** in Āyurvedic medicine, indicated by the translation of its Sanskrit name, 'once again new'. For this purpose ***Punarnavā*** can be taken as a milk decoction, 10–24 grams of the root taken twice daily. The potent rejuvenating properties of ***Punarnavā*** root are also made use of in a variety of rejuvenating formulae, including the famous medicinal confection ***Cyavanaprāśa***. ***Punarnavā***, however, also has a number of more mudane uses, especially for its ability to correct diseases of the urinary tract and treat oedema. As a simple remedy for cystitis the ***svarasa*** or ***cūrṇa*** of ***Punarnavā*** can be taken, 10–15 mL of the juice, or 3–5 grams of the powder, thrice daily until symptoms are gone. In the treatment of oedema 10–15 mL of the fresh juice of the leaves can be mixed with a small amount of ***Marica*** or ***Śūṇṭhī***, taken twice daily for several weeks. The fresh juice is also taken in jaundice and in menstrual disorders. Lt. Col. Chopra found that ***Punarnavā*** was efficacious in the treatment of oedema and ascites due to early cirrhosis and peritonitis, using a liquid extract prepared from either the dry or fresh plant material of ***Svetapunarnavā*** (Nadkarni 1954). Nadkarni (1954) adds that ***Punarnavā*** is equally effective in oedema secondary to heart disease from stenosis of the valves, in pleurisy and in other oedematous conditions. In most cases ***Punarnavā*** is used in polyherbal formulations to treat oedema and other conditions. In the treatment of oedema as well as colic, bloating, flatulence, constipation, haemorrhoids, intestinal parasites, and anaemia, the ***Cakradatta*** recommends ***Punarnavāmaṇḍśra***, composed of equal parts ***Punarnavā***, ***Trivṛt***, ***Śūṇṭhī***, ***Pippalī***, ***Marica***, ***Viḍaṅga***, ***Devadāru***, ***Citraka***, ***Puṣkaramūla***, ***Haridrā***, ***Dañtī***, ***Cavya***, ***Indrayava***, ***Kaṭuka***, ***Pippalīmūla*** and ***Mustaka***, decocted in cow's urine (Sharma 2002). Another formula called ***Punarnavādi taila*** is mentioned by the ***Bhāvaprakāśa*** in the treatment of urinary calculi, muscle pains and hernia associated with the aggravation of ***kapha*** and ***vāta***, used in ***vasti*** (enemata) and internally (Srikanthamurthy 2000). A decoction of ***Punarnavā***, ***Devadāru***, ***Harītakī*** and ***Guḍūcī*** combined with ***Guggulu*** is stated to be effective in abdominal enlargement (***udararoga***), as well as intestinal parasites, obesity, anaemia, oedema and skin diseases (Sharma 2002). Similarly, a combination of ***Punarnavā***, ***Devadāru***, ***Guḍūcī***, ***Pāṭhā***, ***Bilva***, ***Gokṣura***, ***Bṛhatī***, ***Kaṇṭakāri***, ***Haridrā***, ***Dāruharidrā***, ***Pippalī***, ***Citraka*** and ***Vāsaka***, reduced to a fine powder and taken with cow's urine is used in abdominal enlargement secondary to intestinal parasites (Sharma 2002). In ***vāttika*** forms of oedema a combination of ***Punarnavā***, ***Śūṇṭhī***, ***Eraṇḍa*** and ***Bṛhatī*** is stated by the ***Cakradatta*** to be efficacious (Sharma 2002). As a topical therapy for oedema the ***Śāraṅgadhara saṃhitā*** recommends ***Punarnavādi lepa***, prepared by combining equal parts powders of ***Punarnavā***, ***Dāruharidrā***, ***Śūṇṭhī***, ***Siddhārtha*** and ***Śigru*** with rice water (Srikanthamurthy 1984). Given the ability of ***Punarnavā*** to mobilise kidney function and thus promote the elimination of metabolic wastes in joints and muscles, it is also used to treat inflammatory joint disease, including gout and rheumatoid arthritis. To this extent the ***Cakradatta*** recommends a formula called ***Śatyādi kvātha***, consisting of a decoction of ***Punarnavā*** with a paste of ***Śaṭī*** and ***Śūṇṭhī***, taken every day for at least 1 week (Sharma 2002). Similarly, the ***Bhāvaprakāśa*** advocates a complex formula called ***Punarnavā guggulu*** in the treatment of gout, hernia, sciatica, muscular atrophy and inflammatory joint disease (Srikanthamurthy 2000). In the treatment of internal abscesses the ***Śāraṅgadhara saṃhitā*** recommends a decoction of ***Punarnavā*** and ***Varuṇa*** (Srikanthamurthy 1984). ***Punarnavā*** is also valued in ophthalmic disorders, the ***Śāraṅgadhara saṃhitā*** recommending a collyrium (***añjana***) for itching, prepared by mixing the ***cūrṇa*** with milk; mixed with honey to treatment ophthalmic discharges; with ***ghṛta*** for corneal wounds; with ***taila*** for poor vision; and with rice water (***kanjika***) for night blindness (Srikanthamurthy 1984). In the treatment of alcoholism the ***Cakradatta*** recommends a decoction of ***Punarnavā*** to restore ***ojas*** (Sharma 2002). In the treatment of diabetes ***Punarnavā*** can be combined with ***Śilājatu*** and ***Guḍūcī***. ***Punarnavā*** is also consumed as a nourishing vegetable in India, as it is rich in vitamins and minerals, and has undergone investigation for its potential in famine relief (Smith et al 1996).

Dosage:

- ***Cūrṇa***: 3–5 g b.i.d.–t.i.d.
- ***Svarasa***: fresh herb, 10–15 mL b.i.d.–t.i.d.
- ***Kvātha***: dried root, 60–120 mL b.i.d.–t.i.d.
- ***Tincture***: dried root, 1:3, 45%; 2–5 mL b.i.d.–t.i.d.

REFERENCES

Chandan BK, Sharma AK, Anand KK 1991 Boerhavia diffusa: a study of its hepatoprotective activity. Journal of Ethnopharmacology 31(3):299–307

Chude MA, Orisakwe OE, Afonne OJ et al 2001 Hypoglycaemic effect of the aqueous extract of Boerhavia diffusa leaves. Indian Journal of Pharmacology 33:215–216

Dash B 1991 Materia medica of Ayurveda. B. Jain Publishers, New Delhi, p 57–58

Kapoor LD 1990 CRC handbook of Ayurvedic medicinal plants. CRC Press, Boca Raton, p 79

Kirtikar KR, Basu BD 1935 Indian medicinal plants, 2nd edn, vols 1–4. Periodical Experts, Delhi, p 2045–2047

Mehrotra S, Mishra KP, Maurya R et al 2002 Immunomodulation by ethanolic extract of Boerhaavia diffusa roots. International Immunopharmacology 2(7):987–996

Nadkarni KM 1954 The Indian materia medica, with Ayurvedic, Unani and home remedies, revised and enlarged by A.K. Nadkarni. Popular Prakashan PVP, Bombay, p 205, 207

Sharma K, Vali Pasha K, Dandiya PC 1990 Is Boerhavia diffusa linn. (Punarnava) an antistress drug? Indian Pharmacological Society, 23rd Annual Conference, Dec. 6–8, Bombay

Sharma PV 2002 Cakradatta. Sanskrit text with English translation. Chaukhamba, Varanasi, p 118–119, 179, 246, 346, 347, 357

Singh A, Singh RG, Singh RH et al 1986 Effect of Boerhavia diffusa (Punarnava) in experimental pyelonephritis in albino rats. Indian Pharmacological Society, 19th Annual Conference, October 24–26, Srinagar

Smith GC, Clegg MS, Keen CL, Grivetti LE 1996 Mineral values of selected plant foods common to southern Burkina Faso and to Niamey, Niger, West Africa. International Journal of Food Sciences and Nutrition 47(1):41–53

Sohni YR, Bhatt RM 1996 Activity of a crude extract formulation in experimental hepatic amoebiasis and in immunomodulation studies. Journal of Ethnopharmacology 54(2–3):119–124

Srikanthamurthy KR 1984 Śāraṇgadhara saṃhitā: a treatise on Ayurveda. Chaukhamba Orientalia, Varanasi, p 71, 236, 269

Srikanthamurthy KR 2000 Bhāvaprakāśa of Bhāvamiśra, vol 2. Krishnadas Academy, Varanasi, p 408, 481

Srikanthamurthy KR 2001 Bhāvaprakāśa of Bhāvamiśra, vol 1. Krishnadas Academy, Varanasi, p 265

Warrier PK, Nambiar VPK, Ramankutty C (eds) 1994 Indian medicinal plants: a compendium of 500 species, vol 1. Orient Longman, Hyderabad, p 281–283

Williamson EM (ed) 2002 Major herbs of Ayurveda. Churchill Livingstone, London, p 76–77

Yoganarasimhan SN 2000 Medicinal plants of India, vol 2: Tamil Nadu. Self-published, Bangalore, p 547–548

Śālaparṇī, 'leaves like *Śāla*'

BOTANICAL NAME: *Desmodium gangeticum*, Fabaceae

OTHER NAMES: ***Vidarigandhā*** (S); Salpan, Salwan (H); Pulladi, Orila (T)

Botany: ***Śālaparṇī*** is an erect shrub attaining a height of between 60 and 120 cm, with a short woody stem and numerous irregularly angled branches covered in a fine grey pubescence. The leaves are simple, ovate to ovate-lanceolate, acute or acuminate, margins wavy and membranous, glabrous above and mottled with greyish-coloured patches, pale green below with whitish appressed trichomes. The flowers are white to purple in colour, borne in elongated terminal or axillary racemes, giving rise to indehiscent pods with six to eight segments, each segment containing one seed. ***Śālaparṇī*** is found throughout tropical India into the lower portions of the Himalayan range, and it and related species are also found in regions of China (e.g. *Desmodium styracifolium*, *D. pulchellum*), S.E. Asia and Africa (*D. adscendens*). The meaning of its Sanskrit name 'leaves like ***Śala***' suggests that its leaf structure is similar to those of the tree *Shorea robusta* (Kirtikar & Basu 1935, Warrier et al 1994).

Part used: Root.

Dravyguṇa:

- ***Rasa***: *tikta, madhura*
- ***Vīrya***: *uṣṇa, guru*
- ***Karma***: *stambhana, chardinigrahaṇa, jvaraghna, chedana, kāsahara, svāsahara, mūtravirecana, viṣaghna, hṛdaya, rasāyana, tridoṣaghna* (Dash 1991, Kirtikar & Basu 1935, Srikanthamurthy 2001, Warrier et al 1994).

Constituents: The limited amount of constituent information for ***Śālaparṇī*** includes the presence of alkaloids, pterocarpenoids (gangetin, gangetinin and desmodin), triterpenoid glycosides (dehydrosoyasaponin I, soyasaponin I, and soyasaponin III), and flavone and isoflavanoid glycosides (Ghosh & Anandakumar 1981, Govindarajan et al 2003, McManus et al 1993).

Medical research:

- ***In vitro***: antispasmodic (McManus et al 1993), antioxidant (Govindarajan et al 2003), paracidal (Iwu et al 1992).
- ***In vivo***: paracidal (Singh 2005); anti-ulcerogenic (Dharmani et al 2005); anti-anaphylaxis (Addy & Dzandu 1986); CNS depressant (Ghosal & Bhattacharya 1972; Jabbar et al 2001); analgesic (Rathi et al 2004); anti-inflammatory (Ghosh & Anandakumar 1981; Rathi et al 2004); analgesic (Ghosh & Anandakumar 1981; Jabbar et al 2001); hypocholesterolaemic, antioxidant (Kurian et al 2005).

Toxicity: No data found.

Indications: Vomiting, haemorrhoids, diarrhoea, dysentery, intestinal parasites, fever, cough, asthma, tuberculosis, allergies, dysuria, oedema, cardiac debility and cardiopathies, inflammatory joint disease, asthenia and emaciation, diabetes, epilepsy, psychosis, depression, anxiety.

Contraindications: None.

Medicinal uses: ***Śālaparṇī*** is valued in Āyurvedic medicine for its capacity to reduce vitiations of all three ***doṣas***, and is often used in severe conditions such as typhoid fever and tuberculosis when all other treatments fail (Tillotson 2001). To this extent it is used in many formulations to equalise the activities of the different constituents. ***Śālaparṇī*** is particularly valued in asthmatic conditions, which is evidenced by the experimental data, which demonstrate anti-inflammatory, antihistamine and antispasmodic properties. It is also considered an important remedy for the heart, and is a key constituent in ***Daśamūla*** ('ten roots' formula), which has alterative and anti-inflammatory properties, and ***Mahanārāyaṇa taila***, which is used in myalgia, rheumatism and mental disorders. In the treatment of severe ***vāttika*** fever the ***Śāraṅgadhara saṃhitā*** recommends a decoction of equal parts ***Śālaparṇī***, ***Balā***, ***Guḍūcī***, ***Drākṣā***, and ***Sārivā*** (Srikanthamurthy 1984). In the treatment of malabsorptive syndromes with gastrointestinal colic the ***Śāraṅgadhara saṃhitā*** recommends a decoction of equal parts ***Śālaparṇī***, ***Balā***, ***Bilva***, ***Dhānyaka*** and ***Śūṇṭhī*** (Srikanthamurthy 1984). The ***Cakradatta*** mentions the benefit of ***Śālaparṇī*** as an ingredient in ***Balādya ghṛta*** in the treatment of fever, consumption, cough, headache and chest pain, taken with twice its quantity of milk (Sharma 2002). The ***Cakradatta*** also mentions ***Śālaparṇī*** as a constituent of ***Mahāpaiśācika ghṛta***, used in the treatment of psychosis, epilepsy and seizure, and to enhance the intellect and memory in children (Sharma 2002). In ***vāttika*** afflictions of the heart the ***Cakradatta*** recommends that ***Śālaparṇī*** be decocted in milk and taken internally (Sharma 2002). Generally speaking, ***Śālaparṇī*** combines well with botanicals such as ***Arjuna*** and ***Balā*** in diseases of the heart. ***Śālaparṇī*** is said to protect the fetus in threatened miscarriage, and is applied as paste with ***Paruṣaka*** (*Grewia asiatica*) over the umbilical region, pelvis and vulva during labour to ensure an easy delivery (Sharma 2002). In Chinese medicine Guang Jin Qian (*D. styraciflium*) is used in cholelithiasis and jaundice (damp heat of the liver and gall bladder), and Pai Chien Cao (*D. pulchellum*) is used in malaria (Tillotson 2001).

Dosage:

- ***Cūrṇa***: 2–5 g b.i.d.–t.i.d.
- ***Kvātha***: 30–90 mL b.i.d.–t.i.d.
- ***Tincture***: dried root, 1:3, 45%; 2–5 mL b.i.d.–t.i.d.

REFERENCES

Addy ME, Dzandu WK 1986 Dose-response effects of Desmodium adscendens aqueous extract on histamine response, content and anaphylactic reactions in the guinea pig. Journal of Ethnopharmacology 18(1):13–20

Dash B 1991 Materia medica of Ayurveda. B. Jain Publishers, New Delhi, p 20

Dharmani P, Mishra PK, Maurya R et al 2005 Desmodium gangeticum: a potent anti-ulcer agent. Indian Journal of Experimental Biology 43(6):517–521

Ghosal S, Bhattacharya SK 1972 Desmodium alkaloids. II. Chemical and pharmacological evaluation of D. gangeticum. Planta Medica 22(4):434–440

Ghosh D, Anandakumar A 1981 Anti-inflammatory and analgesic activities of gangetin – a pterocarpenoid from Desmodium gangeticum. Indian Journal of Pharmacy 15(4):391–402

Govindarajan R, Rastogi S, Vijayakumar M et al 2003 Studies on the anti-oxidant activities of Desmodium gangeticum. Biological and Pharmaceutical Bulletin 26(10):1424–1427

Iwu MM, Jackson JE, Tally JD, Klayman DL 1992 Evaluation of plant extracts for antileishmanial activity using a mechanism-based radiorespirometric microtechnique (RAM). Planta Medica 58(5):436–441

Jabbar S, Khan MT, Choudhuri MS 2001 The effects of aqueous extracts of Desmodium gangeticum DC. (Leguminosae) on the central nervous system. Die Pharmazie 56(6):506–508

Kirtikar KR, Basu BD 1935 Indian medicinal plants, 2nd edn, vols 1–4. Periodical Experts, Delhi, p 758–759

Kurian GA, Philip S, Varghese T 2005 Effect of aqueous extract of the Desmodium gangeticum DC root in the severity of myocardial infarction. Journal of Ethnopharmacology 97(3): 457–461

McManus OB, Harris GH, Giangiacomo KM et al 1993 An activator of calcium-dependent potassium channels isolated from a medicinal herb. Biochemistry 32(24):6128–6133

Nadkarni KM 1954 The Indian materia medica, with Ayurvedic, Unani and home remedies, revised and enlarged by A.K. Nadkarni. Popular Prakashan PVP, Bombay

Rathi A, Rao CV, Ravishankar B et al 2004 Anti-inflammatory and anti-nociceptive activity of the water decoction Desmodium gangeticum. Journal of Ethnopharmacology 95(2–3):259–263

Sharma PV 2002 Cakradatta. Sanskrit text with English translation. Chaukhamba, Varanasi, p 143, 188, 200, 587

Singh N, Mishra PK, Kapil A et al 2005 Efficacy of Desmodium gangeticum extract and its fractions against experimental visceral leishmaniasis. Journal of Ethnopharmacology 98(1–2):83–88

Srikanthamurthy KR 1984 Śāraṅgadhara saṃhitā: a treatise on Ayurveda. Chaukhamba Orientalia, Varanasi, p 58, 64

Srikanthamurthy KR 2001 Bhāvaprakāśa of Bhāvamiśra, vol 1. Krishnadas Academy, Varanasi, p 232

Tillotson A 2001 The One Earth herbal sourcebook. Twin Streams (Kensington), New York, p 200–201

Warrier PK, Nambiar VPK, Ramankutty C (eds) 1994 Indian medicinal plants: a compendium of 500 species, vol 2. Orient Longman, Hyderabad, p 319

Śaṅkhapuṣpī, 'conch flower'

BOTANICAL NAMES: Various species are cited in various texts for **Śaṅkhapuṣpī**, including *Canscora decussata* (Gentianaceae), *Convolvulus pluricaulis, C. microphyllus* and *Evolvulus alsinoides* (Convolvulaceae), and *Clitoria ternatea* (Papilionaceae).

OTHER NAMES:

- *Canscora decussata:* **Śaṅkhinī** (S); Kalameg, Shankhauli, Shamkhaphuli (H)
- *Convolvulus pluricaulis, C. microphyllus:* **Śaṇkāhvā, Maṅgalyakusumā** (S); Shankhahuli (H)
- *Evolvulus alsinoides:* **Viṣṇukrāṇtā** (S); Shyamakranta (H); Vishnukiranti (T)
- *Clitoria ternatea:* **Girikarṇikā, Aparājitā** (S); Aparjit (H); Kannikkoti, Girikanni (T)

Botany:

- ***Canscora decussata*** is an erect branching annual attaining a height of up 60 cm, the stems four-winged with decussate branches. The leaves are simple, ovate or lanceolate, sessile, and oppositely arranged. The flowers are pink or white, cylindrical and tubular with four lobes, giving rise to cylindrical membranous capsules containing numerous small brown seeds. *C. decussata* is found in moist areas up to 1500 m in elevation, throughout tropical India, Burma, Sri Lanka, Madagascar and Africa (Kirtikar & Basu 1935a, Warrier et al 1994a).
- ***Convolvulus pluricaulis*** is a prostrate or suberect spreading hairy perennial shrub. The leaves are ovate-lanceolate to linear, and the flowers are white or pinkish, solitary or paired. The fruit capsules are oblong-globose, pale brown, containing tiny brown seeds. *C. pluricaulis* is common in dry, rocky or sandy locations (Mahashwari 1963).
- ***Evolvulus alsinoides*** is a small, pubescent procumbent perennial with a small woody root stock, with simple elliptic-oblong or oblong-ovate leaves, alternately arranged. The flowers are light blue in colour, solitary or in pairs, borne in the leaf axils, giving rise to globose four-valved capsules. *E. alsinoides* is found throughout India in exposed areas up to 1800 m in elevation (Kirtikar & Basu 1935b, Warrier et al 1995).
- ***Clitoria ternatea*** is a perennial climber with cylindrical stems and branches, with compound leaves, imparipinnate, with five to seven leaflets. The flowers are blue or white with an orange centre, solitary or axillary, followed by flattened pods containing 6–10 yellowish-brown seeds. *C. ternatea* is found throughout India and SE Asia (Kirtikar & Basu 1935c, Warrier 1994b).

Part used: Root, whole plant.

Dravyguṇa:

Canscora decussata

- ***Rasa***: *tikta, kaṭu, kaśāya*
- ***Vipāka***: *guru*
- ***Vīrya***: *uṣṇa*
- ***Karma***: *dīpana, bhedana, kṛmighna, raktaprasādana, varnya, sandhānīya, kuṣṭhaghna, viṣaghna, medhya, vajīkaraṇa, rasāyana, kaphahara, tridoṣahara* (Kirtikar & Basu 1935a, Warrier et al 1994a).

Convolvulus pluricaulis*, *C. microphyllus

- ***Rasa***: *tikta, kaśāya*
- ***Vipāka***: *guru*
- ***Vīrya***: *uṣṇa*
- ***Karma***: *dīpana, bhedana, kṛmighna, varnya, kuṣṭhaghna, sandhānīya, viṣaghna, medhya, vajīkaraṇa, rasāyana, tridoṣahara* (Srikanthamurthy 2001).

Evolvulus alsinoides
- ***Rasa***: *tikta, kaṭu*
- ***Vipāka***: *guru*
- ***Vīrya***: *śita*
- ***Karma***: *grāhī, jvaraghna, kṛmighna, chedana, varnya, viṣaghna, medhya, vajīkaraṇa, pittahara, tridoṣahara* (Kirtikar & Basu 1935b, Warrier et al 1995).

Clitoria ternatea (blue-flowered variety)
- ***Rasa***: *tikta*
- ***Vipāka***: *kaṭu*
- ***Vīrya***: *śita*
- ***Karma***: *bhedana, kṛmighna, kāsahara, svāsahara, śotahara, viṣaghna, medhya, vajīkaraṇa, cakṣuṣya, pittahara, tridoṣaghna* (Kirtikar & Basu 1935c, Warrier et al 1994b).

Constituents:
- ***Canscora decussata***: Among the limited number of constituents described for *C. decussata* are xanthones, loliolide, gluanone, canscoradione, friedelin and sterols (Ghosal et al 1976, 1978, Yoganarasimhan 2000a).
- ***Convolvulus pluricaulis***: no data found.
- ***Evolvulus alsinoides***: alkaloids (Yoganarasimhan 2000b).
- ***Clitoria ternatea***: The blue-flowered variety contains malonylated flavonol glycosides such as kaempferol, quercetin and myricetin. Unlike the white-flowered variety the blue-flowered Clitoria contains anthocyanins ternatins C_1–C_5, D_3 and preternatins A_3 and C_4) in the flowers. The seeds are stated to contain high levels of oligosaccharides (Kazuma et al 2003a, b, Revilleza et al 1990, Terahara et al 1996).

Medical research:
Canscora decussata
- ***In vitro***: immunostimulant (Madan & Ghosh 2002), antimycobacterial (Ghosal et al 1978).
- ***In vivo***: anticonvulsant (Dikshit et al 1972).

Convolvulus pluricaulis
- ***In vivo***: anti-ulcerogenic (Sairam et al 2001).

Evolvulus alsinoides
- ***In vivo***: anti-inflammatory (Ganju et al 2003).

Clitoria ternatea
- ***In vivo***: nootropic (Jain et al 2003; Rai et al 2001, 2002); anxiolytic, anticonvulsant, anti-ulcerogenic (Jain et al 2003); anti-inflammatory, analgesic (Devi et al 2003).

Toxicity: No data found for any of the species described.

Indications:
- ***Canscora decussata***: Intestinal parasites, fever, tuberculosis, ascites, leucoderma, leprosy, poor memory, epilepsy, psychosis, unconsciousness, spiritual possession, nervous exhaustion, wounds, ulceration.
- ***Convolvulus pluricaulis***: Poor digestion, intestinal parasites, skin diseases, poisoning, epilepsy, poor memory, psychosis.
- ***Evolvulus alsinoides***: Diarrhoea, dysentery, fever, bronchitis, asthma, haemorrhage, poor memory, epilepsy, alopecia, premature greying, debility.
- ***Clitoria ternatea***: Colic, hepatosplenomegaly, intestinal parasites, fever, bronchitis, asthma, tuberculosis, strangury, ascites, skin diseases, skin eruptions, burning sensations, poor memory, headache, otalgia.

Contraindications: All species of ***Śaṅkhapuṣpī*** may interact with antidepressant, antipsychotic and anti-seizure medication.

Medicinal uses: ***Śaṅkhapuṣpī*** provides an interesting challenge for the herbalist given that at least four different species are called such. Although the reasons for this variability are not entirely known, it is likely that these different species are a manifestation of regional availability, and the fact that the term ***Śaṅkhapuṣpī*** is a more or less general term that is synonymous with plants that have a ***medhya*** property, in much the same way that the term ***Brāhmī*** is used to denote the same. In the state of Kerala, for example, local ***vaidyas*** make use of *Clitoria ternatea* as ***Śaṅkhapuṣpī***, even though it also known by other names such as ***Girikarṇikā*** and ***Aparājitā*** (Warrier et al 1994b). In contrast, it is *Convolvulus pluricaulis* that is listed as officinal in the *Ayurvedic Formulary of India* (1978), with *Evolvulus alsinoides* and *Clitoria ternatea* listed as alternatives. Both Warrier et al (1994a) and Kirtikar & Basu (1935a) indicate, however, that only *Canscora decussata* is properly called ***Śaṅkhapuṣpī***, but if we are to take the meaning of ***Śaṅkhapuṣpī*** literally, a comparison of the various flowers would indicate that only *Clitoria ternatea* actually looks like a conch. These inconsistencies are not simply the result of academic error, but are a reflection of actual usage and thus ***Śaṅkhapuṣpī*** will probably continue to mean several different species of plant among Āyurvedic physicians. In one recent study of ***Śaṅkhapuṣpī*** found in the market place in northern India, nine samples were found to be *Convolvulus microphyllus*, one was *Evolvulus alsinoides*, one sample was a mixture of three different species including *E. alsinoides*, *C. microphyllus* and *Amberboa divaricata*, and two samples were *Indigofera cordifolia* (Singh & Viswanathan 2000). Although each plant listed as being ***Śaṅkhapuṣpī*** has ***medhya rasāyana*** properties under their own names, including ***Nīlī***, they also contain different secondary indications and may not be interchangeable. Thus a little caution is recommended when using ***Śaṅkhapuṣpī***, and to ensure strict quality control a botanical voucher should be included with any order. In the ***Cakradatta*** the fresh juice of ***Śaṅkhapuṣpī*** is mixed with the juices of ***Brāhmī***, ***Kūṣmāṇḍa***, ***Vacā*** and ***Kuṣṭha***, mixed with honey and used in the treatment of ***unmāda*** ('psychosis') (Sharma 2002). In the treatment of ***apasmāra*** ('epilepsy') the ***Cakradatta*** recommends ***Brāhmīghṛta***, prepared by cooking one part aged ***ghṛta*** in four parts fresh juice of ***Brāhmī***, mixed with the powders of ***Vacā***, ***Kuṣṭha*** and ***Śaṅkhapuṣpī*** (Sharma 2002). The ***Cakradatta*** also singles out a paste of ***Śaṅkhapuṣpī*** as a particularly potent ***medhya rasāyana***, to enhance the intellect and promote long life, to improve digestion and enhance physical strength, and to improve the voice and lustre of the skin, along with other herbs such as ***Maṇḍūkaparṇī***, ***Guḍūcī and Yaṣṭimadhu*** (Sharma 2002). ***Śaṅkhapuṣpī*** combined with equal parts powders of ***Udīcya***, ***Apāmārga***, ***Viḍaṅga***, ***Vacā***, ***Harītakī***, ***Kuṣṭha*** and ***Śatāvarī***, is stated by the ***Cakradatta*** as making one capable of '... memorizing one thousand stanzas in only three days' (Sharma 2002). Kirtikar & Basu (1935a) state that the fresh juice of *Canscora decussata* is used '... in all cases of insanity, in doses of about one ounce'. Both the root and herb of *Evolvulus alsinoides* is considered to be an important remedy for diarrhoea, the leaf used as an infusion in doses of about 100 mL (Kirtikar & Basu 1935b). The leaf of *E. alsinoides* can also be smoked (***dhūma***) in the treatment of chronic bronchitis and asthma (Kirtikar & Basu 1935b). Kirtikar & Basu (1935c) state that the blue-flowered *Clitoria ternatea* displays all the medicinal properties of the white-flowered variety, but is also ***vajīkaraṇa***. The root of *C. ternatea* is stated to be diuretic and laxative, the root juice used in chronic bronchitis, as ***nasya*** in headache, and as a decoction in irritation of the bladder and urethra (Kirtikar & Basu 1935c). The warmed juice of the leaves of *C. ternatea* mixed with salt is used as an analgesic in otalgia and lymphadenopathy, and the seeds are stated to be cathartic and can cause griping, attributed to the oligosaccharides (Kirtikar & Basu 1935c).

Dosage: general guidelines for the root of all four species.

- ***Cūrṇa***: 3–5 g b.i.d.–t.i.d.
- ***Kvātha***: 30–90 mL b.i.d.–t.i.d.
- ***Tincture***: dried root, 1:3, 45%; 2–5 mL b.i.d.–t.i.d.

REFERENCES

Devi BP, Boominathan R, Mandal SC 2003 Anti-inflammatory, analgesic and antipyretic properties of Clitoria ternatea root. Fitoterapia 74(4):345–349

Dikshit SK, Tiwari PV, Dixit SP 1972 Anticonvulsant activity of Canscora decussata. Indian Journal of Physiology and Pharmacology 16(1):81–83

Ganju L, Karan D, Chanda S et al 2003 Immunomodulatory effects of agents of plant origin. Biomedicine and Pharmacotherapy 57(7):296–300

Ghosal S, Singh AK, Chaudhuri RK 1976 Chemical constituents of Gentianaceae XX: natural occurrence of (-)-loliolide in Canscora decussata. Journal of Pharmaceutical Sciences 65(10):1549–1451

Ghosal S, Biswas K, Chaudhuri RK 1978 Chemical constituents of Gentianaceae XXIV: antimycobacterium tuberculosis activity of naturally occurring xanthones and synthetic analogs. Journal of Pharmaceutical Sciences 67(5):721–722

Jain NN, Ohal CC, Shroff SK et al 2003 Clitoria ternatea and the CNS. Pharmacology, Biochemistry, and Behavior 75(3):529–536

Kazuma K, Noda N, Suzuki M. 2003a Flavonoid composition related to petal color in different lines of Clitoria ternatea. Phytochemistry 64(6):1133–1139

Kazuma K, Noda N, Suzuki M 2003b Malonylated flavonol glycosides from the petals of Clitoria ternatea. Phytochemistry 62(2):229–237

Kirtikar KR, Basu BD 1935a Indian medicinal plants, 2nd edn, vols 1–4. Periodical Experts, Delhi, p 1659, 1660

Kirtikar KR, Basu BD 1935b Indian medicinal plants, 2nd edn, vols 1–4. Periodical Experts, Delhi, p 1738–1739

Kirtikar KR, Basu BD 1935c Indian medicinal plants, 2nd edn, vols 1–4. Periodical Experts, Delhi, p 803
Madan B, Ghosh B 2002 Canscora decussata promotes adhesion of neutrophils to human umbilical vein endothelial cells. Journal of Ethnopharmacology 79(2):229–235
Maheshwari JK 1963 The flora of Delhi. Council of Scientific and Industrial Research, New Delhi p 239
Rai KS, Murthy KD, Karanth KS, Rao MS 2001 Clitoria ternatea (Linn) root extract treatment during growth spurt period enhances learning and memory in rats. Indian Journal of Physiology and Pharmacology 45(3):305–313
Rai KS, Murthy KD, Karanth KS et al 2002 Clitoria ternatea root extract enhances acetylcholine content in rat hippocampus. Fitoterapia 73(7–8):685–689
Revilleza MJ, Mendoza EM, Raymundo LC 1990 Oligosaccharides in several Philippine indigenous food legumes: determination, localization and removal. Plant Foods for Human Nutrition 40(1):83–93
Sairam K, Rao CV, Goel RK 2001 Effect of Convolvulus pluricaulis Chois on gastric ulceration and secretion in rats. Indian Journal of Experimental Biology 39(4):350–354
Sharma PV 2002 Cakradatta: Sanskrit text with English translation. Chaukhamba, Varanasi, p 184, 194, 625, 626
Singh HB, Viswanathan MV 2000 Identification of market samples of crude drug Sankhapushpi. National Seminar on the Frontiers of Research and Development in Medicinal Plants, September 16–18, Lucknow. Central Institute of Medicinal and Aromatic Plants, Council of Scientific and Industrial Research, India
Srikanthamurthy KR 2001 Bhāvaprakāśa of Bhāvamiśra, vol 1. Krishnadas Academy, Varanasi, p 272
Terahara N, Oda M, Matsui T et al 1996 Five new anthocyanins, ternatins A3, B4, B3, B2, and D2, from Clitoria ternatea flowers. Journal of Natural Products 59(2):139–144
Terahara N, Toki K, Saito N et al 1998 Eight new anthocyanins, ternatins C1-C5 and D3 and preternatins A3 and C4 from young clitoria ternatea flowers. Journal of Natural Products 61(11):1361–1367
Warrier PK, Nambiar VPK, Ramankutty C (eds) 1994a Indian medicinal plants: a compendium of 500 species, vol 1. Orient Longman, Hyderabad, p 361
Warrier PK, Nambiar VPK, Ramankutty C (eds) 1994b Indian medicinal plants: a compendium of 500 species, vol 2. Orient Longman, Hyderabad, p 129
Warrier PK, Nambiar VPK, Ramankutty C (eds) 1995 Indian medicinal plants: a compendium of 500 species, vol 3. Orient Longman, Hyderabad, p 11
Yoganarasimhan SN 2000a Medicinal plants of India, vol 2: Tamil Nadu. Self-published, Bangalore, p 100
Yoganarasimhan SN 2000b Medicinal plants of India, vol 2: Tamil Nadu. Self-published, Bangalore, p 223

Śatāvarī, 'one hundred roots'

BOTANICAL NAME: *Asparagus racemosus*, Liliaceae

OTHER NAMES: ***Ābhīru, Bahusutā, Śatāvīryā*** (S); Satavar, Satmuli (H); Kilavari, Satavali (T); Wild Asparagus (E); Tian Men Dong (C)

Botany: ***Śatāvarī*** is a climbing shrub attaining a height of between 1 and 3 m, with a stout and creeping root stock, annual woody cylindrical stems with recurved or straight spines, and succulent tuberous roots that grow in clusters at the base of the stem. The young stems are quite brittle and delicate, and the leaves are actually flattened lateral shoots or scales called cladodes, arranged in tufts of two to six at each node. The flowers are white and fragrant, solitary or in fascicles, simple or branched racemes, giving rise to a globular fruit that is purplish-black when ripe containing seeds with a hard, brittle covering. ***Śatāvarī*** is found throughout tropical India into the Himalayan range up to 1400 m in elevation, extending into SE Asia, Australia and Africa (Kirtikar & Basu 1935, Warrier et al 1994).

Part used: Roots.

Dravyguṇa:

- ***Rasa***: *tikta, madhura*
- ***Vipāka***: *guru*
- ***Vīrya***: *śita, snigdha*
- ***Karma***: *śulapraśamana, stambhana, mūtravirecana, śotahara, stanyajanana, prajāsthāpana, hṛdaya, vedanāsthāpana, cakṣuṣya, medhya, vajīkaraṇa, balya, rasāyana, vātapittahara* (Srikanthamurthy 2001, Warrier et al 1994).

Constituents: ***Śatāvarī*** has been found to contain steroidal glycosides including shatavarins I–IV, as well as diosgenin and various sterols. Other constituents include the alkaloid asparagamine A, flavonoids such as quercitin, rutin and hyperoside, an isoflavone and a mucilage (Saxena & Chourasia 2001; Williamson 2002).

Medical research:

- ***In vitro***: positively ionotropic/chronotropic (Roy et al 1971); antioxidant (Kamat et al 2000); antimicrobial (Mandal et al 2000b).
- ***In vivo***: anti-ulcerogenic (Datta et al 2002; Sairam et al 2003), antitussive (Mandal et al 2000a), bronchodilatory (Roy et al 1971), galactagogue (Sabins et al 1968), dopaminergic antagonist (Dalvi et al 1990); hypotensive (Roy et al 1971), anti-adhesion (Rege et al 1989), hepatoprotective (Muruganadan et al 2000), antitumour (Rao 1981), immunostimulant (Dahanukar et al 1986, Thatte et al 1987).
- ***Human trials***: ***Śatāvarī*** root powder was found to significantly reduce the half-time of gastric emptying in healthy human volunteers, comparable with metoclopramide (Dalvi et al 1990); ***Śatāvarī*** root powder relieved the symptoms of duodenal ulceration in the majority of the patients studied (Singh & Singh 1986). A combination remedy containing ***Śatāvarī*** (Ricalex tablets) was shown to increase milk production in women complaining of deficient milk secretion (Joglekar et al 1967).

Toxicity: The systemic administration of high doses of various extracts of *A. racemosus* did not produce any abnormality in the behaviour pattern of mice and rats (Jetmalani et al 1967). *Asparagus* species may cause delayed-type cell-mediated and IgE-mediated reactions in sensitive individuals (Tabar et al 2003).

Indications: Dyspepsia, gastric and duodenal ulceration, intestinal colic, diarrhoea, hepatitis and hepatomegaly, haemorrhoids, pharyngitis, cough, bronchitis, asthma, tuberculosis, strangury, urethritis, cystitis, nephropathy, leucorrhoea, amenorrhoea, dysmenorrhoea, agalactia, female and male infertility, threatened miscarriage, menopause, epilepsy, fatigue, asthenia, cardiopathies, tumours, surgical adhesions.

Contraindications: ***kaphakopa***, ***agnimāndya*** and ***āma***, due to its ***śita vīrya*** and ***snigdha*** and ***guru*** properties.

Medicinal uses: ***Śatāvarī*** is an important medicament in Āyurvedic medicine to relieve vitiations of ***vāta*** and ***pitta***, combining a nourishing and strengthening activity (***bṛmhaṇa***) with soothing demulcent and emollient properties (***snehana***). ***Śatāvarī*** is thus indicated in any kind of irritation and inflammation in the gastrointestinal, respiratory and urinary tracts. It is particularly indicated in ***amlapitta*** or 'acid gastritis', most notably in the form of a medicated ***ghṛta*** compound called ***Śatāvarī ghṛta***, prepared by decocting a paste of ***Śatāvarī*** root along with an equal quantity of the fresh root juice in milk and ***ghṛta***. The ***Cakradatta*** states that ***Śatāvarī ghṛta*** alleviates ***amlapitta*** caused by vitiations of ***vāta***, ***pitta***, and ***rakta***, and can also be used in the treatment of thirst, fainting, dyspnoea and gout (Sharma 2002). The ***Bhāvaprakāśa*** recommends ***Śatāvarī ghṛta*** in the treatment of passive haemorrhage, gastritis, asthma and consumptive conditions (Srikanthamurthy 2000). For ***vāttika*** fever the fresh juice of ***Śatāvarī*** and ***Guḍūcī*** are mixed with jaggery and taken internally (Sharma 2002). Decocted with goat's milk ***Śatāvarī*** is used in the treatment of ***raktapitta*** and of the passive haemorrhaging of the nose, eyes, ears, mouth, vagina or rectum (Sharma 2002). ***Śatāvarī*** is also an important remedy in consumption and cachexia, used along with botanicals such as ***Aśvagandhā***, ***Balā***, ***Nāgabalā***, ***Gokṣura***, ***Vāsaka***, ***Punarnavā*** and ***Puṣkaramūla***. Combined with equal parts ***Trikaṭu***, ***Triphala***, ***Balā*** and ***Atibalā***, all of which are then combined with equal parts ***lauhabhasma*** (purified iron ore), ***Śatāvarī*** is used in consumptive conditions with severe cachexia, stiffness of the limbs and facial paralysis (Sharma 2002). In the treatment of vertigo ***Śatāvarī*** can be decocted in milk with ***Balā*** and ***Drākṣā*** (Sharma 2002). For epilepsy a simple milk decoction of ***Śatāvarī*** is recommended by the ***Cakradatta*** (Sharma 2002). ***Śatāvarī*** is also an important ingredient in ***Mahānārāyaṇa taila***, used topically in ***abhyaṅga*** in the treatment of angina, muscular spasm, inflammation and pain. Combined with equal parts ***Kaṭuka***, ***Guḍūcī***, ***Triphala*** and ***Paṭola***, ***Śatāvarī*** is used internally in the treatment of gout (Sharma 2002). In the treatment of disease of the heart ***Śatāvarī*** can be used along with botanicals such as ***Arjuna*** and ***Balā***. Prepared as a milk decoction with ***Gokṣura***, and taken with jaggery as an ***anupāna***, ***Śatāvarī*** can be used in the treatment of ***paittika*** variants of dysuria, with burning sensations and haematuria. Although the name ***Śatāvarī*** can be translated as 'one hundred roots', (***śat*** 'one hundred', ***āvarī***-'below') referring to the panicle of roots that is characteristic of the plant's habit, ***Śatāvarī*** has also been translated to mean 'one hundred husbands', indicating its potent ***vajīkaraṇa*** properties, especially in women (Frawley & Lad 1986). ***Śatāvarī*** is a common component of many different Āyurvedic formulations used to treat disorders of the female reproductive tract, used along with botanicals such as ***Balā***, ***Atibalā***, ***Yaṣṭimadhu***, ***Nāgakeśara***, ***Aśvagandhā***, ***Kumārī*** juice, ***Kuranṭaka***, ***Nīlotpala*** and ***Kumuda***. The ***Cakradatta*** suggests that ***Śatāvarī*** is an effective ***vajīkaraṇa rasāyana***, decocted in milk and ***ghṛta*** and taken with honey and ***Pippalī cūrṇa*** (Sharma 2002). To prevent threatened miscarriage (***prajāsthāpana***) the ***Cakradatta*** recommends a milk decoction of ***Śatāvarī***, ***Mañjiṣṭhā***, ***Apāmārga***, and ***Tila***. As a galactagogue (***stanyajanana***) a simple milk decoction of ***Śatāvarī*** is often used, or is part of more complex formulations that include botanicals such as ***Aśvagandhā***, ***Yavānī*** and ***Kuṣṭha***. As a restorative for the male reproductive system and to replenish the ***shukla dhātu***, ***Śatāvarī*** is taken along with botanicals such as ***Aśvagandhā***, ***Balā***, ***Kapikacchū***, ***Gokṣura*** and ***Tila***. To augment the size of the breasts as well as the penis the ***Cakradatta*** recommends a medicated oil to be massaged into these tissues, prepared by decocting ***Śatāvarī***, ***Aśvagandhā***, ***Kuṣṭha***, ***Jaṭāmāmsī*** and ***Bṛhatī*** in milk and sesame oil, until all the milk is evaporated (Sharma 2002). In Chinese medicine a very similar species of *Asparagus* called Tian Men Dong (*Asparagus cochinchinesis*) is used as a kidney and lung yin restorative in the treatment of dryness of the lungs, haemoptysis, thirst, constipation and asthenia (Bensky & Gamble 1993).

Dosage:

- ***Cūrṇa***: 3–15 g b.i.d.–t.i.d.
- ***Kvātha***: 60–120 mL b.i.d.–t.i.d.
- ***Tincture***: recently dried root, 1:3, 25% alcohol, 1–10 mL b.i.d.–t.i.d.

REFERENCES

Bensky D, Gamble A 1993 Chinese herbal medicine materia medica, revised edn. Eastland Press, Seattle, p 359–360
Dahanukar S, Thatte U, Pai N et al 1986 Protective effect of Asparagus racemosus against induced abdominal sepsis. Indian Drugs 24:125–128
Dalvi SS, Nadkarni PM, Gupta KC 1990 Effect of Asparagus racemosus (Shatavari) on gastric emptying time in normal healthy volunteers. Journal of Postgraduate Medicine 36(2):91–94
Datta GK, Sairam K, Priyambada S et al 2002 Antiulcerogenic activity of Satavari mandur: an Ayurvedic herbo-mineral preparation. Indian Journal of Experimental Biology 40(10):1173–1177
Dinan L, Savchenko T, Whiting P 2001 Phytoecdysteroids in the genus Asparagus (Asparagaceae). Phytochemistry 56(6):569–576
Frawley D, Lad V 1986 The Yoga of herbs: an Ayurvedic guide to herbal medicine. Lotus, Santa Fe, p 183
Jetmalani MH, Sabins PB, Gaitonde BB 1967 A study on the pharmacology of various extracts of Shatavari: Asparagus racemosus (Willd). Indian Journal of Medical Research 2:1–10
Joglekar GV, Ahuja RH, Balwani JH 1967 Galactogogue effect of Asparagus racemosus. Indian Medical Journal 61(7):165
Kamat JP, Boloor KK, Devasagayam TP, Venkatacalam SR 2000 Anti-oxidant properties of Asparagus racemosus against damage induced by gamma-radiation in rat liver mitochondria. Journal of Ethnopharmacology 71(3):425–435
Kirtikar KR, Basu BD 1935 Indian medicinal plants, 2nd edn, vols 1–4. Periodical Experts, Delhi, p 2499
Krishnamurthy KM 1991 Wealth of Suśruta. International Institute of Āyurveda, Coimbatore
Mandal SC, Kumar CKA, Mohana Lakshmi S et al 2000a Antitussive effect of Asparagus racemosus root against sulfur dioxide-induced cough in mice. Fitoterapia 71(6):686–689
Mandal SC, Nandy A, Pal M, Saha BP 2000b Evaluation of antibacterial activity of Asparagus racemosus willd. root. Phytotherapy Research 14(2):118–119
Muruganandan S, Garg H, Lal J et al 2000 Studies on the immunostimulant and antihepatotoxic activities of Asparagus racemosus root extract. Journal of Medicinal and Aromatic Plant Sciences 22–23(4A–1A):49–52
Rao AR 1981 Inhibitory action of Asparagus racemosus on DMBA-induced mammary carcinogoenesis in rats. International Journal of Cancer 28(5):607–610
Rege NN, Nazareth HM, Isaac A et al 1989 Immunotherapeutic modulation of intraperitoneal adhesions by Asparagus racemosus. Journal of Postgraduate Medicine 35(4):199–203
Roy RN, Bhagwager S, Chavan SR, Dutta NK 1971 Preliminary pharmacological studies on extracts of root of Asparagus racemosus (Satavari), Willd, N.O. Lilliaceae. Indian Journal of Medical Research 6:132–138
Sabins PB, Gaitonde BB, Jetmalani M 1968 Effect of alcoholic extract of Asparagus racemosus on mammary glands of rats. Indian Journal of Experimental Biology 6:55–57
Sairam K, Priyambada S, Aryya NC, Goel RK 2003 Gastroduodenal ulcer protective activity of Asparagus race-mosus: an experimental, biochemical and histological study. Journal of Ethnopharmacology 86(1):1–10
Saxena VK, Chourasia S 2001 A new isoflavone from the roots of Asparagus racemosus. Fitoterapia 72(3):307–309
Sharma PV 2002 Cakradatta: Sanskrit text with English translation. Chaukhamba, Varanasi, p 12, 124, 137, 178, 192, 234, 236, 458, 653, 654
Singh KP, Singh RH 1986 Clinical trial on Satavari (Asparagus racemosus Willd.) in duodenal ulcer disease. Journal of Research in Āyurveda and Siddha 7:91–100
Srikanthamurthy KR 1984 Śāraṅgadhara saṃhitā: a treatise on Āyurveda. Chaukhamba Orientalia, Varanasi
Srikanthamurthy KR 2000 Bhāvaprakāśa of Bhavamiśhra, vol 2. Krishnadas Academy, Varanasi, p 222
Srikanthamurthy KR 2001 Bhāvaprakāśa of Bhāvamiśra, vol 1. Krishnadas Academy, Varanasi, p 257
Tabar A, Alvarez M, Celay E et al 2003 Allergy to the asparagus. Anales Del Sistema Sanitario de Navarra 26(Suppl 2):17–23
Thatte U, Chhabria S, Karandikar SM, Dahanukar S 1987 Immunotherapeutic modification of E. coli induced abdominal sepsis and mortality in mice by Indian medicinal plants. Indian Drugs 25:95–97
Warrier PK, Nambiar VPK, Ramankutty C (eds) 1994 Indian medicinal plants: a compendium of 500 species, vol 1. Orient Longman, Hyderabad, p 218–223
Williamson EM (ed) 2002 Major herbs of Ayurveda. Churchill Livingstone, London, p 52

Śilājatu, 'to become like stone'

OTHER NAMES: Girija (S); Shilajita (H); Perangyum (T); Mineral pitch (E)

Description: ***Śilājatu*** is a curious resin that can be found exuding from certain steep rock faces in the Himalayan mountain range at altitudes between 1000 and 5000 m. Similar exudates have also been found in other mountain ranges in what is called the Tethyan mountain system, including the Caucasus, Urals, Pamir, Hindu Kush, Karakoram, Tian Shan and Kunlun Shan ranges, and have also been identified as far away as Norway. ***Śilājatu*** is typically found in the summer when the hot sun beats down upon the rocks causing the resin to liquefy and exude, and then harden again upon cooling. As its older common name of bitumen suggests, ***Śilājatu*** was once thought to be the ancient fossilised organic material from what was once the coastline of the tropical Tethys Sea region that existed between the subcontinent of India and Eurasia some 200 million years ago. More recent research, however, has indicated that ***Śilājatu*** is composed primarily of humus with other organic constituents, and is thus likely to be of relatively recent origin. Researchers have found the degraded components of several different medicinal plants in samples of ***Śilājatu***, including *Euphorbia royleana* and *Trifolium repens*, leading to the idea that ***Śilājatu*** is in large part derived from the humification of a variety of resin- or latex-containing plants. The ***Bhāvaprakāśa*** states that there are four types of ***Śilājatu***, classified according to their respective colours, each with a different medicinal activity: ***sauvarṇa*** is reddish; ***rajata*** is yellowish; ***tāmra*** is bluish; and ***lauha*** is blackish. The ***Caraka saṃhitā*** also classifies ***Śilājatu*** based on the morphological features of the rock from which it exudes. Modern research supports these time-honoured perspectives, as it appears that the composition of ***Śilājatu*** is influenced by a variety of factors, including the particular humified plant species involved, the geological nature of the rock, local temperature, humidity and altitude (Phillips 1997, Sharma & Dash 1988, Srikanthamurthy 2001).

Part used: Purified exudate.

Dravyguṇa:

- ***Rasa***: all varieties are *kaṭu* and *tikta; sauvarna* is also *madhura*, and *lauha* is *lavaṇa*
- ***Vipāka***: *kaṭu (sauvarṇa, lauha, tāmra), madhura (rajata)*
- ***Vīrya***: *uṣṇa (tāmra), śita (lauha, sauvarṇa, rajata)*
- ***Karma***: *dīpanapācana, kṛmighna, chedana, kāsahara, svāsahara, kuṣṭhaghna, mūtravirecana, medohara, sandhānīya, viṣaghna, hṛdaya, medhya, vajīkaraṇa, rasāyana, tridoṣaghna* (Nadkarni 1954, Sharma & Dash 1988, Srikanthamurthy 1995, 2001).
- ***Prabhāva***: The *Caraka saṃhitā* states that '... there is no curable disease in the universe that cannot be cured by *Śilājatu*' when administered at the appropriate time, in combination with suitable *dravyas*, and by using the proper method of preparation. Caraka further adds that by taking *Śilājatu* the body becomes strong and sturdy, as if made of stone (Sharma & Dash 1988). The *Cakradatta* states that if a small piece of *Śilājatu* is kept in the mouth it has the ability to give victory in debates and disputes (Sharma 2002).

Constituents: The complex chemistry of ***Śilājatu*** is highly variable, depending upon the where it was collected and processing methods. The early chemical research on crude ***Śilājatu*** indicated a variety of constituents, including a mixture of organic constituents (e.g. benzoic acid, hippuric acid, fatty acids, resins, waxes, gums, albuminoids and vegetable matter) and inorganic constituents (e.g. calcium, potassium, nitrogen, silica, aluminium, magnesium and sodium). Further work concluded that crude ***Śilājatu*** is composed upwards of 80% humus, decaying plant material acted upon by bacteria and fungi, and most notably, fulvic and humic acids. Recent analysis has yielded the presence of biphenyl metabolites, including a benzocoumarin and low-molecular-weight oxygenated dibenzo-α-pyrones, as well as triterpenes, phenolic lipids, and additional trace minerals including antimony, cobalt, copper, iron, lithium, manganese, molybdenum, phosphorous, strontium and zinc (Bucci 2000, Ghosal et al 1988, Nadkarni 1954, Phillips 1997, Tillotson 2001).

Medical research:

- ***In vivo***: nootropic (Jaiswal & Bhattacharya 1992; Schliebs et al 1997); anxiolytic (Jaiswal & Bhattacharya 1992); antiwithdrawal (Tiwari et al 2001); hypolipidaemic, hypoglycaemic (Trivedi et al 2001); anti-ulcerogenic (Goel et al 1990); anti-inflammatory (Goel et al 1990).

Toxicity: Tradition states that humans first became aware of the benefits of ***Śilājatu*** by watching wild animals such as monkeys utilise it as a food source. ***Śilājatu*** is generally regarded as being quite safe, but crude unprocessed ***Śilājatu*** may contain mycotoxins from contaminating fungi such as *Aspergillus niger*, *A. ochraceous* and *Trichothecium roseum*. Unprocessed ***Śilājatu*** may also contain free radicals in the humic constituents that increase in concentration with an increasing pH, and thus certain sources of ***Śilājatu*** that tend to have a higher pH, such as that obtained from Russia, may be a less desirable source (Phillips 1997).

Indications: Dyspepsia, constipation, intestinal parasites, haemorrhoids, hepatits, bronchitis, asthma, consumption, skin diseases, kidney diseases, anaemia, diabetes, obesity, infertility, exhaustion, epilepsy, psychosis, wounds, fractures, arthritis, cancer, ageing.

Contraindications: Caraka states that ***Śilājatu*** is contraindicated with dietary articles that are heavy in nature or promote burning sensations, and with the legume ***Kulattha*** (*Dolichos biflorus*, horse gram) and the meat of ***Kapota*** (pigeon) (Sharma & Dash 1988).

Medicinal uses: ***Śilājatu*** is an exception to every other entry in this text in that it is not directly derived from botanical sources, but its ubiquitous usage among Āyurvedic physicians makes it important to include. ***Śilājatu*** is considered to be an important ***rasāyana***, used both therapeutically in the treatment of a wide number of conditions, to prevent illness and to ward off the effects of old age. As mentioned, there are a variety of types of ***Śilājatu***, and among them the ***Bhāvaprakāśa*** states that ***lauha Śilājatu*** is best; this is black in colour, has an odour resembling cow's urine, and a salty, pungent and bitter taste (Srikanthamurthy 2001). Crude ***Śilājatu***, however, is not considered fit for use as a medicament, and a variety of processing techniques are mentioned in the extant texts to both purify it and modify its therapeutic properties. According to both the ***Cakradatta*** and the ***Śāraṅgadhara saṃhitā*** the crude ***Śilājatu*** is powdered and then macerated in hot water (or a decoction of ***Triphala***) for several hours. The maceration is then filtered and the liquid collected in an earthen plate and exposed to the sun until a scum begins to form on the surface. This scum is then skimmed off the surface of the liquid and dried in the sun until it forms a hard mass (Sharma 2002, Srikanthamurthy 1984). This substance is now considered to be pure and can be processed further or 'impregnated' by macerating the ***Śilājatu*** in the decoction of different ***dravyas*** chosen specifically for their medicinal activities in particular diseases. The ***Caraka saṃhitā*** states the ***Śilājatu*** should be soaked in this decoction and dried in the sun each day for 7 days, then combined with ***lauha bhasma*** (purifed iron) and consumed with cow's milk (Sharma & Dash 1988). Many commercial sources of ***Śilājatu*** probably do not undergo such traditional processing techniques, but may be standardised to fulvic acid and dibenzo-α-pyrone content, which many researchers consider to be the active constituents. ***Śilājatu*** is perhaps best known as a treatment for ***madhumeha*** (diabetes mellitus), and for this purpose the ***Aṣṭāñga Hṛdaya*** recommends that it be macerated in a decoction of herbs from the ***Asanādigaṇa*** group of ***dravyas*** (represented by ***Asana***), used to reduce ***kapha***, diabetes and obesity (Srikanthamurthy 1995). This preparation is taken as part of the diet, along with the meat of desert animals and aged rice, in combination with rigorous exercise. Another commonly used approach in the treatment of diabetes is to combine ***Śilājatu*** with herbs such as ***Triphala*** and ***Guḍūcī***. Its rich mineral content and ***sandhānīya*** ('healing') properties also makes ***Śilājatu*** a good choice when treating musculoskeletal disorders, from osteoarthritis to osteoporosis. It is also used as a specific in the treatment of paralysis, the ***Cakradatta*** recommending a combination of ***Śilājatu***, ***Guggulu*** and ***Pippalī*** with a decoction of ***Daśamūla*** (Sharma

2002). ***Śilājatu*** can be used in any disease, however, and as a ***rasāyana*** has a special ability to treat deficiency conditions, including reproductive problems. It can be used as an adjunct to the primary treatment of conditions such as cancer, or to enhance the potency of other medicaments. The ***Caraka saṃhitā*** recommends that the truly excellent benefits of ***Śilājatu*** are only obtained when it is consumed at the appropriate dosage levels each day for at least 7 weeks (Sharma & Dash 1988).

Dosage:

- ***Cūrṇa***: 1–48 g b.i.d.–t.i.d. The ***Caraka saṃhitā*** states that the lowest potency dose for purified and impregnated ***Śilājatu*** is one ***karṣa*** (12 g) (Sharma & Dash 1988), but many modern Āyurvedic practitioners can be observed to use much lower doses, closer to 2–3 g twice daily.

REFERENCES

Bucci LR 2000 Selected herbals and human exercise performance. American Journal of Clinical Nutrition 72(2):624S–636S

Ghosal S, Singh SK, Kumar Y et al 1988 Anti-ulcerogenic activity of fulvic acids and 4′-methoxy–6-carbomethoxybiphenyl isolated from Shilajit. Phytotherapy Research 2:187–191

Goel RK, Banerjee RS, Acharya SB 1990 Antiulcerogenic and anti-inflammatory studies with shilajit. Journal of Ethnopharmacology 29(1):95–103

Jaiswal AK, Bhattacharya SK 1992 Effects of shilajit on memory, anxiety and brain monoamines in rats. Indian Journal of Pharmacology 24:12–17

Nadkarni KM 1954 The Indian materia medica, with Ayurvedic, Unani and home remedies, revised and enlarged by AK Nadkarni, vol 2. Popular Prakashan PVP, Bombay, p 28–32

Phillips P 1997 Unearthing the evidence. Chemistry in Britain 33(3):32–34. Available: http://www.chemsoc.org/chembytes/ezine/1997/phillips.htm

Schliebs R, Liebmann A, Bhattacharya SK et al 1997 Systemic administration of defined extracts from Withania somnifera (Indian Ginseng) and Shilajit differentially affects cholinergic but not glutamatergic and GABAergic markers in rat brain. Neurochemistry International 30(2):181–190

Sharma PV 2002 Cakradatta: Sanskrit text with English translation. Chaukhamba, Varanasi, p 243, 644, 647

Sharma RK, Dash B 1988 Agnivesa's Caraka Saṃhitā: text with English translation and critical exposition based on Cakrapani Datta's Āyurveda Dipika, vol. 3. Chaukhambha Orientalia, Varanasi, p 50–54

Srikanthamurthy KR 1984 Śāraṅgadhara saṃhitā: a treatise on Ayurveda. Chaukhamba Orientalia, Varanasi, p 156

Srikanthamurthy KR 1995 Vāgbhaṭa's Aṣṭāṅga Hṛdayam, vol 2. Krishnadas Academy, Varanasi, p 388, 403

Srikanthamurthy KR 2001 Bhāvaprakāśa of Bhāvamiśra, vol 1. Krishnadas Academy, Varanasi, p 344–345

Tillotson A 2001 The One Earth herbal sourcebook. Twin Streams (Kensington), New York, p 201

Tiwari P, Ramarao P, Ghosal S 2001 Effects of Shilajit on the development of tolerance to morphine in mice. Phytotherapy Research 15(2):177–179

Trivedi NA, Saxena NS, Mazumdar B et al 2001 Effects of Shilajit on blood glucose, lipid profile and vascular preparation in alloxan induced diabetic rats. Indian Journal of Pharmacology 33:124–145

Śyonāka

BOTANICAL NAME: *Oroxylum indicum*, Bignoniaceae

OTHER NAMES: ***Tuntukah*** (S); Shyona, Sonapatha, Arlu, Pharkhat (H); Palakappayyani, Payyalanta (T); Indian Trumpet tree, Midnight Horror, Tree of Damocles (E); Mu Hu Die (seed) (C)

Botany: ***Śyonāka*** is a small to medium-sized tree between 7.5 and 12 m in height, with a soft, light brown bark with numerous corky lenticels that exudes a green juice when cut. The leaves are two to three times pinnately compound, with five of more pairs of primary pinnae, the leaflets ovate or elliptic, acuminate, glabrous and rounded or cordate at the base. The flowers are numerous, borne in large erect racemes, the campanulate corolla purplish to reddish purple outside and pinkish within, giving way to flattened woody seed capsules up to 1 m long, each containing numerous flattened winged seeds. The common name 'midnight horror' is probably in reference to the fact that the flowers tend to open at night and have a distinctly foul smell. *O. indicum* is found throughout India in moist deciduous forests, as well as in China and SE Asia, and may be found in other locales as a garden plant or in the wild as an escapee (Kirtikar & Basu 1935, Warrier et al 1994).

Part used: Roots, bark, leaves, flowers, seeds.

Dravyguṇa:

- ***Rasa***: *madhura tikta, kaśāya, kaṭu* (root); *tikta, kaṭu, kaśāya* (bark); *madhura, kaśāya* (unripe fruit); *madhura, kaṭu* (ripe fruit)
- ***Vipāka***: *kaṭu*
- ***Vīrya***: *śita*
- ***Karma***: *grāhī, chardinigrahaṇa, kṛmighna, jvaraghna, chedana, kāsahara, svāsahara, mūtravirecana, śotahara, svedana, kuṣṭaghna, vedanāsthāpana, sandhānīya, tridoṣaghna* (root); *pācana, vedan-āsthāpana, vātakopa* (leaf); *dīpanapācana, kṛmighna, chedana, kāsahara, svāsahara, hṛdaya, vātakaphahara* (unripe fruit); *pācana, kṛmighna, hṛdaya* (mature fruit); *recana* (mature seed) (Dash 1991, Kirtikar & Basu 1935, Srikanthamurthy 2001, Warrier et al 1995).

Constituents: The limited amount of chemical research conducted on *O. indicum* indicates the presence of flavones including scutellarein, baicalein, oroxinden, oroxylin A and B and chrysin. Other constituents include the ursolic acid, benzoic acid, several naphthalene related compounds, β-sitosterol, an isoflavone, terpenes, alkaloids, saponins and tannin (Chen et al 2003, Jiwajinda et al 2002, Kapoor 1990, Kizu et al 1994)

Medical research:

- ***In vitro***: antioxidant (Jiwajinda et al 2002), immunostimulant (Laupattarakasem et al 2003), antitumour (Nakahara et al 2001, 2002)

Toxicity: No data found. Products that contain ***Śyonāka*** may be adulterated with other species.

Indications: Anorexia, vomiting, dyspepsia, ulcers, hiccough, flatulent colic, diarrhoea, dysentery, hepatosplenomegaly, intestinal parasites, haemorrhoids, fever, cough, bronchitis, asthma, strangury, oedema, gout, rheumatoid arthritis, neuralgia, headache, sprains, wounds.

Contraindications: Constipation (root).

Medicinal uses: ***Śyonāka*** root is perhaps best known as an ingredient in the ***Daśamūla*** or 'ten roots' formula, but is also found in the famous confection ***Cyavanaprāśa***, and in ***Nārāyaṇa taila***. Apart from being a useful medicinal plant, however, traditional peoples across SE Asia eat the young shoots and unripe fruits. ***Śyonāka*** root, bark and leaf is an important remedy for inflammation of the digestive tract, such as vomiting, ulceration or diarrhoea, used by itself as the freshly collected bark juice or a cold infusion of the root bark powder, or in combination with herbs such as ***Mustaka***, ***Śūṇṭhī*** and ***Yavānī***. ***Śyonāka*** stem bark is also mentioned as a diaphoretic in fever and rheumatic pain (Nadkarni 1954). The fruit specifically is used as an expectorant in Unani medicine (Kirtikar & Basu 1935). The ***Cakradatta*** mentions ***Śyonāka*** among several other plants included in the ***Virataradi*** group, used in the treatment of urinary calculi and dysuria (Sharma 2002). In the treatment of otalgia caused by any of the three ***doṣas*** the ***Śāraṅgadhara saṃhitā*** recommends a medicated oil prepared from the roots of ***Śyonāka***, instilled into the ear (Srikanthamurthy 1984). One researcher reports an apparent cure from nasopharyngeal cancer by use of a decoction of the bark, 1 kg per 5 L of water decocted for 30–40 min, taken in three equal doses with honey on a daily basis. After administration the patient was free of pain within 2 weeks, and despite being considered a terminal case, is reported to be living free of symptoms today (Mao 2002). In Chinese medicine the seeds of *O. indicum* are used to moisten the lungs in the treatment of pharyngitis, cough and hoarseness, to alleviate constrained liver qi, and to promote healing of suppurative ulcers (Bensky & Gamble 1993).

Dosage:

- ***Cūrṇa***: 2–15 g b.i.d.–t.i.d.
- ***Kvātha***: 30–60 mL b.i.d.–t.i.d.
- ***Tincture***: dried root, 1:3, 40%; 2–5 mL b.i.d.–t.i.d.

REFERENCES

Bensky D, Gamble A 1993 Chinese herbal medicine materia medica, revised edn. Eastland Press, Seattle, p 206

Chen LJ, Games DE, Jones J 2003 Isolation and identification of four flavonoid constituents from the seeds of Oroxylum indicum by high-speed counter-current chromatography. Journal of Chromatography (A) 988(1):95–105

Dash B 1991 Materia medica of Ayurveda. B. Jain Publishers, New Delhi, p 18

Jiwajinda S, Santisopasri V, Murakami A et al 2002 Suppressive effects of edible Thai plants on superoxide and nitric oxide generation. Asian Pacific Journal of Cancer Prevention 3(3):215–223

Kapoor LD 1990 CRC handbook of Ayurvedic medicinal plants. CRC Press, Boca Raton, p 252

Kirtikar KR, Basu BD 1935 Indian medicinal plants, 2nd edn, vols 1–4. Periodical Experts, Delhi, p 1839

Kizu H, Habe S, Ishida M, Tomimori T 1994 Studies on the Nepalese crude drugs. XVII. On the naphthalene related compounds from the root bark of Oroxylum indicum. Yakugaku Zasshi 11(7):492–513

Laupattarakasem P, Houghton PJ, Hoult JR, Itharat A 2003 An evaluation of the activity related to inflammation of four plants used in Thailand to treat arthritis. Journal of Ethnopharmacology 85(2–3):207–215

Mao AA 2002 Oroxylum indicum Vent.: a potential anticancer medicinal plant. Indian Journal of Traditional Knowledge 1(1):17–21

Nadkarni KM 1954 The Indian materia medica, with Ayurvedic, Unani and home remedies, revised and enlarged by AK Nadkarni. Popular Prakashan PVP, Bombay, p 876

Nakahara K, Onishi-Kameyama M, Ono H et al 2001 Antimutagenic activity against trp-P–1 of the edible Thai plant, Oroxylum indicum vent. Bioscience, Biotechnology, and Biochemistry 65(10):2358–2360

Nakahara K, Trakoontivakorn G, Alzoreky NS et al 2002 Antimutagenicity of some edible Thai plants, and a bioactive carbazole alkaloid, mahanine, isolated from Micromelum minutum. Journal of Agricultural and Food Chemistry 50(17):4796–4802

Sharma PV 2002 Cakradatta. Sanskrit text with English translation. Chaukhamba, Varanasi, p 317

Srikanthamurthy KR 1984 Śāraṅgadhara saṃhitā: a treatise on Ayurveda. Chaukhamba Orientalia, Varanasi, p 251

Srikanthamurthy KR 2001 Bhāvaprakāśa of Bhāvamiśra, vol 1. Krishnadas Academy, Varanasi, p 231–232

Warrier PK, Nambiar VPK, Ramankutty C (eds) 1995 Indian medicinal plants: a compendium of 500 species, vol 4. Orient Longman, Hyderabad, p 186–190

Trivṛt, 'thricely twisted'

BOTANICAL NAMES: *Operculina turpethum,* Convolvulaceae

OTHER NAMES: Nishoth, Tarbud (H); Shivatai, Kumbham (T); Indian Jalap, Indian Rhubarb, St Thomas Lidpod (E)

Botany: ***Trivṛt*** is a stout perennial climber that exudes a milky juice when cut, with long fleshy roots, and long twisting pubescent stems that are angled, winged and become very tough and brown when old. The leaves are simple, pubescent on both sides, and variable in shape, cordate or truncate at the base, subacute, 5–10 cm long by 1.3–7 cm wide. The flowers are white, tubular-campanulate, sepals long, borne in cymes of a few flowers, giving way to globose capsules enclosed within overlapping brittle sepals. ***Trivṛt*** is found throughout India up to 900 m in elevation, as well as in S.E. Asia, Australia, tropical Africa and it can also be found as an invasive weed in the Americas. The Sanskrit name ***Trivṛt*** or 'thricely twisted' probably refers to the twining habit of this plant (Kirtikar & Basu 1935, Warrier et al 1995).

Part used: Roots.

Dravyguṇa:

- ***Rasa***: *tikta, kaṭu, madhura*
- ***Vipāka***: *kaṭu*
- ***Vīrya***: *uṣṇa*, rūkṣa
- ***Karma***: *dīpanapācana, bhedana, śulapraśamana, virecana, kṛmighna, jvaraghna, chedana, pittakaphahara* (Dash 1991, Kirtikar & Basu 1935, Srikanthamurthy 2001, Warrier et al 1995).

Constituents: ***Trivṛt*** is stated to contain a resin comprising upwards of 9–13% of the crude herb, itself composed of a mixture of the glycosides α- and β-terpethin and terpethinic acids A–E. Other constituents in the herb include scopoletin and other coumarins, rhamnose, fucose, betulin, lupeol, β-sitosterol and glucose (Kapoor 1990, Yoganarasimhan 2000).

Medical research:

- ***In vivo***: anti-inflammatory (Kapoor 1990).

Toxicity: No data found.

Indications: Dyspepsia, constipation, flatulent colic, haemorrhoids, jaundice, hepatosplenomegaly, intestinal parasites, intermittent fever, bronchitis, itching skin, leucoderma, oedema, ascites, myalgia, arthritis, paralysis, obesity, tumours.

Contraindications: Pregnancy, diarrhoea, dysentery, active gastrointestinal inflammation; ***vātakopa***.

Medicinal uses: ***Trivṛt*** is among the most important purgatives in the Indian material medica, although there is some debate as to its botanical origin. The ***Madanapala nighaṇṭu***, for example, lists two varieties: ***Śvetatrivṛt*** ('white' ***Trivṛt***, *O. turpethum*) and ***Krishnatrivṛt*** ('black' ***Trivṛt***, *Ipomoea petaloideschois*), the former being a mild and efficacious purgative, and the latter a violent purgative that irritates the mucosa and is used to restore consciousness and treat states of intoxication (Srikanthamurthy 2001). Generally speaking, the term ***Trivṛt*** refers to ***Śvetatrivṛt***, which is a safe and efficacious purgative in ***pitta*** and ***kaphaja*** conditions, as well as in ***virecana*** in ***pañca karma***, but is stated in several texts to be contraindicated in ***vāttika*** conditions. Texts such as the ***Cakradatta***, however, state that ***Trivṛt*** is an important remedy in the treatment of ***vāttika*** conditions such as ***udāvarta***, or the upward movement of ***vāta***, but is typically combined with botanicals such as ***Triphala***, ***Pippalī***, ***Harītakī***, ***Śūṇṭhī***, ***Ajamodika***, ***Tvak***, and ***Hiṅgu***, as well ***anupāna*** including ***saindhava***, sugar and honey. For constipation with dry faeces and flatus the ***Bhāvaprakāśa*** recommends ***Nāraca cūrṇa***, comprising powdered sugar, ***Trivṛt*** and ***Pippalī*** (Srikanthamurthy 2000). Another preparation is ***Trivṛt lehyam***, prepared by decocting the roots of ***Trivṛt*** and then adding powdered sugar, ***Trivṛt cūrṇa*** and ***Trisugandhā cūrṇa*** ('three aromatics', i.e. ***Elā***, ***Tvak***, ***Patra***) (Nadkarni 1954). In the treatment of ***grahaṇī***, or malabsorption syndromes, the ***Cakradatta*** recommends ***Kalyāṇaguḍa***, a ***lehya*** prepared by decocting 320 g of ***Trivṛt cūrṇa*** with 320 g of sesame oil, 2 kg of jaggery, and 1.92 L of fresh ***Āmalakī*** juice, along with 40 g each of ***Pippalīmūla***, ***Jīraka***, ***Cavya***, ***Gajapippalī***, ***Trikaṭu***, ***Hapuṣā***, ***Ajamodā***, ***Viḍaṅga***, ***Triphala***, ***Yavānī***, ***Pāṭhā***, ***Citraka***, ***Dhānyaka*** and ***saindhava***. This is decocted until it is reduced to a thick jam-like consistency, mixed with 40 g each ***Elā***, ***Tvak*** and ***Patra*** (***Trisugandhā cūrṇa***), and is taken in doses of about 10 g. Cakrapani states that this remedy enhances digestion, promotes proper absorption, relieves cough, dyspnoea and oedema, and is useful in female infertility (Sharma 2002). In the treatment of intestinal parasites ***Trivṛt*** is a common and popular remedy, taken with herbs such as ***Viḍaṅga***, ***Triphala*** and ***Dañtī***. In the treatment of ***paittika pāṇḍu***, a disease often translated as 'anaemia' but in this instance referring more to symptoms of jaundice and hepatic dysfunction, the ***Cakradatta*** recommends ***Trivṛt cūrṇa*** mixed with double its quantity of jaggery, taken in doses of 20 g (Sharma 2002). ***Trivṛt*** is similarly mentioned in the ***nighaṇṭus***, as well as by more modern commentators, as being beneficial in hepatosplenomegaly (***udara roga***), ascites and cirrhosis (Kirtikar & Basu 1935, Sharma 2002). Combined with equal parts ***cūrṇa*** of the dehusked seeds of ***Viḍaṅga***, along with ***Trikaṭu***, ***Citraka***, and ***Dañtī***, ***Trivṛt*** is mixed with jaggery and formed into pills and taken with hot water, used in the treatment of colic and flatulence caused by ***tridoṣa*** (Sharma 2002). Mixed with ***Triphala***, ***Pippalī***, jaggery and honey ***Trivṛt*** is recommended in ***raktapitta***, or innate haemorrhage (Sharma 2002). Prepared as a medicated ***ghṛta Trivṛt*** is used in the treatment of sciatica (Sharma 2002). ***Trivṛt*** also finds its way into formulations used to treat psychosis and epilepsy, particularly when ***pitta*** symptoms are manifest. Mixed with botanicals such as ***Nimba***, ***Haridrā*** and ***Yaṣṭimadhu***, ***Trivṛt*** is stated to be ***sandhānīya***, useful to cleanse wounds and promote healing (Sharma 2002).

Dosage:

- ***Cūrṇa***: 3–7 g b.i.d.–t.i.d.
- ***Kvātha***: 30–90 mL b.i.d.–t.i.d.

REFERENCES

Dash, B. 1991. Materia medica of Ayurveda. B. Jain Publishers, New Delhi, p 38–39

Kapoor LD 1990 CRC handbook of Ayurvedic medicinal plants. CRC Press, Boca Raton, p 251

Kirtikar KR, Basu BD 1935 Indian medicinal plants, 2nd edn, vols 1–4. Periodical Experts, Delhi, p 1730–1731

Nadkarni KM 1954 The Indian materia medica, with Ayurvedic, Unani and home remedies, revised and enlarged by AK Nadkarni. Popular Prakashan PVP, Bombay, p 693

Sharma PV 2002 Cakradatta. Sanskrit text with English translation. Chaukhamba, Varanasi, p 72, 113, 121, 202, 270, 342, 395

Srikanthamurthy KR 2000 Bhāvaprakāśa of Bhāvamiśra, vol. 2. Krishnadas Academy, Varanasi, p 435

Srikanthamurthy KR 2001 Bhāvaprakāśa of Bhāvamiśra, vol 1. Krishnadas Academy, Varanasi, p 258–259

Warrier PK, Nambiar VPK, Ramankutty C (eds) 1995 Indian medicinal plants: a compendium of 500 species, vol 4. Orient Longman, Hyderabad, p 172–178

Yoganarasimhan SN 2000 Medicinal plants of India, vol 2: Tamil Nadu. Self-published, Bangalore, p 386

Uśīra

BOTANICAL NAME: *Vetiveria zizanioides*, Poaceae

OTHER NAMES: ***Sevyah***, ***Sugandhimula***, ***Śitamulaka***, ***Viranamula*** (S); Khas, Ganrar, Panni (H); Vettiver, Viranam (T); Vetiver, Khus (E)

Botany: ***Uśīra*** is a densely tufted perennial grass attaining a height of up to 2 m, with a branching rhizome and spongy aromatic roots, the smaller dissected rootlets providing a higher percentage of essential oil. The leaves are narrow, linear, erect and acute, with compressed sheaths. The inflorescence is borne in sessile and pedicelled spikelets, arranged in a panicle of slender racemes, with each fertilised flower giving rise to an oblong grain. ***Uśīra*** is found throughout India, SE Asia and China, in wetlands and plains up to 1200 m in elevation, and is cultivated in other tropical and subtropical regions including Australia, Africa and South America, as well as in and Mediterranean-type climates including Spain, Italy and southern California. The Sanskrit name ***Uśīra*** is derived from the root word ***Uśi***, referring to an ancient people that used to live in North India. Today ***Uśīra*** is found either as a fertile wild variety that originally hails from northern India or as a predominantly infertile domesticated variety that is propagated by rhizome in southern India. Apart from its medicinal usage, ***Uśīra*** is widely used for erosion control, soil conservation, reclaiming saline and acid sulfate soils, mine rehabilitation, and trapping industrial chemicals used in farming (Kirtikar & Basu 1935, Liao & Luo 2002, Pang et al 2003, Sethi et al 1986, Warrier et al 1996, Yang et al 2003).

Part used: Roots.

Dravyguṇa:

- ***Rasa***: *tikta, madhura*
- ***Vipāka***: *kaṭu*
- ***Vīrya***: *śita, laghu*
- ***Karma***: *pācana, stambhana, chardinigrahaṇa, jvaraghna, chedana, mūtravirecana, mūtraviśodhana, kuṣṭhaghna, dāhapraśamana, raktaprasādana, śoṇitasthāpana, viṣaghna, vātapittahara* (Dash 1991, Kirtikar & Basu 1935, Srikanthamurthy 2001, Warrier et al 1996).

Constituents: There is little constituent information for ***Uśīra*** with the exception of the essential oil, which is obtained by steam distillation. The essential oil is dark brown, olive or amber, with a deep smoky, earthy-woody odour and a sweet persistent undertone. The chemistry of the essential oil is exceedingly complex, including over 150 different sesquiterpenoids such as α-vetivone, β-vetivone, and khusinol, which are often used as chemical markers for the oil. Other constituents in the essential oil include α-amorphene, β-vetivenene, khusimone, zizanal, epizizanol and bicyclo-vetivenol (Duke 2003, Lawless 1995, Yoganarasimhan 2000).

Medical research: No data found.

Toxicity: No data found.

Indications: Nausea and vomiting, gastric reflux, dyspepsia, diarrhoea, flatulent colic, intestinal parasites, fever, burning sensations, extreme thirst, cough, bronchitis, asthma, haemoptysis, epistaxis, dysuria, urethritis, cystitis, skin diseases, ulceration, haemorrhage, migraines, inflammatory joint disease, lumbago, sprains, halitosis, epilepsy, rage, mania, amenorrhoea, dysmenorrhoea.

Contraindications: Pregnancy.

Medicinal uses: ***Uśīra*** has long been valued in India as a fragrant herb with cooling properties, indicated by its synonyms ***Sugandhimūla***, or 'fragrant root', and ***Śitamulaka*** or 'cooling root'. The Tamil name Vettiver refers to the highly dissected rooting structure. Although the medicinal properties of the wild and cultivated varietals are essentially the same, the wild-source essential oil is slightly different and is typically held in higher regard, and as a result is more expensive and more difficult to obtain commercially. The distinctly smoky, woody and earthy aroma of Vetivert, or Khus oil, has long been valued in perfumery, by itself or as a fixative to balance the etheric and deep notes of various perfume blends. Given its earthy and woody scent, Khus oil combines particularly well with oils such as Patchouli, Cinnamon, Sandalwood and Ylang-Ylang, and can be used in aromatherapy to treat ***vāttika*** disorders including anxiety, depression and seizures. The essential oil can also be applied topically over the head to relieve migraines and headaches, and in carrier oil in the treatment of joint inflammation, rheumatism and sprains. The aerial portions of ***Uśīra*** are traditionally used to weave baskets and mats in India, the latter of which are hung over windows and sprinkled with water in the hot weather, causing it to release some of its volatile constituents, and thus providing a unique form of air-conditioning. As a medicinal agent, ***Uśīra*** is pleasant and aromatic with a cooling energy, and thus finds particular application in conditions of heat, including burning sensations, fever, inflammation and irritability. In the digestive tract, ***Uśīra*** is used in the treatment of vomiting, bilious dyspepsia, gastric and duodenal ulceration, diarrhoea and dysentery, all marked by irritability and inflammation. Reduced to a powder and prepared as a cold infusion with ***Mustaka***, ***Candana***, ***Parpaṭa***, ***Śūṇṭhī*** and ***Udīcya***, ***Uśīra*** is used in the treatment of ***paittika*** fever, burning sensations, vomiting and thirst (Sharma 2002). Prepared as a paste with ***Candana***, ***Balāka***, ***Śūṇṭhī*** and ***Vāsaka***, ***Uśīra*** is taken with honey and rice water in the treatment of vomiting (Sharma 2002). In the treatment of poor digestion and weakness of appetite, ***āma***, and diarrhoea associated with severe pain and haemorrhage, the ***Cakradatta*** recommends ***Uśīrādi cūrṇa***, composed of equal parts ***Uśīra***, ***Balāka***, ***Mustaka***, ***Dhānyaka***, ***Śūṇṭhī***, ***Lajjālu***, ***Dhātaki***, ***Lodhra*** and ***Bilva*** (Sharma 2002). In severe thirst caused by a vitiation of ***pitta***, ***Uśīra*** is prepared as a cold infusion along with ***Ghambari*** fruit, ***Candana***, ***Padmaka***, ***Drākṣā***, ***Yaṣṭimadhu*** and powdered sugar (Sharma 2002). Combined with equal parts ***Dūrvā***, ***Kumuda*** stamens, ***Mañjiṣṭhā***, ***Elavāluka***, ***Candana***, ***Mustaka***, ***Raktacandana*** and ***Padmaka***, ***Uśīra*** is decocted in ***ghṛta*** prepared from goat's milk, rice water and goat's milk until only the ***ghṛta*** remains. This formula is stated by the ***Cakradatta*** as being efficacious in the vomiting of blood and epistaxis when taken internally, and is applied locally in passive haemorrhage (Sharma 2002). In burning sensations throughout the body the ***Cakradatta*** recommends a cool bath prepared with the powders of ***Uśīra***, ***Balāka***, ***Padmaka*** and ***Candana*** (Sharma 2002). ***Uśīra*** is also used topically as a ***cūrṇa***, rubbed into the skin to remove foul odours, and when mixed with herbs such as ***Yaṣṭimadhu***, ***Triphala***, ***Dāruharidrā*** and ***Nīlotpala*** is used in the treatment of chicken pox (Sharma 2002). In the treatment of epilepsy ***Uśīra*** can be reduced to a powder and prepared as an incense along with botanicals such as ***Vacā*** and ***Kuṣṭha*** to prevent seizure (Sharma 2002). Prepared as a decoction with ***Nimba***, ***Āmalakī*** and ***Harītakī***, the ***Cakradatta*** states that ***Uśīra*** is effective in the treatment of ***paittika prameha***, a disease characterised by polyuria with a deep coloured urine that has a foul smell, pain in the bladder and genitalia, burning sensations, gastric reflux, and diarrhoea (Sharma 2002). The ***Śāraṅgadhara saṃhitā*** recommends ***Uśīrasava***, a fermented beverage that contains many constituents including ***Uśīra***, in the treatment of innate haemorrhage, skin diseases, diabetes, intestinal parasites and oedema (Srikanthamurthy 1984). ***Uśīra*** is also found as an important constituent in ***Yogarāja guggulu***.

Dosage:

- ***Cūrṇa***: 3–5 g b.i.d.–t.i.d.
- ***Hima***: 60–120 mL b.i.d.–t.i.d.
- ***Tincture***: fresh rootlets, 1:2, 95%; 2–5 mL b.i.d.–t.i.d.

REFERENCES

Dash B 1991 Materia medica of Ayurveda. B. Jain Publishers, New Delhi, p 175

Duke JA (accessed 2003) Chemicals. In: Vetiveria zizanioides (L.) NASH (Poaceae) -Cus-Cus, Cuscus Grass, Vetiver. Dr Duke's phytochemical and ethnobotanical databases. Agricultural Research Service (ARS), United States Department of Agriculture. Available: http://www.ars-grin.gov/duke/plants.html

Kirtikar KR, Basu BD 1935 Indian medicinal plants, 2nd edn, vols 1–4. Periodical Experts, Delhi, p 2671–2672

Lawless J 1995 The illustrated encyclopedia of essential oils. Element, Rockport MA, p 234

Liao X, Luo S 2002 Effects of constructed wetlands on treating with nitrogen and phosphorus in wastewater from hoggery. Ying Yong Sheng Tai Xue Bao 13(6):719–722

Nadkarni KM 1954 The Indian materia medica, with Ayurvedic, Unani and home remedies, revised and enlarged by AK Nadkarni. Popular Prakashan PVP, Bombay

Pang J, Chan GS, Zhang J et al 2003 Physiological aspects of vetiver grass for rehabilitation in abandoned metalliferous mine wastes. Chemosphere 52(9):1559–1570

Sethi KL, Maheshwari ML, Srivastava VK, Gupta R 1986 Natural variability in Vetiveria zizaniodes collections from Bharatpur, part 1. Indian Perfumer 30(2–3):377–380

Sharma PV 2002 Cakradatta. Sanskrit text with English translation. Chaukhamba, Varanasi, p 3, 13, 45, 126, 168, 172, 183, 192, 326, 338, 471

Srikanthamurthy KR 1984 Śāraṅgadhara saṃhitā: a treatise on Ayurveda. Chaukhamba Orientalia, Varanasi, p 139

Srikanthamurthy KR 2001 Bhāvaprakāśa of Bhāvamiśra, vol 1. Krishnadas Academy, Varanasi, p 220

Warrier PK, Nambiar VPK, Ramankutty C (eds) 1996 Indian medicinal plants: a compendium of 500 species, vol 5. Orient Longman, Hyderabad, p 361

Yang B, Shu WS, Ye ZH et al 2003 Growth and metal accumulation in vetiver and two Sesbania species on lead/zinc mine tailings. Chemosphere 52(9):1593–1600

Yoganarasimhan SN 2000 Medicinal plants of India, vol 2: Tamil Nadu. Self-published, Bangalore, p 577

Vacā, 'to speak'

BOTANICAL NAME: *Acorus calamus*, Acoraceae

OTHER NAMES: ***Ugragandhā*** (S); Bach (H); Vashampu (T); Sweet Flag (E)

Botany: ***Vacā*** is a perennial plant with a creeping rhizome about the thickness of a finger, with numerous rootlets, the cortex brown to pinkish brown, the medulla white and spongy. The long, narrow sword-like leathery leaves are bright green, whitish pink at the base, sheathing, up to 1.8 m in length, thickened along the midrib, the other parallel veins barely visible, the margins wavy and the tip acute. The greenish yellow flowers are small, densely packed into a sessile cylindrical spadix about 10 cm long. The entire plant has a characteristic cinnamon-like aroma. The fruits are oblong turbinate berries with a pyramidal top, mostly lacking seeds. ***Vacā*** is found throughout India in wet marshy locations up to elevations of about 1800 m, and is similarly found in other parts of Eurasia and Africa, and has since been introduced into North America. Although *A. calamus* is one of only three species that are generally recognised as being members of the Acoraceae (i.e. *A. calamus*, *A. gramineus*, and recently, *A. americanus*), botanists have further classified *A. calamus* based upon the number of pairs of chromosomes (*n*) found in each genetic species, including hexaploid (6*n*), tetraploid (4*n*), triploid (3*n*) or diploid (2*n*). The Eurasian genetic species of *A. calamus* is stated as being hexaploid, tetraploid or triploid, and is infertile, only reproducing by vegetative means. Dilpoid genetic species of *A. calamus*, as well as the very similar *A. americanus* native to North America are stated to be fertile and reproduce both by seed and rhizome (Kirtikar & Basu 1935, Larry 1973, Warrier et al 1994).

Part used: rhizome and rootlets, best harvested in June (Li & Jiang 1994).

Dravyguṇa:

- ***Rasa***: *kaṭu, tikta*
- ***Vipāka***: *laghu*
- ***Vīrya***: *uṣṇa*
- ***Karma***: *vamana, āsyasravaṇa, dīpanapācana, anulomana, śulapraśamana, kṛmighna, chedana, kāsahara, svāsahara, mūtravirecana, ārtavajanana, medhya, vātakaphahara*
- ***Prabhāva***: *Vacā* is said to stimulate the power of self-expression and to enhance intelligence (Dash 1991, Frawley & Lad 1986, Nadkarni 1954, Warrier et al 1994).

Constituents: ***Vacā*** is noted for its delightfully sweet and pleasing fragrance, a feature of its essential oil, which includes a great variety of constituents including α-asarone and β-asarone, as well as elemicine, *cis*-isoelemecine, *cis* and *trans* eugenol and their methyl esters, camphene, *p*-cymene, β-gurjunene, α-selinene, β-candinene, camphor, α-terpineol, α-calacorene, azulene, calamenene, limonene, linalol, menthol, methylchavicol, sabinene and many others. The potentially toxic β-asarone is stated as being present in all varieties except for the diploid (2*n*) genetic species and the native North American (2*n*) species *(A. americanus)*. Hexaploid species from Kashmir and the triploid European species, however, can contain as little as 5–10% β-asarone, but the tetraploid species most commonly found in India can contain upwards of 75% β-asarone. In regard to the other constituents in ***Vacā*** there is little information: bitter glycosides acorin and acoretin, the flavonoid galangin, the alkaloid choline, oxalic acid, mucilage, resins and tannins (Duke 1985, 2003, Kapoor 1990, Lander & Schreier 1990; Larry 1973; Vashist & Handa 1964; Williamson et al 2002).

Medical research:

- ***In vitro***: immunomodulant (Mehrotra et al 2003), antibacterial (Jain et al 1974), nematocidal (Sugimoto et al 1995).
- ***In vivo***: negatively inotropic/chronotropic (Pancal et al 1989), antispasmodic (Das et al 1962, Opdyke

1977), CNS depressant (Opdyke 1977; Pancal et al 1989); neuroprotective (Shukla et al 2002); anti-ulcerogenic (Rafatullah et al 1994); hypolipidaemic (Parab & Mengi 2002).

Toxicity: Feeding studies in rats using the volatile oil of the Asian species of *A. calamus* has resulted in growth inhibition, hepatic and cardiac abnormalities, serous effusion in abdominal and/or peritoneal cavities, and death (Gross et al 1967; Taylor et al 1967). The LD_{50} for the volatile oil of the Asian species is 777 mg/kg (rat, oral), less than 5 g/kg (guinea pig, dermal), and 221 mg/kg (rat, intraperitoneal). The oil is generally considered to be non-irritating, but is reported to have caused cases of erythema and dermatitis in sensitive individuals (Opdyke 1977).

Indications: Toothache, dyspepsia, hiatus hernia, gastritis, flatulent colic, irritable bowel syndrome, colitis, dysentery, intestinal parasites, upper respiratory tract viral infections, intermittent fever, cough, bronchitis, asthma, sinus headaches, sinusitis, hay fever, urolithiasis, inflammatory joint disease, gout, amenorrhoea, dysmenorrhoea, epilepsy, convulsions, hysteria, depression, shock, loss of memory, deafness, neuralgia, numbness, eczema, general debility.

Contraindications: Caution should be used with the concomitant use of *A. calamus* with benzodiazepines, barbiturates, MAO inhibitors and anticonvulsants (Opdyke 1977). *A. calamus* is an emetic in large doses, and should be avoided in pre-existing cases of nausea and vomiting, and for this reason is also contraindicated in pregnancy. Care should be taken to avoid the use of the Asian (3*n*, 4*n*, 6*n*) species in patients with liver dysfunction, owing to its β-asarone content (Weiss 1988).

Medicinal uses: Across the world Calamus is regarded as a useful bitter-tasting aromatic stomachic, used most commonly in the treatment of disorders marked by coldness, catarrh and spasm, particularly in afflictions of the digestive tract including dyspepsia and bowel spasm. The German physician Rudolf Weiss (1988) considered Calamus to have a "powerful tonic effect on the stomach, encouraging its secretory activity", further adding that he has "seen it used to very satisfactory effect in stomach cancer patients . . . for symptomatic treatment". Āyurvedic medicine, too, confirms the efficacy of ***Vacā*** in digestive disorders, given simply as an infusion or decoction in the treatment of dyspepsia, flatulence and diarrhoea, or in complex polyherbal formulations. In the treatment of ***kaphaja*** colic the ***Cakradatta*** recommends ***Mustādi cūrṇa***, composed of the powders of ***Vacā***, ***Mustaka***, ***Kaṭuka***, ***Harītakī*** and ***Mūrvā*** (Sharma 2002). In the treatment of ***udāvarta***, which is the upward movement of ***apāna vāyu*** causing symptoms including abdominal distension, constipation and dyspnoea, the powders of one part ***Hiṅgu***, two parts ***Kuṣṭha***, four parts ***Vacā***, eight parts ***Śaṭī***, and 16 parts ***Viḍa lavaṇa*** (black salt) are mixed with wine and taken internally (Sharma 2002). In the treatment of ***gulma*** or abdominal tumours the ***Cakradatta*** recommends ***Vacādya cūrṇa***, consisting of equal parts ***Vacā***, ***Harītakī***, ***Hiṅgu***, ***Amlavetasa***, ***Yavānī***, ***Yavakṣāra*** and ***saindhava***, taken with warm water (Sharma 2002). Combined with ***Nimba***, ***Haridrā***, ***Citraka***, ***Kaṭuka*** and purified ***Ativiṣā***, ***Vacā*** is used in ***kaphaja*** fever (Sharma 2002). Combined with ***Mustaka***, ***Devadāru***, purified ***Ativiṣā*** and ***Indrayava***, ***Vacā*** is used in diarrhoea produced by ***vāta*** and ***pitta*** (Sharma 2002). Combined with ***Pippalī***, ***Bilva***, ***Kuṣṭha***, ***Citraka***, ***Devadāru***, ***Yaṣṭimadhu***, ***Śatapuṣpā***, ***Madana***, ***Śaṭī*** and ***Puṣkaramūla***, ***Vacā*** is decocted in oil and milk until all the milk has evaporated to create a medicated oil that is taken internally in the treatment of ***vāttika*** haemorrhoids, as well as in rectal prolapse, dysentery, dysuria, lumbago and lower back weakness (Sharma 2002). Beyond its usage in digestive disorders, ***Vacā*** has other applications, taken alone or in combination with ***Yaṣṭimadhu*** in the treatment of cough, bronchitis and sore throats (Nadkarni 1954). ***Vacā*** is also used in the treatment of gout and skin diseases caused by ***vāta*** and ***kapha***, the ***Cakradatta*** recommending a combination of equal parts ***Vacā***, ***Āmalakī***, ***Harītakī***, ***Bibhītaka***, ***Nimba***, ***Mañjiṣṭhā***, ***Kaṭuka***, ***Guḍūcī*** and ***Dāruharidrā*** called ***Navakārṣika***, used in the treatment of gout and skin diseases (Sharma 2002). In the treatment of ***āmavāta*** or inflammatory joint disease, ***Vacā*** is used in combination with ***Guḍūcī***, ***Śūṇṭhī***, ***Harītakī***, ***Devadāru***, purified ***Ativiṣā*** and ***Śaṭī***, along with a ***kapha*** reducing diet (Sharma 2002). Other indications for ***Vacā*** include cardiac angina, anaemia and jaundice. In the treatment of cardiac angina ***Vacā*** is mixed with equal parts ***Pippalī***, ***Elā***, ***Śūṇṭhī***, ***Ajamodā***, ***Yavakṣāra*** and ***saindhava*** (Sharma 2002). Decocted with ***Triphala***,

Guḍūcī, ***Kaṭuka***, ***Kirātatiktā*** and ***Nimba***, ***Vacā*** is taken with honey in the treatment of anaemia and jaundice (Sharma 2002).

The name ***Vacā*** means 'to speak', referring to its usage in ***apasmāra*** (epilepsy), a condition characterised by seizure, a loss of consciousness and memory loss, allowing the patient to regain the ability to 'speak' and regain normal consciousness. Used in ***nasya***, the 'strongly aromatic' and ***tikṣṇa*** properties suggested by its synonym, ***Ugragandhā***, makes ***Vacā*** an important traditional remedy to restore consciousness. The ***Caraka saṃhitā*** recommends ***Vacādya ghṛta*** in the treatment of epilepsy due to vitiated ***vāta*** and ***kapha***, made simply by decocting one part coarsely ground ***Vacā*** rhizome in four parts ***ghṛta*** and eight parts water until all the water has been evaporated. The resulting preparation may be taken internally in doses of about 5 g, and/or applied in ***nasya*** (Sharma & Dash 1988). In the treatment of convulsion and seizure ***Vacā*** is taken either as a powder or a decoction along with ***Harītakī***, ***Rāsnā***, ***Amlavetasa*** and ***saindhava***, with ***ghṛta*** (Sharma 2002). In a similar vein, ***Vacā*** is considered to be an important remedy in ***unmāda***, or psychosis. The ***Cakradatta*** recommends the fresh juice of ***Vacā***, ***Brāhmī***, ***Kūṣmāṇḍa***, ***Śaṅkhapuṣpī*** and ***Kuṣṭha*** mixed with honey, and taken internally (12–24 g) as a specific treatment for ***unmāda***. Combined with the powders of ***Haridrā***, ***Kuṣṭha***, ***Pippalī***, ***Śūṇṭhī***, ***Jīraka***, ***Yaṣṭimadhu*** and ***saindhava***, ***Vacā cūrṇa*** is also taken with ***ghṛta*** to enhance memory and remove disorders of speech (Sharma 2002). The psychotropic properties of ***Vacā*** have also been utilised in other cultures, among the First Nations people of North America, for example, as well as the Moso shamans of Yunnan China, both groups using it as a spiritual aid (Gilmore 1919; Grinnell 1905, Hart 1981; Miller 1983, Smith 1973). The Bible also mentions the supernatural activities of ***Vacā***, which is included as one of the constituents of a holy unguent that God commands Moses to rub on his body before entering the temple (Exodus 30:22–25). The hallucinogenic properties of ***Vacā*** have been attributed to α-asarone and β-asarone, precursors to 1,2,4-trimethoxy-5-propenylbenzene, a phenylethylamine that is reported to have ten times the potency of mescaline (Miller 1983). The hallucinogenic dose of the whole plant, however, begins at about 25–30 g of the fresh rhizome, and given the aromatic pungency and potentially emetic properties of ***Vacā***, it is a difficult dosage to attain (Miller 1983). As mentioned, the essential oil of the Asian genetic species ($3n$, $4n$, $6n$) of ***Vacā*** contains variable amounts of β-asarone, which has been shown to be carcinogenic in experimental animals. The North American ($2n$) genetic species, however, does not contain β-asarone and can thus be safely used as a substitute (Weiss 1988). Too much concern over the potential carcinogenicity of the Asian species is unwarranted, however, as ***Vacā*** has been used for millennia by peoples all across the world, as both a medicine and a food. Nonetheless, the chronic consumption of the Asian species is not recommended, and should be approached with caution in patients with a history of liver disease. In Chinese medicine the similar but much less fragrant *A. gramineus* rhizome (Shi Chang Pu) is used in much the same way as *A. calamus* is used in Āyurvedic medicine, to open the channels of the body, dispel phlegm and quiet the spirit. It is also stated to harmonise the middle burner, relieving symptoms of epigastric fullness caused by dampness, and is used as an analgesic remedy in joint pain and trauma caused by wind, cold and damp (Bensky & Gamble 1993).

Dosage:

- ***Cūrṇa***: freshly ground dried rhizome, 1–5 g b.i.d–t.i.d; higher doses as an emetic
- ***Phāṇṭa***: dried rhizome, 30–90 mL b.i.d–t.i.d.
- ***Kvātha***: dried rhizome, in milk, 60–90 mL b.i.d–t.i.d
- ***Kalka***: applied externally for headaches, toothache, and in the nasal cavities to treat nasal polyps and sinus congestion; used to promote suppuration in indolent ulcers
- ***Tincture***: fresh rhizome 1:2, 95% alcohol; dried rhizome 1:5, 60% ethanol; 1–3 mL t.i.d.
- ***Ghṛta***: as ***nasya***, 1–3 gtt. in each nostril.

REFERENCES

Bensky D, Gamble A 1993 Chinese herbal medicine materia medica, revised edn. Eastland Press, Seattle, p 415

Das PK, Malhotra CL, Dhalla NS 1962 Spasmolytic activity of asarone and essential oil of Acous calamus, Linn. Archives Internationales de Pharmacodynamie 135:167–177

Dash B 1991 Materia medica of Ayurveda. B. Jain Publishers, New Delhi, p 148

Duke JA 1985 Handbook of medicinal herbs. CRC Press, Boca Raton, p 14–15

Duke JA (accessed 2003) Chemicals. In: Acorus calamus L. (Acoraceae): Calamus, Flagroot, Myrtle Flag, Sweet Calamus, Sweetflag, Sweetroot. Dr. Duke's phytochemical and ethnobotanical databases. Agricultural Research Service (ARS), United States Department of Agriculture. Available: http://www.ars-grin.gov/duke/plants.html

Frawley D, Lad V 1986 The Yoga of herbs: an Ayurvedic guide to herbal medicine. Lotus Press, Santa Fe, p 106

Gilmore MR 1919 Uses of plants by the Indians of the Missouri River Region. SI-BAE Annual Report 33:69–70. In: Moreman, Daniel (accessed 2003) Native American ethnobotany: a database of plants used as drugs, foods, dyes, fibers, and more, by native peoples of North America. University of Michigan, Dearborne. Available: http://herb.umd.umich.edu/

Grinnell GB 1905 Some Cheyenne plant medicines. American Anthropologist 7:37–43. In: Moreman, Daniel (accessed 2003) Native American ethnobotany: a database of plants used as drugs, foods, dyes, fibers, and more, by native peoples of North America. University of Michigan, Dearborne. Available: http://herb.umd.umich.edu/

Gross MA, Jones WI, Cook EL, Biine CC 1967 Carcinogenicity of oil of calamus. Proceedings of the American Association for Cancer Research 8:24

Hart JA 1981 The ethnobotany of the Northern Cheyenne Indians of Montana. Journal of Ethnopharmacology 4:1–55. In: Moreman, Daniel (accessed 2003) Native American ethnobotany: a database of plants used as drugs, foods, dyes, fibers, and more, by native peoples of North America. University of Michigan, Dearborne. Available: http://herb.umd.umich.edu/

Kapoor LD 1990 CRC handbook of Ayurvedic medicinal plants. CRC Press, Boca Raton, p 18

Kirtikar KR, Basu BD 1935 Indian medicinal plants, 2nd edn, vols 1–4. Periodical Experts, Delhi, p 2626–2627

Lander V, Schreier P 1990 Acorenone and gamma-asarone: indicators of the origin of Calamus oils. Flavour and Fragrance Journal 5:75–79

Larry D 1973 Gas-liquid chromatographic determination of beta-asarone, a component of oil of calamus, in flavors and beverages. Journal of the AOAC 56:1281–1283

Madan BR, Arora RB, Kapila K 1960 Anticonvulsant, antiveratrinic and antiarrhythmic actions of Acorus calamus Linn – an Indian indigenous drug. Archives Internationales de Pharmacodynamie 124:201–211

Mehrotra S, Mishra KP, Maurya R et al 2003 Anticellular and immunosuppressive properties of ethanolic extract of Acorus calamus rhizome. International Immunopharmacology 3(1):53–61

Miller RA 1993 The magical and ritual use of herbs. Destiny Books, Rochester, p 58

Nadkarni KM 1954 The Indian materia medica, with Ayurvedic, Unani and home remedies, revised and enlarged by AK Nadkarni. Popular Prakashan PVP, Bombay, p 36, 37

Opdyke DJL 1977 Calamus oil. Food and Cosmetics Toxicology 15:623–626

Pancal GM, Venkatakrishna-Bhatt H, Doctor RB, Vajpayee S 1989 Pharmacology of Acorus calamus L. Indian Journal of Experimental Biology 27(6):561–567

Parab RS, Mengi SA 2002 Hypolipidemic activity of Acorus calamus L. in rats. Fitoterapia 73(6):451–455

Rafatullah S, Tariq M, Mossa JS et al 1994 Antisecretagogue, anti-ulcer and cytoprotective properties of Acorus calamus in rats. Fitoterapia 65:19

Sharma PV 2002 Cakradatta. Sanskrit text with English translation. Chaukhamba, Varanasi, p 15, 55, 88, 114, 199, 200, 236, 246, 263, 283, 294, 302

Sharma RK, Dash B 1988 Agnivesa's Caraka Saṃhitā: text with English translation and critical exposition based on Cakrapani Datta's Āyurveda Dipika, vol 3. Chaukhambha Orientalia, Varanasi, p 447

Shukla PK, Khanna VK, Ali MM et al 2002 Protective effect of Acorus calamus against acrylamide induced neurotoxicity. Phytotherapy Research 16(3):256–260

Smith GW 1973 Arctic Pharmacognosia. Arctic 26:324–333. In: Moreman, Daniel (accessed 2003) Native American ethnobotany: a database of plants used as drugs, foods, dyes, fibers, and more, by native peoples of North America. University of Michigan, Dearborne. Available: http://herb.umd.umich.edu/

Sugimoto N, Goto Y, Akao N et al 1995 Mobility inhibition and nematocidal activity of asarone and related phenylpropanoids on second-stage larvae of Toxocara canis. Biological and Pharmaceutical Bulletin 18(4):605–609

Taylor JM, Jones WI, Hagan EC et al 1967 Toxicity of Oil of Calamus (Jammu variety). Toxicology and Applied Pharmacology 10:405

Vashist VN, Handa KL 1964 A chromatographic investigation of Indian calamus oils. Soap, Perfumery and Cosmetics 37:135–139

Warrier PK, Nambiar VPK, Ramankutty C (eds) 1994 Indian medicinal plants: a compendium of 500 species, vol 1. Orient Longman, Hyderabad, p 51

Weiss R 1988 Herbal medicine. AR Meuss, translator. Beaconsfield Publishers, Beaconsfield, p 44

Williamson EM (ed) 2002 Major herbs of Ayurveda. Churchill Livingstone, London, p 16–18

Vaṃśa

BOTANICAL NAMES: *Bambusa arundinacea, B. bambos,* Bambusaceae

OTHER NAMES: ***Vaṃśarocanā*** (bamboo manna) (S); Bans, Kantabans (H); Veduruppu, Mullumangila, Mungil (T); Thorny Bamboo, Bamboo manna (E)

Botany: ***Vaṃśa*** is a tall thorny bamboo that attains a height of up to 30 m, with a stout tufted rhizome from which many stems or culms arise, each between 15 and 18 cm in diameter. The characteristic growing pattern of bamboos, in which several large culms arise from the same rhizome may be reflected in a possible meaning of ***Vaṃsa's*** Sanskrit name, 'giving out a family'. The stem nodes are prominent, from which both branch complements and stem sheaths arise in an alternating fashion. The lowest node is often found rooting, and usually has two to three short recurved spines approximately 2.5 cm in length. The internodes are between 30 and 45 cm in length, the stem sheath leathery, orange-yellow in colour when young, pubescent outside, shining and ribbed inside. The leaves are borne on secondary branch complements that arise from the node and in turn subdivide, leaflets are linear-lanceolate, linear venation, tip acute, margins entire, glabrous above and pubescent below, up to 20 cm long; the leaf sheaths hairy and small. The flowers are borne in a very large panicle that often occupies the entire stem, the branchlets containing loose clusters of pale, glabrous spikes, giving rise to oblong grains. ***Vaṃśarocanā*** ('bamboo eye') or 'bamboo manna' refers to a whitish to bluish coloured siliceous concretion that progressively accumulates in the internodes until a crack appears in the wood, exposing a part of the secretion, thought to look like an 'eye'. The specific epithet *arundinacea* means 'reed-like'. ***Vaṃśa*** is found throughout the subcontinent of India up to 2100 m in elevation, as well as in other parts of Asia, and is often cultivated (Kirtikar & Basu 1935, Krishnamurthy 1991, Warrier et al 1994).

Part used: Roots, leaves, sprouts, seeds, manna.

Dravyguṇa:

- ***Rasa***: *madhura, kaśāya* (roots, leaves); *kaṭu, tikta, kaśāya* (shoots); *kaṭu, madhura* (seeds); *madhura, kaṭu, kaśāya* (manna)
- ***Vipāka***: *madhura* (root, leaf, manna); *kaṭu* (shoot, seed)
- ***Vīrya***: *śita, rūkṣa* (root, leaf, manna); *uṣṇa, rūkṣa* (shoot, seed)
- ***Karma***: *bhedana, mūtravirecana, raktaprasādana, kuṣṭhaghna, pittakaphahara* (root); *stambhana, jvaraghna, chedana, ārtavajanana, cakṣuṣya, sadhaniya pittahara* (leaf); *bhedana, kṛmighna, mūtravirecana, vidāhi, kaphahara* (shoot); *bhedhana, kṛmighna, mūtravirecana, kaphahara* (seed); *stambhana, jvaraghna, chedana, kāsahara, svāsahara, dāhapraśamana, raktaprasādana, mūtravirecana, kuṣṭhaghna, bṛmhaṇa, vajīkaraṇa, tridoṣaghna* (manna) (Dash 1991, Kirtikar & Basu 1935, Srikanthamurthy 2001, Warrier et al 1994).

Constituents: Researchers report a cyanogenetic glycoside in the young shoots. ***Vaṃśarocanā*** (bamboo manna) consists mostly of silica or a hydrate of silic acid, with traces of iron peroxide, potash, lime, alumina, sodium and other minor constituents including organic plant material (Kapoor 1990, Yoganarasimhan 2000).

Medical research:

- ***In vitro***: insecticidal (Kapoor 1990).
- ***In vivo***: anti-inflammatory (Muniappan & Sundararaj 2003), antifertility (Vanithakumari et al 1989).

Toxicity: No data found.

Indications: Skin diseases and parasitic skin infections, burning sensations, urinary tenesmus, arthritis, debility (root); diarrhoea, haemorrhoids, fever, skin diseases, ophthalmia, amenorrhoea, dysmenorrhoea, lumbago, wounds (leaf); nausea, dyspepsia, ulcers, flatulence, intestinal parasites (shoot); intestinal parasites (seed); vomiting, haematemesis, ulcer, diarrhoea, jaundice, fever, cough, bronchitis, asthma, haemoptysis, tuberculosis, heart disease, burning sensations, haemorrhage, ophthalmia, debility (manna).

Contraindications: ***Vaṃśarocanā*** is contraindicated in constipation and should be used with caution in ***vātakopa*** conditions due its ***śita*** and ***rūkṣa vīrya***. Note, however, that this quality is offset with its more generalised anabolic or ***bṛmhaṇa*** activities. Formulating ***Vaṃśarocanā*** with ***dīpanapācana*** medicaments and using ***snigdha anupāna***, such as milk and ***ghṛta***, are recommended in ***vātakopa*** conditions.

Medicinal uses: All parts of ***Vaṃśa*** are used medicinally, but the most commonly used part of the Thorny Bamboo are the siliceous concretions called ***Vaṃśarocanā***, found accumulating within the internodes of the hollow bamboo stem. While it is possible to obtain ***Vaṃśarocanā*** commercially, Dr K. R. Srikanthamurthy (2001) states that much of what is available in the marketplace is artificial, and thus care should be taken to ensure that the natural product is obtained. Crude ***Vaṃśarocanā*** can be found as small hard white 'rocks' that are very brittle and easy to reduce to a powder. The taste is unremarkable and rather bland ('sweet'), with a slight astringency. ***Vaṃśarocanā*** is a drying herb with a trophorestorative and anti-inflammatory activity in connective tissues and mucus membranes, like other siliceous plants such as Horsetail (*Equisetum arvense*), which is similarly used in Western herbal medicine for consumptive conditions, connective tissue weakness and tissue deficiency. Research has shown that silica is important in the development and mineralisation of connective tissues, and when deficient promotes bone defects and a decline in bone minerals including calcium, phosphorus, and zinc (Reffett et al 2003, Seaborn 2002). Another interesting study showed that silica hydrate (SiOH) initiates calcium phosphate formation in developing bone by providing an acidic surface upon which apatite is nucleated from calcium phosphate solutions found in body fluids (Li et al 1995). The majority of texts indicate that ***Vaṃśarocanā*** is used in ***pitta*** and ***kapha*** disorders, and in some ***vāttika*** diseases such as dysuria (Srikanthamurthy 2001, Warrier et al 1994). Perhaps the most commonly found formula that contains ***Vaṃśarocanā*** is ***Sitopaladi cūrṇa***, consisting of 16 parts ***Sitopala*** (powdered sugar), 8 parts ***Vaṃśarocanā***, 4 parts ***Pippalī***, 2 parts ***Elā*** and 1 part ***Tvak*** bark. ***Sitopaladi cūrṇa*** can be taken by itself, mixed with water or milk, or taken with honey and/or ***ghṛta*** in the treatment of poor appetite, fever, dyspnoea, cough, consumption, haemoptysis and burning sensations (Sharma 2002). There are several other complex formulations that contain ***Vaṃśarocanā*** and are used in the treatment of consumptive diseases (***yakṣmā***), including ***Elādi mantha***, ***Sarpiguḍa*** and ***Cyavanaprāśa***. In the treatment of colic the ***Cakradatta*** mentions a few recipes that include ***Vaṃsarocanā***, along with herbs such as ***Nārikela***, ***Dhānyaka***, ***Pippalī***, ***Jīraka*** and ***Mustaka*** (Sharma 2002). Prepared as a medicated ***ghṛta Vaṃśarocanā*** is used in combination with ***Citraka***, ***Sārivā***, ***Balā***, ***Kālānusārivā***, ***Drākṣā***, ***Viśāla***, ***Yaṣṭimadhu*** and ***Āmalakī*** in the treatment of dysuria and infertility (Sharma 2002). Evidence of its reputed aphrodisiac properties can be found in the ***Cakradatta***, in which ***Vaṃśarocanā*** is mixed with fresh yoghurt, sugar, honey, ***Elā*** and ***Marica***, and is eaten with rice and ***ghṛta*** (Sharma 2002). ***Vaṃśa*** roots are used in eruptive conditions, and are burnt and then applied topically in ringworm, bleeding gums and joint pain (Kirtikar & Basu 1935). The ***Cakradatta*** includes ***Vaṃśa*** in a list of ingredients for a formula called ***Varuṇa ghṛta***, used in the treatment of urinary calculi and dysuria (Sharma 2002). The leaves are traditionally used as an emmenagogue, as an eyewash, and as a ***pittahara*** remedy in conditions such as fever, biliousness, bronchitis, and haemorrhoids (Kirtikar & Basu 1935, Nadkarni 1954). The young shoots are pickled and given in ***agnimāndya***, and are used topically as a poultice or the fresh juice in the treatment of parasitic skin infections (Kirtikar & Basu 1935, Nadkarni 1954). The seeds are stated to have been used as a food by the poorer classes in India, and have antihelminthic activities (Nadkarni 1954, Warrier et al 1994).

Dosage: ***Vaṃśarocanā***

- ***Cūrṇa***: 3–5 g b.i.d.–t.i.d.
- ***Kvātha***: in milk, 60–120 mL b.i.d.–t.i.d.

REFERENCES

Dash B 1991 Materia medica of Ayurveda. B. Jain Publishers, New Delhi, p 127–128

Frawley D, Lad V 1986 The Yoga of herbs: an Ayurvedic guide to herbal medicine. Lotus Press, Santa Fe

Kapoor LD 1990 CRC handbook of Ayurvedic medicinal plants. CRC Press, Boca Raton, p 66

Kirtikar KR, Basu BD 1935 Indian medicinal plants, 2nd edn, vols 1–4. Periodical Experts, Delhi, p 2724–2726

Krishnamurthy KH 1991 Wealth of Suśruta. International Institute of Ayurveda, Coimbatore, p 452

Li P, Ye X, Kangasniemi I et al 1995 In vivo calcium phosphate formation induced by sol-gel-prepared silica. Journal of Biomedical Materials Research 29(3):325–328

Muniappan M, Sundararaj T 2003 Anti-inflammatory and antiulcer activities of Bambusa arundinacea. Journal of Ethnopharmacology 88(2–3):161–167

Nadkarni KM 1954 The Indian materia medica, with Ayurvedic, Unani and home remedies, revised and enlarged by AK Nadkarni. Popular Prakashan PVP, Bombay, p 173–174

Reffitt DM, Ogston N, Jugdaohsingh R et al 2003 Orthosilicic acid stimulates collagen type 1 synthesis and osteoblastic differentiation in human osteoblast-like cells in vitro. Bone 32(2):127–135

Seaborn CD, Nielsen FH 2002 Dietary silicon and arginine affect mineral element composition of rat femur and vertebra. Biological Trace Element Research 89(3):239–250

Sharma PV 2002 Cakradatta. Sanskrit text with English translation. Chaukhamba, Varanasi, p 135, 259, 262, 279, 316, 322, 650–651

Srikanthamurthy KR 2001 Bhāvaprakāśa of Bhāvamiśra, vol 1. Krishnadas Academy, Varanasi, p 176–178, 252, 376

Vanithakumari G, Manonayagi S, Padma S, Malini T 1989 Antifertility effect of Bambusa arundinacea shoot extracts in male rats. Journal of Ethnopharmacology 25(2):173–180

Warrier PK, Nambiar VPK, Ramankutty C (eds) 1994 Indian medicinal plants: a compendium of 500 species, vol 1. Orient Longman, Hyderabad, p 244–246

Yoganarasimhan SN 2000 Medicinal plants of India, vol 2: Tamil Nadu. Self-published, Bangalore, p 69

Vāsaka

BOTANICAL NAMES: *Adhatoda vasica* (syn. *Justicia adhatoda, A. zeylanica*), *A. beddomei, Acanthaceae*

OTHER NAMES: ***Vasa*** (S); Adosa, Adarsa, Adulasa, (H); Adadodi, Kattumurungai (T); Malabar nut (E)

Botany: ***Vāsaka*** is a dense evergreen shrub between 1.2 and 2.4 m high, with long ascending branches covered in a yellowish bark, oppositely arranged. The glabrous leathery leaves are borne on short petioles, elliptic-lanceolate, tip acute, minutely hairy when young. The flowers arise in short, dense terminal pedunculate spikes with large bracts, the corolla white, streaked pink or purple within. The fruit is a small club-shaped capsule with longitudinal channels, containing four to six seeds. ***Vāsaka*** is found wild and cultivated in a diverse range of habitats throughout tropical India and S.E. Asia up to 1300 m in elevation. *A. beddomei* is found primarily in the hilly forest regions of Kerala (Kirtikar & Basu 1935, Warrier et al 1995, Williamson 2002).

Part used: Root, bark, leaf, flower.

Dravyguṇa:

- ***Rasa***: *tikta, kaśāya*
- ***Vipāka***: *kaṭu*
- ***Vīrya***: *śita, laghu, rūkṣa*
- ***Karma***: *chardinigrahaṇa, bhedana, jvaraghna, chedana, kāsahara, svāsahara, śoṇitasthāpana, raktasprasadana, mūtravirecana, śotahara, kuṣṭhaghna, sandhānīya, pittakaphahara* (Dash 1991, Kirtikar & Basu 1935, Srikanthamurthy 2001, Warrier et al 1995).

Constituents: The most widely studied constituents in *A. vasica* are the quinazoline and pyrroloquinazoline alkaloids, of which vasicine (peganine) is the major. Other related alkaloids include vasicinone, adhatodine, adhatonine and vasicoline in the leaves, and vasicinol, vasicinolone, vasicinone, adhatonine and vasicol in the roots. ***Vāsaka*** also contains flavonoids (e.g. apigenin, astragalin, kaempferol and quercitin), the phytosterols β-sitosterol and daucosterol, triterpenes α-amyrin and epitaraxerol, an essential oil containing at least 36 different components including the ketone 4-heptanone, as well as fatty acids and hydrocarbons (Kapoor 1990, Williamson 2002, Yoganarasimhan 2000).

Medical research:
- ***In vitro***: anti-inflammatory (Cakraborty & Brantner 2001).
- ***In vivo***: antitussive (Dhuley 1999); immunostimulant (Grange and Snell 1996), anti-allergenic (Paliwa et al 2000).
- ***Human trials***: an azepinoquinazoline isolated from ***Vāsaka*** was determined to have a potent bronchodilatory effect in humans (Malhotra et al 1988); the alkaloid vasicine isolated from ***Vāsaka*** was found to exert an oxytocic and uterostimulant effect in human volunteers, without negative effects, when injected as a saline solution from the second to eighth day after childbirth (Wakhloo et al 1980).

Toxicity: The compound 7,8,9,10-tetrahydroazepino (2,1-b)-quinazoline-12(6H)-one, isolated from *A. vasica* was determined to have no negative effect upon fertility and reproduction in rats (Pahwa & Zutshi 1993).

Indications: Nausea and vomiting, hepatitis, bleeding diarrhoea, fever, catarrh, cough, asthma, consumption, haemoptysis, menorrhagia, passive haemorrhage, rheumatism, inflammatory joint disease, ophthalmia.

Contraindications: ***vātakopa***; ***Vāsaka*** is contraindicated in pregnancy due to its oxytocic effects, although it may be safely used as a parturient and post-parturient.

Medicinal uses: ***Vāsaka*** is among the most commonly used medicaments in the treatment of respiratory disorders in Āyurvedic medicine, favoured especially in cases marked by haemoptysis, dyspnoea and wasting. The simplest application of ***Vāsaka*** is to simply pluck off a flower bud or the leaves and chew them. As a remedy for cough and bronchitis the fresh juice can be taken in doses of between 10 and 25 mL, mixed with a smaller amount of fresh ***Śuṇṭhī*** juice and honey. An infusion of the leaf or decoction of the root may also be taken with ***Pippalī cūrṇa*** and honey for coughs, bronchitis and asthma. The fresh juice mixed with honey and sugar is used in the treatment of fevers caused by ***pitta*** and ***kapha***, as well as in jaundice (Sharma 2002). In the treatment of hoarseness, haemoptysis and asthma the fresh juice can also be taken with ***Tālīśa*** leaf and honey (Sharma 2002). In the treatment of cough, dyspnoea, haemoptysis, chest wounds, and consumption the ***Cakradatta*** recommends ***Vāsākhaṇḍa***, prepared by decocting 4 kg of ***Vāsaka*** in eight times its volume of water and reducing this to one quarter of its original volume. To this are added sugar (4 kg) and the powders of ***Harītakī*** (2.56 kg) and ***Pippalī*** (80 g). This is decocted further, after which honey (160 g) and ***Caturjāta*** (40 g, comprising equal parts ***Elā***, ***Tvak*** bark, ***Patra*** leaf and ***Nāgakeśara***) are added when cool (Sharma 2002). Decocted with ***Aśvagandhā***, ***Śatāvarī***, ***Daśamūla*** ('ten roots' formula), ***Balā***, ***Puṣkaramūla*** and purified ***Ativiṣā***, ***Vāsaka*** is used in wasting caused by consumptive conditions, taken along with a diet rich in meat and dairy (Sharma 2002). For conditions marked by catarrh ***Vāsaka*** is also recommended in ***dhūma***, and as an emergency remedy for asthma attacks can be smoked in combination with parasympatholytics such as ***Dhattūra***. In the treatment of vomiting the ***Cakradatta*** recommends a paste of ***Vāsaka***, ***Candana***, ***Uśīra***, ***Balāka***, and ***Śuṇṭhī***, taken with rice water (Sharma 2002). A poultice of the leaves and decoction of the root is also used in rheumatic afflictions and joint pain. Decocted with ***Guḍūcī*** and ***Āragvadha***, and taken with castor oil, the ***Cakradatta*** states that ***Vāsaka*** is taken as a general remedy for ***vātarakta*** (gout) (Sharma 2002).

Noted for its oxytocic effects ***Vāsaka*** root is highly regarded as a parturient in stalled labour, and can help to check post-partum haemorrhage. The antihaemorrhagic properties also indicates ***Vāsaka*** in other diseases marked by passive hemorrhage (***rakta pitta***), including bleeding diarrhoea, menorrhagia and epistaxis, taken in various forms as well as a medicated ***ghṛta*** (Sharma 2002). In combination with ***Harītakī***, ***Nimba***, ***Āmalakī***, ***Mustaka***, ***Bibhītaka***, and ***Kupīlu***, Vaidya Mana Bajracharya (1997) indicates that ***Vāsaka*** is useful in formulations used to treat dacryohaemorrhoea and dacryoblenorrhoea. In the treatment of wounds, insect and snake bites the fresh plant poultice is applied externally, the fresh juice or infusion taken internally at the same time (Kirtikar & Basu 1935). ***Vāsaka*** has also been traditionally used as an insecticide, and can be applied as a medicated oil of the root with ***Nimba*** and ***Haridrā*** in the treatment of scabies, and when mixed with ***Śaṅka bhasma*** the fresh juice is used to remove foul body odours (Nadkarni 1954).

Dosage:

- ***Svarasa***: 10–25 mL b.i.d.–t.i.d.
- ***Cūrṇa***: 2–5 g b.i.d.–t.i.d.
- ***Kvātha***: 30–120 mL b.i.d.–t.i.d.
- ***Tincture***: root and bark, 1:3, 50%; 2–5 mL b.i.d.–t.i.d.

REFERENCES

Bajracharya M, Tillotson A, Abel R 1997 Ayurvedic ophthalmology: a recension of the Shalakya Tantra of Videhadhipati Janaka. Piyushabarshi Aushadhalaya Mahabouddha, Kathmandu, p 66–67

Cakraborty A, Brantner AH 2001 Study of alkaloids from Adhatoda vasica Nees on their anti-inflammatory activity. Phytotherapy Research 15(6):532–534

Dash B 1991 Materia medica of Ayurveda. B. Jain Publishers, New Delhi, p 127

Dhuley JN 1999 Antitussive effect of Adhatoda vasica extract on mechanical or chemical stimulation-induced coughing in animals. Journal of Ethnopharmacology 67(3):361–365

Grange JM, Snell NJ 1996 Activity of bromhexine and ambroxol, semi-synthetic derivatives of vasicine from the Indian shrub Adhatoda vasica, against Mycobacterium tuberculosis in vitro. Journal of Ethnopharmacology 50(1):49–53

Kapoor LD 1990 CRC handbook of Ayurvedic medicinal plants. CRC Press, Boca Raton, p 216

Kirtikar KR, Basu BD 1935 Indian medicinal plants, 2nd edn, vols 1–4. Periodical Experts, Delhi, p 1899–1902

Malhotra S, Koul SK, Sharma RL et al 1988 Studies on some biologically active azepinoquinazolines: Part I, an approach to potent bronchodilatory compounds. Indian Journal of Chemistry 27B:937–940

Nadkarni KM 1954 The Indian materia medica, with Ayurvedic, Unani and home remedies, revised and enlarged by AK Nadkarni. Popular Prakashan PVP, Bombay, p 42

Pahwa GS, Zutshi U 1993 Short communication effect of 7,8,9,10-tetrahydroazepino(2,1-b)-quinazoline-12(6H)-one, a new anti-asthmatic compound on reproduction in rat and rabbit. Indian Journal of Pharmacology 25(2):101–102

Paliwa JK, Dwivedi AK, Singh S, Gutpa RC 2000 Pharmacokinetics and in-situ absorption studies of a new anti-allergic compound 73/602 in rats. International Journal of Pharmaceutics 197(1–2):213–220

Sharma PV 2002 Cakradatta: Sanskrit text with English translation. Chaukhamba, Varanasi p 19, 123, 127, 131, 134, 168, 233

Srikanthamurthy KR 2001 Bhāvaprakāśa of Bhāvamiśra, vol 1. Krishnadas Academy, Varanasi, p 241

Wakhloo RL, Girija K, Gupta OP, Atal CK 1980 Short communication safety of vasicine hydrochloride in human volunteers. Indian Journal of Pharmacology 12(2):129–131

Warrier PK, Nambiar VPK, Ramankutty C (eds) 1995 Indian medicinal plants: a compendium of 500 species, vol 3. Orient Longman, Hyderabad, p 268–271

Williamson EM (ed) 2002 Major herbs of Ayurveda. Churchill Livingstone, London, p 20

Yoganarasimhan SN 2000 Medicinal plants of India, vol 2: Tamil Nadu. Self-published, Bangalore, p 22

Viḍaṅga, 'skilful'

BOTANICAL NAME: *Embelia ribes,* Myrsinaceae

OTHER NAMES: ***Vellah*** (S)*;* Baberang, Viranga (H); Vayuvilanga, Vilal, Kattukodi (T); Embelia (E)

Botany: ***Viḍaṅga*** is a large climbing shrub with long slender branches, long internodes, and the bark studded with lenticels. The leathery leaves are simple, alternate, elliptic-lanceolate, obtusely acuminate, shiny green and glabrous above, silvery below, with scattered, minute sunken glands. The small white to greenish white flowers are borne in terminal and axillary panicled racemes, the calyx five-lobed, the corolla hairy with five stamens. The fruit is a smooth globose berry, consisting of a thin reddish coloured pericarp containing a single seed. ***Viḍaṅga*** is found in forested hilly areas, from the Himalayas southwards into Tamil Nadu, Kerala and Sri Lanka, as well as throughout S.E. Asia (Kirtikar & Basu 1935 Warrier et al 1994).

Part used: Fruit, leaves, root.

Dravyguṇa: Fruit

- ***Rasa***: *kaśāya, kaṭu*
- ***Vipāka***: *laghu*
- ***Vīrya***: *uṣṇa, rūkṣa, laghu*
- ***Karma***: *dīpanapācana, bhedana, kṛmighna, jvaraghna, mūtravirecana, raktaprasādana, kuṣṭhaghna, vedanāsthāpana, sandhānīya, kaphavātahara* (Dash 1991, Kirtikar & Basu 1935, Srikanthamurthy 2001, Warrier et al 1994).

Constituents: The most studied chemical in ***Viḍaṅga*** is embelin (embolic acid), or rather, potassium embelate (2,5-dihydroxy,3-undecyl-1,4-benzoquinone). A related quinone found in ***Viḍaṅga*** is vilangin, a structure of two embelin mocules attached with a CH_2 bridge. Other constituents include the alkaloid christembine, a volatile oil, quercitol, tannins and fatty acids (Kapoor 1990, Yoganarasimhan 2000).

Medical research:

- ***In vitro***: antibacterial (Chitra et al 2003).
- ***In vivo***: antifertility (Agrawal et al 1986, Seth et al 1982); analgesic (Atal et al 1984, Zutshi et al 1989); hypoglycaemic, hypolipidaemic (Bhandari et al 2002); antitumour (Chitra et al 2003).
- ***Human trials***: ***Viḍaṅga*** has been found to be safe and effective as a female contraceptive, with encouraging results in phase-I clinical trials (Sharma et al 2001); a 400 mg tablet of ***Viḍaṅga*** given each morning for 10 days beginning on the fifth day of menstruation in fertile women was found to be an effective contraceptive agent, without side-effects (Shah 1971).

Toxicity: *Embelia ribes* has been reported to possibly cause optic atrophy among the Ethiopian population. Researchers examined this potential by feeding newly born chicks the crude herb in both high doses (5 g/kg per day) and low doses (0.5 g/kg per day), along with regular chick feed. Treatment with *E. ribes* was found to dose-dependently reduce the peripheral field of vision, and interfered with visual discrimination tasks. Researchers compared these effects with the administration of purified embelin isolated from *E. ribes*, and found that these effects were mimicked, suggesting that embelin may be responsible for the visual defects. Anatomical evidence of degeneration of ganglion cells was found in retinae exposed to high doses of *E. ribes* but no retinal lesions were detected in chicks following treatment with cumulative doses of less than 5 g/kg per day (Low et al 1985). Potassium embelate, or 2,5-dihydroxy,3-undecyl-1,4-benzoquinone, isolated from *Embelia ribes* was subjected to toxicity evaluation which included subacute, chronic, reproductive toxicity testing and teratological investigations in laboratory mice, rats and monkeys. The results did not indicate adverse effects, suggesting that potassium embelate is a safe compound (Johri et al

1990). Researchers report that equal parts powders of *Embelia ribes*, *Piper longum* and borax fed to pregnant rats resulted in low birth weights, with cases of herniation of the intestines into the umbilical cord and mothers gaining less weight during gestation (Chaudhury et al 2001).

Indications: Poor appetite, tooth decay, dyspepsia, flatulence, colic, constipation, intestinal parasites, fever, cough, asthma, cardiac debility, skin diseases, skin infection, tumour, psychosis, debility and weakness.

Contraindications: ***Pittakopa***; pregnancy, diarrhoea, bowel inflammation.

Medicinal uses: ***Viḍaṅga*** has many uses in Āyurvedic medicine but most importantly is used to dispel intestinal worms and fungal pathogens such as ringworm. It is, however, a comparatively pleasant remedy, and the dried fruit could even be chewed like pumpkin seeds if it were not for the acrid, burning sensation that occurs in the back of the throat shortly after ingestion, reminiscent of black pepper. In most instances about 8–12 g of the seed will be powdered and administered with honey, followed with a little warm water, taken first thing in the morning on an empty stomach. No food is taken for the entire day, and the next morning castor oil is taken to expel the dead worms. One recipe that is reputed to 'destroy all worms as a thunderbolt does demons' is ***Viḍaṅga ghṛta***, prepared by decocting 24 parts ***Triphala***, eight parts ***Viḍaṅga*** and one part ***Daśamūla*** in 128 parts water until the quantity of water is reduced to one-fourth of its original volume. The decoction is then strained and mixed with eight parts ***ghṛta*** and some ***saindhava*** added in for good measure, and decocted until there is no water remaining (Sharma 2002), 3–6 g b.i.d.–t.i.d., taken with warm water. In the treatment of heart pain caused by parasitic infection the ***Cakradatta*** recommends a fermented gruel of barley mixed with the powders of ***Viḍaṅga*** and ***Kuṣṭha*** (Sharma 2002). In the treatment of ringworm ***Viḍaṅga*** can be prepared in mustard oil or applied as a paste, and applied topically. Beyond its use in parasitic infections, however, ***Viḍaṅga*** is an important remedy in both ***vāttika*** and ***kaphaja*** conditions, used in dryness of the bowels, constipation, colic and flatulence as well as in ***kaphaja*** polyuria and obesity. Due to its pungent properties ***Viḍaṅga*** is an effective sialagogue and digestive stimulant, both the roots and fruit used in anorexia as well as a powder in the treatment of dental caries as a dentifrice. As a digestive stimulant used especially in inflammatory joint disease (***āmavāta***) the ***Cakradatta*** recommends a combination of ***Viḍaṅga***, ***Śatapuṣpā***, ***Marica*** and ***saindhava*** taken with warm water (Sharma 2002). In the treatment of severe colic the dehusked ***Viḍaṅga*** seed is reduced to a powder and taken along with equal parts powders of ***Trikaṭu***, ***Trivṛt***, ***Dañtī*** and ***Citraka***, mixed into balls with jaggery, taken in the morning in doses of 3–5 g with warm water (Sharma 2002). In the treatment of constipation marked by hardness of the bowels, flatulence, colic and abdominal pain the ***Cakradatta*** recommends a ***cūrṇa*** composed of five parts ***Viḍaṅga***, four parts ***svarjika kṣāra*** (an alkali containing sodium bicarbonate), three parts ***Kuṣṭha***, two parts ***Vacā*** and one part ***Hiṅgu*** (Sharma 2002). Mixed with equal parts ***Trikaṭu***, ***Citraka***, ***Bhallātaka***, ***Tila*** and ***Harītakī***, ***Viḍaṅga*** is used in the treatment of haemorrhoids, skin diseases, oedema, constipation, intestinal parasites, anaemia and poisoning (Sharma 2002). In the treatment of abdominal tumours (***gulma***) the ***Cakradatta*** recommends a medicated ***ghṛta*** prepared by decocting ***Viḍaṅga*** with equal parts ***Trikaṭu***, ***Triphala***, ***Dhānyaka***, ***Cavya***, and ***Citraka***, in milk and ***ghṛta*** until only the ***ghṛta*** remains (Sharma 2002). In the treatment of splenomegaly (***plīhan***) the ***Cakradatta*** recommends ***Viḍaṅga dikṣāra***, composed of equal parts ***Viḍaṅga***, ***Citraka***, ***Vacā*** and flour, mixed with ***ghṛta*** and reduced to ash, taken with milk (Sharma 2002). Mixed with equal parts ***Harītakī***, ***Śūṇṭhī***, ***Trivṛt***, ***Marica*** and ***saindhava***, ***Viḍaṅga*** is mixed with cow's urine and used as a purgative in ***virecana*** therapy (Sharma 2002). Although used mostly for its ***bhedana*** properties, ***Viḍaṅga*** mixed with purified ***Ativiṣā***, ***Mustaka***, ***Devadāru***, ***Pāṭhā*** and ***Indrayava***, with six parts ***Marica***, is used in the treatment of diarrhoea with oedema (Sharma 2002). The root and bark of ***Viḍaṅga*** are used similarly to the seed, applied topically as a counter-irritant in joint disease, rheumatism and lung congestion. The freshly chopped leaves or leaf juice can be applied topically in the treatment of skin diseases and wounds.

Dosage: fruit, root, bark

- ***Cūrṇa***: 3–12 g b.i.d.–t.i.d.

- ***Kvātha***: 1:4, 30–90 mL
- ***Taila***: topically, as needed.

REFERENCES

Agrawal S, Chauhan S, Mathur R 1986 Antifertility effects of embelin in male rats. Andrologia 18(2):125–131

Atal CK, Siddiqui MA, Zutshi U et al 1984 Non-narcotic orally effective, centrally acting analgesic from an Ayurvedic drug. Journal of Ethnopharmacology 11(3):309–317

Bhandari U, Kanojia R, Pillai KK 2002 Effect of ethanolic extract of Embelia ribes on dyslipidemia in diabetic rats. International Journal of Experimental Diabetes Research 3(3):159–162

Chaudhury MR, Chandrasekaran R, Mishra S 2001 Embryotoxicity and teratogenicity studies of an Ayurvedic contraceptive: pippaliyadi vati. Journal of Ethnopharmacology 74(2):189–193

Chitra M, Devi CS, Sukumar E 2003 Antibacterial activity of embelin. Fitoterapia 74(4):401–403

Dash B 1991 Materia medica of Ayurveda. B. Jain Publishers, New Delhi, p 149

Johri RK, Dhar SK, Pahwa GS et al 1990 Toxicity studies with potassium embelate, a new analgesic compound. Indian Journal of Experimental Biology 28(3):213–217

Kapoor LD 1990 CRC handbook of Ayurvedic medicinal plants. CRC Press, Boca Raton, p 174

Kirtikar KR, Basu BD 1935 Indian medicinal plants, 2nd edn, vols 1–4. Periodical Experts, Delhi, p 1478

Low G, Rogers LJ, Brumley SP, Ehrlich D 1985 Visual deficits and retinotoxicity caused by the naturally occurring anthelmintics, Embelia ribes and Hagenia abyssinica. Toxicology and Applied Pharmacology 81(2):220–230

Seth SD, Johri N, Sundaram KR 1982 Antispermatogenic effect of embelin from Embelia ribes. Indian Journal of Pharmacology 14(2):207–211

Shah NK 1971 A study of an indigenous drug Maswin as an oral contraceptive. Current Medical Practice 15(2):614–616

Sharma PV 2002 Cakradatta. Sanskrit text with English translation. Chaukhamba, Varanasi, p 47, 83, 112, 249, 270, 286, 296, 305, 350, 672

Sharma RS, Rajalakshmi M, Jeyaraj DA 2001 Current status of fertility control methods in India. Journal of Biosciences 26(4 Suppl):391–405

Srikanthamurthy KR 2001 Bhāvaprakāśa of Bhāvamiśra, vol 1. Krishnadas Academy, Varanasi, p 177

Warrier PK, Nambiar VPK, Ramankutty C (eds) 1994 Indian medicinal plants: a compendium of 500 species, vol 2. Orient Longman, Hyderabad, p 368–371

Yoganarasimhan SN 2000 Medicinal plants of India, vol 2: Tamil Nadu. Self-published, Bangalore, p 211

Zutshi U, Johri RK, Atal CK 1989 Possible interaction of potassium embelate, a putative analgesic agent, with opiate receptors. Indian Journal of Experimental Biology 27(7):656–657

Yavānī

BOTANICAL NAMES: *Trachyspermum ammi, T. copticum, Carum copticum, C. ajowan, Ptychotis ajowan,* Apiaceae

OTHER NAMES: ***Yavānī, Agnivardhana*** (S); Ajmud, Ajwain (H); Ashamtavomam, Omam (T); Bishop's Weed (E)

SIMILAR SPECIES: ***Ajamodā*** (*Trachyspermum roxiburghianum,* Apiaceae)

Botany: ***Yavānī*** is an erect annual herb that attains a height of between 60 and 90 cm, with striate stems, the leaves pinnately divided two to three times. The white flowers are borne in compound umbels, the fruits small, ridged and compressed. ***Yavānī*** is found throughout the subcontinent of India, mostly as a cultivated herb, a natural range that extends westwards into the Middle East and Europe (Kirtikar & Basu 1935, Warrier et al 1996).

Part used: Seeds.

Dravyguṇa:

- ***Rasa***: *kaṭu, tikta*
- ***Vipāka***: *kaṭu*
- ***Vīrya***: *uṣṇa, laghu, rūkṣa*
- ***Karma***: *dīpanapācana, anulomana, kṛmighna, svāsahara, kaphavātahara* (Srikanthamurthy 2001, Warrier et al 1996).

Constituents: ***Yavānī*** seeds contain an essential oil comprising *p*-cymene, dipentene, α- and β-pinenes, γ-terpinene, thymol, camphene, myrcene, δ-3-carene, limonene, carvascrol and others. In 2001 Ishikawa et al isolated 25 different water-soluble constituents, including two monoterpenoids, eight light monoterpenoid glucosides, one alkyl glucoside, three aromatic glucosides, two nucleosides and eight glucides. ***Yavānī*** also contains a fixed oil containing resin acids, palmatic acid, petroselenic acid, oleic acid and linoleic acid, and nutrients riboflavin, thiamin, nicotinic acid, carotene, calcium, chromium, cobalt, copper, iodine, iron, manganese, phosphorus, and zinc (Ishikawa et al 2001, Williamson 2002, Yoganarasimhan 2000).

Medical research:

- ***In vitro***: antiviral (Hussein et al 2000), antithrombotic (Srivastava 1988).
- ***In vivo***: antispasmodic, antihistamine (Boskabady & Shaikhi 2000); antibacterial (Singh et al 2002).

Toxicity: Duke states that ***Yavānī*** contains between 3633 and 33 000 p.p.m. of thymol, which is stated to have an oral LD_{50} of 0.98 g/kg in rats and 0.88 g/kg in guinea pigs. ***Yavānī***, however, is a commonly used culinary spice and is generally recognised as safe (Duke 2005, Williamson 2002).

Indications: Dyspepsia, flatulent colic, intestinal parasites, cough, bronchitis, asthma, rheumatism, urinary tenesmus.

Contraindications: ***pittakopa***.

Medicinal uses: ***Yavānī*** is a popular household remedy for poor digestion, and when taken in sufficient quantities imparts a pleasant sensation of warmth and relaxation in cases of dyspepsia and flatulent colic. For this purpose a simple infusion can be made, along with ***Śūṇṭhī*** and ***Dhānyaka***, or the seed can be ground into a powder and consumed with one-quarter part ***saindhava***. The essential oils in ***Yavānī*** act as an antispasmodic, and thus the herb finds use in intestinal and urinary spasm, and is often added along with ***virecana dravyas*** to inhibit spasm. Combined with herbs such as Wild Yam (*Dioscorea villosa*) and Fringe Tree (*Chionanthus virginicus*), ***Yavānī*** is an effective remedy in cholecystalgia. ***Yavānī*** is the chief constituent in ***Yavānī cūrṇa***, a formulation

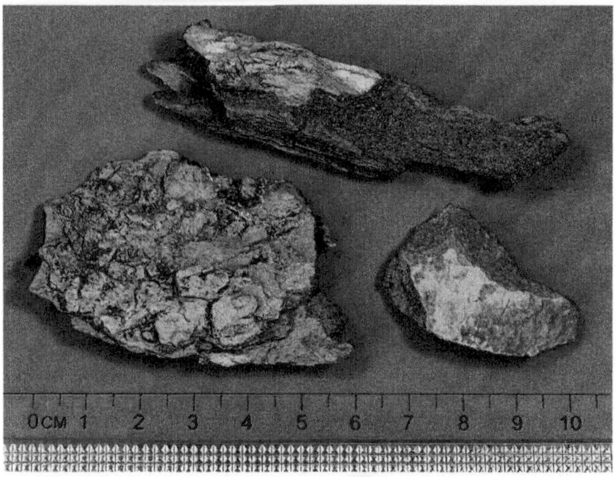

Figure 1

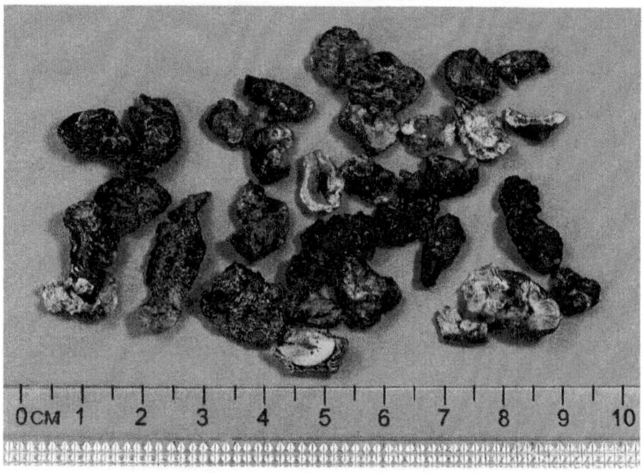

Figure 2

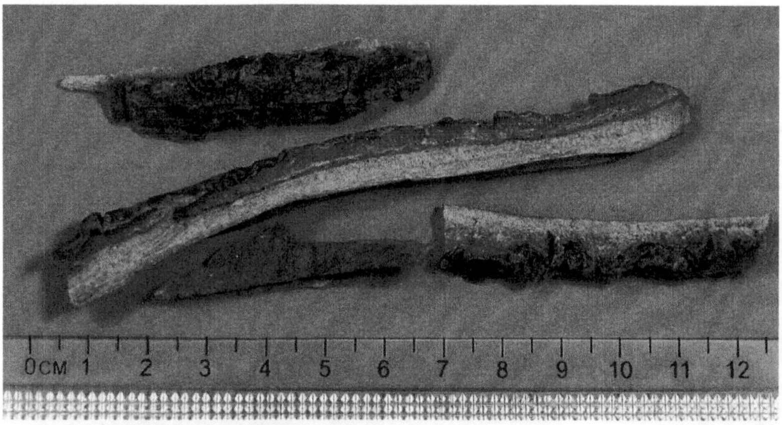

Figure 3

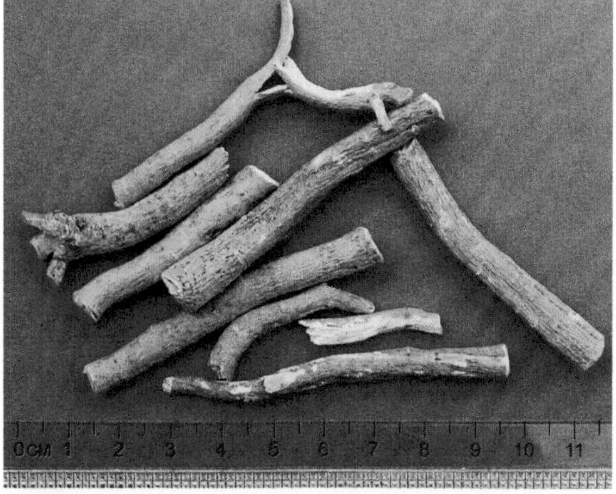

Figure 4

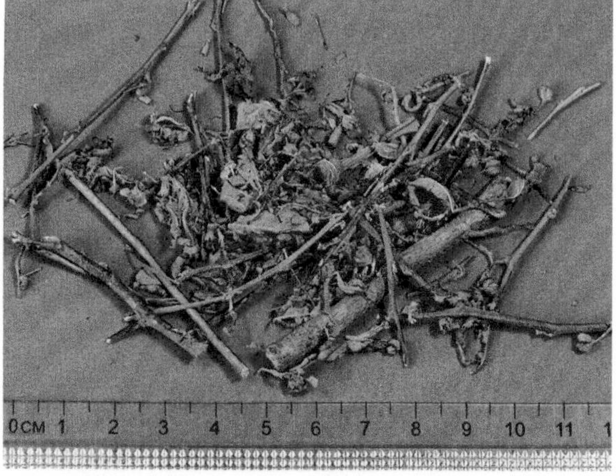

Figure 5

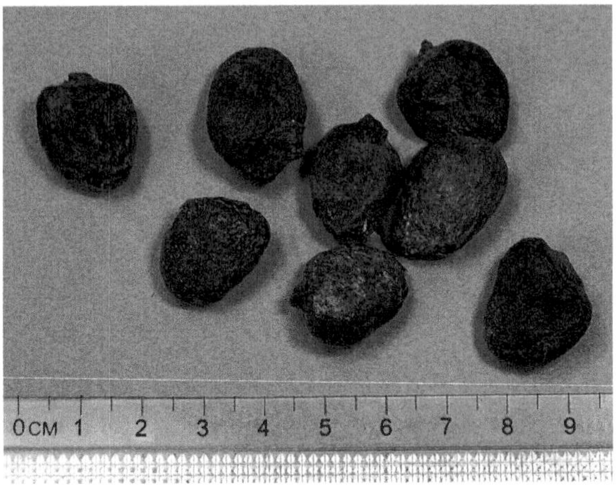

Figure 6

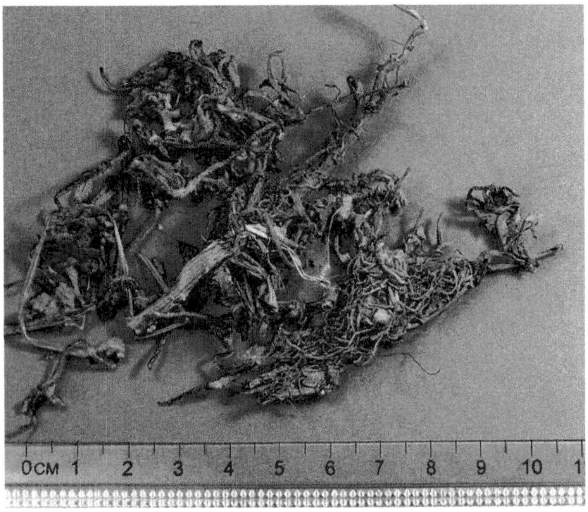

Figure 7

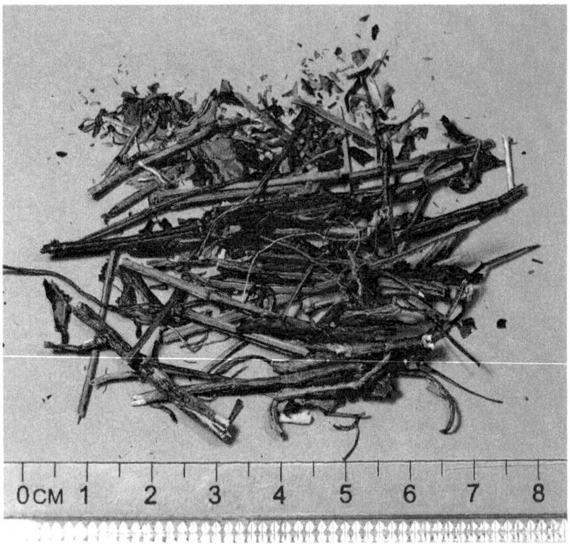

Figure 8

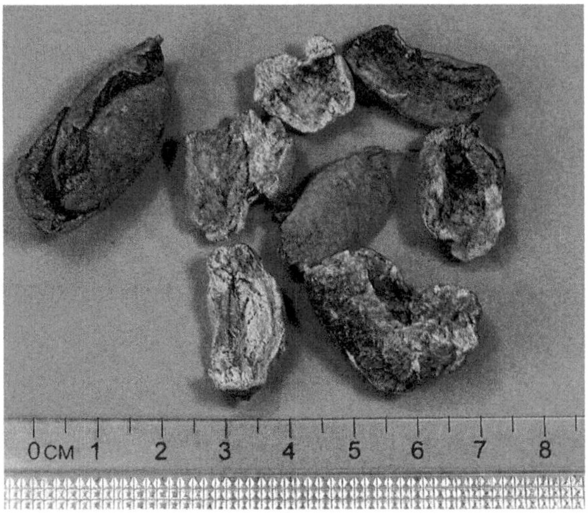

Figure 9

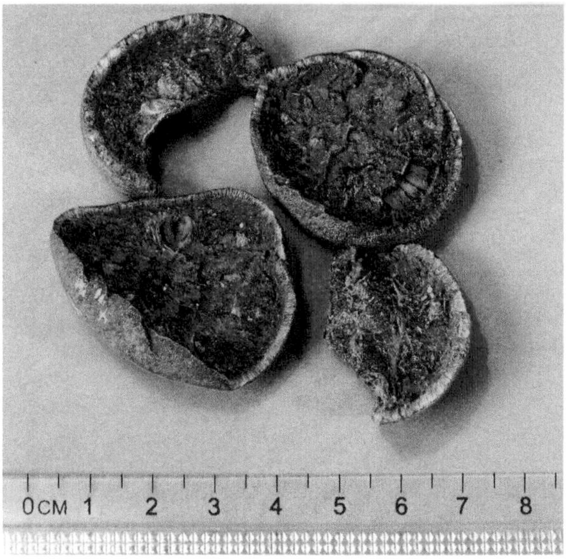

Figure 10

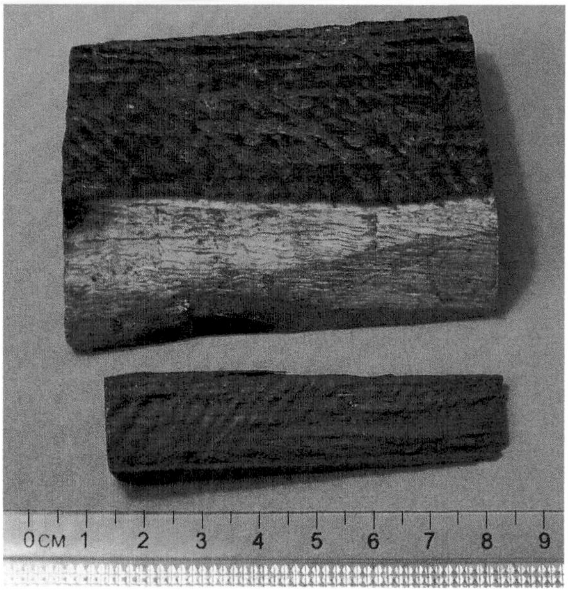

Figure 12

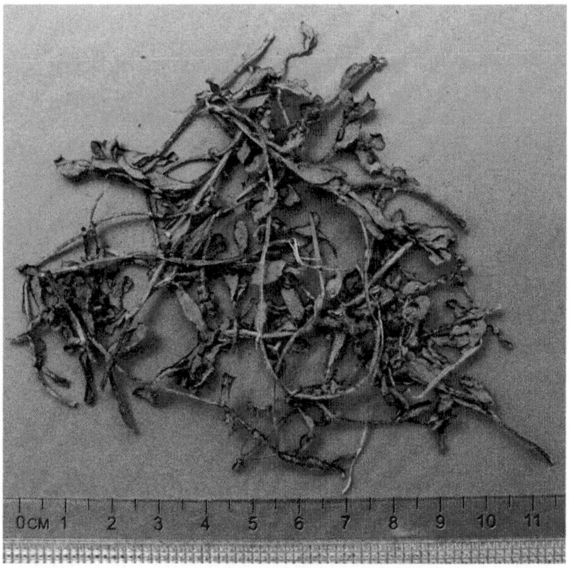

Figure 11

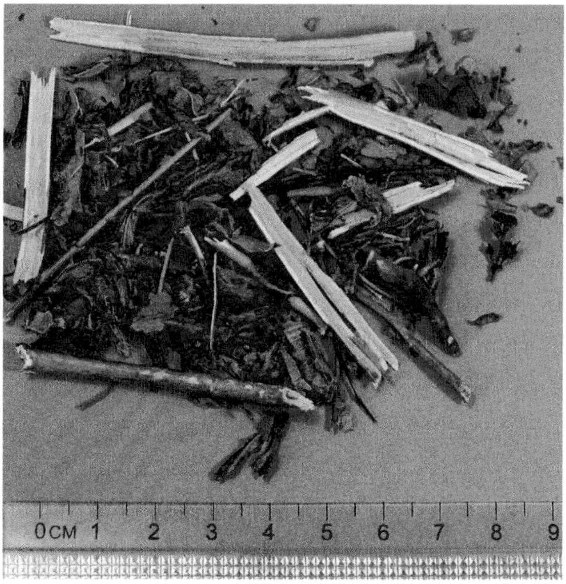

Figure 13

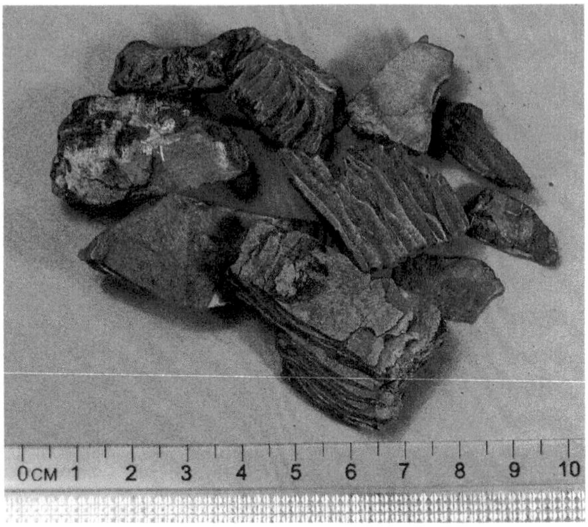

Figure 14

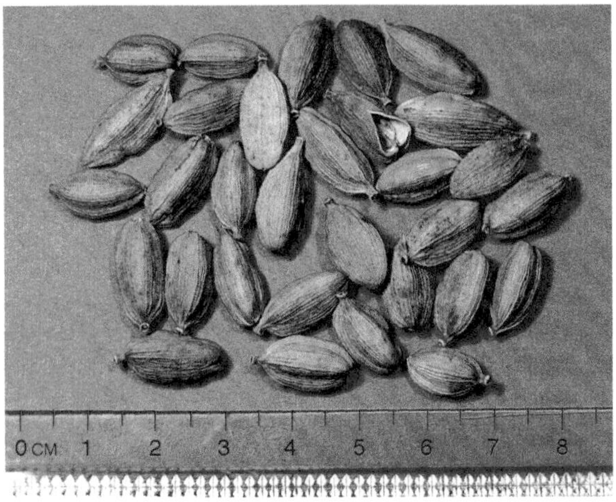

Figure 15

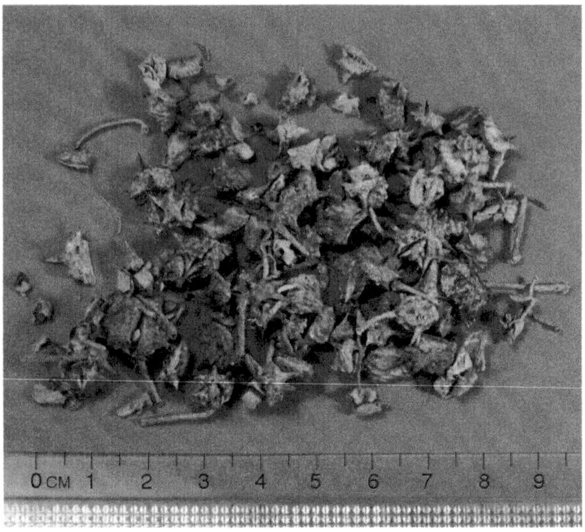

Figure 16

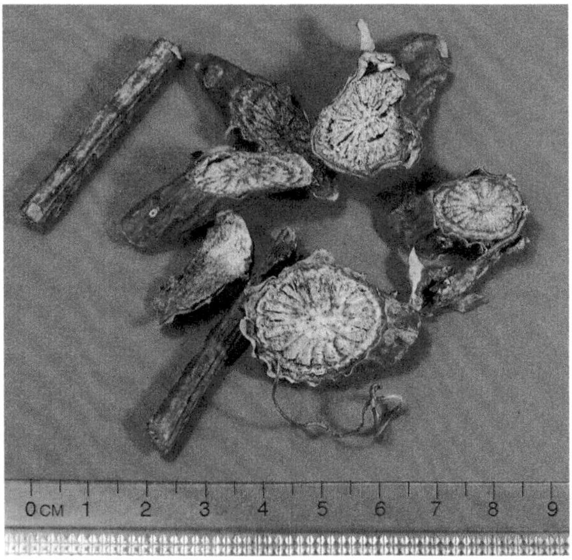

Figure 17

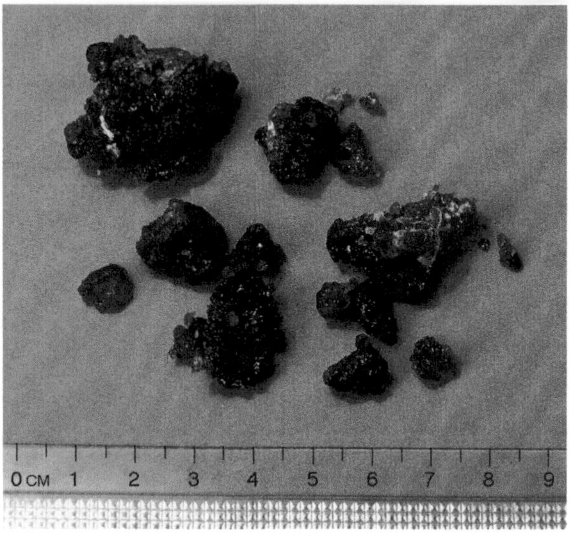

Figure 18

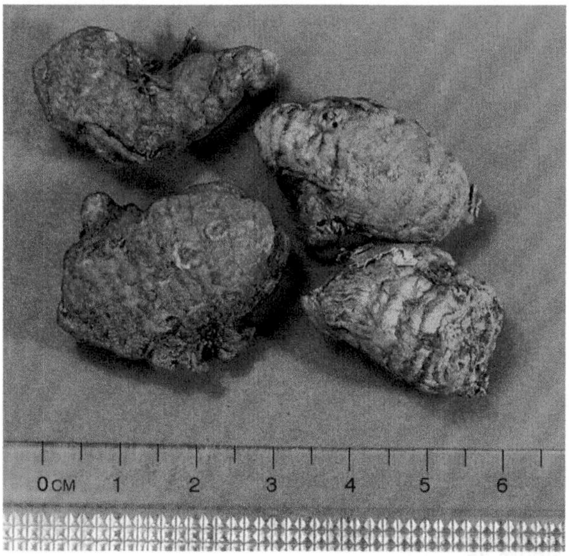

Figure 19

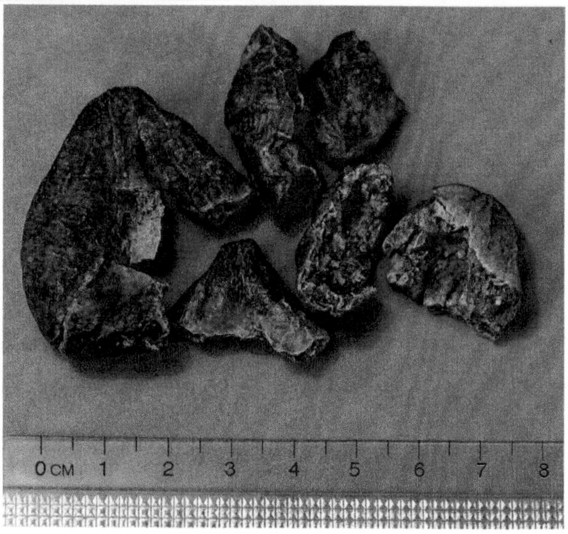

Figure 20

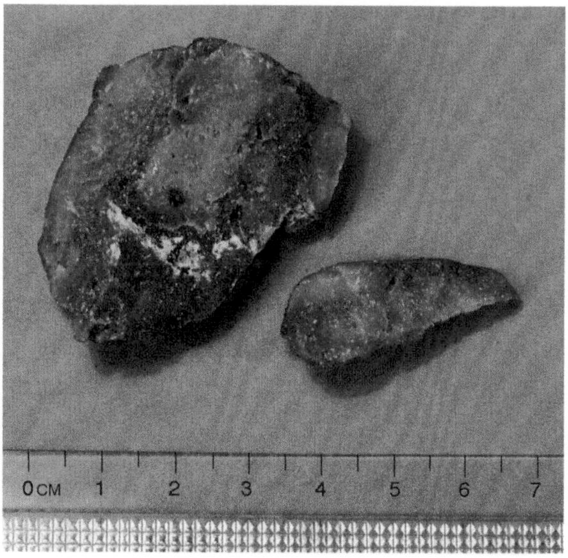

Figure 21

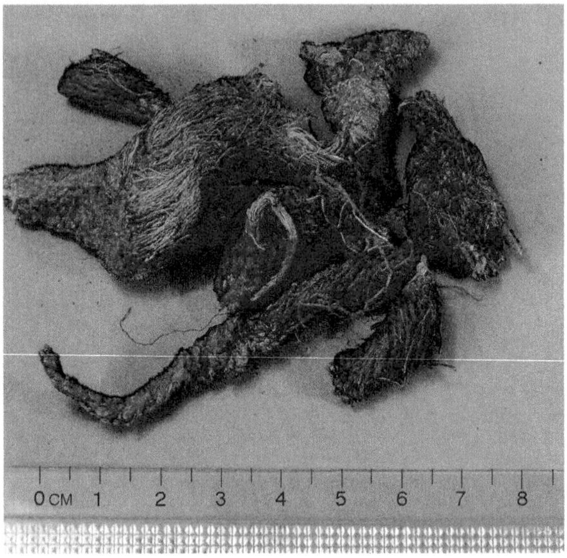

Figure 22

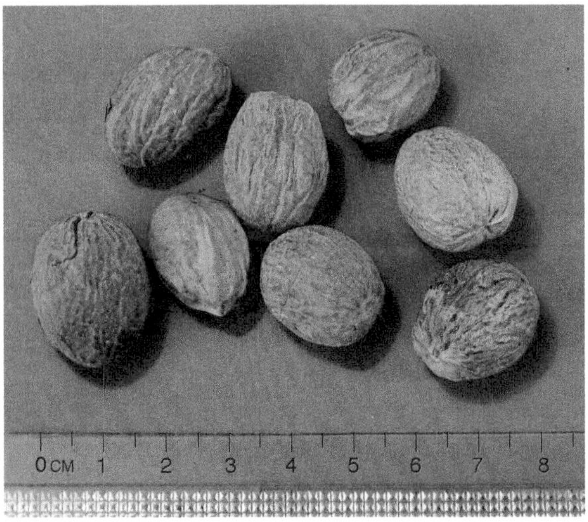

Figure 23

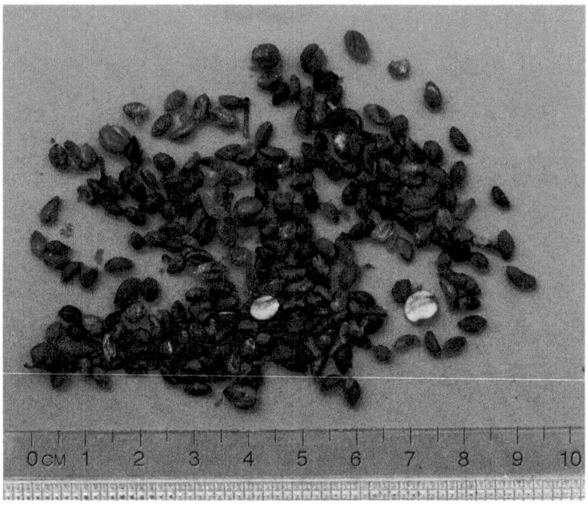

Figure 24

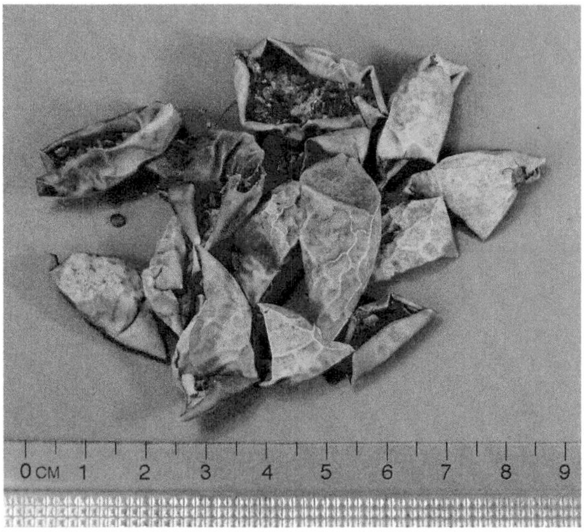

Figure 25

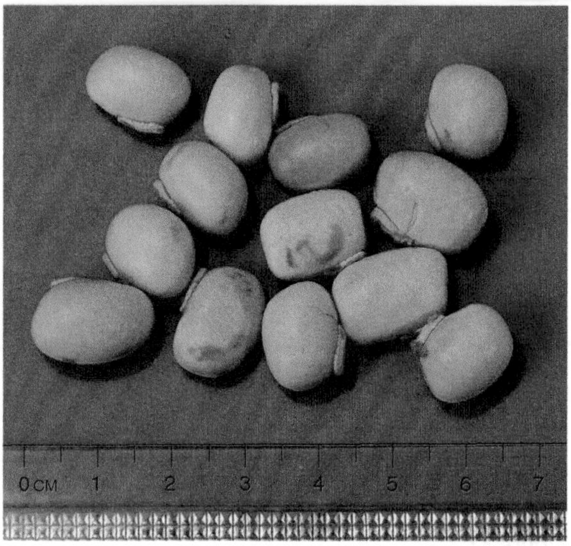

Figure 26

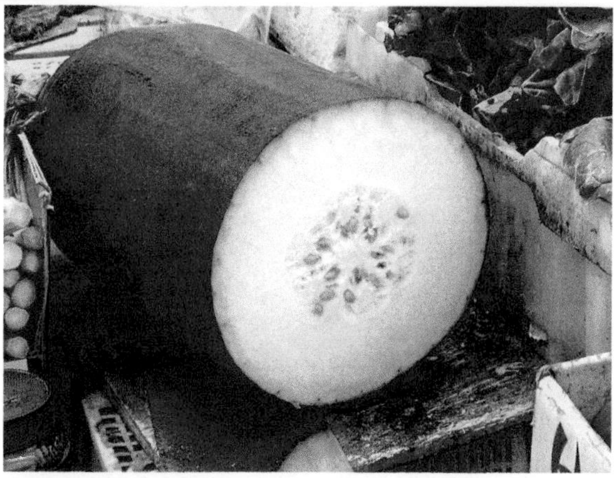

Figure 28

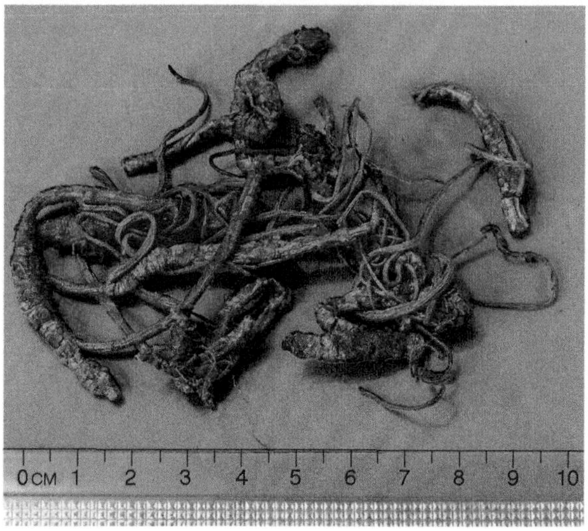

Figure 27

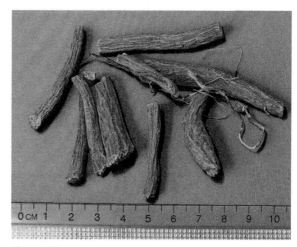

Figure 29

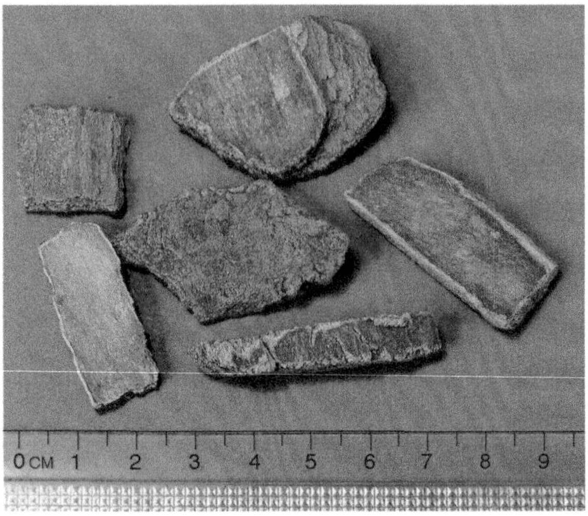

Figure 30

Figure 31

Figure 32

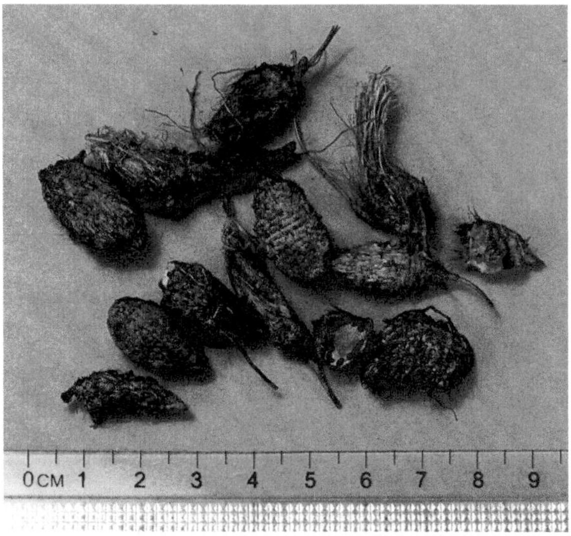

Figure 33

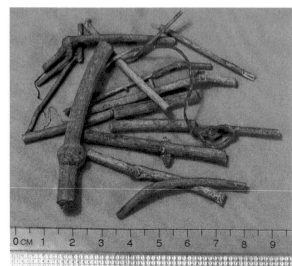

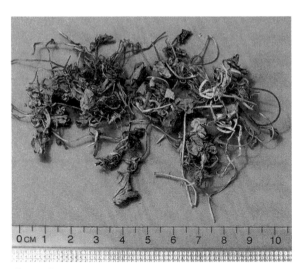

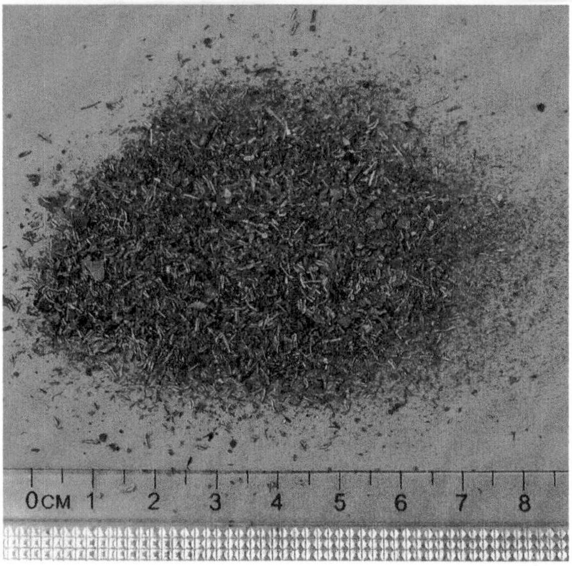

Figure 34

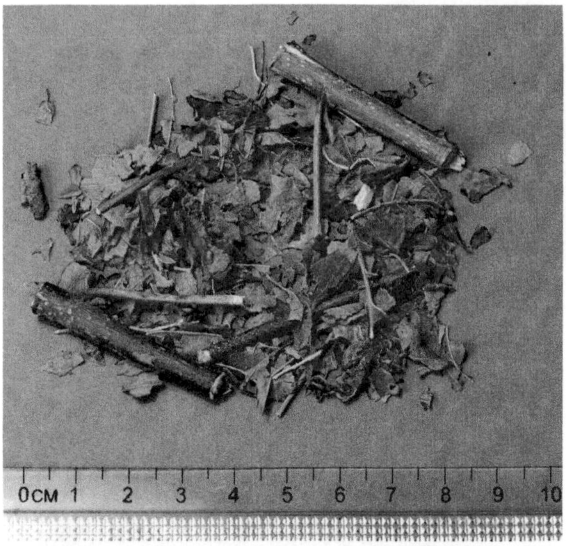

Figure 35

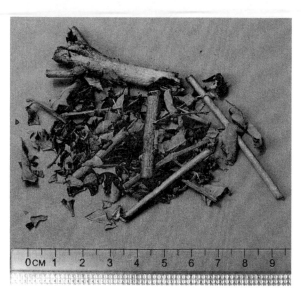

Figure 36

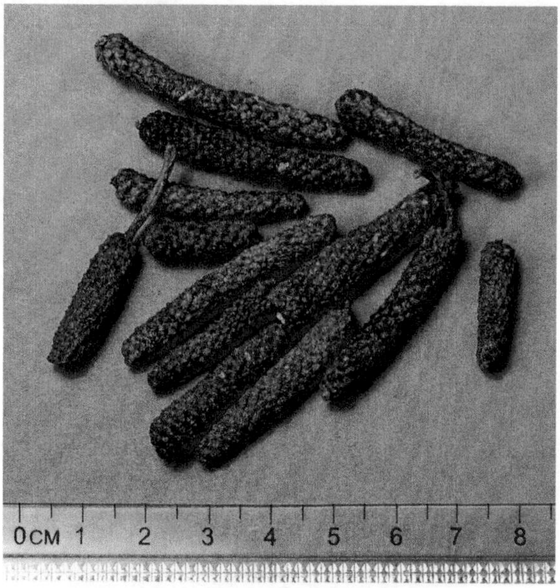

Figure 37

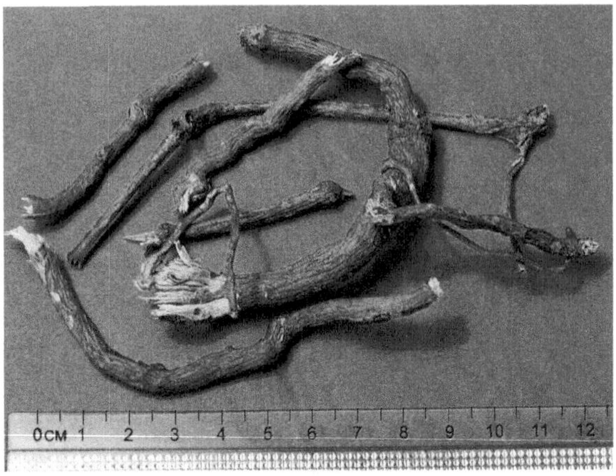

Figure 38

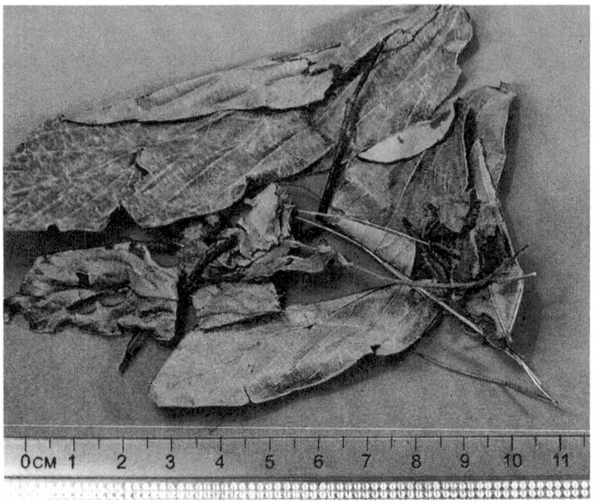

Figure 39

Figure 40

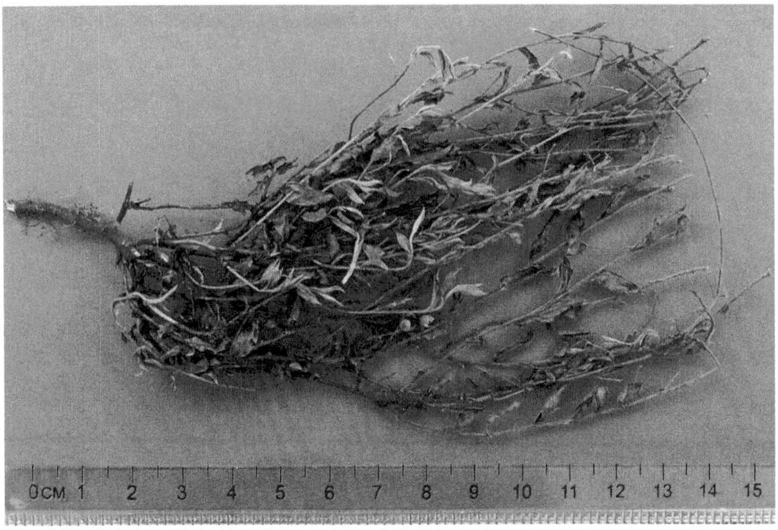

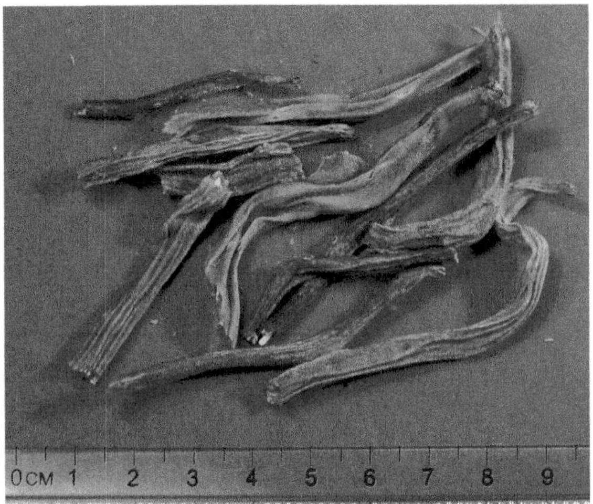

Figure 41

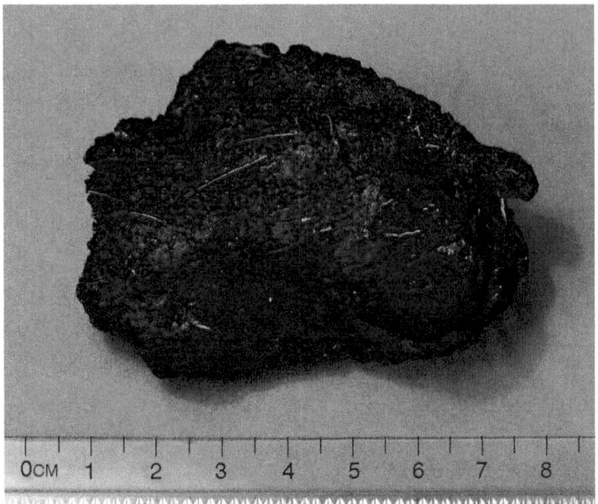

Figure 42

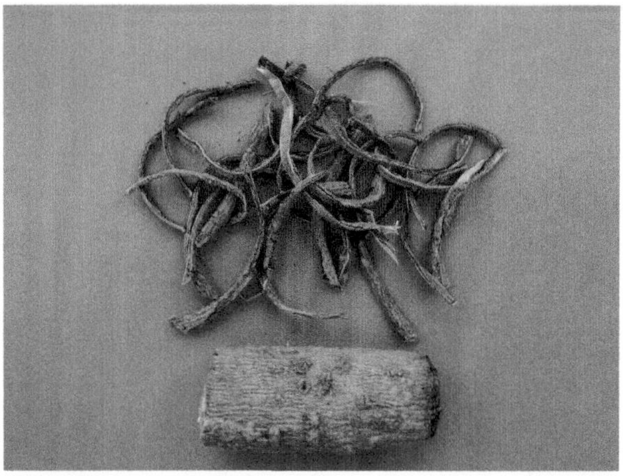

Figure 43

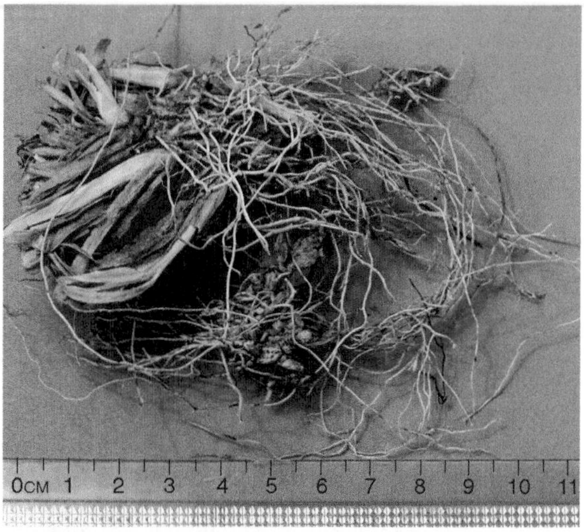

Figure 45

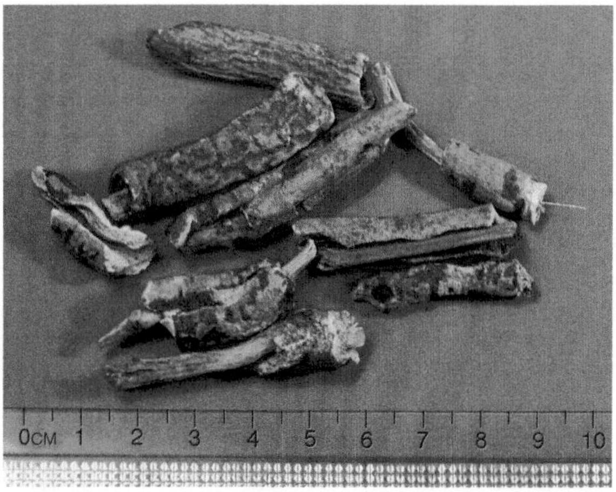

Figure 44

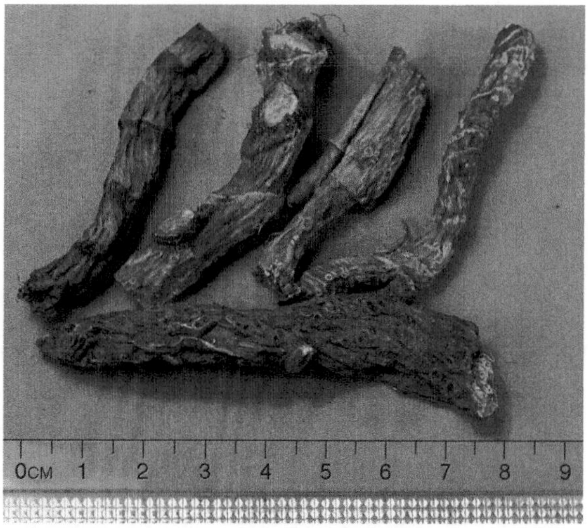

Figure 46

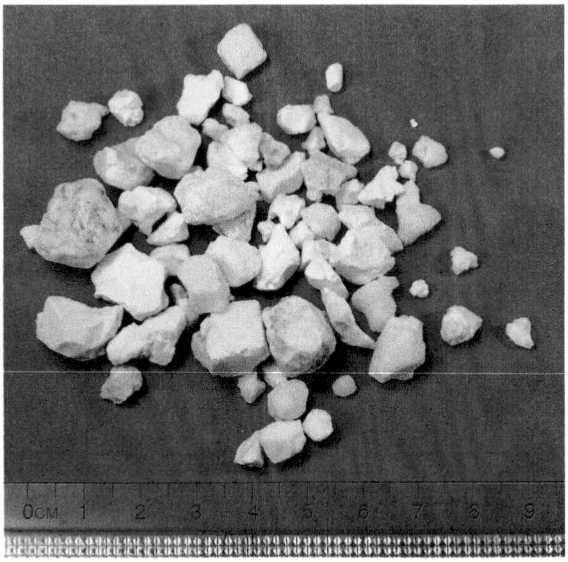

Figure 47

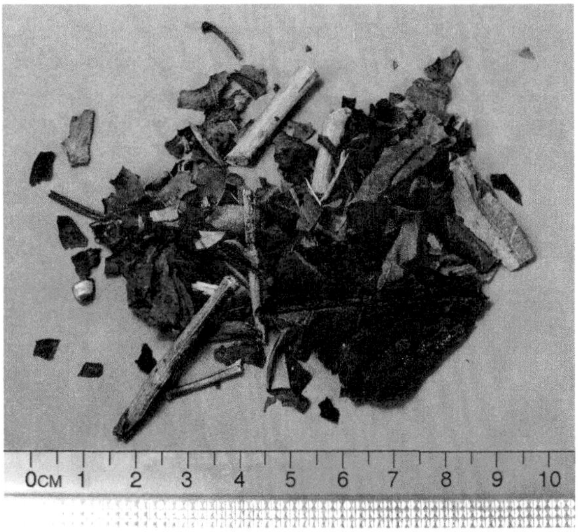

Figure 48

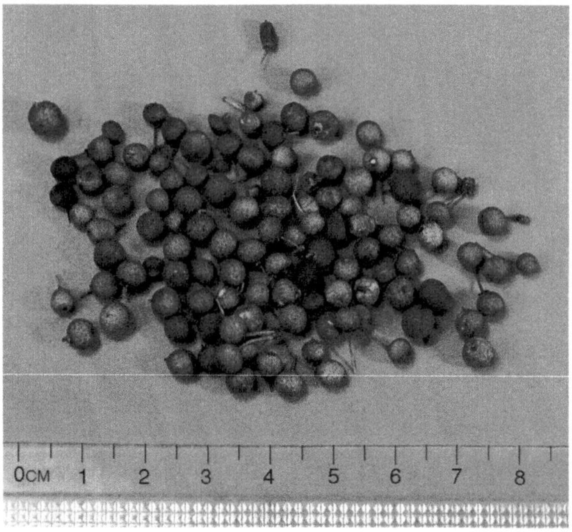

Figure 49

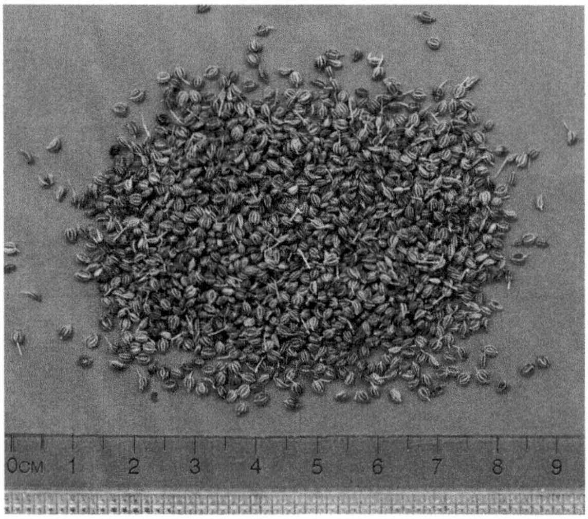

Figure 50

mentioned by the ***Śārańgadhara saṃhitā*** in the treatment of colic, oedema, sciatica and rheumatoid arthritis. Taken with equal parts freshly powdered ***Harītakī*** and one half-part powder each ***Pippalī*** seed, ***Hińgu*** resin, and ***saindhava***, ***Yavānī*** is fried in ***ghṛta***, and eaten with a little rice over a period of weeks in the treatment of intestinal parasites and to improve digestion. In infantile colic a weak decoction is made from the seeds and sweetened with a little sugar, in much the same way as gripe water made from Dill seed. To this end ***Yavānī*** is commonly prescribed in lactating women, drunk as a decoction along with other similar herbs (e.g. Ginger, Fennel, Coriander seed) to prevent infantile colic, and as a galactagogue. Nadkarni (1954) mentions a decoction of equal parts ***Yavānī*** seeds, ***Vāsaka*** leaves, ***Pippalī*** seeds and Poppy capsules (*Papaver* spp.) as an effective antitussive and expectorant in the treatment of chronic bronchitis and lung congestion. Applied topically, both the freshly ground seed and the essential oil act as counter-irritants, best used in ***vāta*** or ***kapha*** forms of arthritis and rheumatism, as well as over the chest in bronchitis marked by coldness and debility.

Dosage:

- ***Cūrṇa***: 3–5 g b.i.d.–t.i.d.
- ***Kvātha***: 1:4, 30–90 mL b.i.d.–t.i.d.
- ***Tincture***: 1:5, 50% alcohol, 3–5 mL

REFERENCES

Boskabady MH, Shaikhi J 2000 Inhibitory effect of Carum copticum on histamine (H1) receptors of isolated guinea-pig tracheal chains. Journal of Ethnopharmacology 69(3):217–227

Duke JA (accessed 2005) Chemicals. In: Trachyspermum ammi (L.) SPRAGUE ex TURRILL (Apiaceae): Ajwan. Dr. Duke's phytochemical and ethnobotanical databases. Agricultural Research Service (ARS), United States Department of Agriculture. Available: http://www.ars-grin.gov/duke/plants.html

Hussein G, Miyashiro H, Nakamura N et al 2000 Inhibitory effects of sudanese medicinal plant extracts on hepatitis C virus (HCV) protease. Phytotherapy Research 14(7):510–516

Ishikawa T, Sega Y, Kitajima J 2001 Water-soluble constituents of ajowan. Chemical and Pharmaceutical Bulletin (Tokyo) 49(7):840–844

Kirtikar KR, Basu BD 1935 Indian medicinal plants, 2nd edn, vols 1–4. Periodical Experts, Delhi, p 1204–1205

Nadkarni KM 1954 The Indian materia medica, with Ayurvedic, Unani and home remedies, revised and enlarged by AK Nadkarni. Popular Prakashan PVP, Bombay, p 1030

Singh G, Kapoor IP, Pandey SK et al 2002 Studies on essential oils: part 10; antibacterial activity of volatile oils of some spices. Phytotherapy Research 16(7):680–682

Srikanthamurthy KR 2001 Bhāvaprakāśa of Bhāvamiśra, vol 1. Krishnadas Academy, Varanasi, p 170–171, 202

Srivastava KC 1988 Extract of a spice shows antiaggregatory effects and alters arachidonic acid metabolism in human platelets. Prostaglandins, Leukotrienes, and Essential Fatty Acids 33(1):1–6

Warrier PK, Nambiar VPK, Ramankutty C (eds) 1996 Indian medicinal plants: a compendium of 500 species, vol 5. Orient Longman, Hyderabad, p 299–303

Williamson EM (ed) 2002 Major herbs of Ayurveda. Churchill Livingstone, London, p 306–309

Yoganarasimhan SN 2000 Medicinal plants of India, vol 2: Tamil Nadu. Self-published, Bangalore, p 551

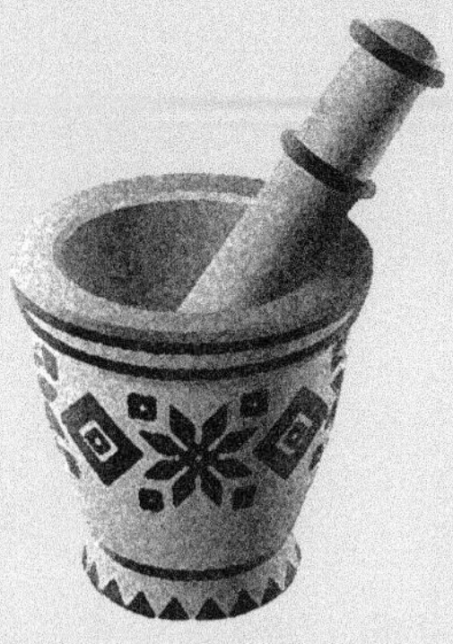

PART 3

APPENDICES

PART 3

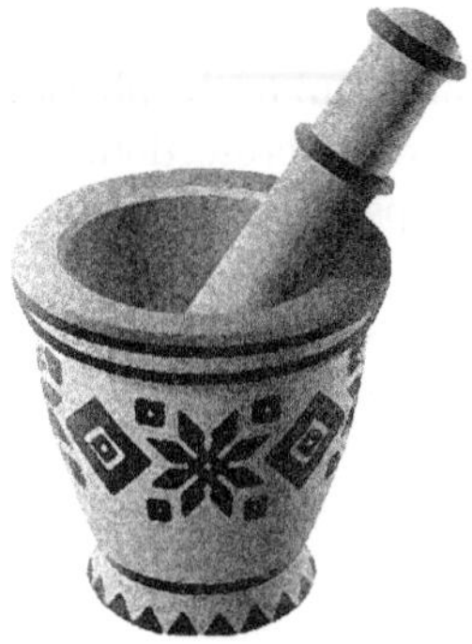

Appendix 1

DIETARY AND LIFESTYLE REGIMENS

The following is a list of dietary and lifestyle recommendations that can be used to balance and pacify increased or vitiated ***doṣas***; for two or more ***doṣas*** the appropriate regimens may be combined. The following regimens, however, are not meant to be applied rigidly in otherwise healthy and balanced individuals – such persons may select from a cornucopia of healthy and beneficial influences, in context with their age, the season and the climate.

DIETARY AND LIFESTYLE REGIMEN FOR *vātaja* CONDITIONS

General guidelines

The nature of ***vāta*** is cold, dry, light, unstable and erratic and therefore herbs, foods, beverages and lifestyle habits used to pacify ***vāta*** should be opposite in nature, i.e. warming, moistening, heavy, stable and grounding.

Foods to emphasise

Fruits: most local seasonal fruits, in moderation; baked fresh fruits (e.g. apples, pears) and cooked dried fruits (e.g. prunes, figs, raisins etc.); tropical fruits including mango, papaya, pineapple, banana, sweet oranges.
Vegetables: all cooked vegetables, especially root vegetables and squash, preferably steamed, boiled or baked; well-cooked onions and garlic; leafy green vegetables prepared with spicy herbs and fat.
Grains and cereals: oats, basmati rice, jasmine rice, brown rice, quinoa, amaranth, khus khus (couscous), whole-wheat pasta, whole-wheat chapati or tortilla.
Legumes: adzuki, mung, tofu, tempeh miso; in small amounts, cooked well with herbs such as ginger and garlic and consumed with warm broth.
Nuts and seeds: most nuts and seed in moderation, including sesame, almonds, pumpkin, walnut, cashew, sunflower, coconut, pecan, filbert, brazil, hemp, flax.
Dairy: butter, ***ghṛta***, yogurt, full fat cream, goat cheese, in small amounts.
Meat and animals products: most animal products, including eggs, chicken, beef, pork, goat, lamb, fatty fish, buffalo, ostrich, wild game.
Oils and fats: most oils and fats, including olive oil, butter, ghee, coconut oil, sesame oil, hemp oil.
Spices and condiments: most spices in moderation, including cardamom, nutmeg, hing (asafoetida), ginger, cumin, cinnamon, garlic, ***saindhava***, basil, rosemary, oregano, tamari, five-spice, black bean, soy sauce, nutritional yeast, vinegar.
Beverages: warm water, herbal teas that have a sweet, warming and spicy flavour (e.g. licorice, cinnamon and ginger), fresh vegetable juices, almond milk, wine, dark beers.
Sweeteners: fresh honey, maple syrup, jaggery, molasses.

Foods to avoid

Fruits: dried fruit (uncooked); bitter-tasting fruits such as cranberries, lemon, limes; unripe fruits.
Vegetables: raw vegetables.
Grains and cereals: granola, muesli, corn, millet, bread, popcorn, rice cakes, potatoes.
Legumes: most legumes should be avoided.
Nuts and seeds: none, except in excess.
Dairy: ice cream, cold milk.

Meat and animal products: none.
Oils and fats: margarine, lard, corn, canola, peanut.
Spices and condiments: chili, black pepper, mustard, horseradish, salt to excess.
Beverages: cold water, ice water, soy milk, coffee, spirits.
Sweeteners: white sugar; any sweetener to excess.

Lifestyle habits to emphasise

As the nature of ***vāta*** is unstable, erratic and changeable it is important to emphasise ritual and routine, with regular hours for eating, sleeping and working. Slow meditative exercises such as ***hatha yoga*** and tai chi are helpful, as are anaerobic, muscle-building exercises. Time should be spent in the natural world, in the mountains and forests, with children and animals, investigating creative and healing abilities. The home and work space should be well-ventilated, warm, safe, quiet, comfortable and nurturing.

Lifestyle habits to avoid

Excessive travel, excessive media influence (TV, radio, newspapers), excessive exposure to electromagnetic radiation (e.g. computer monitors), inadequate sleep, irregular hours, exposure to wind and cold, excessive sexual activity, exposure to noxious or stimulating odours.

Aromatherapy

Fragrances and scents to balance ***vāta*** should be warming, soothing and clearing, such as chamomile, lavender, rose, geranium, neroli, vetivert, rosemary, lemon balm, peppermint, basil, sweet marjoram, bergamot, hyssop, lemon, clary sage, myrrh, frankincense, sandalwood, aniseed, cinnamon, eucalyptus and camphor.

Colours

Most colours are good for ***vāta*** but natural pastel colours should be emphasised, not overly stimulating, bright (neon), dark or metallic colours. Examples include small amounts of yellow, orange, red, with moderate amounts of maroon, purple, blue, green, hazel, tan, khaki and ivory.

Meditation

The goal of meditation in ***vāttika*** conditions is to create an internal balance between the male and female energies, reconnect the spirit and soul to the physical body and develop an aura of spiritual protection. This can be realised by the use of psychophysical techniques such as ***prāṇayama***, meditating upon and ritually using sacred objects, and visualising beneficent deities to ask for their assistance. Modern day examples of paths that utilise these techniques include ***vajrayāna*** and ***bhakti yoga***.

DIETARY AND LIFESTYLE REGIMEN FOR *pittaja* CONDITIONS

General guidelines

The nature of ***pitta*** is hot, light, ascending and fast, and therefore herbs, foods, beverages and lifestyle habits used to pacify ***pitta*** should be opposite in nature, i.e. cooling, heavy, descending and relaxing.

Foods to emphasise

Fruits: all local fruits, in season, especially cooling fruits such as pear, grapes and melon; tropical fruits.
Vegetables: most vegetables, consumed raw and steamed, especially leafy green and cruciferous vegetables; cooling vegetables such as cucumber and cilantro.
Grains and cereals: most cereals and grains, including oats, basmati rice, jasmine rice, brown rice, quinoa, amaranth, khus khus (couscous), chapati.
Legumes: all legumes in moderation.
Nuts and seeds: cooling nuts and seeds including coconut, pumpkin, and melon; small amounts of other seeds, including almond, brazil, cashew, filbert.
Dairy: milk, unripened cheeses, buttermilk, ghee, butter.
Meat and animal products: most animal products, consumed in small to moderate amounts, including eggs, poultry, cold-water fish, rabbit, wild game; small amounts of goat, mutton and lamb.
Oils and fats: flax, hemp, ghee, butter, coconut, sunflower, olive.
Spices and condiments: cooling or neutral spices such as turmeric, mint, cumin, coriander, fennel, cilantro, cardamom; ***saindhava*** in moderation.
Beverages: cool spring water daily, kukicha (twig) tea, any herbal tea except those made with spicy herbs such as cinnamon and ginger, fresh vegetable and fruit juices, rice and almond milk.

Sweeteners: most sweeteners, in small amounts, jaggery, maple syrup and treacle.

Foods to avoid

Fruits: all sour-tasting fruits, including sour citrus fruits (e.g. lemons, grapefruit, sour oranges); warming fruits including papaya, sour mango and strawberry.
Vegetables: raw onions and garlic; chilies, tomatoes, peppers, potatoes, eggplant (aubergine), radish, daikon, watercress, mustard greens.
Grains and cereals: fermented grains, e.g. sourdough bread, idli.
Legumes: peanut; fermented soy products.
Nuts and seeds: most nuts tend to be warming in nature and should be avoided to excess.
Dairy: sharp and pungent cheeses, yogurt, sour cream.
Meat and animal products: tropical fish, red meat, pork, shellfish.
Oils and fats: canola, peanut, sesame.
Spices and condiments: warming spices, including chili, black pepper, mustard, horseradish, ginger, clove and cinnamon; vinegar, catsup (ketchup).
Beverages: coffee, alcohol.
Sweeteners: molasses, old honey.

Lifestyle habits to emphasise

As the nature of ***pitta*** is hot, light and sharp, emotions such as impatience, ambition, aggression and anger tend to dominate. It is thus important to emphasise a balanced, calm and relaxing lifestyle to counter these qualities, cultivating patience, friendliness, empathy and compassion. Exercise can be helpful to discharge excess energy, but should be performed with a routine of mental discipline that promotes self-control, such as the martial arts or ***hatha yoga***. Such activities should be balanced with social pursuits, contributing to the welfare of society, enjoying social outings, listening to music, laughing and telling stories with friends. Time should be spent next to rivers and lakes, in gardens of flowers and other delightful places, bathing in the moonlight, and in the company of women and gentle individuals. The home and work space should be well-ventilated and cool, decorated in cooling colours and fresh cut flowers.

Lifestyle habits to avoid

Excessive expression of anger, sarcasm and criticism, competitive relationships, excessive physical activity in warm weather and direct exposure to the hot sun.

Aromatherapy

Fragrances and scents to balance ***pitta*** should be cooling, soothing and grounding in nature. Floral fragrances are particularly useful for ***pitta***. Examples include chamomile, lavender, rose, gardenia, honeysuckle, ylang-ylang, vetivert, jasmine and sandalwood.

Colours

Emphasise colours that have a cooling energy, including white and off-whites, pale colours, pastels, and blues and greens. Overtly bright colours should be avoided, as should many in the red to yellow spectrum as they are too heating and aggravating to ***pitta***. Black, greys and browns can also be used, but to a lesser extent.

Meditation

Meditation techniques to pacify ***pitta*** increase and balance the lunar qualities of the psyche, emphasising as introspection, intuition, forgiveness and compassion. Techniques should be chosen for their directness and simplicity, rather than elaborate rituals. The most effective approaches include mindfulness of breath (***ānapānasati bhāvanā***), the development of insight (***vipassanā***) and self-inquiry (***vedānta***), coupled with compassion for all living beings (***mettā bhāvanā***).

DIETARY AND LIFESTYLE REGIMEN FOR ***kaphaja*** CONDITIONS

General guidelines

The nature of ***kapha*** is cold, heavy, smooth, moist and dull and therefore herbs, foods, beverages and lifestyle habits used to pacify ***kapha*** should be opposite in nature, i.e. warming, light, rough, dry and sharp.

Foods to emphasise

Fruits: sour and mildly sweet fruits, including apple, cranberry, grapefruit, lemon, lime, papaya, pineapple; dried fruits in small amounts.
Vegetables: most vegetables, eaten steamed or baked.
Cereals and grains: grains and cereals with a dry and light quality, including millet, long grain brown rice, quinoa, amaranth, granola, buckwheat, barley, corn, popped grains.
Legumes: most legumes, cooked with spicy and warming herbs such as ginger, including mung, lentil, split pea, soy and kidney bean.
Nuts and seeds: dry and light seeds in moderation, including sunflower and pumpkin.
Dairy: old ghee, aged cheese, goat cheese: all in small amounts.
Meats and animal products: lean animal products, in small to moderate amounts, including fish, poultry, rabbit, mutton, goat, ostrich, and wild meat.
Oils: mustard oil, olive oil, sesame oil, used in small amounts.
Spices and condiments: all spices are indicated; vinegars; small amounts of salt.
Beverages: warm water squeezed with lemon or lime, any herbal tea, green tea, coffee.
Sweeteners: old honey.

Foods to avoid

Fruits: most fruits are generally avoided because of their excessive water content and cooling nature.
Vegetables: raw vegetables, fried vegetables, avocado.
Cereals and grains: flour products; heavy and moistening grains such as wheat and oats.
Legumes: oily and heavy legumes, such as peanut and black gram.
Nuts and seeds: most nuts and seeds, including cashew, filbert, walnut, macadamia and almond.
Dairy: dairy should be avoided because of its heavy and congesting nature, including milk, ice cream, cream, unripened cheeses, yogurt.
Meat and animal products: most meats are too heavy and greasy for ***kapha***, including beef, fatty fish, pork, and shellfish.
Oils and fats: most oils, due to their heavy and congesting nature.
Spices and condiments: table salt, toppings, dressings, mayonnaise.
Beverages: excessive water, cold water, rice and almond milk.
Sweeteners: white sugar, molasses, raw sugar, jaggery, maple syrup, treacle.

Lifestyle habits to emphasise

As the nature of ***kapha*** is cold, heavy and wet, there is a tendency towards dullness, apathy and lethargy. It is thus important to emphasise lifestyle patterns that are active, energetic and stimulating to break up the stagnation of ***kapha***. This includes regular saunas, vigorous exercise and manual labour, as well as busying oneself with volunteering and charitable work, enabling others to find fulfillment. Time should be spent in open, dry locations, under the influence of the warm sun and breeze, in the company of men, children and dynamic individuals. The home and work space should be a well-ventilated, warm, and dry, decorated in warm, stimulating colours.

Lifestyle habits to avoid

Inactivity, laziness, excessive sleeping, day sleep, sleeping until late morning, exposure to cold and damp.

Aromatherapy

Essential oils for ***kapha*** should be warming, stimulating and clearing in nature. Balsamic, pungent and musky odours are best, including cedar, pine, rosemary, basil, frankincense, myrrh, eucalyptus, cajeput, camphor, ginger and clove.

Colours

Colours that have a warming energy such as yellow, orange, gold or red are useful for ***kapha***, as is brown, grey and black. Soft, pale, cool and pastel colours should be avoided.

Meditation

Meditation techniques to pacify ***kapha*** increase and balance the solar qualities of the psyche, enhancing motivation, will power and independence. Techniques should be chosen for their energetic and active qualities, rather than techniques that involve extended periods of sitting and stillness. The most effective approach is typified by ***bhakti*** and ***karma yogas***, which encourage active forms of worship and humanitarian service.

PART 3

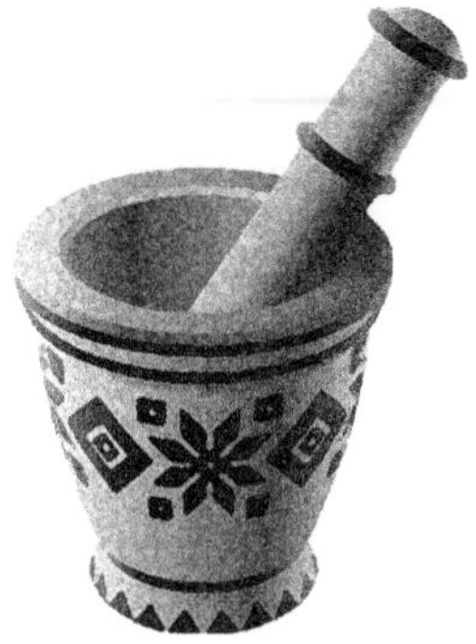

Appendix 2

ĀYURVEDIC FORMULATIONS

The following is a list of some of the more important or commonly used formulas in Āyurveda, including ***kvātha*** (decoctions), ***cūrṇa*** (powders), ***guggulu*** (resins), ***guṭikā*** and ***vaṭī*** (pills), ***avalehya*** (confections), ***taila*** (medicated oils), ***ghṛta*** (medicated clarified butters), ***asava/ariṣṭam*** (natural fermentations) and ***bhasma*** (purified calcinations). A listing of the ingredients is provided, as well as the ***prakṣepa dravyas*** that are added during the course of preparation and the ***anupāna*** taken with each medicament. These are the original formulas in the extant literature, which may or may not be representative of commercially produced products with the same name. In a few cases where the original ingredient listed in the formula is unclear substitutes will often be used.

Kvātha (DECOCTION)

Āragvadhādi kvātha

Ingredients: ***Āragvadha*** fruit, ***Indrayava*** seed, ***Pāṭalā*** root, ***Kākatikta*** root, ***Nimba*** stem bark, ***Guḍūcī*** stem, ***Mūrvā*** root, ***Sruvavṛkṣa*** herb, ***Pāṭhā*** root, ***Bhūnimba*** herb, ***Sairyaka*** herb, ***Paṭola*** leaf, ***Karanja*** seed, ***Saptacchada*** stem bark, ***Citraka*** root, ***Kālājālī*** fruit, ***Madanaphala*** fruit, ***Sahacara*** herb, ***Ghoṇṭā*** seed.
Indications: vomiting, intoxication, fever, diabetes, ulcer, itching, skin disease; reduces ***kapha***.
Dosage: 48 g.

Cāturbhadra kvātha

Ingredients: ***Guḍūcī*** stem, purified ***Ativiṣā*** root, ***Śuṇṭhī*** rhizome, ***Mustaka*** rhizome.
Prakṣepa dravyas: ***Śuṇṭhī*** rhizome, ***Jiraka*** seed.
Indications: ***āma***, digestive weakness.
Dosage: 48 g.

Daśamūla kvātha

Ingredients: ***Śālaparṇi*** root, ***Pṛśniparṇī*** root, ***Bṛhatī*** root, ***Kaṇṭakāri*** root, ***Gokṣura*** root, ***Bilva*** root, ***Agnimañtha*** root, ***Śyonāka*** root, ***Gambhārī*** root, ***Pāṭalā*** root.
Prakṣepa dravyas: ***Pippalī cūrṇa***.
Indications: colic, fever, cough, dyspnoea.
Dosage: 48 g.

Drākṣādi kvātha

Ingredients: ***Drākṣā*** fruit, ***Madhūka*** flower, ***Yaṣṭīmadhu*** root, ***Rodhra*** stem bark, ***Gambhārī*** fruit, ***Sārivā*** root, ***Mustaka*** rhizome, ***Āmalakī*** fruit pulp, ***Hṛībera*** root, ***Padma*** stamens, ***Padmaka*** wood, ***Mṛṇāla*** stem, ***Candana*** wood, ***Uśīra*** root, ***Nīlotpala*** flower, ***Parūṣaka*** fruit, ***Jātī*** flower.
Prakṣepa dravyas: honey.
Indications: vomiting, burning sensations, fever, passive haemorrhage, fainting.
Dosage: 48 g.

Ghandharvahastādi kvātha

Ingredients: ***Eraṇḍa*** root, ***Ciribilva*** seed or leaves, ***Hutāśa*** root, ***Śuṇṭhī*** rhizome, ***Punarnavā*** root, ***Durālabhā*** herb, ***Tālamūla*** root.
Prakṣepa dravyas: ***saindhava***, jaggery.
Indications: digestive weakness, anorexia, constipation.
Dosage: 48 g.

Nimbādi kvātha

Ingredients: ***Nimba*** stem bark, ***Śuṇṭhī*** rhizome, ***Guḍūcī*** stem, ***Devadāru*** root, ***Śaṭī*** rhizome, ***Bhūnimba*** herb, ***Pauṣkara*** root, ***Pippalī*** fruit, ***Gajapippalī*** fruit, ***Bṛhatī*** root.
Prakṣepa dravyas: honey.
Indications: fever, respiratory congestion.
Dosage: 48 g.

Nyagrodhādi kvātha

Ingredients: ***Nyagrodha*** stem bark, ***Aśvattha*** stem bark, ***Udumbara*** stem bark, ***Lodhra*** (***śābara***, ***pattika***) stem bark, ***Jambū*** (***mahā***, ***kṣudra***) stem bark, ***jambū*** stem bark, ***Arjuna*** stem bark, ***Āmrātaka*** stem bark, ***Kaṭphala*** stem bark, ***Plakṣa*** stem bark, ***Āmra*** stem bark, ***Vetasa*** stem bark, ***Piyāla*** stem bark, ***Palāśa*** stem bark, ***Aśvattha*** stem bark, ***Badara*** stem bark, ***Kadamba*** stem bark, ***Viralā*** stem bark, ***Yaṣṭīmadhu*** root, ***Madhūka*** flower.
Indications: malabsorption syndromes, thirst, burning sensations, passive haemorrhage, ulcer.
Dosage: 48 g.

Paṭolādi kvātha

Ingredients: ***Paṭola*** leaf, ***Kaṭuka*** rhizome, ***Candana*** wood, ***Mūrva*** root, ***Guḍūcī*** stem, ***Pāṭhā*** root.
Prakṣepa dravyas: ***Pippalī cūrṇa***, honey.
Indications: poor appetite, vomiting, fever, jaundice, skin disease.
Dosage: 48 g.

Saptasāra kvātha

Ingredients: ***Punarnavā*** root, ***Bilva*** root, ***Khalva*** seed, ***Eraṇḍa*** root, ***Sahacara*** herb, ***Śuṇṭhī*** rhizome, ***Agnimañtha*** root.
Prakṣepa dravyas: ***Pippalī cūrṇa***, jaggery, ***saindhava***.
Indications: digestive weakness, constipation, abdominal distension, ascites, splenomegaly, dysmenorrhoea, angina pectoris.
Dosage: 48 g.

Vāsāguḍūcyādi kvātha

Ingredients: ***Vāsaka*** root, ***Guḍūcī*** stem, ***Harītakī*** fruit pulp, ***Bibhītaka*** fruit pulp, ***Āmalakī*** fruit pulp, ***Kaṭukī*** rhizome, ***Bhūnimba*** herb, ***Nimba*** stem bark.
Prakṣepa dravyas: honey
Indications: anaemia, passive haemorrhage, jaundice.
Dosage: 48 g.

Cūrṇa (POWDER)

Avipattikāra cūrṇa

Ingredients: ***Śuṇṭhī*** rhizome, ***Marica*** fruit, ***Pippalī*** fruit, ***Harītaki*** fruit, ***Harītakī*** fruit pulp, ***Bibhītaka*** fruit pulp, ***Āmalakī*** fruit pulp, ***Mustaka*** rhizome, ***Viḍa lavaṇa***, ***Viḍaṅga*** fruit, ***Sthūla elā*** fruit, ***Tejapatra*** leaf, ***Lavaṅga*** flower, ***Trivṛt*** root, sugar.
Anupāna dravyas: honey, water, milk.
Indications: digestive weakness, poor appetite, dyspepsia, constipation, haemorrhoids, dysuria.
Dosage: 3–6 g.

Bhāskaralavaṇa cūrṇa

Ingredients: ***Sāmudra lavaṇa***, ***Sauvarcala lavaṇa***, ***Viḍa lavaṇa***, ***saindhava lavaṇa***, ***Dhānyaka*** fruit, ***Pippalī*** fruit, ***Pippalīmūla*** root, ***Kṛṣṇajīraka*** fruit, ***Patra*** leaf, ***Nāgakeśara*** flower, ***Tālīsa*** flower, ***Amlavetasa*** fruit, ***Marica*** fruit, ***Śvetajīraka*** fruit, ***Śuṇṭhī*** rhizome, ***Dāḍima*** seed, ***Tvak*** stem bark, ***Elā*** fruit.
Anupāna dravyas: whey, buttermilk, wine, warm water.
Indications: digestive weakness, poor appetite, nausea, bloating, colic, malabsorption.
Dosage: 3 g.

Elādi cūrṇa

Ingredients: ***Elā*** fruit, ***Lavaṅga*** flower, ***Nāgakeśara*** flower, ***Kolamajja*** fruit pulp, ***Lāja***, ***Priyaṅgu*** flower, ***Mustaka*** rhizome, ***Candana*** wood, ***Pippalī*** fruit.
Anupāna dravyas: honey, sugar.
Indications: vomiting, cough, dyspnoea, asthma.
Dosage: 2–4 g.

Hiṅgvāṣṭaka cūrṇa

Ingredients: ***Śuṇṭhī*** rhizome, ***Marica*** fruit, ***Pippalī*** fruit, ***Ajamodā*** fruit, ***saindhava***, ***Śvetajīraka*** fruit, ***Kṛṣṇajīraka*** fruit, ***Hiṅgu*** resin.
Anupāna dravyas: clarified butter.

Indications: digestive weakness, poor appetite, colic, malabsorption, bowel disorders, bloating.
Dosage: 1–3 g.

Nārāyaṇa cūrṇa

Ingredients: ***Yavāni*** fruit, ***Hapuṣā*** root, ***Dhānyaka*** fruit, ***Śatapuṣpā*** fruit, ***Upakuñcika*** fruit, ***Kṛṣṇajīraka*** fruit, ***Pippalīmūla*** root, ***Ajagandhā*** seed, ***Śaṭhī*** rhizome, ***Vacā*** rhizome, ***Citraka*** root, ***Jīraka*** seed, ***Śuṇṭhī*** rhizome, ***Marica*** fruit, ***Pippalī*** fruit, ***Svarṇakṣīrī*** root, ***Harītakī*** fruit pulp, ***Bibhītaka*** fruit pulp, ***Āmalakī*** fruit pulp, ***Yavakṣāra***, ***Svarjikṣāra***, ***Paṣkaramūla*** root, ***Kuṣtha*** root, ***Sauvarcala lavaṇa***, ***saindhava lavaṇa***, ***Viḍa lavaṇa***, ***Sāmudra lavaṇa***, ***Aubhida lavaṇa***, ***Dantī*** fruit, ***Viḍaṅga*** fruit, ***Trivṛt*** root, ***Indravāruṇī*** root, ***Sātalā*** herb.
Anupāna dravyas: buttermilk, warm water, ***Badara*** juice, beer, whey, ***Vṛksāmla*** juice, ***Dāḍima*** juice.
Indications: fever, digestive weakness, malabsorption, bowel disorders, intestinal obstruction, haemorrhoids, anal fistula, cough, dyspnoea, heart diseases, anaemia, splenomegaly, ascites, oedema.
Dosage: 1–3 g.

Puṣyānuga cūrṇa

Ingredients: ***Pāṭha*** root, ***Jambu*** dehusked seed, ***Āmra*** dehusked seed, ***Pāṣāṇabheda*** rhizome, ***Rasāñjana***, ***Ambaṣṭhakī*** root, ***Kunduru*** exudate, ***Mañjiṣṭhā*** stem, ***Padmakeśara*** stamens, ***Kuṇkuma*** style/stigma, purified ***Ativiṣā*** root, ***Mustaka*** rhizome, ***Bilva*** stem bark, ***Lodhra*** stem bark, ***Gairika***, ***Kaṭphala*** fruit, ***Marica*** fruit, ***Śuṇṭhī*** rhizome, ***Drākṣā*** fruit, ***Raktacandana*** wood, ***Araluka*** stem bark, ***Kuṭaja*** stem bark, ***Śvetasārivā*** root, ***Dhātakī*** flower, ***Yaṣṭīmadhu*** root, ***Arjuna*** stem bark.
Anupāna dravyas: honey.
Indications: leucorrhoea, metrorrhagia, menorrhagia, diarrhoea, dysentery, haemorrhage.
Dosage: 1–3 g.

Sitopalādi cūrṇa

Ingredients: Sugar candy, ***Vaṃśarocanā***, ***Pippalī*** fruit, ***Sthūla elā*** fruit, ***Tvak*** stem bark.
Anupāna dravyas: honey, ***ghṛta***.
Indications: poor appetite, cough, laryngitis, pharyngitis, bronchitis, fever.
Dosage: 1–3 g.

Sudarśana cūrṇa

Ingredients: ***Aguru*** wood, ***Haridrā*** rhizome, ***Devadarū*** wood, ***Vacā*** rhizome, ***Mustaka*** rhizome, ***Harītakī*** fruit, ***Yavāsa*** root, ***Śṛṅgī*** gall, ***Kaṇṭakāri*** herb, ***Śuṇṭhī*** rhizome, ***Trāyantī*** herb, ***Parpaṭa*** herb, ***Nimba*** stem bark, ***Pippalīmūla*** root, ***Hrīvera*** root, ***Śaṭī*** rhizome, ***Puṣkaramūla*** root, ***Pippalī*** fruit, ***Mūrvā*** root, ***Kuṭaja*** stem bark, ***Yaṣṭīmadhu*** root, ***Śigrū*** seed, ***Indrayava*** seed, ***Śatāvarī*** root, ***Dāruharidrā*** root, ***Raktacandana*** wood, ***Padmaka*** wood, ***Sarala*** wood, ***Uśīra*** root, ***Tvak*** stem bark, ***Saurāṣṭrī***, ***Śālaparṇī*** root, ***Yamāṇī*** fruit, purified ***Ativiṣā*** root, ***Bilva*** stem bark, ***Marica*** fruit, ***Prasāraṇī*** leaf, ***Āmalakī*** fruit pulp, ***Gūḍūcī*** stem, ***Kaṭuka*** rhizome, ***Citraka*** root, ***Paṭola*** leaf, ***Pṛśniparṇī*** root, ***Kirātatikta*** herb.
Anupāna dravyas: warm water.
Indications: disease of the liver and spleen, fever, intermittent fevers, prolonged fevers.
Dosage: 2–4 g.

Trikaṭu cūrṇa

Ingredients: ***Pippalī*** fruit, ***Marica*** fruit, ***Śuṇṭhī*** rhizome.
Anupāna dravyas: warm water, honey.
Indications: ***āma***, weak digestion, anorexia, cough, catarrhal conditions, poor circulation, skin diseases.
Dosage: 1–3 g.

Triphala cūrṇa

Ingredients: ***Harītakī*** fruit pulp, ***Bibhītaka*** fruit pulp, ***Āmalakī*** fruit pulp.
Anupāna dravyas: warm water, honey, ***ghṛta***.
Indications: flatulence, diabetes, eye diseases.
Dosage: 3–6 g.

Guggulu: RESIN

Kāñcanāra guggulu

Ingredients: ***Kāñcanāra*** stem bark, ***Harītakī*** fruit pulp, ***Bibhītaka*** fruit pulp, ***Āmalakī*** fruit pulp, ***Śuṇṭhī*** rhizome, ***Marica*** fruit, ***Pippalī*** fruit, ***Varuṇa*** stem bark, ***Sthūla elā*** fruit, ***Tvak*** stem bark, ***Patra*** leaf, ***Guggulu*** resin.
Anupāna dravyas: warm water.

Indications: abdominal distension, anal fistula, ulcer, skin diseases, cervical adenitis, scrofula, tumours.
Dosage: 3 g.

Kaiśora guggulu

Ingredients: ***Guggulu*** resin, ***Harītakī*** fruit pulp, ***Bibhītaka*** fruit pulp, ***Āmalakī*** fruit pulp, ***Gūḍūcī*** stem, ***Śuṇṭhī*** rhizome, ***Marica*** fruit, ***Pippalī*** fruit, ***Viḍaṅga*** fruit, ***Trivṛt*** root, ***Dantī*** root, clarified butter.
Anupāna dravyas: milk.
Indications: weakness of digestion, inflammatory joint disease, sciatica, otorrhoea, scrofula, ulcers, boils, anal fistula.
Dosage: 3 g.

Gokṣurādi guggulu

Ingredients: ***Gokṣura*** fruit, ***Guggulu*** resin, ***Harītakī*** fruit pulp, ***Bibhītaka*** fruit pulp, ***Āmalakī*** fruit pulp, ***Śuṇṭhī*** rhizome, ***Marica*** fruit, ***Pippalī*** fruit, ***Mustaka*** rhizome.
Anupāna dravyas: warm water, decoctions of ***Mustaka***, ***Uśīra*** or ***Pāṣāṇabheda***.
Indications: menorrhagia, prostatitis, impotence, dysuria, urinary calculi, diabetes.
Dosage: 3 g.

Triphala guggulu

Ingredients: ***Harītakī*** fruit pulp, ***Bibhītaka*** fruit pulp, ***Āmalakī*** fruit pulp, ***Pippalī*** fruit, ***Guggulu*** resin.
Anupāna dravyas: warm water.
Indications: oedema, anal fistula, haemorrhoids, arthritis.
Dosage: 3 g.

Yogarāja guggulu

Ingredients: ***Citraka*** root, ***Pippalīmūla*** root, ***Yamāni*** seed, ***Kṛṣṇajīraka*** fruit, ***Viḍaṅga*** fruit, ***Ajamodā*** fruit, ***Śvetajīraka*** fruit, ***Devadāru*** wood, ***Cavya*** stem, ***Elā*** seed, ***saindhava***, ***Kuṣṭha*** root, ***Rāsnā*** leaf and root, ***Gokṣura*** fruit, ***Dhānyaka*** fruit, ***Harītakī*** fruit pulp, ***Bibhītaka*** fruit pulp, ***Āmalakī*** fruit pulp, ***Mustaka*** rhizome, ***Śuṇṭhī*** rhizome, ***Marica*** fruit, ***Pippalī*** fruit, ***Tvak*** stem bark, ***Uśīra*** root, ***Yavakṣāra***, ***Tālīśa patra*** leaf, ***Patra*** leaf, ***Guggulu*** resin, clarified butter.
Anupāna dravyas: warm water, honey, ***Laśuna*** juice.
Indications: inflammatory joint disease, joint weakness, myalgia, obesity.
Dosage: 3 g.

Guṭikā AND *vaṭī*: PILL

Agnituṇḍi vaṭī

Ingredients: ***Pārada***, ***Vatsanābha*** rhizome, ***Gandhaka***, ***Ajamodā*** fruit, ***Harītakī*** fruit pulp, ***Bibhītaka*** fruit pulp, ***Āmalakī*** fruit pulp, ***Svarjikṣāra***, ***Yavakṣāra***, ***Citraka*** root, ***saindhava***, ***Jīraka*** fruit, ***Sauvarcala***, ***Viḍaṅga*** fruit, ***Sāmudra lavaṇa***, ***Ṭaṅkaṇa***, ***Viṣamuṣṭī*** fruit, ***Jambīrāmla*** juice.
Anupāna dravyas: lime juice, warm water.
Indications: weakness of digestion, ***āma***, fever.
Dosage: 125–250 mg.

Kastūryādi guṭikā

Ingredients: ***Kaṣtūrī***, ***Kirātatikta*** herb, ***Rāsnā*** root and leaf, ***Gandhamārjāra vīrya***, ***Loha bhasma***, ***Karpūra*** exudate, ***Jātīphala*** seed, ***Yavakṣāra***, ***Sarjikākṣāra***, ***Harītakī*** fruit pulp, ***Bibhītaka*** fruit pulp, ***Āmalakī*** fruit pulp, ***Tvak*** stem bark, ***Elā*** seed, ***Patra*** leaf, ***Hiravī***, ***Śvetajīraka*** fruit, ***Kṛṣnajīraka*** fruit, ***Ajamodā*** fruit, ***Ākāra karabha***, ***Śatapuṣpā*** flower, ***Yaṣṭīmadhu*** root, ***Karayāmpu*** fruit, ***Gairika***, ***Hrīvera*** root, ***Rasa sindūra***, ***Pāraṅki*** stem bark, ***Paśupāśi*** stem bark, ***Candana*** wood, ***Vacā*** rhizome, ***Kaṅkola*** fruit, ***Śuṇṭhī*** rhizome, ***Marica*** fruit, ***Pippalī*** fruit, ***Ṭaṅkaṇa***, ***Srotāñjana***, ***Vatsanābha*** rhizome, ***Manaḥśilā***, ***Candrikā*** seed, ***Hiṅgula***, ***Bhṛṅgarāja*** juice.
Anupāna dravyas: ***Jīraka*** fruit ***kvātha***.
Indications: fever, dyspnoea.
Dosage: 125 mg.

Khadirādi guṭikā

Ingredients: ***Khadira*** wood, ***Arimeda*** stem bark, ***Candana*** wood, ***Padmaka*** wood, ***Uśīra*** root, ***Mañjiṣṭhā*** stem, ***Dhātakī*** flower, ***Mustaka*** rhizome, ***Prapuaṇḍarīka*** stem, ***Yaṣṭīmadu*** root, ***Tvak*** stem

bark, ***Elā*** seed, ***Padma*** flower, ***Nāgakeśara*** flower, ***Lākṣā*** exudate, ***Rasāñjana***, ***Jaṭāmāṁsī*** rhizome, ***Harītakī*** fruit pulp, ***Bibhītaka*** fruit pulp, ***Āmalakī*** fruit pulp, ***Lodhra*** stem bark, ***Hrīvera*** root, ***Haridrā*** rhizome, ***Dāruharidrā*** stem, ***Priyaṅgu*** flower, ***Lajjālu*** herb, ***Kaṭphala*** fruit, ***Vacā*** rhizome, ***Yavāsā*** root, ***Agaru*** wood, ***Pattaṅga*** root, ***Gairika***, ***Srotāñjana***, ***Lavaṅga*** flower, ***Nakha***, ***Kaṅkola*** rhizome, ***Jātipatrī*** aril, ***Karpūra*** exudate.
Anupāna dravyas: honey.
Indications: bad breath, apthous stomatitis, toothache, dental caries, hoarseness.
Dosage: 2 g, dissolved in mouth.

Candraprabhā vaṭī

Ingredients: ***Karpūra*** (***Candraprabhā***) leaf, ***Vacā*** rhizome, ***Mustaka*** rhizome, ***Bhūnimba*** herb, ***Guḍūcī*** stem, ***Devadāru*** wood, ***Haridrā*** rhizome, purified ***Ativiṣā*** root, ***Dāruharidrā*** stem, ***Pippalīmūla*** root, ***Citraka*** root, ***Dhānyaka*** fruit, ***Harītakī*** fruit pulp, ***Bibhītaka*** fruit pulp, ***Āmalakī*** fruit pulp, ***Cavya*** stem, ***Viḍanga*** fruit, ***Gajapippalī*** fruit, ***Śuṇṭhī*** rhizome, ***Marica*** fruit, ***Pippalī*** fruit, ***Svarna mākṣika bhasma***, ***Yavakṣāra***, ***Sarjikṣāra***, ***Saindhava lavaṇa***, ***Sauvarcala lavaṇa***, ***Viḍa lavaṇa***, ***Trivṛt*** root, ***Dantī*** root, ***Tejapatra*** leaf, ***Tvak*** stem bark, ***Patra*** leaf, ***Elā*** seed, ***Vaṃśarocanā***, ***Lauha bhasma***, sugar, ***Śilājatu***, ***Guggulu*** resin.
Anupāna dravyas: water, milk, sesame seed powder.
Indications: flatulence, colic, anaemia, jaundice, dysuria, urinary calculi, gout, haemorrhoids, diabetes, chicken pox, fevers, itching.
Dosage: 250–500 mg.

Citrakādi guṭikā

Ingredients: ***Citraka*** root, ***Pippalīmūla*** root, ***Yavakṣāra***, ***Sarjikṣāra***, ***Sauvarcala lavaṇa***, ***Saindhava lavaṇa***, ***Viḍa lavaṇa***, ***Audbhida lavaṇa***, ***Sāmudra lavaṇa***, ***Śuṇṭhī*** rhizome, ***Marica*** fruit, ***Pippalī*** fruit, ***Ajamodā*** fruit, ***Cavya*** stem, ***Mātuluṅga*** juice.
Anupāna dravyas: warm water, buttermilk.
Indications: digestive weakness, ***āma***, flatulence, malabsorption syndromes.
Dosage: 500 mg.

Gorocanāḍī vaṭī

Ingredients: ***Gorocana***, ***Mṛgaśṛṅga***, ***Ruḍrākṣa*** seed, ***Candana*** wood, ***Vacā*** rhizome, ***Aklāri*** fruit, ***Uśīra*** root, ***Kamala*** flower, ***Gandha mājara virya***, ***Nāga bhasma***, ***Kṛṣna mṛgasṛṅga***, ***Gosṛṇga***, ***Varāhasṛṇga***, ***Ajāśṛṅga***, ***Māhiśṛṅga***, ***Kirātatikta*** herb, ***Svarṇa bhasma***, ***Pravāla bhasma***, ***Srotāñjana***, ***Karpūra*** leaves, ***Jīraka*** fruit, ***Droṇapuṣpī*** herb, ***Kārpāsa*** seed, ***Apāmārga*** seed, ***Laśuna*** bulb, ***Cirabilva*** wood, ***Śuṇṭhī*** rhizome, ***Marica*** fruit, ***Pippalī*** fruit, ***Agnimañtha*** root, ***Pitacandana*** wood, ***Pāṭhā*** root, ***Śaṅkhapuṣpa*** herb, ***Nīlinī*** herb, ***Harītakī*** fruit pulp, ***Bibhītaka*** fruit pulp, ***Āmalakī*** fruit pulp, ***Jātīphala*** seed, ***Māyāphala***, ***Śatapuṣpī*** flower, ***Ajālī*** fruit, ***Mustaka*** rhizome, ***Kṛṣnajīraka*** fruit, ***Ambara*** fruit, ***Ādraka*** juice.
Anupāna dravyas: ***Ādraka*** juice, ***Nāgavallī*** juice, ***Tulasī*** juice.
Indications: fever, cough, dyspnoea, diseases of the throat, disorders of the liver.
Dosage: 125 mg.

Mānasamitra vaṭaka

Ingredients: ***Balā*** root, ***Nāgabalā*** root, ***Bilva*** root, ***Śālaparṇī*** root, ***Pravāla*** herb, ***Śaṅkhapuṣpī*** herb, ***Tāmra***, ***Svarṇa bhasma***, ***Puṣkaramūla*** root, ***Mṛgaśṛṅga bhasma***, ***Vacā*** rhizome, ***Mākṣika bhasma***, ***Candana*** wood, ***Raktacandana*** wood, ***Muktā***, ***Aguru bhasma***, ***Yaṣṭīmadhu*** root, ***Tvak*** stem bark, ***Pippalī*** fruit, ***Karpūra***, ***Elāvāluka*** seed, ***Viśāla*** herb, ***Aklāri*** herb, ***Nirguṇḍi*** root, ***Mustaka*** rhizome, ***Rāsnā*** root and leaf, ***Rajata bhasma***, ***Śilājatu***, ***Gojivhā*** herb, ***Padma*** aril, ***Jīvaka*** root, ***Ṛṣabhaka*** root, ***Kākolī*** root, ***Kṣīrakākolī*** root, ***Bṛhatī*** root, ***Kaṇṭakāri*** herb, ***Muṇḍitikā*** herb, ***Bhūnimba*** herb, ***Āragvadha*** stem bark, ***Parūṣaka*** root, ***Harītakī*** fruit pulp, ***Bibhītaka*** fruit pulp, ***Āmalakī*** fruit pulp, ***Guḍūcī*** stem, ***Śvetasārivā*** root, ***Kṛṣnasārivā*** root, ***Jīvantī*** root, ***Somalatā*** herb, ***Aśvagandhā*** root, ***Haridrā*** rhizome, ***Uśīra*** root, ***Drākṣā*** fruit, ***Yaṣṭyāhvaya*** root, ***Ṛddhi*** tuber, ***Dūrvā*** root, ***Haṃsapādī*** herb, ***Mustaka*** rhizome, ***Lavaṇga*** flower, ***Tulasī*** leaf, ***Kastūri***, ***Kuṅkuma*** style/stigma, ***Trāyamāṇā*** leaf juice, ***Śaṅkhapuṣpī*** herb, ***Vacā*** rhizome, ***Śvetasārivā*** root, ***Lakṣmaṇa*** root, ***Bilva*** root, ***Balā*** root, ***Somavallī*** juice, breast milk, cow's milk.

Anupāna dravyas: milk.
Indications: mental diseases, insanity, psychosis, mental retardation.
Dosage: 1000 mg.

Laśunādi vaṭī

Ingredients: ***Laśuna*** bulb, ***Jīraka*** fruit, ***saindhava***, ***Gandhaka***, ***Śuṇṭhī*** rhizome, ***Marica*** fruit, ***Pippalī*** fruit, ***Hiṅgu*** exudate, ***Nimbu*** leaf juice.
Anupāna dravyas: warm water.
Indications: indigestion, diarrhoea, gastroenteritis.
Dosage: 1000 mg.

Śaṅkha vaṭī

Ingredients: ***Ciñcākṣāra***, ***Sauvarcala lavaṇa***, ***Saindhava lavaṇa***, ***Viḍa lavaṇa***, ***Audbhida lavaṇa***, ***Sāmudra lavaṇa***, ***Śaṅkha bhasma***, ***Śuṇṭhī*** rhizome, ***Marica*** fruit, ***Pippalī*** fruit, ***Pārada***, ***Vatsanābha*** rhizome, ***Gandhaka***.
Anupāna dravyas: honey, warm water, buttermilk.
Indications: digestive weakness, anorexia, colic, malabsorption, bowel disorders.
Dosage: 250–500 mg.

Śivā guṭikā

Ingredients: ***Kuṭaja*** bark, ***Harītakī*** fruit pulp, ***Bibhītaka*** fruit pulp, ***Āmalakī*** fruit pulp, ***Nimba*** stem bark, ***Paṭola*** herb, ***Mustaka*** rhizome, ***Śuṇṭhī*** rhizome, ***Śilājatu***, sugar, ***Vaṃśarocana***, ***Pippalī*** fruit, ***Karkaṭaśṛṅgī*** gall, ***Kaṇṭakārī*** root and fruit, ***Tvak*** stem bark, ***Elā*** seed, ***Patra*** leaf, ***Drākṣā*** fruit, ***Kharjūra*** fruit, ***Gambhārī*** fruit, ***Lauha bhasma***, ***Abhraka bhasma***.
Anupāna dravyas: warm water.
Indications: anaemia, skin diseases, fever, asthma, hepatomegaly, haemorrhoids, dysuria, consumption, tumours.
Dosage: 6 g, at least 2–3 hours before or after meals.

Avaleha: CONFECTION

Agastyaharītakī rasāyana

Ingredients: ***Bilva*** root, ***Śyonaka*** root, ***Gambhāri*** root, ***Pāṭalā*** root, ***Agnimañtha*** root, ***Śālaparṇī*** root, ***Pṛśniparṇī*** root, ***Bṛhatī*** root, ***Kaṇṭakārī*** root, ***Gokṣura*** root, ***Kapikacchū*** seed, ***Śaṅkhapuṣpī*** herb, ***Śaṭī*** rhizome, ***Balā*** root, ***Gajapippalī*** fruit, ***Apāmārga*** root, ***Pippalīmūla*** root, ***Citraka*** root, ***Bhārṅgī*** root, ***Puṣkaramūla*** root, ***Yava*** seed, ***Harītakī*** fruit, ***Pippalī*** fruit, jaggery, clarified butter, sesame oil, honey.
Anupāna dravyas: warm water, milk.
Indications: as a ***rasāyana***; hiccough, cough, dyspnoea, consumption, weakness, fever.
Dosage: 6–12 g.

Aśvagandhādi lehya

Ingredients: ***Aśvagandhā*** root, ***Sārivā*** root, ***Jīraka*** fruit, ***Madhusnuhī*** rhizome, ***Drākṣā*** fruit, ***Elā*** seed clarified sugar, butter, honey, water.
Anupāna dravyas: milk.
Indications: as a ***rasāyana***; consumption, weakness, infertility.
Dosage: 6–12 g.

Bilvādi lehya

Ingredients: ***Bilva*** root, ***Mustaka*** rhizome, ***Dhānyaka*** fruit, ***Jīraka*** fruit, ***Elā*** seed, ***Tvak*** stem bark, ***Nāgakeśara*** flower, ***Śuṇṭhī*** rhizome, ***Marica*** fruit, ***Pippalī*** fruit, aged jaggery.
Anupāna dravyas: milk, water.
Indications: anorexia, weakness of digestion, vomiting, dyspnoea.
Dosage: 6–12 g.

Brahma rasāyana

Ingredients: ***Āmalaki*** fruit pulp, ***Bilva*** root, ***Gambhāri*** root, ***Pāṭalā*** root, ***Agnimañtha*** root, ***Śālaparṇī*** root, ***Pṛśniparṇī*** root, ***Bṛhatī*** root, ***Kaṇṭakārī*** root, ***Gokṣura*** root, ***Balā*** root, ***Punarnavā*** root, ***Eraṇḍa*** root, ***Māṣaparṇī*** herb, ***Mudgaparṇī*** herb, ***Śatāvarī*** root, ***Medā*** root, ***Jīvantī*** root, ***Jīvaka*** root, ***Ṛṣabhaka*** root, ***Śālī*** root, ***Kāśa*** root, ***Śara*** root, ***Darbha*** root, ***Ikṣu*** root, ***Tvak*** stem bark, ***Elā*** seed, ***Mustaka*** rhizome, ***Haridrā*** rhizome, ***Pippalī*** fruit, ***Agaru*** wood, ***Candana*** wood, ***Maṇḍūkaparṇī*** herb, ***Nāgakeśara*** flower, ***Śaṅkhapuṣpī*** herb, ***Vacā*** rhizome, ***Yaṣṭīmadhu*** root, ***Viḍaṅga*** fruit, rock sugar, clarified butter, sesame oil, honey.
Anupāna dravyas: milk, water.

Indications: as a ***rasāyana***; memory loss, senility, insomnia, headache, mental diseases, cough, weakness and fatigue, male infertility.
Dosage: 12 g.

Cyavanaprāśa

Ingredients: ***Āmalaki*** fresh fruit, ***Bilva*** root, ***Agnimañtha*** root, ***Śyonaka*** root, ***Gambhāri*** root, ***Pāṭalī*** root, ***Balā*** root, ***Śālaparṇī*** root, ***Pṛśniparṇī*** root, ***Māṣaparṇī*** root, ***Mudgaparṇī*** root, ***Pippalī*** fruit, ***Gokṣura*** root, ***Bṛhatī*** root, ***Kaṇṭakārī*** root, ***Śṛṅgī*** gall, ***Bhūmyāmalakī*** herb, ***Drākṣā*** fruit, ***Jīvantī*** root, ***Puṣkara*** root, ***Agaru*** wood, ***Harītakī*** fruit pulp, ***Guḍūcī*** stem, ***Ṛddhi*** root, ***Jīvaka*** root, ***Ṛṣabhaka*** root, ***Śaṭī*** rhizome, ***Mustaka*** rhizome, ***Punarnavā*** root, ***Medā*** root, ***Elā*** seed, ***Candana*** wood, ***Utpala*** flower, ***Vidārikanda*** tuber, ***Vāsāmūla*** root, ***Kākolī*** root, ***Kākanāsikā*** fruit, ***Vaṃśarocanā***, ***Tvak*** stem bark, ***Patra*** leaf, ***Nagakeśara*** flower, clarified butter, sesame oil, honey, sugar.
Anupāna dravyas: milk, water.
Indications: as a ***rasāyana***; cough, dyspnoea, asthma, consumption, weakness and fatigue, diseases of the heart, premature ageing.
Dosage: 12–24 g.

Daśamūla Harītakī

Ingredients: ***Śālaparṇi*** root, ***Pṛśniparṇī*** root, ***Bṛhatī*** root, ***Kaṇṭakāri*** root, ***Gokṣura*** root, ***Bilva*** root, ***Agnimañtha*** root, ***Śyonāka*** root, ***Gambhārī*** root, ***Pāṭalā*** root, ***Harītakī*** fruit pulp, ***Tvak*** stem bark, ***Elā*** seed, ***Patra*** leaf, ***Śuṇṭhī*** rhizome, ***Marica*** fruit, ***Pippalī*** fruit, ***Yavakṣāra***, jaggery, honey.
Anupāna dravyas: milk, water.
Indications: anorexia, dyspnoea, ascites, splenomegaly, abdominal distension, dysuria, oedema, inflammatory joint disease.
Dosage: 6–12 g.

Drākṣāvaleha

Ingredients: ***Drākṣā*** fruit, ***Pippalī*** fruit, ***Yaṣṭīmadhu*** root, ***Śuṇṭhī*** rhizome, ***Vaṃśarocanā***, ***Āmalakī*** fruit juice, sugar, honey.
Anupāna dravyas: milk, water.
Indications: anaemia, jaundice, hepatitis.
Dosage: 6–12 g.

Kūṣmāṇḍaka rasāyana

Ingredients: ***Kūṣmāṇāṇḍa*** fruit, ***Pippalī*** fruit, ***Śuṇṭhī*** rhizome, ***Jīraka*** fruit, ***Tvak*** stem bark, ***Elā*** seed, ***Patra*** leaf, ***Marica*** fruit, ***Dhānyaka*** fruit, honey, sugar, clarified butter.
Anupāna dravyas: milk, water.
Indications: hiccough, cough, dyspnoea, chest injuries, fever.
Dosage: 6–12 g.

Madhusnuhī rasāyana

Ingredients: ***Śuṇṭhī*** rhizome, ***Pippalī*** fruit, ***Marica*** fruit, ***Harītakī*** fruit pulp, ***Bibhītaka*** fruit pulp, ***Āmalakī*** fruit pulp, ***Tvak*** stem bark, ***Elā*** seed, ***Tejapatra*** leaf, ***Jātīphala*** seed, ***Jātīpatrī*** aril, ***Citraka*** root, ***Lavaṅga*** flower, ***Dhānyaka*** fruit, ***Śvetajīraka*** fruit, ***Kṛṣṇajīraka*** fruit, ***Vanyajīraka*** fruit, ***Viḍaṅga*** fruit, ***Cavya*** stem, ***Kuṣṭha*** root, ***Trivṛtā*** root, ***Pippalīmūla*** root, ***Aśvagandhā*** root, ***Bhārṅgi*** root, ***Tejoī*** seed, ***Nāgakeśara*** flower, ***Gandhaka***, ***Guggulu*** exudate, ***Madhusnuhī*** rhizome, clarified butter, sugar, honey.
Anupāna dravyas: milk, water.
Indications: diseases of the throat, anal fistula, gout, skin diseases, ulcers, diabetic carbuncles, cervical adenitis, tumour.
Dosage: 12 g.

Śatāvarī guḍa

Ingredients: ***Śatāvarī*** root, ***Śuṇṭhī*** *rhizome*, ***Elā*** seed, ***Musalī*** tuber, ***Pāṭhā*** root, ***Gokṣura*** fruit, ***Śvetasārivā*** root, ***Kṛṣṇasārivā*** root, ***Bhūmyāmalakī*** root, ***Vidārī*** tuber, ***Pippalī*** fruit, ***Yaṣṭīmadhu*** root, ***Gomūtra šilājatu***, ***Vaṃśarocanā***, sugar, jaggery, clarified butter.
Anupāna dravyas: milk, water.
Indications: dysuria, passive haemorrhage, hepatitis, weakness, consumption, chest injuries, burning sensations in the feet, female reproductive disorders.
Dosage: 12 g.

Taila (MEDICATED OIL)

Aṇu taila

Ingredients: ***Jīvantī*** root, ***Hrīvera*** root, ***Devadāru*** wood, ***Mustaka*** rhizome, ***Tvak*** stem bark, ***Uśīra*** root,

Sārivā root, ***Candana*** wood, ***Dāruharidrā*** stem, ***Yaṣṭīmadhu*** root, ***Mustaka*** rhizome, ***Agaru*** wood, ***Śatāvarī*** root, ***Kamala*** flower, ***Bilva*** stem bark, ***Utpala*** flower, ***Bṛhatī*** root, ***Kaṇṭakāri*** herb, ***Rāsnā*** root, ***Śālaparṇī*** herb, ***Pṛśniparṇī*** herb, ***Viḍaṅga*** fruit, ***Tejapatra*** leaf, ***Elā*** seed, ***Reṇuka*** seed, ***Kamala*** stamens, goat milk, sesame oil.
Indications: headache, rhinitis, sinusitis.
Dosage: as ***nasya***.

Balāguḍūcyādi taila

Ingredients: ***Balā*** root, ***Gūḍūcī*** stem, ***Devadāru*** wood, ***Jaṭāmāṃsī*** rhizome, ***Kuṣṭha*** root, ***Candana*** wood, ***Kunduru*** exudate, ***Tagara*** root, ***Aśvagandhā*** root, ***Sarala*** root, ***Rāsnā*** root, sesame oil.
Indications: pain, burning sensation, inflammatory joint disease.
Dosage: topically, as needed.

Balāshvagandalākṣādi taila

Ingredients: ***Balā*** root, ***Aśvagandhā*** root, ***Lākṣā*** exudate, ***Dadhimastu***, ***Rāsnā*** root, ***Candana*** wood, ***Mañjiṣṭhā*** stem, ***Dūrvā*** root, ***Yaṣṭīmadhu*** root, ***Coraka*** herb, ***Sāriva*** root, ***Uśīra*** root, ***Mustaka*** rhizome, ***Kuṣṭha*** root, ***Agaru*** wood, ***Devadarū*** wood, ***Haridrā*** rhizome, ***Kumudā*** rhizome, ***Reṇukā*** seed, ***Śatapuṣpā*** flower, ***Padma*** stamens, sesame oil.
Indications: fever, cough, dyspnoea, psychosis, emaciation.
Dosage: topically, as needed.

Bhṛṅgarāja taila

Ingredients: ***Bhṛṅgarāja*** leaf juice, ***Mañjiṣṭhā*** stem, ***Padmaka*** wood, ***Lodhra*** stem bark, ***Candana*** wood, ***Gairika***, ***Balā*** root, ***Haridrā*** rhizome, ***Dāruharidrā*** stem, ***Nāgakeśara*** flower, ***Priyaṅgu*** flower, ***Yaṣṭīmadhu*** root, ***Kamala*** root, ***Sārivā*** root, sesame oil.
Indications: mental disorders, ear diseases, eye diseases, headache, alopecia.
Dosage: topically, as needed; as ***nasya***.

Candanādi taila

Ingredients: ***Candana*** wood, ***Hrīvera*** root, ***Nakha***, ***Haridrā*** rhizome, ***Yaṣṭīmadhu*** root, ***Śaileya*** herb, ***Padmaka*** wood, ***Mañjiṣṭha*** stem, ***Sarala*** root, ***Devadāru*** wood, ***Śaṭī*** rhizome, ***Elā*** seed, ***Jātī*** flower, ***Nāgakeśara*** flower, ***Tejapatra*** leaf, ***Bilva*** stem bark, ***Uśīra*** root, ***Kaṅkola*** rhizome, ***Raktacandana*** wood, ***Mustaka*** rhizome, ***Haridrā*** rhizome, ***Dāruharidrā*** stem, ***Śvetasārivā*** root, ***Kṛṣnasārivā*** root, ***Kaṭuka*** rhizome, ***Lavaṅga*** flower, ***Aguru*** wood, ***Kuṅkuma*** stigma/style, ***Tvak*** stem bark, ***Reṇukā*** seed, ***Nalikā*** stem bark, ***Lākṣā*** juice, sesame oil, honey.
Indications: burning sensations, passive haemorrhage, consumption, epilepsy, psychosis, disease of the eye.
Dosage: topically, as needed.

Kṣīrabalā taila

Ingredients: ***Balā*** root, milk, sesame oil.
Anupāna: milk, warm water.
Indications: neuromuscular diseases.
Dosage: 12 g; topically, as needed; ***nasya***.

Murivenna taila

Ingredients: ***Karañja*** bark, ***Nāgavallī*** leaf, ***Kumārī*** leaf, ***Pāribhadra*** leaf, ***Palāṇḍu*** bulb, ***Śigru*** leaf, ***Madanaghaṇṭī*** herb, ***Śatāvarī*** root, coconut oil.
Indications: pain, fractures, injuries, infections, burns, ulcerations.
Dosage: topically, as needed.

Nārāyaṇa taila

Ingredients: ***Bilva*** root, ***Agnimañtha*** root, ***Śyonāka*** root, ***Pāṭalā*** root, ***Pāribhadra*** root, ***Prasāraṇī*** root, ***Aśvagandhā*** root, ***Bṛhatī*** root, ***Kaṇṭakārī*** herb, ***Balā*** root, ***Atibalā*** root, ***Gokṣura*** fruit, ***Punarnavā*** root, ***Śatapuṣpā*** flower, ***Devadāru*** wood, ***Jaṭāmāṁsī*** rhizome, ***Śaileya*** herb, ***Vacā*** rhizome, ***Candana*** wood, ***Tagara*** root, ***Kuṣṭha*** root, ***Elā*** seed, ***Śālaparṇī*** root, ***Pṛśniparṇī*** root, ***Mudgaparṇī*** root, ***Māṣaparṇī*** root, ***Rāsnā*** root and leaf, ***Śatāvarī*** root juice, ***saindhava***, sesame oil, milk.
Anupāna: milk, warm water.
Indications: mental diseases, pain, paralysis, arthritis, sciatica, emaciation, hernia, diseases of the head, impotency.
Dosage: 6 g; topically, as needed; ***nasya***.

Nīlībhṛṅgādi taila

Ingredients: ***Nīlī*** leaf juice, ***Bhṛṅgarāja*** leaf juice, ***Indravāruṇī*** leaf, ***Āmalakī*** fruit juice, ***Yaṣṭīmadhu*** root, ***Guñjā*** root, ***Añjana***, goat milk, water buffalo milk, cow milk, coconut water, sesame oil.
Indications: hair loss, alopecia.
Dosage: topically, as needed.

Piṇḍa taila

Ingredients: ***Mañjiṣṭhā*** stem, ***Sarja*** exudate, ***Sārivā*** root, beeswax, sesame oil.
Indications: burning sensations, inflammatory joint disease.
Dosage: topically, as needed; ***nasya***.

Ghṛta (MEDICATED *ghṛta*)

Amṛtā ghṛta

Ingredients: ***Gūḍūcī*** stem, ***Śuṇṭhī*** rhizome, clarified butter.
Anupāna: milk, warm water.
Indications: inflammatory joint disease, parasites, ulcers, haemorrhoids, abdominal distension, skin conditions.
Dosage: 12 g.

Brāhmī ghṛta

Ingredients: ***Brāhmī*** leaf juice, ***Śuṇṭhī*** rhizome, ***Marica*** fruit, ***Pippalī*** fruit, ***Kṛṣṇatrvṛt*** root, ***Śvetatrvṛt*** root, ***Dantī*** root, ***Śaṅkhapuṣpī*** herb, ***Āragvadha*** fruit, ***Saptalā*** herb, ***Viḍaṅga*** fruit, clarified butter.
Anupāna: milk, warm water.
Indications: epilepsy, psychosis, infertility, skin disease.
Dosage: 12 g.

Dāḍimādi ghṛta

Ingredients: ***Dāḍima*** seed, ***Dhānyaka*** fruit, ***Citraka*** root, ***Śṛṅgavera*** rhizome, ***Pippalī*** fruit, clarified butter.
Anupāna: milk, warm water.
Indications: weakness of digestion, anaemia, abdominal distension, haemorrhoids, heart disease, disorders of pregnancy.
Dosage: 48 g.

Dhānvantara ghṛta

Ingredients: ***Bilva*** root, ***Śyonāka*** root, ***Gambhārī*** root, ***Pāṭalā*** root, ***Agnimañtha*** root, ***Śālaparṇī*** root, ***Pṛśniparṇī*** root, ***Bṛhatī*** root, ***Kaṇṭakārī*** root, ***Gokṣura*** root, ***Śaṭī*** rhizome, ***Dantī*** root, ***Devadāru*** wood, ***Śvetapunarnavā*** root, ***Raktapunarnavā*** root, ***Snuhī*** root, ***Arka*** root, ***Harītakī*** fruit pulp, ***Muṇḍitikā*** root, ***Bhallātaka*** fruit, ***Karañja*** root, ***Varuṇa*** root, ***Pippalimūla*** root, ***Puṣkaramūla*** root, ***Yava*** seed, ***Kola*** seed, ***Kulattha*** seed, ***Pippalī*** fruit, ***Gajapippalī*** fruit, ***Cavya*** stem, ***Vacā*** rhizome, ***Jalavetasa*** herb, ***Rohiṣā*** root, ***Trivṛt*** root, ***Viḍanga*** fruit, ***Kampilla*** stem, ***Bhārṅgī*** root, clarified butter.
Anupāna: warm water.
Indications: vomiting, cough, consumption, abdominal distension, oedema, haemorrhoids, anaemia, diabetes, skin diseases, psychosis, epilepsy.
Dosage: 48 g.

Jātyādi ghṛta

Ingredients: ***Jātīpatra*** aril, ***Nimba*** leaf, ***Paṭola*** leaf, ***Kaṭuka*** rhizome, ***Dārvī*** stem, ***Haridrā*** rhizome, ***Sārivā*** root, ***Mañjṣṭhā*** stem, ***Uśīra*** root, ***Tuttha***, ***Yaṣṭīmadhu*** root, ***Karañja*** fruit, beeswax, clarified butter.
Anupāna: water.
Indications: ulcers, burns, fractures, pain, skin diseases.
Dosage: topically, as needed.

Mahātikta ghṛta

Ingredients: ***Saptaparṇa*** stem bark, purified ***Ativiṣā*** root, ***Āragvadha*** fruit, ***Kaṭukā*** rhizome, ***Pāṭhā*** root, ***Mustaka*** rhizome, ***Uśīra*** root, ***Harītakī*** fruit pulp, ***Bibhītaka*** fruit pulp, ***Āmalakī*** fruit pulp, ***Paṭola*** leaf, ***Nimba*** stem bark, ***Parpaṭa*** herb, ***Dhanvayāsa*** herb, ***Raktacandana*** wood, ***Pippalī*** fruit, ***Gajapippalī*** fruit, ***Padmaka*** wood, ***Haridrā*** rhizome, ***Dāruharidrā*** stem, ***Vacā*** rhizome, ***Indravāruṇī*** herb, ***Śatāvarī*** root, ***Śvetasārivā*** root, ***Kṛṣṇasārivā*** root, ***Indrayava*** seed, ***Vāsaka*** root, ***Mūrvā*** root, ***Gūḍūcī*** stem, ***Kirātatiktā*** herb, ***Yaṣṭīmadhu*** root, ***Trāyamāṇā*** herb, clarified butter.
Anupāna: warm water, milk.

Indications: dyspepsia, anaemia, jaundice, passive haemorrhage, herpes, abscesses, skin diseases, malabsorption, haemorrhoids, epilepsy.
Dosage: 6 g; applied topically, as needed.

Nārasimha ghṛta

Ingredients: ***Khadira*** wood, ***Citraka*** root, ***Śimśapā*** stem bark, ***Asana*** stem bark, ***Harītakī*** fruit pulp, ***Viḍaṅga*** fruit, ***Bhallātaka*** fruit, ***Lauha***, ***Bhṛṅgarāja*** leaf juice, ***Bibhītaka*** fruit pulp, ***Āmalakī*** fruit pulp, milk, butter.
Anupāna: honey, sugar, milk, cool water.
Indications: as a ***rasāyana***; infertility, hair loss, weakness, emaciation.
Dosage: 12 g.

Sārasvāta ghṛta

Ingredients: ***Harītakī*** fruit pulp, ***Śuṇṭhī*** rhizome, ***Marica*** fruit, ***Pippalī*** fruit, ***Pāṭhā*** root, ***Vacā*** rhizome, ***Śigru*** root bark, ***saindhava***, goat's milk, clarified butter.
Anupāna: warm water, warm milk.
Indications: weakness of voice, hoarseness, poor memory, difficulty learning, weak digestion.
Dosage: 12 g.

Sukumāra ghṛta

Ingredients: ***Punarnavā*** root, ***Bilva*** root, ***Śyonāka*** root, ***Gambhārī*** root, ***Paṭalā*** root, ***Agnimañtha*** root, ***Śālaparṇī*** root, ***Pṛśniparṇī*** root, ***Bṛhatī*** root, ***Kaṇṭakārī*** root, ***Gokṣura*** root, ***Kṣīrakākolī*** root, ***Aśvagandhā*** root, ***Eraṇḍa*** root, ***Śatāvarī*** root, ***Darbha*** root, ***Kuśa*** root, ***Śara*** root, ***Kāśa*** root, ***Ikṣu*** root, ***Poṭagala*** root, ***Pippalī*** fruit and root, ***Yaṣṭīmadhu*** root, ***Kāṣṭhasāra*** wood, ***Drākṣā*** dried fruit, ***Yavānī*** fruit, ***Śuṇṭhī*** rhizome, ***saindhava***, castor oil, milk, clarified butter, jaggery.
Anupāna: warm water, warm milk.
Indications: constipation, haemorrhoids, hernia, splenomegaly, abdominal distension, oedema, dysmenorrhoea, abscesses, weakness, fatigue.
Dosage: 12 g.

Triphala ghṛta

Ingredients: ***Harītakī*** fruit pulp, ***Bibhītaka*** fruit pulp, ***Āmalakī*** fruit pulp, ***Śuṇṭhī*** rhizome, ***Marica*** fruit, ***Pippalī*** fruit, ***Drākṣā*** fruit, ***Yaṣṭīmadhu*** root, ***Kaṭuka*** rhizome, ***Prapuaṇḍarīka*** flower, ***Sūkṣmailā*** seed, ***Viḍaṅga*** fruit, ***Nāgakeśara*** fruit, ***Nīlotpala*** flower, ***Śvetasārivā*** root, ***Kṛṣṇasārivā*** root, ***Candana*** wood, ***Haridrā*** rhizome, ***Dāruharidrā*** stem, clarified butter, milk.
Anupāna: warm water, milk.
Indications: jaundice, eye diseases, erysipelas, tumours, menorrhagia.
Dosage: 12 g.

Asava AND *ariṣṭa*: (NATURAL FERMENTATIONS)

Abhayāriṣṭa

Ingredients: ***Harītakī*** fruit pulp, ***Drākṣā*** fruit, ***Viḍaṅga*** fruit, ***Madhūka*** flower, ***Gokṣura*** fruit, ***Trivṛt*** root, ***Dhānyaka*** fruit, ***Dhātakī*** flower, ***Indravāruṇī*** root, ***Cavya*** stem, ***Śatapuṣpā*** fruit, ***Śuṇṭhī*** rhizome, ***Dantī*** root, ***Kunduru*** exudate, jaggery, water.
Indications: digestive weakness, haemorrhoids, constipation, malabsorption, bowel disorders, abdominal distension, parasites, emaciation, shock.
Dosage: 12–24 mL.

Aśokāriṣṭa

Ingredients: ***Aśoka*** stem bark, ***Dhātakī*** flower, ***Ajālī*** fruit, ***Mustaka*** rhizome, ***Śuṇṭhī*** rhizome, ***Dārvī*** stem, ***Utpala*** flower, ***Harītakī*** fruit pulp, ***Bibhītaka*** fruit pulp, ***Āmalakī*** fruit pulp, ***Āmra*** seed, ***Jīraka*** fruit, ***Vāsaka*** root, ***Candana*** wood, jaggery, water.
Indications: haemorrhage, dysmenorrhoea, leucorrhoea, menorrhagia, diabetes, haematuria.
Dosage: 12–24 mL.

Aśvagandhādyariṣṭa

Ingredients: ***Aśvagandhā*** root, ***Musalī*** root, ***Mañjiṣṭhā*** stem, ***Harītakī*** fruit pulp, ***Haridrā*** rhizome, ***Dāruharidrā*** stem, ***Yaṣṭīmadhu*** root, ***Rāsnā*** root, ***Vidārī*** tuber, ***Arjuna*** stem bark, ***Mustaka*** rhizome, ***Trivṛt*** root, ***Sārivā*** root, ***Kṛṣṇasārivā*** root, ***Candana*** wood, ***Raktacandana*** wood, ***Vacā*** rhizome, ***Dhātakī*** flower, ***Śuṇṭhī*** rhizome, ***Marica*** fruit, ***Pippalī*** fruit, ***Tvak*** stem bark, ***Tejapatra*** leaf, ***Priyaṅgu*** fruit, ***Nāgakeśara*** flower, honey, water.

Indications: digestive weakness, fainting, vertigo, psychosis, epilepsy.
Dosage: 12–24 mL.

Balāriṣṭa

Ingredients: ***Balā*** root, ***Aśvagandhā*** root, ***Dhātakī*** flower, ***Kṣīrakākolī*** root, ***Eraṇḍa*** root, ***Rāsnā*** root, ***Elā*** seed, ***Prasāparṇī*** leaf, ***Lavaṅga*** flower, ***Uśīra*** root, ***Gokṣura*** fruit, jaggery, water.
Indications: digestive weakness, infertility, asthenia.
Dosage: 12–24 mL.

Daśamūlāriṣṭa

Ingredients: ***Śālaparṇi*** root, ***Pṛśniparṇī*** root, ***Bṛhatī*** root, ***Kaṇṭakāri*** root, ***Gokṣura*** root, ***Bilva*** root, ***Agnimañtha*** root, ***Śyonāka*** root, ***Gambhārī*** root, ***Pāṭalā*** root, ***Citraka*** root, ***Puṣkaramūla*** root, ***Lodhra*** stem bark, ***Gūḍūcī*** root, ***Āmalakī*** fruit pulp, ***Durālabhā*** herb, ***Khadira*** wood, ***Bījasāra*** wood, ***Harītakī*** fruit pulp, ***Kuṣṭha*** root, ***Mañjiṣṭhā*** stem, ***Devadāru*** wood, ***Viḍaṅga*** fruit, ***Yaṣṭīmadhu*** root, ***Bhārṅgī*** root, ***Kapittha*** fruit pulp, ***Bibhītaka*** fruit pulp, ***Punarnavā*** root, ***Cavya*** stem, ***Jaṭāmāṁsī*** root, ***Priyaṅgu*** fruit, ***Sārivā*** root, ***Kṛṣṇajīraka*** fruit, ***Trivṛt*** root, ***Reṇukā*** seed, ***Rāsnā*** leaf and root, ***Pippalī*** fruit, ***Pūga*** seed, ***Śaṭī*** rhizome, ***Haridrā*** rhizome, ***Satapuṣpā*** fruit, ***Padmaka*** stem, ***Nāgakeśara*** flower, ***Mustaka*** rhizome, ***Indrayava*** seed, ***Śṛṅgī*** gall, ***Jivaka*** root, ***Ṛṣabhaka*** root, ***Medā*** root, ***Mahāmedā*** root, ***Kākolī*** root, ***Kṣīrakākolī*** root, ***Ṛddhi*** tuber, ***Vṛddhikā*** tuber, ***Drākṣā*** fruit, ***Dhātaki*** flower, ***Kaṅkola*** seed, ***Hrīvera*** root, ***Candana*** wood, ***Jātīphala*** seed, ***Lavaṅga*** fruit, ***Tvak*** stem bark, ***Elā*** seed, ***Tejapatra*** leaf, ***Kastūrī***, ***Kataka*** seed, jaggery, honey, water.
Indications: cough, asthma, anorexia, vomiting, abdominal distension, malabsorption, bowel disorders, haemorrhoids, anal fistula, jaundice, diabetes, dysuria, urinary calculi, emaciation, weakness, infertility, postpartum.
Dosage: 12–24 mL.

Drākṣāriṣṭa

Ingredients: ***Drākṣā*** fruit, ***Tvak*** stem bark, ***Elā*** seed, ***Tejapatra*** leaf, ***Nāgakeśara*** flower, ***Priyaṅgu*** fruit, ***Marica*** fruit, ***Pippalī*** fruit, ***Viḍaṅga*** fruit, ***Dhātakī*** flower, jaggery, water.
Indications: digestive weakness, constipation, cough, dyspnoea, laryngitis, chest injuries, anaemia, emaciation, weakness, infertility.
Dosage: 12–24 mL.

Kumāryāsava

Ingredients: ***Kumārī*** leaf juice, ***Śuṇṭhī*** rhizome, ***Marica*** fruit, ***Pippalī*** fruit, ***Lavaṅga*** flower, ***Tvak*** stem bark, ***Elā*** seed, ***Tejapatra*** leaf, ***Nāgakeśara*** flower, ***Citraka*** root, ***Pippalī mūla*** root, ***Viḍaṅga*** seed, ***Gajapippalī*** fruit, ***Cavya*** stem, ***Dhānyaka*** fruit, ***Pūga*** seed, ***Kaṭukā*** rhizome, ***Mustaka*** rhizome, ***Harītakī*** fruit pulp, ***Bibhītaka*** fruit pulp, ***Āmalakī*** fruit pulp, ***Rāsnā*** root, ***Devadāru*** wood, ***Haridrā*** rhizome, ***Dāruharidrā*** stem, ***Mūrvā*** root, ***Gūḍūcī*** stem, ***Dantī*** root, ***Puṣkaramūla*** root, ***Balā*** root, ***Atibalā*** root, ***Kapikacchū*** seed, ***Gokṣura*** fruit, ***Śatapuṣpā*** seed, ***Hiṅgu*** leaf, ***Ākārakarabha***, root, ***Uṭiṅgaṇa*** seed, ***Śvetapunarnavā*** root, ***Raktapunarnavā*** root, ***Lodhra*** stem bark, ***Dhātakī*** flower, ***Mākṣika bhasma***, ***Loha bhasma***, jaggery, honey, water.
Indications: weakness of digestion, colic, abdominal distension, liver disorders, dysuria, diabetes, psychosis, epilepsy, weakness, passive haemorrhage.
Dosage: 12–24 mL.

Kuṭajāriṣṭa

Ingredients: ***Kuṭaja*** root bark, ***Drākṣā*** fruit, ***Madhūka*** flower, ***Gambhārī*** stem bark, ***Dhātakī*** flower, jaggery, water.
Indications: malabsorption, gastroenteritis, dysentery, fever.
Dosage: 12–24 mL.

Lohāsava

Ingredients: ***Loha cūrṇa***, ***Śuṇṭhī*** rhizome, ***Marica*** fruit, ***Pippalī*** fruit, ***Harītakī*** fruit pulp, ***Bibhītaka*** fruit pulp, ***Āmalakī*** fruit pulp, ***Yavānī*** fruit, ***Viḍaṅga*** fruit, ***Mustaka*** rhizome, ***Citraka*** root, ***Dhātakī*** flower, honey, jaggery, water.
Indications: anaemia, oedema, abdominal distension, splenomegaly, malabsorption, haemorrhoids, anal fistula, skin diseases, cough, dyspnoea, heart disease.
Dosage: 12–24 mL.

Vāsakāsava

Ingredients: ***Vāsaka*** herb, ***Dhātakī*** flower, ***Tvak*** stem bark, ***Elā*** seed, ***Tejapatra*** leaf, ***Nāgakeśara*** flower, ***Kaṅkola*** fruit, ***Śuṇṭhī*** rhizome, ***Marica*** fruit, ***Pippalī*** fruit, ***Hrīvera*** root, jaggery, water.
Indications: cough, passive haemorrhage, fever, oedema, consumption.
Dosage: 12–24 mL.

Bhasma (PURIFIED CALCINATIONS)

Abhraka bhasma

Ingredients: purified mica.
Anupāna: honey, clarified butter, ***Triphala*** decoction, ***Guḍūcī*** stem juice.
Indications: used as a ***rasāyana***; weakness of digestion, malabsorption, bowel disorders, cough, dyspnoea, passive haemorrhage, diabetes, anaemia.
Dosage: 125–375 mg.

Lauha bhasma

Ingredients: purified iron.
Indications: dyspepsia, colic, diarrhoea, ascites, splenomegaly, anaemia, jaundice, parasites, obesity, diabetes, oedema, dyspnoea, skin diseases.
Anupāna: honey, clarified butter, ***Trikaṭu cūrṇa***, ***Triphala cūrṇa***, ***Haridrā*** rhizome juice.
Dosage: 125–250 mg.

Pravāla bhasma

Ingredients: purified coral.
Indications: cough, dyspnoea, fever, oedema, dysuria, nephritis, cardiac arrhythmia, weakness, consumption, passive haemorrhage.
Anupāna: ***Gokṣura kvātha***, ***Śatāvarī kvātha***, honey.
Dosage: 250 mg.

Gandhaka bhasma

Ingredients: purified sulphur.
Indications: poor digestion, malabsorption, intestinal parasites, splenomegaly, itching, skin diseases, consumption, weakness.
Anupāna: honey.
Dosage: 125 mg.

Śaṅkha bhasma

Ingredients: purified conch shell.
Indications: indigestion, dyspepsia, colic, malabsorption, bowel disorders, hepatosplenomegaly, poisoning.
Anupāna: clarified butter, honey.
Dosage: 250–300 mg.

Śṛṅga bhasma

Ingredients: purified deer horn.
Indications: hiccough, cough, dyspnoea, colic, pleurisy, angina pectoris.
Anupāna: honey, clarified butter, ***Trikaṭu cūrṇa***, ***Triphala cūrṇa***, ***Haridrā*** rhizome juice.
Dosage: 250–500 mg.

Svarṇa bhasma

Ingredients: purified gold.
Indications: fever, consumption, emaciation, mental deficiencies, epilepsy, poisoning, diseases of the heart, diseases of the eye, immunodeficiency.
Anupāna: honey, butter.
Dosage: 15.5–62.5 mg.

Tāmra bhasma

Ingredients: purified copper.
Indications: poor digestion, gastritis, abdominal distension and pain, cough, dyspnoea, disorders of the liver, vitiligo, poisoning, diseases of the eye, consumption.
Anupāna: honey, clarified butter, ***Trikaṭu cūrṇa***, ***Triphala cūrṇa***, ***Haridrā*** rhizome juice.
Dosage: 31.25–62.5 mg.

Vajra bhasma

Ingredients: purified diamond.
Indications: anaemia, ascites, splenomegaly, oedema, consumption, eye diseases, tumours.
Anupāna: honey.
Dosage: 8 mg.

Yaśada bhasma

Ingredients: purified zinc.
Indications: malabsorption, cough, dyspnoea, consumption, diabetes, anaemia, diseases of the eye.
Anupāna: honey, ***Gūḍūcī*** stem ***kvātha***, ***Trikaṭu kvātha***.
Dosage: 125 mg.

PART 3

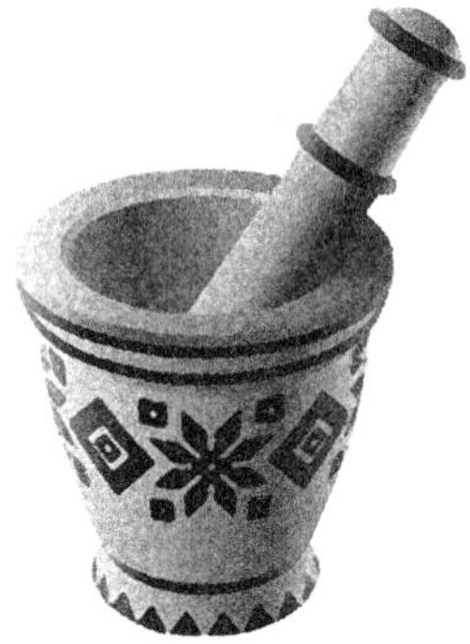

Appendix 3

GLOSSARY OF ĀYURVEDIC HERBS, MINERALS AND ANIMAL PRODUCTS

BOTANICALS AND BOTANICAL PRODUCTS

Ābhā	*Acacia arabica*
Āḍhakī	*Cajanus cajan*
Agnimañtha	*Premna integrifolia, P. micronata*
Aguru	*Aquilaria agallocha*
Ahiphena	*Papaver somniferum*
Ajagandhā	*Gynandropsis gynandra*
Ajamodā	*Trachyspermum roxburghianum, Apium graveolens*
Ākārakarabha	*Anacyclus pyrethrum*
Aklāri	*Lodoicea maldivica*
Akṣoḍa	*Juglans regia*
Āmalaka	*Emblica officinalis*
Ambaṣṭhākī	*Hibiscus sabdariffa*
Amlavetasa	*Garcinia pedunculata, Rheum emodi*
Āmra	*Mangifera indica*
Āmrātaka	*Spondias pinnata*
Apāmārga	*Achyranthes aspera*
Aparājitā	*Clitoria ternatea*
Āragvadha	*Cassia fistula*
Araluka	*Ailanthus excelsa*
Ārdraka (fresh form)	*Zingiber officinalis*
Arimeda	*Acacia leuocophloea*
Arjuna	*Terminalia arjuna*
Arka	*Calotropsis procera*
Āsana	*Pterocarpus marsupium*
Aṣmantaka	*Bauhinia variegata*
Aśoka	*Saraca asoca, S. indica*
Āsphoṭa	*Hemidesmus indicus*
Asthisamhṛta	*Cissus quadrangularis*
Aśvagandhā	*Withania somnifera*
Aśvakarṇa	*Dipterocarpus alatus, Terminalia tomentosa*
Aśvattha	*Ficus religiosa*
Atasī	*Linum usitatissimum*
Atibalā	*Abutilon indicum*
Ativiṣā	*Aconitum heterophyllum*
Ātmaguptā	*Mucuna prurita*
Babūla	*Acacia arabica*
Bākucī	*Psorolea corylifolia*
Bakula	*Mimusops elengi*
Balā	*Sida cordifolia*
Balāka	*Coleus vettiveroides*
Basthāntri	*Argyreia speciosa*
Bhallātaka	*Semecarpus anacardium*
Bhāṅga	*Cannabis sativa*
Bhārṅgī	*Clerodendrum serratum*
Bhṛhatgokṣura	*Pedalium murex, Acacia suma*
Bhṛṅgarāja	*Ecipta alba, E. prostata*
Bhūmyāmalakī	*Phyllanthus amarus, P. niruri*
Bhūrja	*Betula utilis*
Bhūtika	*Cymbopogon ciratus*
Bibhītaka	*Terminalia belerica*
Bījapūra	*Citrus medica*
Bilva	*Aegle marmelos*
Bimbī	*Coccinia indica*
Bola	*Commiphora myrrha*
Brāhmī	*Bacopa monniera*
Bṛhatī	*Solanum indicum*
Campaka	*Michelia champaca*
Caṇaka	*Cicer arientinum*
Caṇḍā	*Angelica archangelica*
Candana	*Santalum album*
Candrikā	*Lepidium sativum*
Cāṅgerī	*Oxalis corniculata*
Cavya	*Piper chaba*
Chāgakarṇa	*Vateria indica*
Ciñcā	*Tamarindus indica*
Cirabilva	*Holoptelea integrifolia*
Citraka	*Plumbago zeylanica*
Coraka	*Angelica glauca*
Dāḍima	*Punica granatum*
Dantī	*Baliospermum montanum*
Darbha	*Imperata cylindrica*
Dāruharidrā	*Berberis aristata, B. asiatica*

Dārvī	*Berberis aristata*
Devadāru	*Cedrus deodar*
Dhanvayāsa	*Fagonia cretica*
Dhānyaka	*Coriandrum sativum*
Dhātakī	*Woodfordia fruticosa*
Dhattūra	*Datura* spp.
Dhava	*Anogeissus latifolia*
Drākṣā	*Vitis vinifera*
Dravantī	*Jatropha glandulifera*
Droṇapuṣpa	*Leucas cephalotes*
Dugdhikā	*Euphorbia thymifolia, E. prostrata*
Durālabhā	*Fagonia cretica*
Dūrvā	*Cynodon dactylon*
Elā	*Elettaria cardamomum*
Elavāluka	*Prunus avium, P. cerasus*
Eraṇḍa	*Ricinus communis*
Ervāru	*Cucumis melo var. utilissimus*
Gajapippalī	*Scindapsus officinalis*
Gambhārī	*Gmelia arborea*
Gaṇḍhādūrvā	*Cyperus rotundus*
Gaṇgerukī	*Grewia populifolia*
Ghoṇṭā	*Zizyphus xylopyra*
Gojivhā	*Onosma bracteatum*
Gokṣura	*Tribulus terrestris*
Granthiparṇa	*Leonotis nepetaefolia*
Guḍūcī	*Tinospora cordifolia*
Guggulu	*Commiphora mukul*
Guñjā	*Abrus precatorius*
Haṃsapadī	*Adiantum lunulatum*
Hapuṣā	*Juniperus communis*
Haridrā	*Curcuma longa*
Harītakī	*Terminalia chebula*
Himsrā	*Capparis spinosa*
Hiṅgu	*Ferula foetida*
Hṛddhātrī	*Smilax china*
Hrīvera	*Coleus vettiveroides*
Ikṣu	*Saccharum officinarum*
Ikṣura bīja	*Astercantha longifolia* seed
Indravāruṇī	*Citrullus colocynthis* variety
Indrayava	*Holarrhena antidysenterica* seed
Īśvarī	*Aristolochia indica*
Jalakarṇā	*Lippia nodiflora*
Jalavetasa	*Salix tetrasperma*
Jambū	*Syzygium cumini*
Japā	*Hibiscus rosa sinensis*
Jaṭāmāmsī	*Nardostachys jatamansi*
Jātī	*Jasminum officinale*
Jātīphala	*Myristica fragrans*
Jayanti	*Sesbania sesban*
Jayapāla	*Croton toglium*
Jīraka	*Cuminum cyminum*
Jīvaka	*Microstylis muscifera*
Jīv˜antī	*Leptadenia reticulata*
Jyotiṣmatī	*Celastrus paniculatus*
Kadalī	*Musa paradisiaca*
Kadaṃba	*Anthocephalus cadamba*
Kadara	*Acacia suma*
Kākajaṅghā	*Peristrophe bicalyculata*
Kākamācī	*Solanum nigrum*
Kākanāsikā	*Pentatropsis microphylla*
Kākatiktā	*Cardiospermum halicacabum*
Kākolī	*Lilium polyphyllum*
Kālanusārivā	*Valeriana wallachi*
Kamala	*Nelumbo nucifera*
Kampilla	*Mallotus philippinensis*
Kāñcanāra	*Bauhinia variegata*
Kaṅkola	*Piper cubeba*
Kaṇṭakāri	*Solanum xanthocarpum*
Kapittha	*Feronia limonia*
Karañja	*Pongamia pinnata*
Kāravall	*Momordica charantia*
Karavīra	*Nerium indicum*
Karcūra	*Curcuma zedoaria*
Kariṅkāra	*Carissa carandas*
Karkaṭaśṛṅgī	*Pistacia integerrima*
Kārpāssa	*Gossypium herbaceum*
Karpūra	*Cinnamomum camphora*
Kāśa	*Saccharum spontaneum*
Kaśeru	*Scirpus kysoor*
Kastūrilatikā	*Hibiscus esculentus*
Kataka	*Strychnos potatorum*
Kaṭphala	*Myrica nagi*
Kaṭuka	*Picrorrhiza kurroa**
Ketakī	*Pandanus tectorius, P. odoratissimus*
Khadira	*Acacia catechu*
Kharjūra	*Phoenix dactylifera, P. sylvestris*
Kirātatiktā	*Swerta chirata*
Kodrava	*Paspalum scrobiculatum*
Kokilākṣa	*Astercantha longifolia*
Kola	*Zizyphus jujuba*
Kolamajja	*Zizyphus jujuba* seed
Kośātakī	*Luffa acutangula*
Kṛṣṇajīraka	*Carum carvi*
Kṛṣṇasārivā	*Cryptolepis buchanani*
Kṛṣṇatrivṛt	*Ipomoea petaloideschois*
Kṣīrakākolī	*Fritillaria roylei*
Kṣīravidārī	*Ipomoea digitata*
Kulattha	*Dolichos biflorus*
Kumārī	*Aloe barbadensis*
Kumuda	*Nymphaea alba*
Kuñduru	*Boswellia serrata*
Kuṅkuma	*Crocus sativa*
Kupīlu	*Strychnos nux vomica*
Kuraṇṭaka	*Barleria prionitis*

Kuśa	*Desmostachya bipinnata*
Kūṣmāṇḍa	*Benincasa hispida*
Kuṣṭha	*Saussurea lappa**
Kusumbha	*Carthamus tinctorius*
Kuṭaja	*Holarrhena antidysenterica*
Lājā	Fried rice paddy
Lajjālu	*Mimosa pudica*
Lakṣmaṇā	*Solanum xanthocarpum*
Lakuca	*Artocarpus lakoocha*
Lāmajjaka	*Cymbopogon jwarancusa*
Lāṅgalī	*Gloriosa superba*
Laśuna	*Allium sativum*
Latākarañja	*Caesalpinia crista*
Lavaṅga	*Syzygium aromaticum*
Lodhra	*Symplocos racemosa*
Madana	*Randia dumetorium*
Madanaghaṇṭī	*Borreria hispida*
Madayantī	*Lawsonia inermis*
Mādhavī	*Hiptage benghalensis*
Madhūka	*Maduca indica*
Madhusnuhī	*Smilax chinesis*
Mahābalā	*Sida rhombifolia*
Mahāmedā	*Polygonatum cirrhifolium*
Maṇḍūkaparṇī	*Centella asiatica*
Mañjiṣṭhā	*Rubia cordifolia*
Marica	*Piper nigrum*
Markandika	*Cassia angustifolia*
Māṣa	*Phaseolus mungo*
Māṣaparṇī	*Teramnus labialis*
Masūra	*Lens culinaris*
Mātuluṅga	*Citrus medica*
Māyakku	*Quercus infectoria*
Medā	*Polygonatum cirrhifolium*
Meṣaśṛgī	*Gymnema sylvestre*
Methi	*Trigonella foenum graecum*
Mudga	*Phaseolus radiatus*
Mudgaparṇi	*Phaseolus trilobus*
Mūlaka	*Raphanus sativus*
Muṇḍitikā	*Sphaeranthus indicus*
Muni	*Sesbania grandiflora*
Murā	*Selinium tenufolium*
Mūrva	*Marsdenia tenacissima*
Mūṣākarṇi	*Merremia emarginata*
Musalī	*Chlorophytum tuberosum, Asparagus adescendens*
Mustaka	*Cyperus rotundus*
Nāgabalā	*Sida veronicaefolia, Grewia hirsute*
Nāgakeśara	*Mesua ferrea*
Nāgavallī	*Piper betle*
Nalikā	*Cinnamomum tāmala*
Nandī	*Ficus arnottiana*
Nārikela	*Cocos nucifera*
Nata	*Valeriana wallachi*
Nicula	*Barringtonia acutangula*
Nīlī	*Indigofera tinctoria*
Nīlotpala	*Nymphaea stellata*
Nimba	*Azadirachta indica*
Nimbū	*Citrus limon*
Nirguṇḍī	*Vitex negundo*
Nyagrodha	*Ficus bengalensis*
Padma	*Nelumbo nucifera*
Padmaka	*Prunus cerasoides*
Palāṇḍu	*Allium cepa*
Palāśa	*Butea monosperma*
Pāraṅkī	*Garuga pinnata*
Pārasikayavānī	*Hyocyamus niger*
Pāribhadra	*Erythrina indica*
Parpaṭa	*Fumaria parviflora*
Parūṣaka	*Grewia asiatica*
Pāṣāṇabheda	*Bergenia ligulata*
Paśupāśi	*Myristica malabarica*
Pāṭalāi	*Stereospermum suaveolens*
Pāṭalī	*Schrebera swietenoides*
Pāṭhā	*Cissampelos pareira*
Paṭola	*Trichosanthes dioica*
Patra	*Cinnamomum tamala*
Pattaṅga	*Caesalpinia sappan*
Phalgu	*Ficus hispida*
Pīlu	*Salvadora persica*
Pippalī	*Piper longum*
Pitacandana	*Coscinium fenestratum*
Plakṣa	*Ficus lacor*
Ponnāṅgāṇī	*Alternanthera triandra*
Poṭagala	*Typha elephantina*
Prapuaṇḍarīka	*Nelumbo nucifera*
Prapunnāḍa	*Cassia tora*
Prasāriṇī	*Paederia foetida*
Prativiṣā	*Aconitum palmatum*
Priyāla	*Buchanania lanzen*
Priyaṅgu	*Callicarpa macrophylla*
Pṛśniparṇī	*Uraria picta*
Pūga	*Areca catechu*
Pullāni	*Calycopteris floribunda*
Puṣkara	*Inula racemosa*
Puṣkaramūla	*Inula racemosa* root
Pūtikā	*Caesalpinia crista*
Raktacandana	*Pterocarpus santalinus**
Raktapunarnavā	*Boerhavia diffusa, B. repens*
Rāmaśitalikā	*Amaranthus tricolor*
Rasāñjana	Solid extract of *Daruharidrā*
Rāsnā	*Pluchea lanceolata, Alpina galanga*
Ṛddhi	*Habenaria intermedia*
Reṇukā	*Vitex agnus castus*

Rohiṣā *Cymbopogon martini, C. schoenanthus*
Rohitaka *Tecomella undulata, Aphanamixis polystachya*
Ṛṣabhaka *Microstylis wallichii**
Rudrākṣa *Elaeocarpus ganitrus*
Sahacara *Barleria prionitis*
Sahadevī *Vernonia cinerea*
Śaileya *Parmelia perlata*
Śāka *Tectona grandis*
Śākhoṭaka *Streblus asper*
Śāla *Shorea robusta, Vateria indica*
Śālaparṇī *Desmodium gangeticum*
Śāli *Oryza sativa*
Śālmalī *Salmalia malabarica*
Śaṇa *Crotalaria juncea*
Śaṅkhapuṣpī *Convolvulus pluricalis, Evolvulus alsinoides, Clitoria ternatea, Canscora decussata*
Śaṅkhinī *Ctenolepis cerasiformis*
Saptāla *Euphorbia dracunculoides*
Saptaparṇa *Alstonia scholaris*
Śara *Saccharum munja*
Sarala *Pinus roxburghii*
Sarjasa *Vateria indica*
Sarpagandhā *Rauwolfia serpentina*
Sarṣapa *Brassica campestris*
Śatapatrikā *Rosa centifolia*
Śatapuṣpā *Foeniculum vulgare, Anethum graveolens*
Śatāvarī *Asparagus racemosa*
Śaṭī *Hedychium spicatum*
Siddhārtha *Brassica campestris*
Śigru *Moringa pterygosperma*
Śilājatu Derived from the humification of a variety of resin or latex-containing plants
Śiṃśapā *Dalbergia sissoo*
Śirīṣa *Albizzia lebbeck*
Snuhī *Euphorbia nerifolia*
Somavallī *Sarcostemma brevistigma, Ephedra gerardiana*
Spṛkkā *Schizachyrum exile, Delphinium zalil*
Śriveṣṭaka *Pinus longifolia* resin
Śṛṅgāṭaka *Trapa bispinosa*
Sruvavṛkṣa *Flacourtia indica, Gymnosporia spinosa*
Sthauṇeya *Taxus baccata*
Sthūla elā *Amomum subulatum*
Śūṇṭhī *Zingiber officinale*
Sūraṇa *Amorphophallus campanulatus*
Svarṇapatrī *Cassia angustifolia*
Śvetacandana *Santalum album*
Śvetajīraka *Cuminum cyminum*
Śvetapunarnavā *Boerhavia repens*
Śvetasārivā *Hemidesmus indicus*
Śyonāka *Oroxylum indicum*
Tagara *Valeriana wallachi*
Takkola *Illicium verum*
Tāla *Borassus flabellifer*
Tālamūlī *Curculigo orchioides*
Tālīśa *Abies webbiana*
Tāmalakī *Phyllanthus niruri*
Tāmrucūḍa pādikā *Adiantum lunulatum*
Tejanī *Zanthoxylum alatum*
Tejapatra *Cinnamomum tamala*
Tejovaṭī *Zanthoxylum alatum*
Tila *Sesamum indicum*
Timira *Curcuma longa*
Tiniśa *Ougeinia dalbergioides*
Tintiḍīka *Rhus parviflora*
Trapusa *Cucumis sativus*
Trāyāmāṇā *Gentiana kuroo*
Trivṛt *Ipomoea turpethum*
Tulasī *Ocimum sanctum*
Tumbinī *Lagenaria siceraria*
Turuṣka *Liquidambar orientalis*
Tuvaraka *Hydnocarpus laurifolia, H. kurzii*
Tvak *Cinnamomum zeylanicum*
Udīcya *Coleus vettiveroides*
Udumbara *Ficus racemosa*
Upakuñcika *Nigella sativa*
Uśīra *Vetiveria zizanioides*
Uṭiṅgaṇa *Blepharis edulis*
Utpala *Nymphaea stellata*
Vacā *Acorus calamus*
Vaṃśa *Bambusa bambos, B. arundinaceae*
Vaṃśarocanā *Vaṃśa* manna
Vāñjulā *Salix caprea*
Vanyajīraka *Centratherum anthelminticum*
Vārāhi *Dioscorea bulbifera*
Varṣābhu *Trianthema portulacastrum*
Varuṇa *Crataeva nurvala*
Vāsaka *Adhatodha vasica*
Vasuka *Osmanthus fragrans, Calotropis procera*
Vatsanābha *Aconitum chasmanthum*
Viḍaṅga *Embelia ribes*
Vidārī *Pueraria tuberosa*
Viralā *Diospyros tomentosa*
Viśāla *Citrullus colocynthis* variety
Viṣamuṣṭi *Strychnos nux vomica*
Vṛddhadāruka *Ipomoea petaloidea*
Vṛddhi *Habenaria intermedia, Dioscorea bulbifera*

Vṛkṣāmla	*Garcinia indica*
Vṛścikālī	*Tragia involucrata*
Vyāghranakha	*Capparis zeylanica*
Yaṣṭimadhu	*Glycyrrhiza glabra*
Yava	*Hordeum vulgare*
Yavakṣāra	alkaline *Yava* ash, prepared by calcination
Yavānī	*Trachyspermum ammi*
Yavāsaka	*Alhagi pseudalhagi*

*Listed in the database of the Convention on International Trade in Endangered Species of Wild Fauna and Flora (CITES) for India and/or Nepal.

MINERALS

Abhraka	mica
Añjana	antimony sulfide
Aubhida Lavaṇa	a kind of salt obtained from saline soil
Gairika	red ochre
Gandhaka	sulfur
Godañta	gypsum
Gomeda	hesonite
Gṛhadhūma	soot
Haritāla	arsenic (yellow variety)
Hiṅgula	cinnabar
Hīraka	diamond
Hiravī	magnesium silicate
Jasada	zinc
Kāṃsya	brass
Kāsīsa	iron sulfate
Kharpara	calamite
Khaṭī	chalk
Kṛṣṇa Lavaṇa	black salt
Loha	iron
Mākṣika	copper pyrite
Malla	arsenic
Manaḥśilā	realgar
Maṇḍūra	iron oxide
Māṇikya	ruby
Marakatamaṇi	emerald
Mayūragrīvaka	copper sulfate
Mṛddāraśṛṅga	lead monoxide
Nāga	lead
Narasāra	ammonium chloride
Nīla	sapphire
Pañca Lavaṇa	**saindhava, sāmudra, audbhida, sauvarcala, and viḍa lavaṇa**
Pārada	mercury
Pīta Loha	bronze
Puṣpāñjana	zinc oxide
Puṣparāga	topaz
Rajata	silver
Rājavarta	lapis lazuli
Raṅga	tin
Rasa	mercury
Rūpya	silver
Saindhava Lavaṇa	(pink) rock salt
Sāmudra Lavaṇa	sea salt
Sarjīkākṣāra	sodium carbonate
Saurāṣṭrī	alum
Sauvarcala Lavaṇa	sonchal salt (sodium chloride + sodium sulfate)
Sauvīra	lead sulfide
Sauvīrāñjana	antimony sulfide
Sindūra	red oxide of lead
Sīsa	lead
Soraka	salt pewter
Sphaṭika	alum
Srotāñjana	galena
Suvarṇa	gold
Suvarṇamākṣika	copper pyrite
Svarṇa	gold
Tāmra	copper
Ṭaṅkaṇa	borax
Tārkṣya	emerald
Tuttha	copper sulfate
Vaiḍūrya	cat's eye
Vaikrānta Dhātu	magnesium oxide
Vaikrānta Ratṇa	tourmaline
Vaṅga	tin
Viḍa Lavaṇa	black salt
Vimala	iron pyrite
Yaśda	zinc

ANIMAL PRODUCTS

Ajā, Chāga	goat
Ākhu	rat
Ambara	ambergris, intestinal concretion of *Physeter catodon**
Aṇḍa	egg
Aśva	horse
Avi	sheep
Barhi	peacock
Basta	sheep
Bhūnāga	earthworm
Carma	animal hide
Danti	teeth, tusk (elephant)
Dugdha, Kṣīra	milk
Eṇa	antelope (*Antilope cervicapra*)*
Gaja, Hasti	elephant (*Elephas maximus*)*
Gandhamārjāra	civet cat musk, derived from

Vīrya	*Viverra zibetha* and *Viverra civettina**
Go	cow
Godha	iguana
Gorocana	ox gall, ox bile
Gṛdhra	vulture (*Gyps* spp., *Neophron percnopterus*, *Sarcogyps calvus*, *Aegypius calvus*)*
Jalaukā	leech
Kāka	crow
Kañka	heron
Kapota	pigeon
Karabha, Uṣṭra	camel
Karṇamala	ear wax
Kaṣṭūrī, Mṛgamada	musk, derived from *Moschus moschiferus**
Khara	donkey
Kīta	insects
Kṛkavāku	rooster
Kukkuṭa	hen
Kuramasī	hoof
Kūrma	tortoise (*Geochelone elegans*, *Indotestudo elongata*, *Indotestudo forstenii*, *Manouria emys*)*
Kuruñga	monkey (*Macaca* spp., *Pygathrix roxellana*, *Semnopithecus entellus*, *Trachypithecus* spp.)*
Lākṣā	lac
Madhu	honey
Madhūcchiṣṭha	beeswax
Mahiṣa	water buffalo
Majja	marrow
Māmsa	flesh
Markoṭa	ants
Mastu	yogurt water
Matsya, Jhaṣa	fish
Mesa	ram
Mṛga	deer (*Axis porcinus*, *Cervus* spp.)*
Muktā, Mauktika	pearl
Muktāsphoṭa	mother of pearl
Mūtra	urine
Nakha	snail shell, nails, claws
Nārīkṣīra, Stanya	breast milk
Pakṣa, Picchā	feather
Pitta	bile
Pravāla	coral
Purīṣa	dung
Rakta	blood
Ṛkṣa	bear (*Ailurus fulgens*, *Helarctos malayanus*, *Melursus ursinus*, *Ursus* spp.)*
Roma	wool, hair
Śakṛt, Viṭ	dung
Salyaka	porcupine
Samudraphena	cuttlefish bone
Śaṅkha	conch shell
Sarpa, Ahi	snake
Śaśa	rabbit
Simha	lion (*Panthera leo*)*
Śṛṇga	horn
Śukti	oyster shell
Takra	buttermilk
Varāha	pig
Vasā	fat
Vṛṣa	ox
Vṛṣcika	scorpion
Vyāghri	tiger (*Panthera tigris*)*

*Listed in the database of the Convention on International Trade in Endangered Species of Wild Fauna and Flora (CITES) for India and/or Nepal.

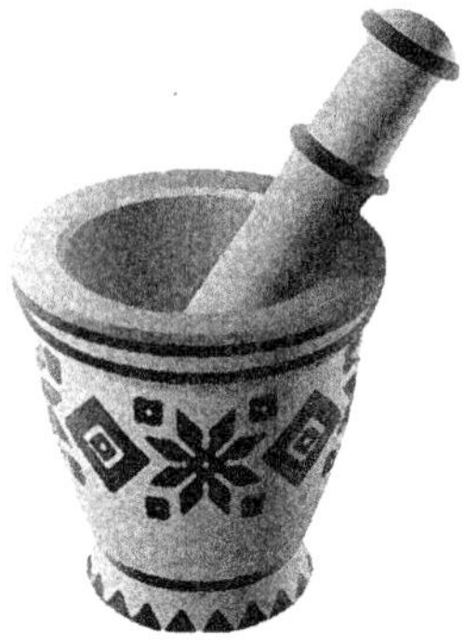

Appendix 4

ĀYURVEDIC WEIGHTS AND MEASURES

Smaller units	Larger units	Mass (metric)	Volume (metric)
	1 *trasareṇu*	0.0362 mg	0.0362 μL
6 *trasareṇu*	1 *marīci*	0.22 mg*	0.22 μL*
6 *marīci*	1 *rājika*	1.3 mg*	1.3 μL*
3 *rājika*	1 *sarṣapa*	3.91 mg*	3.91 μL*
8 *sarṣapa*	1 *yava*	31.25 mg	31.25 μL
4 *yava*	1 *guñja*	125 mg	125 μL
8 *guñja*	1 *māṣa*	1 g	1 mL
4 *māṣa*	1 *ṣāṇa*	4 g	4 mL
12 *māṣa*	1 *karṣa*	12 g	12 mL
2 *karṣa*	1 *śukti*	24 g	24 mL
2 *śukti*	1 *pala*	48 g	48 mL
2 *pala*	1 *prasṛta*	96 g	96 mL
2 *prasṛta*	1 *kuḍava*	192 g	192 mL
2 *kuḍava*	1 *mānika*	384 g	384 mL
2 *mānika*	1 *prastha*	768 g	768 mL
4 *prastha*	1 *āḍhaka*	3.072 kg	3.072 L
100 *pala*	1 *tula*	4.8 kg	4.8 L
4 *āḍhaka*	1 *droṇa*	12.288 kg	12.288 L
2 *droṇa*	1 *śūrpa*	24.576 kg	24.576 L
2 *śūrpa*	1 *droṇi*	49.152 kg	49.152 L
20 *tula*	1 *bhāra*	96 kg	96 L
4 *droṇi*	1 *khari*	196.608 kg	196.608 L

* Approximately (rounded to second decimal).

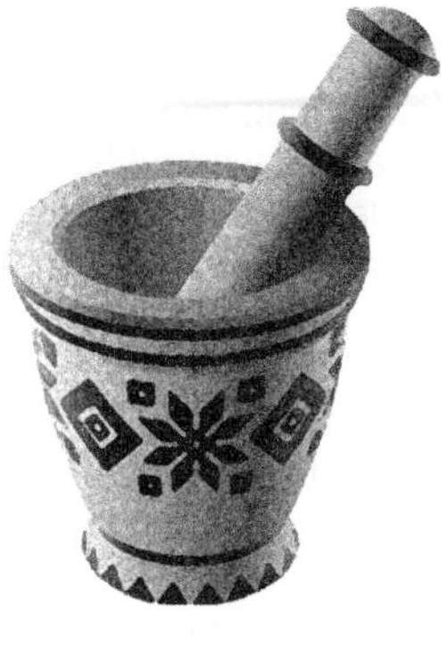

Appendix 5

GLOSSARY OF ĀYURVEDIC TERMS

abhiṣyandī ***dravyas*** which by their ***guru*** and ***picchila*** nature block the ***srotāṃsi*** causing heaviness and congestion

abhyaṅga oleation, full-body oil massage

ācaryā learned person, sage

agni lord of fire, home and hearth; the digestive capacity of the patient (digestive fire); part of the ***daśavidha parīkṣā*** (ten methods of examination); ascending male energy, opposite of ***soma***

agnimāndya poor digestion

Agniveśa student of Ātreya, author of the ***Agniveśa saṃhitā***

ahaṃkāra ego complex

āhāra the dietary habits of the patient; part of the ***daśavidha parīkṣā***, or ten methods of examination

ājñā sixth ***cakra***, the third eye

ākāśa 'ether', the principle of pervasiveness

akṛti observation of the build and general physical characteristics in the ***aṣṭāsthāna parīkṣā***

ālocaka pitta one of the five sub-***doṣas*** of ***pitta***

āma 'undigested food', toxins

āmaśaya upper digestive tract (stomach, liver/gall bladder, pancreas, small intestine)

amla sour

amṛta nectar of immortality

anāhata fourth ***cakra***, the heart ***cakra***

ānanda bliss

ānandamaya kośa 'bliss sheath' in the ***pañca kośa***

aṇḍāṇu ovum; female reproductive essence

āñga limb

agnimāndya weak digestion

añjana medicinal agent introduced to eyes; collyrium

annamaya kośa 'food sheath', synonymous with the ***sthūla śarira***

añtarmārga inner pathway of disease

antra colon

anulomana ***dravyas*** that assists in digestion and promotes normal bowel movement

anupāna a food, beverage, or condiment used to modify the effects of a medicinal agent; e.g. ***ghṛta***, honey, water, etc.

anupaśaya knowledge by error, see ***upaśaya***

anurasa secondary ***rasa***(s) (tastes)

anuvāsana vasti enema with medicated oil

ap element of water, the principle of cohesion

apāna one of the five sub-***doṣas*** of ***vāta***; the downward moving force responsible for menstruation, ejaculation and the discharge of urine and faeces

apara ojas extrinsic vitality

ariṣṭa fermented medicinal beverage, heated during preparation

arogya absence of disease

ārtavajanana ***dravyas*** that correct menstruation

artha 'purpose'

āsana ***hatha yoga*** posture

āsava fermented medicinal beverage, not heated during preparation

Aṣṭāñga Hṛdaya 'the heart of the eight limbs' of Āyurveda; authored by Vāgbhaṭa; forms the ***bṛhat trayī*** (greater triad), along with the ***Caraka*** and ***Suśruta saṃhitās***

aṣṭāñga yoga 'the eight limbs of ***yoga***'

aṣṭāsthāna parīkṣā 'eight methods of diagnosis'
Aśvini Kumāras the twin celestial physicans
asranut antihaemorrhagic, stypic
asthi bone **dhātu**
Atharva veda one of the four sacred canons in Hinduism; a collection of hymns on various subjects, including magic, healing and philosophy
ātman the universal soul; synonymous with **puruṣa**
Ātreya Punarvasu Ātreya; teacher of Agniveśa and student of Bharadvāja
avagāham bath
avalambaka one of the sub-**doṣas** of **kapha**; associated with respiratory function and serosal membranes of viscera
avaleha 'to lick', a thick medicinal confection prepared with honey, sugar and **ghṛta**
āyus 'life'
bāhya rogāyana external channel
balā 'strength', tissue resistance
Bāla cikitsā treatment of children
balām the strength of the patient; part of the **daśavidha parīkṣā** (ten methods of examination)
balya **dravyas** which increase strength
bhakti devotion
Bharadvāja the first human proponent of Āyurveda
bhasma a substance reduced to ash through the intense and prolonged application of heat
bhedana **dravyas** which forcibly expel the contents of the bowel
bhrājaka pitta one of the sub-**doṣas** of **pitta**
bhukti physical pleasure
bhūta element
bhūtāgnis sub-sets of **agni** responsible for the assimilation and metabolism of the **pañcabhūtas**
bodhaka one of the sub-**doṣas** of **kapha**; associated with the functions of the tongue and satiety
Brahmā Lord of Creation
brāhmamuhūrta period of time before sunrise conducive to study and meditation
brahman the 'vast expanse', synonymous with **puruṣa**
bṛmhaṇa anabolic; stoutening therapies
bṛmhaṇa nasya **nasya** for relieving **vāta**
buddha one who has realised **buddhi**
buddhi higher intellect, unclouded by the desire and machinations of the ego (**ahaṃkāra**)
cakra 'wheel', vortex of spiritual energy arranged hierarchically
cala movement, instability
Caraka author of the **Caraka saṃhitā**
Caraka saṃhitā the most revered text of Āyurveda, compiled by Caraka; said to be based upon a much older work called the **Agniveśa saṃhitā**; redacted by Dṛḍhabala
caya increase, accumulation
chedana **dravyas** that 'scrape' out **kapha** for elimination
cikitsā 'treatment'
citta consciousness; the mind suffused with **saṃskāras**
cūrṇa finely sieved powder
dadhi curd, similar to yogurt or kefir
daha, **dahi** burning sensations
Dakṣa Prajāpati protector of all living beings
dakṣiṇāyana period of time between summer and winter solstice
Daṃṣṭrā cikitsā treatment of animal-inflicted wounds, poisoning, toxicology
darśana viewpoint or perspective; illumination
deśa the environment in which the patient lives; part of the **daśavidha parīkṣā**
deva 'to shine'; beings that have transcended a corporeal existence
Dhanvantari the god of Āyurveda, as an incarnation of Viṣṇu and teacher of Suśruta; Kasiraja Divodāsa
dhara a **snehana** technique in which a continuous stream of warm medicated oil is poured in a specific area of the body
dharma law, righteousness, duty, morality
dhātu structural support system of the body; principle of structure vis. **rasa**, **rakta**, **māṃsa**, **medas**, **asthi**, **majjā**, and **śukra/aṇḍāṇu**
dhātvāgni subtype of **agni** that attends to the metabolic function of a specific **dhātu**

dhūma 'smoke'; specifically, the therapeutic inhalation of smoke
dinācaryā 'daily regimen'
dīpana ***dravyas*** that enkindle ***agni***
doṣa 'blemish'; bodily humour
doṣapradusana ***doṣa***-increasing effect
doṣapraśamana ***doṣa***-deacreasing effect
drava liquid
dravya 'substance'; medicament
dravyguṇa 'knowledge of substance', Āyurvedic pharmacology; the study of the biological effects of a food or medicament upon the body
Dṛḍhabalā the redactor of the ***Caraka saṃhitā***
dṛk eyes; examination of the eyes and eye-sight in the ***aṣṭāsthāna parīkṣā*** (eight methods of diagnosis)
dukha sorrow, unhappiness, pain, discontentment
dūṣya the state of the ***doṣas***, ***dhātus*** and ***malas***; part of the ***daśavidha parīkṣā*** (ten methods of examination)
eka one; e.g. ***eka doṣa*** (one ***doṣa***)
gandhā 'smell'
gaṇḍūṣa dhāraṇā gargling
ghṛta clarified butter
Graha cikitsā treatment of spiritual possession; medical astrology
grāhī ***dravyas*** that dry up the excessive moisture in the body and are ***dīpanapācana***
griṣma summer
guḍa jaggery; unrefined solidified cane sugar juice
guṭikā pill
guṇa quality
guru 'heavy'; venerated teacher
gurvādi guṇas the 'ten pairs of opposite qualities'
Hatha yoga limb (***āñga***) of Vedic science that deals with doctrines and practices orientated towards spiritual liberation through physical perfection
hemañta early winter
hima cold infusion
hṛdaya 'heart'; ***dravyas*** which strengthen the heart
ida nāḍī the 'channel of comfort'; located to the left of the ***suṣumnā nāḍī***, terminating in the left nostril; equated with the feminine aspect of physicality
Indra 'ruler'; the king of the gods in the Vedic pantheon
Jarā cikitsā treatment of ageing; rejuvenative therapies
jaṭharāgni the digestive fire
jihvā 'tongue'; examination of the tongue in the ***aṣṭāsthāna parīkṣā***
jīva 'life'
jīvanīya life-giving
jīvātman individual soul
jñāna pure knowledge
jñāna indriyās 'organs of knowledge'; i.e. the five senses
jvara 'fever', the archetype of many pathogenic processes described in Āyurveda
jyotiṣ Vedic astrology
kāla the staging or progression of the condition; part of the ***daśavidha parīkṣā*** (ten methods of examination)
Kali the fearsome 'black' goddess; consort of Śiva; destroyer of illusion and self-limitation
kalka bolus
kānda 'bulb'; source of the 72 000 ***nāḍīs***; located in the umbilical region
kapha one of the three ***doṣas***; phlegm; congestion
kaphaja of ***kapha***
kāraṇa 'cause'; the ***kāraṇa śarira*** (syn. ***ānandamaya kośa***) is the originator of all the ***kośa*** (sheaths) of the body
karma action; work; therapeutic effect
karma indriyās 'organs of action', i.e. hands, mouth, arms, legs, anus and genitalia
karṇa tarpaṇam application of a medicated oil in the ears
kaśāya decrease; astringent; decoction
kaṭhiṇa 'hard'
kati vasti a ***snehana*** technique in which a medicated oil is allowed to seep into the skin over the lumbar region of the back
kaṭu 'pungent'
Kāya cikitsā general internal medicine

kāyakarma infractions of bodily action
khara rough, brittle
kledaka kapha one of the five sub-**doṣas** of **kapha**; associated with the mucosal secretions of the gastrointestinal tract and electrolyte balance
kledana moistening
kopa vitiation
kṛmi parasites
kṛmighna antihelminthics
kṛṣna 'black'
kundalinī cosmic feminine principle that lies coiled in the **mūlādhāra cakra**; rises to unite with the cosmic masculine principle in the **sahasrāra cakra** with spiritual liberation
kuṭīprāveśika 'to enter into the hut'; rejuventation therapies performed on an in-patient basis
kvātha decoction
laghu 'light'
lakṣaṇas symptoms
Lakṣmī goddess of abundance and prosperity
langhana catabolic; decreasing therapies
lavaṇa salty
lekhana to dry up excessive moisture in the body
madakārī to cause intoxication
madhu honey
madhura sweet
madya wine
madhyama rogamārga the 'medial' pathway of disease
mahābhūtas the 'great' elements, vis. **pṛthvī**, **ap**, **tejas**, **vāyu**, **ākāśa**
mahat cosmic law
majjā marrow
mala waste, impurity; faeces; examination of faeces in the **aṣṭāsthāna parīkṣā** (eight methods of diagnosis)
māṃsa muscle **dhātu**
manas the lower mind, interfacing with the **jñāna indriyās**, and under control of the **ahaṃkāra**
manda slow, dull
mañdāgni weak digestion
maṇipūra 'wheel of the jewelled city'; the third **cakra**
manomaya kośa **kosha** located between the **prāṇāmaya kośa** and the **vijñānamaya kośa** in the **sūkṣma sarira**; the lower mind
marśa **nasya** used for therapeutic administration
masala a mixture of spices
māyā self-developed illusion
medas 'adipose tissue' **dhātu**
medhya **dravyas** that promote **buddhi**
medohara to reduce **medas**
Mīmāṃsā teachings of the Vedas that relate to ritual and **mantra**
mokṣa liberation
mṛdu 'soft'
mūlādhāra the 'root' **cakra**
mūtra 'urine'; examination of urine in the **aṣṭāsthāna parīkṣā** (eight methods of diagnosis)
mūtravirecana diuretic
nāḍī subtle energy channel; examination of the pulse in the **aṣṭāsthāna parīkṣā** (eight methods of diagnosis)
Nāgārjuna buddhist sage, alchemist and physician; at least four different personages throughout history
nasya errhine, medicament for nasal administration
navanīta butter
neti nasal administration of a liquid medication with a small, teapot-shaped vessel
nidāna aetiology, pathology, diagnosis
nirāma 'without **āma**'
nirūha vasti enema with herbal decoction
nirvāṇa cessation of suffering
Nyāya darśana teachings of the Vedas that relate to logical procedures
ojas vital energy, often equated with immunological and neuroendocrinal mechanisms
oṃ the unstruck sound
pācaka pitta one of the five sub-**doṣas** of **pitta**
pācana **dravyas** that 'cook' or denature the food which has been consumed
paittika of **pitta**
pañca 'five'
pañca karma five methods of purification (**śodhana**), vis. **vamana**, **virecana**, **vasti**, **rakta mokṣaṇa**, **nasya**
pañca kośa the 'five sheaths' of existence

pañcabhūtas the 'five elements'
pāṇḍu anaemia
panir unripened cheese
para ojas instrinsic vitality
phāṇṭa warm infusion
picchila 'slippery'
picu a **snehana** technique in which a cloth soaked in medicated oil is applied over a specific area of the body
piṇḍa sveda the use of a medicated grain–herb combination wrapped in linen, soaked in warm oil, and applied to the body
pingalā nāḍī the 'tawny current'; one of the two principle **nāḍīs** located to the right of the **suṣumnā nāḍī**, terminating in the right nostril; equated with the masculine principle of the body
pitta one of the three **doṣas**; 'bile', inflammation
pittaja of **pitta**
pizhichil a **snehana** technique in which a medicated oil is wrung from cloths over a specific area of the body
prabhāva inexplicable; the activity of a medicament that cannot be rationalised; spiritual energy; ritual methods in the preparation of a medicament
prajñaparādha 'crimes against wisdom'
prakṛti matrix, the Goddess, nature; also the constitution of the patient, part of the **daśavidha parīkṣā**
prāmana quantity
pramāthi **dravyas** that remove the accumulated **doṣas** from the **srotāṃsi**
prāṇa one of the five sub-**doṣas** of **vāta**; the vital force, governing cardiopulmonary function
prāṇāmaya kośa the lowest sheath within the **sūkṣma śarira**; residence of **prāṇa**
prāṇayama yogic breathing techniques
pratimarśa **nasya** used on a daily basis, in small volumes
pṛthvī 'earth', the principle of inertia
pūja worship; sacred ritual
purīṣa 'faeces'
puruṣa in the **prakṛti-puruṣa** dualism, the transcendant unknowable aspect from which all things arise; cosmic male principle, synonymous with **ātman**
pūrva karmas preparatory methods; i.e. **snehana** and **svedana**, performed prior to the **pañca karmas**
pūrvarūpa prodromal symptoms
Rāja yoga synonymous with **aṣṭāñga yoga**, or referring to the higher, meditative aspects of **hatha yoga** practices
rajas the quality of 'movement' and 'colour'
rakta 'blood' **dhātu**
raktaprasādana **dravyas** that purify **rakta**
ranjaka pitta one of the five sub-**doṣas** of **pitta**; governs the hepatobiliary system, the spleen, and the haematopoiesis (red blood cell formation)
rasa 'taste'; the first **dhātu**; mercury; juice
rasahala pharmacy
rasāyana **dravyas** that ward off old age and disease; rejuvenative
recana **dravyas** that forcibly expel the contents of the bowel in liquid form
Ṛg veda the most ancient of the Hindu vedas; the basis of brahmanical practices
rogamārga pathway of disease, comprising the **añtarmārga** (inner), **bāhya rogayana** (outer) and **madhyama rogamārga** (medial) pathways
ṛtusandhi seasonal transitions
rūkṣa 'dry'
rūkṣana drying therapies
rūpa 'sight'; symptoms
ṛtucaryā seasonal regimen
śabda 'sound'; examination of the voice in the **aṣṭāsthāna parīkṣā** (eight methods of diagnosis)
sādhaka pitta one of the five sub-**doṣas** of **pitta**; associated with sensory perception
sadvṛtta conduct, moral observance, behaviour
sahasrāra the crown **cakra**
saindhava rock salt

sākṣi 'witness'
sākṣi bhava na bearing witness, a form of meditation
Śakti consort of Śiva; in its diminutive form (**śakti**) it means 'power'
salya cikitsā treatment requiring the use of a knife; surgery
sama in balance, normal, equal
Sāma veda 'knowledge of songs'; one of the four vedas associated with sacred hymns
samāna one of the five sub-**doṣas** of **vāta**; associated with digestion
śamana pacificatory therapies, subduing **doṣas** by indirect means
śamana nasya **nasya** for relieving **pitta**
saṃhitā 'collected sayings'; authoratative text
saṃprāpti pathogenesis, how a disease comes to be
saṃsāra 'wheel' of birth, life, death and rebirth
saṃsarga two **doṣas** in combination
samśamana **doṣa** pacification
saṃskāras 'activators', sometimes referring to rituals, but in the yogic tradition referring to imprints upon the psyche that cause one to perpetuate **karma**
sandhana galenical
sāñdra 'solid'
Sāṅkhya a form of ontology that classifies existance into 24 different categories, and the spiritual path that rejects all things except for **puruṣa**
sannipāta three **doṣas**, in combination
sapta dhātus the seven **dhātus**
śarat hot and humid weather after the monsoon
śarira 'body'
śāstra 'teaching'
sātmya that which is normal, or habitual; the lifestyle habits of the patient; one of the aspects of the **daśavidha parīkṣā** (ten methods of examination)
sattva the quality of harmony; the mental and emotional state of the patient; part of the **daśavidha parīkṣā** (ten methods of examination)
śiro dhārā a **snehana** technique in which a continuous stream of warm medicated oil is poured across the forehead
śiro vasti a **snehana** technique in which a leather band is placed around the patient's head to make a vessel, and a medicated oil is poured into this vessel and allowed to seep into the patient's head
śiro lepana application of a herbal paste on the forehead
śirīṣa late winter
śita 'cold'
Śiva a major diety in Hinduism, the personified aspect of the transcendent reality
ślakṣna smooth and sticky
śloka verse
śodhana 'killing', a method of **dravya** purification; **dravyas** which dislodge the **malas** from their respective locations in either an upward or downward direction
śoṇita 'blood'
śukra 'semen'
siddhi occult powers obtained through meditation and other psychospiritual practices
śleṣaka kapha sub-**doṣa** of **kapha** said to be concentrated in the synovium of the joints; concerned with lubrication and maintanence of structure
snāna bathing
sneha oil or fat; medicated fats for internal administration
snehana oleation therapies
snehapāna internal administration of a medicated oil or non-medicated oil
snigdha greasy, moist, oily
soma opposite of **agni**, the lunar essence; magical elixir
soṣana absorbing
sparśa touch; palpation in the **aṣṭāsthāna parīkṣā** (eight methods of diagnosis)
srota channel
srotāṃsi channels
srotorodha congestion; blockage of the **srotāṃsi**
stambhana 'cooling'; **dravyas** that inhibit bowel movements
sthāna seat of influence, location

sthira 'stable'
sthūla overt, gross
sthūla śarira the 'gross body', also called the ***annamaya kośa***
sukha happiness, pleasure, satisfaction
sūkṣma 'subtle'
sūkṣma dravyas ***dravyas*** that enter into even the most minute channel of the body
sūkṣma rasa subtle essence that feeds the mind, obtained upon digestion of food, medicaments and beverages
sūkṣma śarira the 'subtle body'; composed, collectively, of the ***prāṇāmaya***, ***manomaya*** and ***vijñānamaya kośas***
surā beer
suṣumnā nāḍī the 'central channel', the path through which ***kundalinī*** ascends
svādhiṣṭhāna the second ***cakra***
sveda 'sweat'
svedana diaphoretic and heating therapies
svarasa fresh juice extract
svasthahita ***doṣa***-balancing effect
svedana 'heating'; sudation (sweating) therapies
taila sesame oil
takra buttermilk
tamas the quality of 'inertia'
tanmātrās subtle aspects of the material universe perceived by the five ***jñāna indriyās***
Tantra yoga canon of literature associated with worship of Śiva and Śakti; concerned with the awakening of ***kundalinī***
tarpaka kapha sub-***doṣa*** of ***kapha***; concentrated in the spinal column, said to have an inhibitory effect upon the waking state
tejas 'fire', the principle of radiance
tikṣṇa 'sharp'
tikta 'bitter'
tila sesame seed
tridoṣa the three ***doṣas***
triguṇa the three primordial qualities, vis. ***sattva***, ***rajas*** and ***tamas***
tṛṣṇā 'thirst'
upaśaya knowledge by trial, see ***anupaśaya***
Urdhvāñga cikitsā treatment of the head and neck
uṣṇa 'hot'
uttaravasti douche
uttarāyaṇa period of time between winter and summer soltice
vācīkarma infractions of speech
Vāgbhaṭa the author of the ***Aṣṭāñga Hṛdaya*** and the ***Aṣṭāñga Sangraha***; scholars are not sure if the author of these two works is the same person
vaisamya abnormal state of the ***doṣas***
Vaiśeṣika darśana one of the six schools (***darśanas***) of Hindusim, concerned with logic and the differences between things
vajīkaraṇa sexual virilisation, fertility enhancer
vamana ***dravyas*** which remove ***kapha*** and ***pitta*** through the mouth by force (i.e. vomiting)
varna colour, complexion
varṣa 'autumn'
vasanta 'spring'
vasti 'bladder', also enema (referring to the usage of an animal bladder used to contain the medicated liquid)
vāta one of the three ***doṣas***; flatus, degeneration
vātātapika 'wind and sun' therapy; rejuvenation therapies performed on an out-patient basis
vāttika, ***vātaja*** of ***vāta***
vayaḥ the age of the patient; part of the ***daśavidha parīkṣā*** (ten methods of examination)
vāyu 'wind' element, the principle of vibration
vedanāsthāpana analgesics
Vedānta one of the six schools (***darśanas***) of Hindusim; an esoteric approach to meditation that favours a non-dualistic orientation (***advaita***), that there is only one Reality or one being, called the ***ātman***
Vedas the 'knowledges'; sacred canon of Hindu, consisting of the ***Rig Veda***, ***Atharva Veda***, ***Yajur Veda*** and ***Sāma Veda***
vidāhi burning sensations
vijñānamaya kośa 'sheath of knowledge', the residence of ***ahaṃkāra*** and ***buddhi*** in the psychospiritual body
vikara 'disease'
vikṛti disease tendency

vipāka post-digestive effect
virecana nasya ***nasya*** for relieving ***kapha***
vīrya 'energy'; energetic property of a ***dravya***
viśada 'friction'
viśuddha the fifth ***cakra***
vṛddhi 'increase'
Vṛṣa cikitsā treatment of impotence and sterility; virilisation
vyāna one of the five sub-***doṣas*** of ***vāta***; moves in the body in spiral currents, often correlated with the cardiovascular system
vyavāyi ***dravyas*** that act very quickly first by spreading all over the body
vyāyāma 'exercise'
yāga 'sacrifice'
Yajur veda 'knowledge of sacrifice', one of the four Vedas orientated towards brahmanical practices such as ***pūja*** (worship)
Yoga 'union', one of the six schools (***darśanas***) of Hinduism
yoga deśa 'yogic body'
yogavāhī an agent that enhances the potency of a ***dravya***
yogin male ***yoga*** practitioner
yogini female ***yoga*** practitioner
yukti 'rationale'

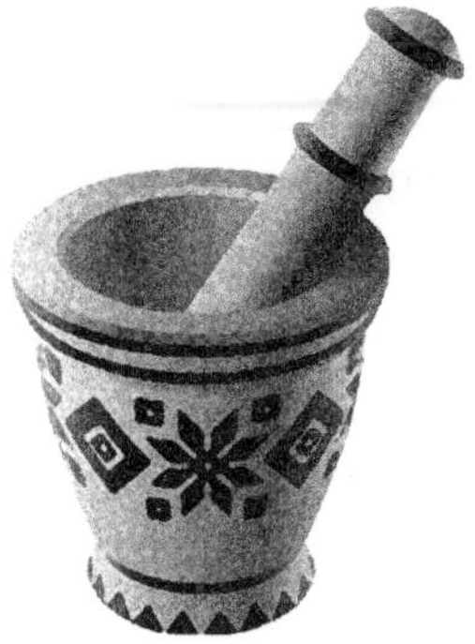

Appendix 6

ĀYURVEDIC RESOURCES

The following is a list of various Āyurvedic resources, including professional associations, educational institutes, manufacturers and booksellers. For recent updates please direct your internet browser to http://www.toddcaldecott.com.

ĀYURVEDIC ASSOCIATIONS (INDIA)

National Institute of Āyurveda
Department of Ayurveda, Yoga & Naturopathy, Unani, Siddha and Homoeopathy
Ministry of Health & Family Welfare, Government of India,
Madhav Vilas Palace, Amer Road
Jaipur 302002, India
Tel: 0091-141-2635709,2635816
Fax: 0091-141-2635709
Email: nia@raj.nic.in
Web: www.nia.nic.in

Central Council of Indian Medicine (CCIM)
Central Council for Research in Ayurveda & Siddha (CCRAS)
Ministry of Health and Family Welfare, Govt. of India
Jawahar Lal Nehru Bhartiya Chikitsa Avam Homoeopathy Anusandhan Bhawan
61–65, Institutional Area, Janakpuri
New Delhi 110058, India
Tel (CCIM): 0091-11-25610978
Tel (CCRAS): 0091-011-25614970
Web: www.ccimindia.org
Web: www.ccras.org

Central Research Institute
Dr T.V. Menon
Cheruthuruthy, Trichur
Kerala 679531, India
E-mail: criachy@sancharnet.in

Ayurveda Foundation
5, Wonderland, 7, M. G. Road
Pune 411 001, India
Tel: 0091-020-56010618
Fax: 0091-020-26335541
Web: www.nanalfoundation.org

Foundation for Revitalisation of Local Health Traditions
74/2, Jarakbande Kaval
Post: Attur, Via Yelahanka
Bangalore 560 064, India
Tel: 0091 80 2856 8000
Fax: 0091 80 2856 5873
Email: info@frlht.org.in
Web: www.frlht-india.org

ĀYURVEDIC ASSOCIATIONS (EUROPE)

Ayurvedic Medical Association U.K.
59, Dulverton Road, South Croydon, Surrey
CR2 8PJ, United Kingdom
Tel: 0044(0)20 8657 6147
Fax: 0044(0)20 8333 7904
Web: www.londonhealth.co.uk/ayurvedicmedicine.asp

British Ayurvedic Medical Council (BAMC)
British Association of Accredited Ayurvedic Practitioners (BAAAP)
47 Nottingham Place, London W1M 3FE, United Kingdom
Tel: 0044(0)207 7224 6070

European Herbal Practitioners Association
8 Lion Yard, Tremadoc Road
London SW4 7NQ, UK
Tel: 0044(0)20 7627 2680
Fax: 0044(0)20 7627 8947
Email: info@euroherb.com
Web: www.users.globalnet.co.uk/~ehpa/

ĀYURVEDIC ASSOCIATIONS (AMERICAS)

National Ayurvedic Medical Association
620 Cabrillo Avenue,
Santa Cruz, CA 95065, USA
Email: info@ayurveda-nama.org
Web: www.ayurveda-nama.org

The National Institute of Ayurvedic Medicine
584 Milltown Road Brewster
New York 10509, USA
Tel: 001-845-278-8700
Fax: 001-845-278-8215
Web: www.niam.com/corp-web/index.htm

American Herbalists Guild
1931 Gaddis Road
Canton, GA 30115, USA
Tel: 001-770-751-6021
Fax: 001-770-751-7472
Email: ahgoffice@earthlink.net
Web: www.americanherbalistsguild.com

ĀYURVEDIC EDUCATION (INDIA)

Gujarat Ayurved University
Administrative Bhawan
Post Bag No.4
Jamnagar 361008, India
Tel: 0091-288-2677324
Fax: 0091-288-2555966
E-mail: Info@ayurveduniversity.com
Website: www.ayurveduniversity.com

Chakrapani Global Center for Training & Research in Ayurveda
A 33, Prabhu Marg, Tilak Nagar
Jaipur – 302004, India
Tel: 0091-141-2624003
Fax: 0091-141-2620746
web: www.chakrapaniayurveda.com

Ayurveda India
Dr Raghunandan Sharma M.D.(Ayu)
H-38; South Extension I
New Delhi 110049, India
Tel: 0091-11-24641132
Fax: 0091-11-24648034
Email: ayur@ayurplanet.com
Web: www.ayurplanet.com

International Academy of Ayurved
Ātreya Rugnalaya, M.Y. Lele Chowk
Erandawana, Pune 411 004, India
Tel/fax: 0091 20 2567 8532
Email: avilele@hotmail.com
Web: www.ayurved-int.com

Kerala Ayurveda Pharmacy Ltd
Athani Post, Ernakulam District
Kerala 683585, India
Tel: 0091 484 2476301
Fax: 0091 484 474376
E-mail: response@ayurvedagram.com
Web: www.kaplayurveda.com

The Arya Vaidya Pharmacy (Coimbatore) Limited
Arsha Yoga Vidya Peetam
326, Perumal Koil Street, Ramanathapuram
Coimbatore – 641 045, India
Tel: 0091-422-2315412
Fax: 0091-422-2314953
E-mail: ayurveda@vsnl.com
Web: www.avpayurveda.com

Jiva Ayurveda
Dr Partap S. Chauhan
1144, Sector 19, Faridabad – 121002, Haryana, India
Tel: 0091-129-229 6174
Fax: 0091-129-229 5547
Web: www.ayurvedic.org

ĀYURVEDIC EDUCATION (EUROPE)

The Ayurveda Institute UK
461 Brighton Rd, South Croydon
Surrey C2R 6EW, United Kingdom

Tel/fax: 02084054407
Email: ayurveda@blueyonder.co.uk
Web: www.ayurvedainstitute.co.uk

The Manipal Ayurvedic University Of Europe
81 Wimpole Street
London W1G 9RF, United Kingdom
Tel: 0044(0)207 224 6070
Fax: 0044(0)207 224 6080
Email: info@unifiedherbal.com
Web: www.ayurvedagb.com/ayurvediccollege/home.htm

European Institute of Vedic Studies
BP 18 30610 Sauve, France
Tel: 0033 (0)466 53 76 87
Fax: 0033 (0)466 53 76 88
Email: atreya@atreya.com
Web: www.atreya.com

Ayur Yoga
Gerd Ziegler
Unter Ibach 21
79837 Ibach, Germany
Tel: 0049(0)7672-906215
Fax: 0049(0)89-2443-30325
Email: mail@ayuryoga.de
Web: http://www.ayuryoga.de

Shakti Ayurveda
Ave. Meridiana 358, 4b
08027 Barcelona, Spain
Tel: 0034655 400 306
Email: info@shaktiayurveda.com
Web: www.shaktiayurveda.com

Joytinat International College of Ayurveda & Yoga
via Balbi 33/29
Genova, Italy
Tel/fax: 0039(0)10-2758507
Email: info@joytinat.it
Web: www.joytinat.it

ĀYURVEDIC EDUCATION (AMERICAS)

Wild Rose College of Natural Healing
Traditional Ayurvedic Medicine (TAM) correspondence course
400 – 1228 Kensington Rd NW, Calgary
Alberta T2N 3P9, Canada
Tel: 001-403-270-0936
Fax: 001-403-283-0799
Email: coordinators@wrc.net
Web: www.wrc.net

The East West School of Herbology
P.O. Box 275
Ben Lomond, CA 95005, USA
Tel: 001-800-717-5010
Fax: 001-831-336-4548
Email: herbcourse@planetherbs.com
Web: http://www.planetherbs.com

The American University of Complementary Medicine
Ayurvedic Medicine Certificate (660 hours)
MS & PhD Ayurvedic Medicine
11543 Olympic Blvd, Los Angeles, California, 90064, USA
Tel: 001-310-914-4116
Web: www.aucm.org

Ayurveda Institute of America
Dr Jay Apte
561 Pilgrim Drive Suite B
Foster City, CA 94404, USA
Tel: 001-650-341-8400
Fax: 001-650-341-8440
Email: jayapte@ayurvedainstitute.com

California College of Ayurveda
Dr Marc Halpern
1117A East Main St, Grass Valley
CA 95945, USA
Tel: 001-886-541-6699
Email: info@ayurvedacollege.com
Web: www.ayurvedacollege.com

Ganesha Institute
Pratichi Mathur
1111 West Camino Real, Suite 109, PMB 211
Sunnyvale, CA 94087, USA
Tel: 001-800-924-6815
Email: info@healingmission.com

Diamond Way Ayur Veda
Melanie and Robert Sachs
P.O.Box 13753
San Luis Obispo, CA 93406, USA

Tel/Fax: 001-805-543-9291
Toll free: 001-866-303-3321
Email: ayurveda8@earthlink.net

Ayurveda Healing Arts Institute of the Medicine Buddha Healing Center
Michael Kreuzer, D. Ayur
2427 McKinley Avenue, Suite 1
Berkeley, California 94703, USA
Tel: 001-510-843-0163

Ayurvedic Certification Course
Pat Hansen, MA
3660 S. Glencoe St
Denver, Colorado 80237, USA
Tel: 001-303-512-0819
Email: padmashakt@aol.com

Rocky Mountain School of Yoga & Ayurveda
Sarasvati Buhrman, PhD
P.O. Box 1091
Boulder, Colorado 80306, USA
Tel: 001-303-499-2910, 443-6923
Email: rmiya@earthnet.net

Alandi School of Ayurveda
Alandi Ashram
1705 14th St, PMB 392
Boulder, CO 80302, USA
Tel: 001-303-786-7437
Fax: 001-303-494-7308
Email: alandi_ashram@yahoo.com

Florida Vedic College
Drs Light and Bryan Miller
2017 Fiesta Drive
Sarasota, Florida 34231, USA
Tel: 001-941-929-0999
Web: www.ayurvedichealers.com

Hindu University of America
113 N. Econlockhatchee Trail
Orlando, FL 32825-3732, USA
Tel: 001-407-275-0013
Email: staff@hindu-university.edu

College of Maharishi Ayur-Ved
Maharishi International University
1603 North Fourth Street Building # 144
Fairfield, IA 52556, USA
Tel: 001-641-472-4600

Kripalu Center
Hilary Garivaltis
P.O. Box 793
West Street, Route 183
Lenox, MA 01240, USA

Golden Lotus, Center for Health Resources
8793 A, Waters Street
Montague, MI 49437, USA
Tel: 001-231-894-6778

American School of Ayurveda
460 Ridgedale Ave
East Hanover, NJ 07936, USA
Tel: 001-973-887-8828
Fax: 001-973-887-3088
Web: ayurvedawisdom@aol.com

New Jersey Institute of Ayurveda
Dr Aparna Bapat
356 Bloomfield Avenue
Montclair, NJ 07042, USA
Tel: 001-973-783-1036
Email: info@starseedyoga.com

Ayurvedic Holistic Center
Swami Sada Shiva Tirtha
82A Bayville Avenue
Bayville, NY, USA
Tel: 001-800-452-1798, 516-628-8200
Web: www.ayurvedahc.com

The National Institute of Ayurvedic Medicine
Scott Gerson, MD
584 Milltown Road Brewster,
New York 10509, USA
Tel: 001-888-246-NIAM
Fax: 001-914-278-8700

The Ayurvedic Institute
Dr Vasant Lad
11311 Menaul Blvd, NE Albuquerque
NM 87112, USA
Tel: 001-505-291-9698
Fax: 001-505-294-7572
Web: www.ayurveda.com

American Institute of Vedic Science
Dr David Frawley
PO Box 8357, Santa Fe
NM 87504-8357, USA
Tel: 001-505-983-9385
Fax: 001-505-982-5807
Web: www.vedanet.com

Vinayak Ayurveda and Panchakarma Research Foundation
Dr Sunil Joshi
2509 Virginia NE Suite D
Albuquerque, New Mexico 87110, USA
Tel: 001-505-296-6522
Fax: 001-505-298-2932
Email: vac@vinayakayurveda.com

Maharishi Vedic Medicine
2721 Arizona St. NE Albuquerque
NM 87110, USA
Tel: 001-505-830-0415, 001-800-811-0550
Fax: 001-989-803-6000
Email: MCVMNM@aol.com

Wise Earth School of Ayurveda
Swamini Mayatitananda
Wise Earth Hermitage
70 Canterfield Lane
Candler, North Carolina 28715, USA
Tel: 001-828-258-9999
Web: www.wisearth.org

Blue Lotus School of Ayurveda
P. O. Box 8044 Asheville
NC 28814-8044, USA
Tel: 001-828-250-1039

Ojas Ayurveda & Yoga Institute, Inc., Ayurveda Health Center
Dr Shekhar Annambhotla
3340 Cove Landing Macungie, PA, USA
Tel: 001-610-966-9403
Web: www.ojas.us

Green Mountain Institute
Fred Duncan, D. Ayur
49 School Street
Hartford, Vermont, USA
Tel: 001-802-295-6629
Web: www.greenmountaininstitute.com

Ayurvedic Academy & Natural Medicine Clinic
Dr Vivek Shanbhag
819 NE 65th Street
Seattle, Washington 98115, USA
Tel: 001-206-729-9999
Web: www.ayurvedaonline.com

Ayurvedic Academy of Canada
347 Bay Street
Suite 101, Toronto
Ontario M5H 2R7 Canada

Fundación de Salud Ayurveda Prema
Centro Colaborativo Gujarat Ayurved University
Santa Fe 3373 6° B (1425)
Buenos Aires, Argentina
Tel: 0054-11 4824-1574/4827-4590
Email: info@medicinaayurveda.org
Web: www.medicinaayurveda.org

ĀYURVEDIC EDUCATION (AUSTRALIA)

Australian College of Ayurvedic Medicine
19 Bowey Avenue
Enfield SA 5085, Australia
Tel/fax: 011-618-83497303
Email: suchi-karma@picknowl.com.au

ĀYURVEDIC HOSPITALS (INDIA AND NEPAL)

Arya Vaidya Sala
Kottakkal, Kerala
India 676 503
Tel: 0091 483 2742216
Fax: 0091 483 2742210
E-mail: mail@aryavaidyasala.com
Web: http://www.aryavaidyasala.com

Ayurinstitute – Centre for Ayurveda & Panchakarma Therapy and Eye Care Clinic
F-15, Sector 1 Market, Vashi, Navi Mumbai
Maharashtra, India 400703
Tel: 0091-022-27823588 / 27826155
Email: ayurinstitute@yahoo.com
Website: www.ayurvision.com

Ayurveda Health Home
Pioneer Panca-Karma Centre of Nepal
Tilingatar (Near Shahanshah Hotel)
Dhapasi-7, Kathmandu, Nepal
Tel: 00977-1-4358761, 00977-1-4355144
P.O.Box: 2869, Kathmandu, Nepal
Email: info@ayurveda.com.np
Web: www.ayurveda.com.np

Piyushabarshi Aushadhalaya
9/35, Masangalli, Mahabouddha
Kathmandu, Nepal
Tel: 00977-1-4223960
Fax: 00977-1-4428743
Email: bajra@ayurvedicclinic.net
Web: www.ayurvedicclinic.net

Kerala Ayurveda Pharmacy Ltd
Athani Post, Ernakulam District
Kerala 683585, India
Tel: 0091 484 2476301
Fax: 0091 484 474376
E-mail: response@ayurvedagram.com
Web: www.kaplayurveda.com

The Arya Vaidya Pharmacy (Coimbatore) Limited
326, Perumal Koil Street, Ramanathapuram
Coimbatore – 641 045, India.
Tel: 0091 422 – 2315412
Fax: 0091 422 – 2314953
E-mail: ayurveda@vsnl.com
Web: www.avpayurveda.com

Harivihar
Bilathikulam, Calicut
Kerala 673006, India
Tel: 0091 495 2765865
Email: admin@harivihar.com
Web: http://www.harivihar.com

CNS Chikitsalayam
Mezhathur, Tritala
Palakkad District 679534 Kerala, India
Tel: 0091 492 672055
Fax: 0091 492 612509
E-mail: cns_ayurveda@vsnl.com
Web: http://www.cnschikitsalayam.org

Sitaram Ayurveda Pharmacy Ltd
Thrissur, Pin–680 001
Kerala, India
Tel: 0091(0)487 2448570, 2448540, 2420198
Fax: 0091(0)487 2448814
Res: 0091(0)487 2382971
Cell: 0091 98460 20540
E-mail: chyavana@sancharnet.in
Web: www.sitaramayurveda.com

ĀYURVEDIC PRODUCTS (INDIA AND NEPAL)

Arya Vaidya Sala
Kottakkal, Kerala,
India 676 503
Tel: 0091 483 2742216
Fax: 0091 483 2742210
E-mail: mail@aryavaidyasala.com
Web: http://www.aryavaidyasala.com

Piyushabarshi Aushadhalaya
9/35, Masangalli, Mahabouddha
Kathmandu, Nepal
Tel: 00977-1-4223960
Fax: 00977-1-4428743
Email: bajra@ayurvedicclinic.net
Web: www.ayurvedicclinic.net

Kerala Ayurveda Pharmacy Ltd
Athani Post, Ernakulam District
Kerala 683585, India
Tel: 0091 484 2476301
Fax: 0091 484 474376
Email: response@ayurvedagram.com
Web: www.kaplayurveda.com

The Arya Vaidya Pharmacy (Coimbatore) Limited
326, Perumal Koil Street, Ramanathapuram
Coimbatore – 641 045, India.
Tel: 0091 422 – 2315412
Fax: 0091 422 – 2314953
E-mail: ayurveda@vsnl.com
Web: www.avpayurveda.com

Sitaram Ayurveda Pharmacy Ltd
Thrissur, Pin – 680 001
Kerala, India
Tel: 0091(0)487 2448570, 2448540, 2420198
Fax: 0091(0)487 2448814
Res: 0091(0)487 2382971
Cell: 0091 98460 20540
E-mail: chyavana@sancharnet.in
Web: www.sitaramayurveda.com

Charak Pharma Pvt Ltd
Evergreen Industrial Estate, 2nd Floor Shakti Mills Lane,
Dr.E. Moses Road Mahalaxmi, Mumbai
Maharashtra 400011, India
Email: charak@vsnl.com
Web: www.charak.com

Dabur
Kaushambi, Ghaziabad
Uttar Pradesh 201010, India
Tel: 0091 (0120) 3982000/3001000
Web: www.dabur.com

The Himalaya Drug Company
Makali, Bangalore 562 123, India
Tel: 0091 080 2371 4444
Fax: 0091-080 2371 4474
Web: www.himalayahealthcare.com

Murali B N Khandige Herbs & Plantations Pvt Ltd
46/1, Jaraganahalli, Kanakapura Main Road
Bangalore 560045, India
Tel: 0091 80 5449116
Fax: 0091 80 5445408
Email: pureherbs@vsnl.net

Zandu Pharmaceuticals Works
Gokhale Road (S) Dadar
Mumbai 400025, India
Web: http://www.zanduayurveda.com/

AayurMed Biotech P. Ltd
31, New Silver Home
15, New Kantwadi Road
Bandra (West)
Mumbai 400050, India
Tel: 0091-26421551
Email: nikmo@vsnl.com

ĀYURVEDIC PRODUCTS (EUROPE)

Pukka Herbs Ltd
Tel: 0044 (0)1275 461950 teas, finance
Tel: 0044 (0)1275 461950 bulk sales, herbs
Email: sebastian@pukkaherbs.com, tim@pukkaherbs.com

Indigo Herbal Ltd
PO Box 22317 London W13 8WE, UK
Tel/fax: 0044 (0)20 8621 3633
Email: info@indigoherbal.co.uk

ĀYURVEDIC PRODUCTS (AMERICAS)

Banyan Botanicals
6705 Eagle Rock Ave. NE
Albuquerque, NM 87113, USA
Tel: 001-888-829-5722, 001-505-821-5083
Email: info@banyanbotanicals.com
Web: www.banyanbotanicals.com

Bazaar of India Imports
1810 University Ave., Berkeley CA 94703-1516, USA
00-261-SOMA (800-261-7662)
001-510-548-4110

Om Organics
3245 Prairie Avenue Suite A, Boulder
CO 80301, USA
Tel: (888) 550-VEDA, 001-720-406 3940
Email: herbs@omorganics.com
Web: www.omorganics.com

Herbs for Health, Harmony and Healing
2475 Robb Dr. #413
Reno NV 89523, USA
Tel: 001775 624 6254
Fax: 001509 356 3106

Planetary Formulas
PO Box 533
Soquel, CA 95073, USA

Tel: 001-800-606-6226, 001-831 438-1700
Fax: 001-831-438-7410
Web: www.planetaryformulas.com

Ayu Products
819 NE 65th Street, Seattle
Washington 98115, USA
Tel: 001-206-729-9999
E-mail: drs@ayurvedaonline.com

Yogi Tea
2545 Prairie Rd, Eugene
OR 97402, USA
Tel: 001-800-964-4832, 001-541-461-2160
Fax: 001-541-461-2191
Email: customerservice@yogitea.com
Web: www.yogitea.com

Ayush Herbs Inc
2239, 152nd Ave. NE
Redmond, WA 98052, USA
Tel: 001-800-925-1371, 001-425-637-1400
Fax: 001-425-451-2670
Email: ayurveda@ayush.com
Web: www.ayush.com

Tattva's Herbs LLC
1127 33rd Ave E.
Seattle, WA 98112, USA
Tel: 001-206-380-2633
Fax: 001-206-568-3169
Email: tattvasherbs@comcast.net
Web: www.tattvasherbs.com

Maharishi Ayurveda Products International, Inc
1068, Elkton Drive, Colorado Springs
CO 80907, USA
Tel: 001-800-345-8332, 001-719-260-5500
Email: questions@mapi.com
Web: www.mapi.com

ĀYURVEDIC PRODUCTS (AUSTRALIA)

Yatan Holistic Ayurvedic Centre
38A Cecil St, Gordon
NSW 2072, Australia
Tel: 0061-(0)2-9499 7164
Fax: 0061-(0)2-9499 7619
Email: vaidya@yatan-ayur.com.au
Web: www.yatan-ayur.com.au

ĀYURVEDIC BOOKSELLERS (ONLINE)

Vedams Books
http://www.vedamsbooks.com

Bagchee Associates
http://www.bagchee.com

Motilal Banarsidass
http://www.mlbd.com

South Asia Books
http://www.SouthAsiaBooks.com/

Twenty-First Century Book Store
http://www.21stbooks.com

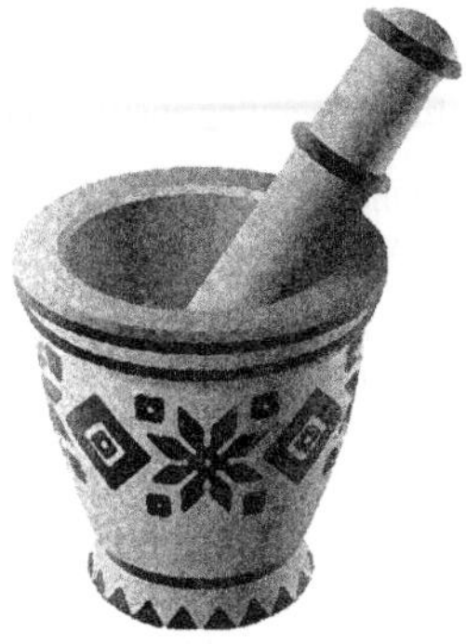

Bibliography and references

Aruna R, Balasubramanian AV, Sujatha V 1991 Nidaana: diagnosis in traditional medicine. Lok Swasthya Parampara Samvardhan Samiti, Madras

Bajracharya, MB 1995 The real facts of Ayurveda. Piyushabarshi Aushadhalaya Mahabouddha, Kathmandu

Basham AL 1959 The wonder that was India: a survey of the culture of the Indian sub-continent before the coming of the Muslims. Grove Press, New York

Bensky D, Gamble A 1993 Chinese herbal medicine materia medica. Revised edition. Eastland Press, Seattle

Bhishagratna KKL 1907 An English translation of the Susruta Samhita. Wilkins Press, Calcutta

Chopra Col. Sir RN 1958 Chopra's indigenous drugs of India, 2nd edn. U.N. Dhur, Calcutta

Dash B 1991 Materia medica of Ayurveda. B. Jain Publishers, New Delhi

Dash B 1994 Encyclopedia of Tibetan medicine: being the Tibetan text of Rgyud Bzi and Sanskrit restoration of Amṛta Hṛdaya Aṣṭāṅga Guhyopadeśa Tantra and expository translation in English, vols 1 and 2. Sri Satguru, Delhi

Dash B, Junius M 1983 A handbook of Ayurveda. Concept Publishing, New Delhi

Dastur JF 1962 Medicinal plants of India and Pakistan, 2nd edn. D. B. Taraporevala, Bombay

Desikachar TKV 1999 The heart of Yoga: developing a personal practice. Inner Traditions, Rochester VT

Feuerstein G 1997 The Shambhala encyclopedia of Yoga. Shambhala, Boston, p 230

Finckh E 1988 Studies in Tibetan medicine. Snow Lion, Ithaca NY

Frawley D 1989 Ayurvedic healing: a comprehensive guide. Passage Press, Salt Lake City

Frawley D 1996 Ayurveda and the mind. Lotus, Twin Lakes WI

Frawley D, Lad V 1986 The Yoga of herbs: an Ayurvedic guide to herbal medicine. Lotus Press, Santa Fe

Goldstein J 1994 Insight meditation. Shambhala, Boston

Goswami SS 1996 Laya Yoga. Inner Traditions, Rochester VT

Gupta LP 1996 Essentials of Āyurveda. Chaukhamba Sanskrit Pratishthan, Varanasi

Huynh HK, Seifert GM 1981 Pulse diagnosis by Li Shi Zhen. Paradigm, Brookline MA

India. Ministry of Health and Family Planning. 1978. The Ayurvedic formulary of India. Part 1. 1st edn. Delhi

Jain SK 1968 Medicinal plants, 2nd edn. National Book Trust, New Delhi

Johari H 2000 Chakras: energy centers of transformation. Destiny Books, Rochester VT

Kirtikar KR, Basu BD 1993 Indian medicinal plants, 2nd edn, vols 1–4. 1935. Reprint. Periodical Experts, Delhi

Krishna G 1971 Kundalini: the evolutionary energy in man. Shambhala, Boulder, p 12–13

Krishnamurthy KH 1991 Wealth of Suśruta. International Institute of Āyurveda, Coimbatore

Krishnamurthy KH 2003 Bhela-Saṃhitā: text with English translation, commentary and critical notes. Chaukhambha Visvabharati, Varanasi

Kumar V 1997 Ayurvedic clinical medicine. Sri Satguru, Delhi

Lad V 1996 Secrets of the pulse: the ancient art of Ayurvedic pulse diagnosis. Ayurvedic Press, Albuquerque

Leung AY, Foster S 1996 Encyclopedia of common natural ingredients used in food, drugs and cosmetics, 2nd edn. John Wiley, New York

Nadkarni KM 1976 The Indian materia medica, with Ayurvedic, Unani and home remedies. Revised and enlarged by A.K. Nadkarni, 1954. Reprint. Bombay Popular Prakashan PVP, Bombay

Nyanatiloka 1982 Path to deliverance. Buddhist Publication Society, Kandy

Perry LM, Metzger J 1980 Medicinal plants of East and Southeast Asia: attributed properties and uses. MIT Press, Cambridge MA

Qaiser S, Qaiser M 1978 Combretaceae. Flora of West Pakistan No. 122. University of Karachi, Karachi

Rey L 2003 Thermoluminescence of ultra-high dilutions of lithium chloride and sodium chloride. Physica Acta 323: 67–74

Scudder JM 1874 Specific diagnosis: a study of diseases. Reprint. Eclectic Medical Publications, Sandy OR, p139

Sen SP, Khosla RL 1968 Effect of Sodhana on the toxicity of aconite (vatsnava). Current Medical Practice 12

Sharma AJ 2002 The Pañcakarma treatment of Āyurveda, including Keraliya Pañcakarma. Sri Satguru, Delhi

Sharma PV 1976 Introduction to Dravyguṇa (Indian pharmacology). Chaukhambha Orientalia, Varanasi, p 9, 10, 23, 88–89

Sharma PV 1992 History of medicine in India. Indian National Science Academy, New Delhi, p 185

Sharma PV 1999 Suśruta saṃhitā: with English translation of text and Ḍalhaṇa's commentary along with critical notes, vol 1. Chaukhambha Orientalia, Varanasi, p iv

Sharma PV 2002 Cakradatta (text with English translation). Chaukhambha, Varanasi

Sharma RK, Dash B 1985–88 Agnivesa's Caraka Saṃhitā (text with English translation and critical exposition based on Cakrapani Datta's Āyurveda Dipika) vols 1–3. Chaukhambha Orientalia, Varanasi, p 596

Sikdar JC trans 1988 Nadivijnanam and Nadiprakasa: Old Sanskrit treatise on the science of pulse with English translation. Prakrit Bharti Academy, Jaipur

Singhal SN, Tripathi SN, Sharma KR 1985 Mādhavakara: Ayurvedic clinical diagnosis. Singhal Publications, Varanasi

Srikanthamurthy KR 1983 Clinical methods in Ayurveda. Chaukhamba Orientalia, Varanasi

Srikanthamurthy KR trans 1984 Sarnagadhar-saṃhita: a treatise on Ayurveda. Chaukhambha Orientalia, Varanasi

Srikanthamurthy KR 1994–5 Vāgbhaṭa's Astāñga Hṛdayam (text, English translation, notes, appendices and indices) vols 1–3. Krishnadas Academy, Varanasi

Srikanthamurthy KR 1995 Mādhava Nidānam: Roga Viniscaya of Mādhavakara. Chaukhambha Orientalia, Varanasi

Srikanthamurthy KR 2000–1 Bhāvaprakāśa of Bhāvamiśra (text, English translation, notes, appendices and index). vol 1–2. Krishnadas Academy, Varanasi

Svoboda R 1992 Ayurveda: health, life and longevity. Penguin Books, London

Tarabilda E 1997 Ayurveda revolutionized: integrating ancient and modern Ayurveda. Lotus Press, Twin Lakes

Tewari PV 2002 Kāśyapa-saṃhitā or Vṛddhajīvakīya tantra: text with English translation and commentary. Chaukhambha Visvabharati, Varanasi

Thorat S, Dahanukar S 1991 Can we dispense with Āyurvedic samskaras? Journal of Postgraduate Medicine 37 (3): 157–159

Tierra M, Frawley D (eds) 1988 Planetary herbology: an integration of Western herbs into the traditional Chinese and Ayurvedic systems. Lotus Press, Twin Lakes

Varier PS 1994–96 Indian medicinal plants: a compendium of 500 species. vol 1–5. Orient Longman, Hyderabad

Weiss R 1988 Herbal medicine. Translatd by A.R. Meuss. Beaconsfield Publishers, Beaconsfield, England

Zysk KG 1998 Asceticism and healing in ancient India: medicine in the Buddhist monastery. Motilal Banarsidass, Delhi

Subject Index

An asterisk following a page number indicates an entry in the Glossary. Where the letter 'n' follows a page number it refers to the relevant endnote.

A

B

N

O

P

R

Index of Plants

Page numbers in **bold** indicate where full treatment can be found in Part 2 of the book.

Printed and bound by CPI Group (UK) Ltd, Croydon, CR0 4YY
03/10/2024
01040363-0003